CLINICAL PSYCHOPHARMACOLOGY

CLINICAL PSYCHOPHARMACOLOGY

Principles and Practice

S. Nassir Ghaemi, MD, MPH

Professor of Psychiatry and Pharmacology

Tufts University School of Medicine

Lecturer on Psychiatry

Harvard Medical School

Boston, Massachusetts

OXFORD
UNIVERSITY PRESS

OXFORD
UNIVERSITY PRESS

Oxford University Press is a department of the University of Oxford. It furthers the University's objective of excellence in research, scholarship, and education by publishing worldwide. Oxford is a registered trade mark of Oxford University Press in the UK and certain other countries.

Published in the United States of America by Oxford University Press
198 Madison Avenue, New York, NY 10016, United States of America.

Library of Congress Cataloging-in-Publication Data
Names: Ghaemi, S. Nassir, author.
Title: Clinical psychopharmacology : principles and practice / by S. Nassir Ghaemi.
Description: New York, NY : Oxford University Press, [2019] | Includes index.
Identifiers: LCCN 2018029138 | ISBN 9780199995486 (pbk.)
Subjects: | MESH: Psychotropic Drugs—pharmacology |
Psychopharmacology—methods | Mental Disorders—drug therapy
Classification: LCC RM315 | NLM QV 77.2 | DDC 615.7/88—dc23
LC record available at https://lccn.loc.gov/2018029138

10 11

Printed by Marquis, Canada

I thank the following publications for granting permission to reproduce excerpts from previously published articles:

CHAPTER 1
Excerpt reprinted with permission from Wolters Kluwer. SN Ghaemi, A new psychopharmacology nomenclature. J Clin Psychopharmacol. 2015 Aug;35(4):428–33. A New Nomenclature for Psychotropic Drugs.

CHAPTER 4
Adapted with permission from Cambridge University Press. S. Nassir Ghaemi, *A Clinician's Guide to Statistics and Epidemiology in Mental Health, Measuring Truth and Uncertainty* © S. N. Ghaemi 2009, published by Cambridge University Press.

CHAPTER 5
Adapted with permission from John Wiley and Sons. Ghaemi SN. The case for, and against, evidence-based psychiatry. Acta Psychiatrica Scandinavica.

CHAPTER 6
Adapted with permission from Cambridge University Press. Ghaemi, SN, Selker, HP. Maintenance efficacy designs in psychiatry: Randomized discontinuation trials-enriched but not better. Journal of clinical and Translational Science.

CHAPTER 7
Adapted with permission of BMJ Publishing Group Ltd. SN Ghaemi, Evid Based Ment Health. The failure to know what isn't known: negative publication bias with lamotrigine and a glimpse inside peer review. 2009 Aug;12(3):65–8.

CHAPTER 16
Adapted with permission from SAGE Publications, Inc. Journals. S. Nassir Ghaemi MD MPH, Toward a Hippocratic Psychopharmacology. Canadian journal of psychiatry. 2008 Mar;53(3):189–96.

CHAPTER 25
Adapted with permission from SAGE Ltd. Permissions Team. Amerio A, Gálvez JF, Odone A, Dalley SA, Ghaemi SN. Carcinogenicity of psychotropic drugs: A systematic review of US Food and Drug Administration-required preclinical in vivo studies. Aust N Z J Psychiatry. 2015 Aug;49(8):686–96.

CHAPTERS 33 AND 34
Adapted with permission from Taylor and Francis Group LLC Books. S. Nassir Ghaemi MD MPH. Polypharmacy in Psychiatry. New York: Marcel Dekker, 2002. 1–34, 311–334.

CHAPTER 36
Adapted with permission of The John Hopkins University Press. SN Ghaemi, Postmodern medicine: an analysis of the pharmaceutical industry and its critics. Perspect Biol Med. 2013 Spring;56(2):223–35

CHAPTER 43
Adapted from Ghaemi SN, Goodwin FK. The ethics of clinical innovation in psychopharmacology: Challenging traditional bioethics. Philos Ethics Humanit Med. 2007 Nov 8;2:26. Open access.

Appendix II
Adapted with permission of Blackwell Munksgard. Ghaemi SN, Dalley S, Catania C, Barroilhet S. Bipolar or borderline: a clinical overview. Acta Psychiatr Scand. 2014 Aug;130(2):99–108.

DISCLOSURE

Since October 2017, Nassir Ghaemi has been employed as a Director of Translational Medicine-Neuroscience in early drug discovery and development at Novartis Institutes for Biomedical Research in Cambridge, MA. The bulk of this text was completed before he began that employment. The views expressed here are solely his own, and do not reflect those of his employers. Carbamazepine (Tegretol), clozapine (Clozaril), and methylphenidate (Ritalin) are marketed by Novartis.

To Frederick K. Goodwin, MD -friend and mentor

In diseases of the mind . . . it is an art of no little importance to administer medicines properly; but, it is an art of much greater importance and more difficult acquisition to know when to suspend or altogether omit them.

—Philippe Pinel, 1806

All drugs are toxic; only their dosing and indication makes them therapeutic.

—adapted from Paracelsus, 1538

Drugs [are] the most uncertain element in our art.

—William Osler, 1921

SELECTED REFERENCES

P. Pinel, A Treatise on Insanity, 1806, reprinted 1983, Birmingham, Alabama, Classics of Medicine Library, Gryphon Editions Ltd, p. 10.

Paracelsus, Four Treatises. Translated C. Lilian Temkin, Edited by Henry E. Sigerist. Baltimore: Johns Hopkins University Press, 1941, p. 22: "All things are poison . . . the Dosis alone makes a thing not a poison".

William Osler, Counsels and Ideals, edited Humphrey Milford, London: Oxford University Press, 2nd edition, 1921, p 116.

Contents

SECTION III: CLINICAL PSYCHOPHARMACOLOGY OF DRUG CLASSES

SECTION IV: CLINICAL PSYCHOPHARMACOLOGY OF DISEASES AND SYNDROMES

SECTION V: SPECIAL TOPICS IN PSYCHOPHARMACOLOGY

APPENDICES: DIAGNOSTIC CONTROVERSIES

Preface

This kind of textbook of clinical psychopharmacology—directly focused on minimizing symptomatic treatment and maximizing disease-oriented treatment—has not been written previously.

It is a different kind of textbook of psychopharmacology, not meant to reflect the common consensus of what most clinicians believe or practice. It is not a mere compendium of commonly accepted views. In that sense, it is not a textbook, as typically conceived, but a challenge. Truth is not a matter of majority vote, Henry David Thoreau said. What is the status quo, or the mainstream view, is not necessarily true, including in clinical medicine. This textbook seeks to present what is true, as best as its author can divine, irrespective of popularity or commonality. Doubtless there will be mistakes that the future might correct, but they will not be driven by preference for conventional wisdom. It is hoped that readers will seek such an approach, even if it challenges or conflicts with some of their own viewpoints, and that they might use this textbook accordingly, not merely to accept it as a whole, nor to reject it as a whole, but rather to use it to think about their assumptions and beliefs, so as to become better clinicians.

Clinical psychopharmacology is practiced today in a manner opposed to the rest of the medical profession. Psychiatric practice tends to a non-Hippocratic approach (the Galenic approach), which the rest of medicine put aside a century ago (Chapter 16). Other textbooks of psychopharmacology unconsciously and without apology teach the Galenic, non-Hippocratic approach. In this view, biological theories are the basis for decision-making. One of the best aspects of reliance on biological theory primarily is that facts can be distorted to fit the theory. It matters little whether one uses four humors, or three monoamines, or the ego and the id—many facts can be distorted to justify a favored theory.

In contrast, the Hippocratic approach prioritized clinical observation over biological theory. It focused on symptoms in real clinical practice, not speculations about bodily causes. Over time, this clinical approach inspired the founders of clinical research in medicine, leading to the use of statistics to revolutionize clinical medicine, as with the discovery of the method of randomization to prove or disprove treatment efficacy.

Yet biology always has been seductive, and clinical research can appear pedestrian. Research publications and funding are much greater in the former topic than the latter. In the end, biological research still needs to be translated into clinical practice. Biological speculation itself fails to achieve that translation.

Truths of theory are transient. Not only is Galen out of date, but so are many biological theories of recent vintage, like the catecholamine hypothesis of depression or the dopamine hypothesis of schizophrenia. Clinical observation and research, in contrast, is steadier: the same melancholia that Hippocrates described can be discerned in depression today; the same mania that Arateus of Cappadocia explained in the second century A.D. is visible in current mania.

Clinical research is the solid ground of medicine; biological theory is a necessary but changing superstructure. If these relations are reversed, then mere speculation takes over, and the more solid ground of science is lost. This textbook will take that clinical approach, explicitly eschewing the common standard biological theory approach to teaching psychopharmacology.

In non-Hippocratic medicine, many treatments are provided aggressively at high doses and for indefinite durations, and all symptoms are treated in this aggressive manner equally. In Hippocratic medicine, there is a scientifically and clinically sound rationale for when to be aggressive with dosing and type of medication (for diseases) and when to be more conservative and cautious (for non-diseases). Hence the wisdom of Paracelsus, who can be paraphrased to say that: all medications are toxic; it is only their dosing and indication which makes them therapeutic.

This textbook will try to do two things: One—identify and differentiate psychiatric diseases from symptoms and from "clinical pictures," which, although receiving psychiatric attention, are not diseases. Two—teach the practice of psychopharmacology of diseases based on examination of the clinical research evidence, not through biological speculation about neurotransmitter systems.

Above all, this textbook of psychopharmacology will be clinical; it will not treat all symptoms equally and advocate aggressive indefinite treatment with many different medications based on biological speculations drawn from animal studies of questionable relevance to humans. The recommendations made here will be based primarily on human studies, on direct clinical research that shows benefit or harm, and will differentially emphasize caution versus more aggressive treatment of symptoms versus diseases, respectively.

The goal is to help psychiatrists to practice not just in a modern manner, but in a more ethically and scientifically sound manner than has been the case previously. Many proposals in this text will no doubt have shortcomings and will need correction and revision, but even with those inevitable limitations, one can hope that they represent an advance on the status quo.

S. Nassir Ghaemi, MD, MPH
Professor, Psychiatry and Pharmacology
Tufts University School of Medicine
Lecturer, Psychiatry
Harvard Medical School
Boston, Massachusetts

Prolegomena

Ten Fallacies and Ten Truths of Psychopharmacology

TEN FALLACIES OF PSYCHOPHARMACOLOGY

1. More is better. (If a low dose helps a little, a higher dose helps more. Not so.)
2. What gets you well keeps you well. (Happily ever after: but many drugs work acutely but not preventively, and vice versa.)
3. Treat to remission. (If one drug helps somewhat, and two drugs help more, keep going until all symptoms are gone completely; they rarely do, but side effects increase inevitably.)
4. Polypharmacy is good. (A variant on the first fallacy: If one drug helps somewhat, two drugs will help more.)
5. Make one change at a time. (Clinical practice isn't research; one can go too slowly.)
6. Four to eight weeks is a sufficient trial of a drug. (Possibly correct for some acute trials, but not for maintenance trials.)
7. Dose low, go slow. (If common, this approach produces undue suffering).
8. Always taper a drug. (Sometimes very harmful effects call for immediate discontinuation; not all drugs have withdrawal syndromes.)
9. Treat the most severe symptom. (This often has no relationship to the underlying disease.)
10. Always incorporate the patient's preference. (The patient can be wrong.)

TEN TRUTHS OF PSYCHOPHARMACOLOGY

1. Your treatment is as good as your diagnosis.
2. Treat diseases, not symptoms.

3. All drugs are guilty until proven innocent. (The default position is: Do not prescribe; you must have proven benefits that exceed harms to prescribe.)
4. All drugs are toxic; only the dosing and indication makes them therapeutic.
5. Always have an exit strategy. (Do not prescribe acutely, and assume indefinite treatment. Have an endpoint in mind, or a strong scientific rationale for long-term use).
6. Most current psychotropic drugs have symptomatic benefits, but are not disease-modifying. The clearest exception is lithium.
7. Older drugs are more effective than newer drugs.
8. Newer drugs are more tolerable than older drugs.
9. Treatment 'resistance' usually reflects either misdiagnosis or an invalid diagnosis.
10. Course, not symptoms, reveals the diagnosis.

Readers can turn to Chapter 49 for further explanation of these fallacies and truths of psychopharmacology.

SECTION I

Basic Psychopharmacology

A New Psychopharmacology Nomenclature

AN INNOVATIVE TEXTBOOK OF PSYCHOPHARMACOLOGY WOULD FAIL IF IT continued to use false and outdated terminology for drug classes. Antidepressants are not antidepressants; antipsychotics are not just for psychosis; anxiolytics are not just anxiolytic; stimulants don't stimulate; "mood stabilizer" has no scientific meaning.

All these terms began as clinical shorthand in the 1960s for possible clinical effects of an exciting new crop of medications, most of whose mechanisms were unknown. The uneducated guesses of that era have been reified into phrases that patients and clinicians use as if they are true. In fact, half a century later, this clinical shorthand has been disproven, either as simply false, or as insufficiently clear, or sometimes as simply not meaningful scientifically. It's time to start a textbook of psychopharmacology with clear, scientifically sound terms for drug classes.

In contrast to the parroted repetition of drug class names for half a century, the psychiatric profession has been obsessed for over three decades with how to classify its diagnoses. Centered around revisions of the American Psychiatric Association's (APA) *Diagnostic and Statistical Manual of Mental Disorders* (DSM, various editions), much of this debate has been about the practical implications of how we diagnose mental illnesses. It is presumed frequently that if a condition has an official DSM diagnosis, then it will be treated more assiduously, often with medications, and, depending on whether one likes or dislikes psychotropic drugs, interest groups array themselves for or against proposed diagnostic revisions.

In contrast, the classification of psychotropic medications has been ignored until recently. The terms used for psychotropic drug classes are imprecise and misleading: "antidepressants," "antipsychotics," "anxiolytics," "stimulants." "Antidepressants" often are ineffective for many depressive conditions; "antipsychotics" are often effective in many non-psychotic conditions; "antidepressants" are often as effective for anxiety symptoms as "anxiolytics." And the terms "mood stabilizer" and "stimulant" are devoid of scientific meaning altogether, as will be shown in this chapter.

Current psychiatric drug classification is based on clinical terms devised and popularized over half a century ago, with codification by a special committee of the World Health Organization in 1967. It's certainly time for an update.

In the last few years, the main psychopharmacology organizations in the United States and Europe (the American College of Neuropsychopharmacology [ACNP] and the European College of Neuropsychopharmacology [ECNP]) convened a task force for just such an update. The conclusions of that task force were that drug class definitions should be based on their biological mechanism, not clinical purpose. The rationale for this approach is that clinical purposes can vary and change, but biological mechanisms, once identified, are fixed.

This textbook agrees with this basic notion, but differs from the ACNP/ECNP task force approach because the latter seeks to identify drugs in great detail, based on their biological mechanisms, and, further, to connect such mechanisms to DSM-based clinical indications. Such detailed biological definitions will be too clumsy and inefficient for clinicians. Furthermore, the problem with too much emphasis on biological mechanisms is that each drug has many biological mechanisms, not just one. Serotonin reuptake inhibitors (SRIs) also are cytokine inhibitors, and clotting factor inhibitors, and nitric oxide inhibitors, and so on. How do we know which biological mechanism is the most important?

The view taken here is that biological mechanisms should be used, but in a broad and flexible way. It may turn out that some biological mechanisms that are useful for defining a drug class are not the actual mechanisms of clinical effect. For instance, tricyclic antidepressants (defined by their chemical structure) have effects on neuropathic pain that may have to do with their impact on blocking sodium and calcium channels peripherally, not their effects on norepinephrine and serotonin.

So biological mechanisms may be better than clinical definitions, but the former can lead to confusion too if overdone. Furthermore, drug class definitions should have nothing to do with DSM diagnostic definitions, because, as discussed in Chapter 16, the latter can change as well, and, more importantly, they are weak in their scientific validity. The proposed new drug nomenclature in this chapter will be based on biological mechanism, but with the broadest such definitions, both for clinical utility and for flexibility in relation to the range of specific mechanisms that each drug may have for different clinical uses.

CURRENT USAGE: FIVE DRUG CLASSES

In current usage, there are five major drug classes in the traditional psychopharmacology nomenclature: antidepressants, antipsychotics, mood stabilizers, anxiolytics, and stimulants. A major problem with current usage is that the phrases used are not accurate scientifically, and can be misleading in their uses, as described in Box 1.1.

BOX 1.1
PROBLEMS WITH THE CURRENT PSYCHOPHARMACOLOGY NOMENCLATURE

1. Based on clinical terms ("antidepressant") that are not directly related to diagnoses (different types of depression exist);
2. Therapeutically, nonspecific (antidepressants are anxiolytic; antipsychotics are antimanic);
3. Sometimes too narrow (antipsychotics can work for non-psychotic conditions; antidepressants can work for non-depressive conditions);
4. Sometimes too broad (antidepressants are ineffective for some depressive conditions);
5. Sometimes defined by the pharmaceutical industry (origin of the term "mood stabilizer");
6. Can be associated with stigma ("antipsychotic");
7. May mislead patients ("mood stabilizer" can imply not being allowed to have a range of moods);
8. May bias research ("mood stabilizers" may not be seen as "antidepressants" worthy of study for depressive conditions).

Source: S. N. Ghaemi, "A New Nomenclature for Psychotropic Drugs," Journal of Clinical Psychopharmacology: *2015;35(4). Reprinted with permission of Wolters Kluwer.*

These five classes of drugs tend to have typical corresponding diagnoses for usage: "major depressive disorder" (MDD), schizophrenia, bipolar illness, anxiety diagnoses, and attention deficit disorder (ADD). Each common class is examined in Table 1.1, along with background regarding their historical origins, secondary indications, and biological mechanisms.

As can be seen in Table 1.1, it seems to be the case in general that primary indications for the drug classes do not demonstrate more efficacy than secondary indications. Two of five drug classes had relatively consistent pharmacological structures. All but two (amphetamines and sedating agents) had relatively consistent biological mechanisms.

This analysis finds that a drug's biological mechanism is the most consistent method for classifying psychotropic medications. The two exceptions involved either pharmacological structure (amphetamines) and/or clinical effect (sedating agents).

A NEW NOMENCLATURE

Table 1.2 provides an alternative nomenclature based on broad biological mechanism. These mechanisms apply to all drugs in each class, although subclasses and specific agents may differ from each other in having or not having other mechanistic effects.

TABLE 1.1 Traditional Psychopharmacology Nomenclature

	Antidepressants	Antipsychotics	Mood stabilizers	Anxiolytics/Hypnotics	Stimulants
Main corresponding diagnosis	MDD	Schizophrenia	Bipolar illness	Anxiety diagnoses	ADD
Efficacy in main corresponding diagnosis	Moderate	Moderate	Marked	Marked	Marked
Secondary diagnoses treated	Anxiety diagnoses	Mania, Bipolar depression, MDD	MDD	Insomnia	MDD, Sexual dysfunction, Weight loss
Efficacy in secondary diagnoses	Marked	Moderate to marked	Moderate	Marked	Marked
Consistent pharmacological structure	No	No	No	Mostly (benzodiazepines)	Mostly (amphetamines)
Consistent biological mechanism	Mostly (increased monoamine activity)	Mostly (dopamine blockade)	Mostly (second messenger regulation)	Mostly (GABA agonism)	Mostly (dopamine agonism)
Historical basis	1950s mania in hospitalized schizophrenia	1960s benefit in schizophrenia	1950s combined amphetamine-barbiturate treatment	1940s–1950s benzodiazepine effect	1930s treatment of depression

TABLE 1.2 A Proposed Scientific Psychopharmacology Nomenclature

	Monoamine agonists	Dopamine blockers	Second messenger modifiers	GABAergic agonists	Amphetamines	Other
Clinical efficacy	Unipolar depression and anxiety syndromes	Schizophrenia and mania	Prevention of mood episodes	Anxiety syndromes and/or insomnia	ADD and unipolar depression	Antihistamines, Adrenergic blockers, and Melatonin agonists are effective for anxiety symptoms and/or insomnia
Scientific basis	All drugs that improve depression and anxiety in this class increase dopamine, norepinephrine, and/or serotonin activity	All drugs that treat psychosis block dopamine receptors	All proven drugs that prevent mood episodes in bipolar disorder affect second messenger systems extensively, with little primary neurotransmitter effect	All proven drugs for anxiety symptoms in most cases along with insomnia, or only in insomnia for some agents	All drugs that produce immediate stimulant effects for cognition or mood are dopamine agonists	All proven drugs for anxiety symptoms and/or insomnia

"Antidepressants": Monoamine Agonists

The term "antidepressant" is perhaps the most misleading term in all psychopharmacology. As will be shown, if by "antidepressant" is meant efficacy for depressive states, then this class of medications is not antidepressant, since it is ineffective for many depressive states (Table 1.3).

Few realize that these medications were discovered initially not because they took patients from a depressive state to a normal one, but rather because they took patients from a non-manic state to a manic state. In short, the first observations were that they caused mania, not that they treated depression. Perhaps they should be called "promanic" drugs, instead of antidepressant drugs.

The discovery was made by Roland Kuhn, a Swiss psychiatrist trained in the existential/phenomenological tradition. Geigy, a pharmaceutical company, had developed an agent that was similar in structure to chlorpromazine, the first antipsychotic. The new drug, which would be imipramine, the first tricyclic antidepressant, was expected to treat psychosis in schizophrenia. Kuhn was given the medication for its first trials. He found

TABLE 1.3 Nomenclature for Monoamine Agonists (Formerly Called "Antidepressants")

Subclass	Specific agents
SRI	Citalopram
	Escitalopram
	Paroxetine*
	Venlafaxine*
	Fluvoxamine
	Trazodone
	Vilazodone
NRI	Desipramine, Nortriptyline, Atomoxetine
SRI/NRI	Duloxetine
	Venlafaxine*
	Fluoxetine
	Paroxetine*
	Clomipramine
	Amitriptyline
	Doxepin
	Imipramine
SRI/DRI	Sertraline
Serotonin/norepinephrine agonist	Mirtazapine
Serotonin agonist/antagonist	Buspirone

SRI = serotonin reuptake inhibitor, NRI = norepinephrine reuptake inhibitor, DRI = dopamine reuptake inhibitor.

**These agents are pure SRIs at low dose, but have NRI activity added at usual doses.*

that it did not improve delusions or hallucinations in a number of patients with schizophrenia, but one patient, who was delusional but quiet and relatively low in affect, suddenly became excited and ran around and became very active. Kuhn correctly judged that the sudden increase in energy was the manic effect of imipramine. This earliest clinical observation happened in patients putatively diagnosed with schizophrenia in the 1950s (an era in which many such patients instead often had manic-depressive illness). Dr. Alan Broadhurst of Geigy, who was involved in those initial observations, recounted what happened in an oral history:

> Some patients began to deteriorate with increasing agitation and a few went into frank hypomania.
>
> One gentleman, in such a state, managed to obtain a bicycle and rode in his nightshirt to a nearby village, singing merrily, much to the alarm of the inhabitants. This was not very good PR either for the hospital or for Geigy.... [It was] so exciting that a drug should produce mood changes like this. We were simply at a loss to explain it . . . we began to wonder if the flattened affect of schizophrenia was somehow elevated by the drug to hypomania, might a similar elevation of mood be possible in patients with depression. (From "Psychopharmacology to neuropsychopharmacology in the 1980s and the story of CINP as told in autobiography." Thomas A. Ban, Budapest: Animula Publishing House, 2010, p 339)

The Geigy researchers and Kuhn didn't know that his patient was probably a misdiagnosed patient with manic-depression, with imipramine revealing the underlying susceptibility to mania, but they appreciated that the manic effect of imipramine suggested potential benefit for depression, rather than for schizophrenia. Kuhn conducted the first systematic trial in depression in 1956, and noted benefit in severe melancholia.

Given the clear mania-inducing effects of these drugs, the term "mood elevator" would have been clinically appropriate, or perhaps "psychic energizer" as suggested by some. Eventually the term "antidepressant," in an analogy to "antibiotic," caught on most. It was thought that antidepressants would treat all kinds of depressive states, just as antibiotics treated all kinds of infections. This assumption has been proven untrue, but the name persists and continues to give patients and clinicians the same false impression that if you are depressed, then you should take an "antidepressant." It sounds logical in English; it's just false scientifically.

This is so because the efficacy of "antidepressants" as a class has been disproven in bipolar depression, acutely in most studies, and for maintenance prevention even more definitively. The "antidepressant" class is also disproven as effective in MDD with mild baseline depressive severity, based on a meta-analysis of all extant published and unpublished Food and Drug Administration (FDA) data. About one-half of all antidepressant randomized clinical trials of acute depression have been negative. In vascular depression, and depression in the setting of cardiovascular disease, antidepressants often are found to be ineffective compared to placebo (see Chapter 19).

In contrast to the irregular and often absent benefit of so-called antidepressants for a range of depressive states, this class of medications is most consistently effective for improvement of anxiety symptoms. Such is the case for studies of generalized anxiety, panic, and often obsessions or compulsions. Based on their best consistent clinical benefits, "antidepressants" should be called "anxiolytics" instead.

The pharmacological structure of antidepressants varies. The only subgroup defined by its pharmacological structure is the tricyclic antidepressant (TCA) class. Yet other agents that are similar in tricyclic structure, like chlorpromazine and carbamazepine, do not have notable benefits for depressive states.

Biological mechanism is the most consistent finding in this drug class; namely, monoamine agonism. These agents increase activity of one or more of the three monoamines: dopamine, serotonin, and norepinephrine. They may do so through direct receptor stimulation, or indirectly via blockade of reuptake pumps in the synapse. Whatever the mechanism, the result is to increase activity of one or more of the monoamines. Hence, the proposed drug class name for these medications is "monoamine agonists."

Further specification by biological mechanism can occur, since some SRIs are also noradrenergic (fluoxetine, venlafaxine, duloxetine) or dopaminergic (sertraline), and some TCAs are have both serotonin and norepinephrine reuptake inhibition (NRI; tertiary agents) and some only have NRI (desipramine, nortriptyline). Another pure NRI is atomoxetine, despite technical FDA indication for non-depression uses (adult attention-deficit hyperactivity disorder [ADHD]). Bupropion has very mild dopamine agonist and norepinephrine agonist effects, but the potency of these effects is small (much less than sertraline for dopaminergic effects). Bupropion also has an amphetamine structure; hence, on this schema it will be categorized as an amphetamine, which, as noted later, is the only drug class in this proposed nomenclature in which the pharmacological structure is retained as its main classifying feature. Mirtazapine is an alpha-2 adrenergic receptor antagonist, which increases norepinephrine availability; it is also a serotonin-2 and -3 receptor blocker, which increases serotonin-1 neurotransmission, thought to exert antidepressant effects. Hence it can be classified as a norepinephrine/serotonin agonist, as are SRI/NRI agents.

"Antipsychotics": Dopamine Blockers

In the early 1950s, chlorpromazine was found to reduce agitation in hospitalized patients with schizophrenia. This general anti-agitation effect led to the drug class name of "major tranquilizers," in contrast to the benzodiazepines, which had come to the market a few decades beforehand, termed "minor tranquilizers." Soon, it was noted that chlorpromazine and its analogues produced extrapyramidal side effects, which were used to define the class as "neuroleptics" ("breaking neurons," in Latin). This terminology was more common in France, but psychiatrists in the United States and United Kingdom preferred to use a phrase that didn't relate to side effects, and thus the term "antipsychotic" gained vogue. It was first introduced by the Canadian psychiatrist Heinz Lehmann in the 1960s, and gained increasing usage. Lehmann was aware that the term was based on limited evidence: "In 1956, when I was addressing the Canadian Medical Association, I introduced the term 'antipsychotic' apologetically, and more as a metaphor than a designation." Time has proven Lehmann more correct than he knew: these agents work for psychotic symptoms; they also benefit non-psychotic mania and sometimes non-psychotic depressive states. The term "neuroleptic" is more consistent clinically because all agents in this class have at least some extrapyramidal side effects. However, using side effects for class names would be expected to produce negative attitudes toward those agents. The "antipsychotic" label is imprecise though, since these agents are effective in non-psychotic states, like mania, and they are most widely used for bipolar illness and depressive conditions (Table 1.4).

If one had to choose among these class names, the term "neuroleptic" is more valid, since all these agents have extrapyramidal side effects (EPS), while the "antipsychotic" term does not capture the frequent use of these agents in non-psychotic conditions. The "neuroleptic" class name also has more validity, given that animal models of antipsychotic effect are based on the motor effects of dopamine blockade (catalepsy).

If one turns to biological mechanism, all drugs in this class have been blockers of dopamine receptors, to a greater or lesser degree, with one recent exception (pimavanserin). Hence, the term "dopamine blocker" is proposed here as the best consistent and neutral term for the definition of this drug class. This dopamine blockade is strongest for D1 and D2 receptors, but it can also affect other receptors. Prior attempts to develop pure dopamine blockers that excluded D1 or D2, such as the pure D4 blocker remoxipride, failed to produce clinical efficacy for psychosis. Again, specific agents in the class differ widely in pharmacological structure; early agents were phenothiazines in structure, but others (like haloperidol) were butyrophenones, and still others (like clozapine and olanzapine) dibenzodiazepines; other complex structures also abound.

Subclasses with the overall dopamine-blocking class can be identified most prominently on whether or not there is also substantial serotonin-2 receptor blockade, a feature

TABLE 1.4 Nomenclature for Dopamine Blockers (Formerly Called "Antipsychotics")

Subclass	Specific agents
Dopamine blockers*	Haloperidol
	Chlorpromazine
	Thiothixene
	Trifluoperazine
	Thioridazine
Dopamine/serotonin blockers	Clozapine
	Olanzapine
	Risperidone
	Quetiapine
	Asenapine
	Iloperidone
	Lurasidone
	Cariprazine
Dopamine/serotonin blockers with partial agonism	Aripiprazole
	Brexpiprazole
	Ziprasidone

of the second generation of antipsychotics in the last two decades. The term "atypical" is used for that class, but given that it is used much more frequently than the original ("typical") class, and that now more second-generation than first-generation agents exist, it would seem odd to call "atypical" what is now standard and typical. More importantly, some differences exist in biological mechanisms among specific agents in the dopamine/serotonin blockers. Specifically, aripiprazole and brexpiprazole display some dopamine agonism; ziprasidone has notable SRI/NRI effects; and lurasidone is a serotonin agonist.

"Mood Stabilizers": Second Messenger Modifiers

The phrase "mood stabilizer" has no scientific meaning. It was used colloquially in the 1950s for the combined prescription of an "upper," dextroamphetamine, and a "downer," phenobarbital. This amphetamine/barbiturate combination obviously has nothing to do with lithium and benefits for bipolar illness. Rather, the therapeutic concept involved raising and lowering moods simultaneously and symptomatically (Table 1.5). This idea doesn't capture lithium's effect of preventing future manic and depressive episodes, while having few immediate symptomatic effects.

In fact, for many years, the term "mood stabilizer" wasn't used much in psychiatry, nor applied to bipolar illness, since lithium was the only agent available for this condition from the 1960s into the 1980s. When carbamazepine was developed in the 1980s, and then valproate was marketed for mania in the early 1990s, the term "mood stabilizer" began to be used for the class, driven primarily by marketing of valproate by its manufacturer. This usage obfuscated the fact that lithium's main efficacy was in prevention of future episodes, not treatment of current symptoms, as the phrase "mood stabilizer" implied.

Later, pharmaceutical companies obtained indications for most new antipsychotics for acute mania as well. Since most such agents were widely used in bipolar disorder, the term "mood stabilizer" was applied to them, despite absence of evidence of prophylactic efficacy.

If agents in this class are limited to the drugs that have efficacy in prevention of manic or depressive episodes, then included agents would be lithium, valproate, carbamazepine, and lamotrigine. The dopamine blockers would be excluded since their maintenance prevention studies may be invalid due to a biased "enriched" design, where only drug-responsive patients are preselected to enter maintenance studies, as described in Chapter 6.

If this clinical definition is accepted, and these four agents (lithium and three anticonvulsants: valproate, carbamazepine, and lamotrigine) are included as a class

TABLE 1.5 Nomenclature for Second Messenger Modifiers (Formerly Called "Mood Stabilizers")

Subclass	Specific agents
Second messenger modifiers	Lithium
	Valproate
	Carbamazepine
Other	*Glutamate blocker:* Lamotrigine

together for preventive treatment of bipolar illness, then one can ask whether they share any pharmacological or biological properties. Their pharmacological structures are extremely variable even among this limited group of agents, ranging from a single ion (lithium), to a simple carbohydrate structure (valproate), to a tricyclic structure (carbamazepine), to a complex molecule (lamotrigine).

Biological mechanisms were largely unknown in this class until the 1980s, when it became clear that lithium had manifold and powerful second messenger intracellular effects, which had major neuroprotective effects, and ultimately caused changes in gene activity leading to neuroplastic alteration of axonal connections. Valproate and carbamazepine were also found to have some second messenger effects, though not as extensive as lithium's (affecting proteins like protein kinase C for valproate, and cyclic adenosyl monophosphate [AMP] activity for carbamazepine).

Thus, the most consistent finding is that the biological mechanism for those three agents involves second messengers. The class therefore could be defined as "second messenger modifiers," since these agents appear to all modify second messenger pathways without much activity in synaptic neurotransmitters and their receptors. The exception is lamotrigine, which is a potent glutamate receptor antagonist.

"Anxiolytics/Hypnotics": GABAergic Agonists

The term "anxiolytics/hypnotics" is used mainly for the benzodiazepine drug class, which was initially introduced in the 1930s and 1940s (Table 1.6). They were viewed as "minor

TABLE 1.6 Nomenclature for GABAergic Agonists and Other Drug Classes with Anxiolytic or Sedating Effects

Subclass	Specific agents
GABAergic agonists:	Benzodiazepines (diazepam, lorazepam, alprazolam, clonazepam, among others)
	Gabapentin
	Zolpidem
	Zaleplon
Other	*Antihistamines:*
	Quetiapine*
	Doxepin*
	Diphenhydramine
	Hydroxyzine
	Adrenergic blockers:
	Propanolol
	Clonidine
	Melatonin agonist:
	Ramelteon

* *Predominant mechanism at low dose.*

tranquilizers," with milder anti-agitation effects than the antipsychotics'. Barbiturates had been used previously, and continued to be used, for anxiolytic effects. But barbiturates were more dangerous than benzodiazepines in overdose, and also more addictive. Nonetheless, benzodiazepines could still be fatal in overdose and proved addictive in their own right. After a major increase in benzodiazepine usage in the 1970s and 1980s, SRIs were developed and found to have good anxiolytic effect, without risk of fatal overdose or addiction. In the last few decades, SRIs have become the primary class of medication used for anxiolytic effect, especially over the long term, although benzodiazepines continue to be used as well, especially for immediate benefit. SRIs were marketed in the United States and Europe primarily as "antidepressants," despite their clear anxiolytic profile, mainly because their manufacturers saw more commercial marketing success in competing against TCAs for the depression market, as opposed to benzodiazepines for the anxiety market. Some direct serotonin receptor agonists, like buspirone, have been developed specifically for anxiety conditions. Antihistamines also have anxiolytic effects.

Anxiolytic agents also tend to be "hypnotic": they induce sleep. This is the case with benzodiazepines and barbiturates, but it is a difference with SRIs, which can worsen sleep patterns. Agents specifically developed for insomnia, besides some benzodiazepines, tend to have GABAergic agonistic mechanisms (zolpidem, zaleplon, eszoplicone).

The pharmacological structures of these classes of agents (benzodiazepines, SRIs, antihistamines) differ widely, as do their biological mechanisms. The most consistent biological mechanism for anxiolytic effect, though, involves GABAergic agonism, which is found with all benzodiazepines and many non-benzodiazepine agents used for anxiety (gabapentin, pregabalin) or sleep (zolpidem, zaleplon, eszoplicone).

In short, though differing biological mechanisms exist for anxiolytic effects, the most consistent mechanism involves GABA agonism. Other agents either have other biological mechanisms previously described (SRIs are monoamine agonists), or can be listed separately in a miscellaneous class of agents with nonspecific sedating properties (antihistamines, anti-adrenergic agents, melatonin agonists).

"Stimulants": Dopamine Agonists

The term "stimulant" also is devoid of scientific meaning. It appears to refer to the direct symptomatic affect of feeling "stimulated" in some way; but this subjective experience is not a scientific phenomenon either in the brain or in terms of psychopathology. Rather, this term tends to be used in an attempt to imply that a person will have better attention and focus and productivity when using these agents (Table 1.7). Most such agents are amphetamines, and are used for ADD. Some treatments for ADD are not amphetamines, like atomoxetine, which is an NRI. It is not generally called a "stimulant" because it doesn't appear to have immediate energizing effects, unlike amphetamines. Modafinil, another "stimulant" used to increase energy and attention, is similar in structure to amphetamines.

In sum, the term "stimulant" appears to be applied mainly to amphetamines, or agents with amphetamine-like structures. In this case, the pharmacological structure of the class is consistent, but so is the biological mechanistic effect: dopamine agonism. Some agents

TABLE 1.7 Nomenclature for Amphetamines (Formerly Called "Stimulants")

Subclass	Specific agents
Dextroamphetamine-based	Dexedrine (dextroamphetamine)
	Adderall (racemic mix)
	Vyvanse (Lisdexamphetamine)
Methylphenidate-based	Ritalin, Ritalin ER
	Focalin (dexmethylphenidate)
	Concerta (methylphenidate ER)
Amphetamine-like	Bupropion
	Modafinil

also have norepinephrine agonism, like methylphenidate, but most also have dopamine agonism. (The only exception is atomoxetine).

It is noteworthy that pure NRIs, such as desipramine or atomoxetine, show benefit for ADHD, but are not viewed clinically as "stimulants" because they do not exercise immediate energy-increasing effects and have delayed cognition-enhancing effects, in contrast to dopamine agonists, such as amphetamines. Thus, instead of using the vaguer symptomatic term, this class of medications could be termed "dopamine agonists," which would be a subtype of the larger monoamine agonist class, described in the preceding as a replacement for "antidepressant" terminology. This usage would be consistent with the fact that amphetamines are potent "antidepressants," and in fact, from the 1930s into the 1970s, they were the first modern class of medications used for depression.

CONCLUSIONS

The current classification of psychotropic drugs is vague, incomplete, out-of-date, and sometimes just meaningless scientifically. Instead of this misleading list of drug class names, this textbook proposes more precise terms based on common biological mechanisms, described broadly and without excessive detail. It is understood that these biological mechanisms are not exhaustive, and may not be directly related to specific clinical uses, but they are valid, as stated, and provide a scientifically accurate and clinically neutral way of referring to medications. The specific rationale for using medications for clinical uses will depend on clinical studies proving or disproving such use, as opposed to false beliefs for or against using medications based on these vague English words.

This approach would allow clinicians, researchers, and patients to get beyond common misconceptions. Instead of asking, "Why should I not take an antidepressant for depression?" a patient would realize that taking a monoamine agonist may or may not be effective for a depressive condition, depending on what the clinical research shows. Instead of asking, "Why should I take a mood stabilizer for depression?" or "Why should a I take an antipsychotic for depression?" or "Why should I take an antidepressant for anxiety?" patients and clinicians would use more neutral terms that would not prejudge those situations. Again, clinical research would and should be the arbiter, not presumptions based on linguistic usage.

The culture is already suffused with these terms: most patients have heard of serotonin and dopamine. A small amount of further education can define the meaning of "monoamines" and "second messengers."

With this new nomenclature, clinicians will learn to study the clinical research evidence separate from drug classification before making judgments about which drugs should be given clinically for which conditions. Increased attention to clinical research evidence, now often underappreciated in psychopharmacology teaching that is solely focused on biological mechanism combined with linguistic convention, would be a positive result of the proposed classification system.

It can be said that knowledge of pharmacodynamic mechanisms is weak: drugs within a class vary, and their direct relationship to clinical efficacy is not proven (and perhaps even theoretically unprovable). One could challenge the monoamine agonism consistently found in "antidepressants" and point to the huge literature on immunomodulating effects. The proposed nomenclature doesn't claim that the selected pharmacodynamic mechanisms are the proven causes of clinical efficacy, but rather that the selected pharmacodynamic mechanisms are simply present to a consistent degree. The key classification question is not whether the biological mechanism is central to the illness it treats, but rather whether it defines the class consistently and coherently.

There is accepted precedent for this proposal. The monoamine oxidase inhibitor drug class has always been defined by its pharmacodynamic mechanism. The class has proven efficacy for many depressive conditions (though not bipolar depression), many anxiety conditions, and some other uses (e.g., early Parkinson disease for selegiline). The proposal here is to generalize from the monoamine oxidase inhibitor nomenclature to all drug classes and use their pharmacodynamic mechanisms for classification more generally.

Years ago, Rudolph Virchow said that scientific drug treatment would occur when we could combine clinical data with biological mechanisms. This new drug nomenclature would help achieve this goal.

In summary, the proposed new nomenclature is more scientifically valid than our current clinical usage and would allow for more meaningful and accurate communication between clinicians and patients. In this book, standard current usage will be combined with use of the new proposed terms in an effort to encourage readers to begin to transition to the new drug classification provided here.

SELECTED REFERENCES

Broadhurst, A. (1996). Before and after imipramine. In D. Healy (Ed.), The *Psychopharmacologists* (Vol. 1, pp. 111–134). London: Chapman and Hall.

Ghaemi, S. N. (2015). A new nomenclature for psychotropic drugs. *Journal of Clinical Psychopharmacology, 35*, 428–433.

King, C., & Voruganti, L. N. (2002). What's in a name? The evolution of the nomenclature of antipsychotic drugs. *Journal of Psychiatry & Neuroscience, 27*, 168–175.

2

Fundamentals of Neurobiology

THE PREVIOUS CHAPTER DISCUSSED HOW SOME OF THE BIOLOGICAL mechanisms of drugs could be used as the basis for giving them names that are more scientific than the names currently used (e.g., antipsychotics, antidepressants, mood stabilizers). The biology of drugs is complicated, though, and all drugs have multiple mechanisms. In this chapter, more detail will be provided on the neurobiology of the major drugs used in psychopharmacology, as relevant to clinical practice. This discussion will have three parts: pharmacodynamics (biological effects on chemical function in the brain), pharmacokinetics (absorption and metabolism and drug interactions), and neuroanatomy (structure of the brain as relevant to clinical psychopharmacology).

NEUROANATOMY FOR THE PSYCHOPHARMACOLOGIST

Besides knowing *what* drugs do to certain chemicals or proteins in the brain, it is important to know *where* drugs affect those chemicals or proteins. There is some basic knowledge about neuroanatomy that is relevant to the clinical practice of psychopharmacology.

One basic observation has to do with the distribution of two major groupings of neurotransmitters. The monoamines—serotonin, dopamine, and norepinephrine—are specifically distributed, mostly in the midbrain. In contrast, the inhibitory agent GABA and the excitatory agent glutamate—which are not monoamines—are nonspecifically distributed throughout the neocortex. In other words, the monoamine system has just a few tracts of connections, which involve the limbic system, the main area of the brain that regulates emotion. In contrast, GABA and glutamate are present in the entire surface of the neocortex and affect higher cognitive functions, as well as motor and sensory activity.

Neuroanatomy of the Monoamine Systems

The three major neurotransmitters are dopamine, serotonin, and norepinephrine. They each originate in midbrain nuclei and transmit mainly to the limbic and frontal lobes (Figure 2.1).

Dopamine is produced in cells whose nuclei are in the substantia nigra and in the ventral tegmental area (VTA). The nigrostriatal projections are limited to the basal ganglia, and thus affect involuntary movements. They are thought to be involved with extrapyramidal symptoms (EPS) of Parkinsonian tremor/rigidity, dystonia, akathisia, and tardive dyskinesia. The VTA projections join the median forebrain bundle (MFB) and are distributed to limbic structures: amygdala, temporal lobe, and the frontal lobe (Figure 2.2).

Norepinephrine is produced in cells whose nuclei are in the locus ceruleus (LC) in the upper midbrain. The LC projections join the MFB and are distributed to limbic structures: the amygdala, temporal lobe, and frontal lobe (Figure 2.3).

Serotonin is produced in cells whose nuclei are in the median raphe nuclei of the lower midbrain. The raphe projections go in two directions. Their upward projections join the MFB and are distributed to limbic structures: the amygdala, temporal lobe, and frontal lobe. Their downward projections extend to the substantia gelatinosa of the spinal cord, where they are thought to mediate pain response.

An important observation is that the MFB carries all three major monoamine neurotransmitter projections to limbic and frontal regions that mediate emotion. Since those projections are closely intermingled in the MFB, they interdigitate and have multiple interaxonal connections. In other words, they communicate with each other

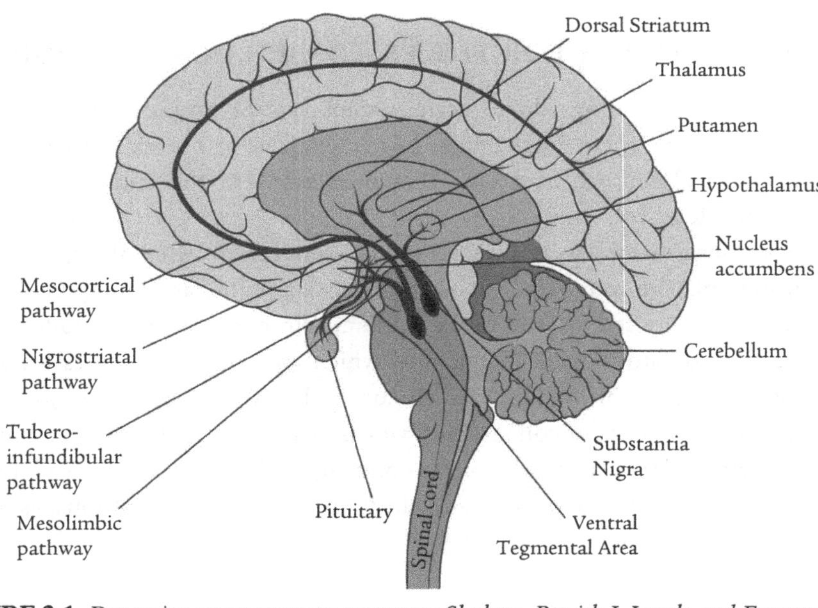

FIGURE 2.1 *Dopamine neuroanatomy.* SOURCE: *Slashme, Patrick J. Lynch, and Fvasconcellos on Wikipedia. https://commons.wikimedia.org/wiki/File:Dopaminergic_pathways.svg.*

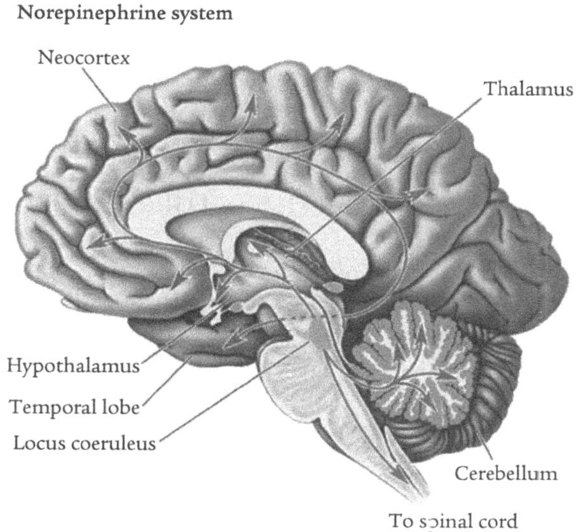

FIGURE 2.2 *Norepinephrine neuroanatomy.* SOURCE: *Bear, M. F., Connors, B. W., Parasido, M. A. Neuroscience: Exploring the Brain, 2nd ed. Philadelphia: Lippincott Williams & Wilkins, 2001. Reprinted with permission from Lippincott Williams & Wilkins.*

in the MFB before they reach their ultimate limbic destinations. Hence it is impossible to affect one of the monoamines without affecting the others. If the LC is stimulated, noradrenergic neurons will communicate with serotonergic neurons in the MFB and cause changes in serotonergic activity; and vice versa. This is a major reason why there is no truly "selective" serotonin reuptake inhibitor (SSRI); hence the acronym SSRI is a marketing tool that has no valid scientific meaning. These drugs are "SRIs," but they

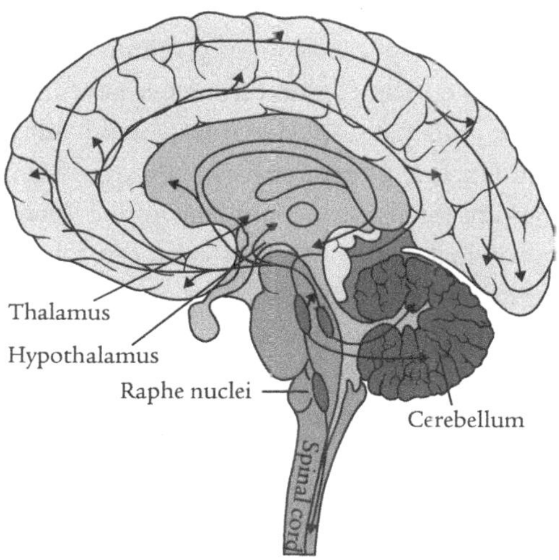

FIGURE 2.3 *Serotonin neuroanatomy.* SOURCE: *DO11.10 and Fvasconcellos on Wikipedia. https://commons.wikimedia.org/wiki/File:Serotonergic_neurons.svg.*

are not selective, because they produce changes in noradrenergic and dopaminergic function, indirectly, through the MFB. (Furthermore, as we'll see, most "SSRIs" are not selective because they *directly* affect other neurotransmitters, besides serotonin, in the synapse).

Neuroanatomy of the Neocortex: GABA and Glutamate

The monoamines are limited in scope, emerging from a small area of the midbrain in a few nuclei, and projecting specifically to limbic regions that mediate emotion. In contrast, GABA and glutamate are promiscuous, being made in many small nuclei all throughout the entire neocortex, in all regions, not just frontal and temporal, but also parietal and occipital.

Where there is GABA, there is glutamate. Where there is glutamate, there is GABA. They are the yin and yang of the brain. GABA inhibits neurotransmission; glutamate enhances neurotransmission. They counterbalance each other, in a careful waltz of the brain's homeostasis. Too much glutamate activity leads to neuronal death: excitotoxicity. Too much GABA activity leads to neuronal dormancy and lack of function.

GABA and glutamate are by far the most common neurotransmitters in the brain; they are much more prevalent than monoamines. GABA acts via its own GABA receptors, which are connected to chloride ion channels. When GABA is stimulated, it opens chloride ion channels. Glutamate is mediated by N-methyl d-Aspartate (NMDA) receptors, without any ion channel mechanisms. Ion channels produce immediate effects, while complex protein receptors have delayed effects, as will be discussed. This is why GABA receptor stimulation with benzodiazepines produces immediate clinical effects of anxiolysis, while drugs that affect glutamate tend to require days or longer for any initial clinical effects.

Other Neurotransmitters

For the practice of clinical psychopharmacology, given most of the psychotropic drugs in current use, the preceding knowledge about those five neurotransmitters—dopamine, serotonin, norepinephrine, glutamate, and GABA—should suffice. However, there are many other neurotransmitters in the brain, and even though we may not have drugs that affect them currently, they are still relevant to understanding how neurobiology relates to clinical psychiatric practice. In some cases, drugs exist, or probably will exist, that affect these systems. The other neurotransmitters to be discussed are acetylcholine, histamine, steroids, opiates, and nitric oxide.

Acetylcholine (AcH) is produced by cells in the nucleus accumbens, in the basal forebrain, which project in two directions: upward to the temporal and frontal lobes, and downward to the basal ganglia. The downward projection is involved in involuntary movements, and thus interacts with nigrostriatal dopaminergic projections to influence extrapyramidal function. In general, stimulation of AcH seems to diminish abnormal extrapyramidal clinical effects (i.e., less Parkinsonian tremor with dopamine blockers). The upward projection appears to affect cognitive function, with AcH blockade being associated with memory impairment and confusion of the sensorium.

Histamine is diffusely produced in the neocortex, and its actions are mediated by histamine-1 (H-1) receptors. Like the diffusely distributed GABA, histamine stimulation appears to produce generalized cognitive effects of reduced clinical anxiety. Since histamine receptors are not tied to ion channels, these effects are delayed, rather than immediate as with benzodiazepines. There is some evidence that H-1 receptor stimulation may lead to increased appetite.

Steroids are produced by glands of the body (thyroid and adrenal mainly), and enter the brain from the peripheral bloodstream. Steroids are small molecules that do not utilize any receptors but directly diffuse into neurons and enter the nuclei of neurons to produce genetic changes in transcription, without any mediation by receptors or second messengers. Hence their effects, though not immediate via ion channels, are very fast and extensive.

Opiates are produced by neurons and stimulate opiate-specific receptors, especially in the spinal cord and limbic regions, which reduce pain sensitivity.

Nitric oxide (NO) is a unique and novel neurotransmitter because, unlike all the others mentioned, it is not a chemical protein but a gas. It diffuses between cells without any receptor mediation and directly affects second messengers. Its effects are not well understood, but some researchers speculate that NO may produce clinical benefits for depression. Some SRIs, like paroxetine, are potent inhibitors of NO synthase, the enzyme that produces NO.

PHARMACOLOGICAL STRUCTURE AND BIOSYNTHESIS OF SELECTED NEUROTRANSMITTERS

The monoamines have structures that are similar. Their biosynthesis occurs from amino acids present in the diet. This is why some alternative medicine advocates recommend amino acids like tryptophan, the precursor to serotonin, to treat depression. Some relate the effect of diet on mood to these amino acids: turkey is said to be high in tryptophan, and thus causes sleepiness through its serotonergic effects. There appears to be some relevance: experiments with tryptophan-depleted diets seem to show increased depression in research subjects, at least short-term. The effects appear to be transient, though, and probably have little if any influence on those who have the genetics of manic-depressive disease: their disease produces severe recurrent episodes of depression; the highest-tryptophan diet in the world would never stop the disease, albeit perhaps modifying temporarily the severity of any single episode within the disease course.

Another limitation to the natural medicine approach of taking amino acid pills for depression is that these amino acids are partially degraded in the stomach, and only a partial amount will survive the gut, enter the blood, then traverse the blood–brain barrier (BBB) to have any effect in the end organ. Pharmacological drugs, like SRIs, produce the same biological effects in the brain more effectively, efficiently, and reliably than amino acid supplements.

Synaptic versus Postsynaptic Neurotransmission

Most clinicians and teachers of psychopharmacology focus almost exclusively on the neuronal synapse. Hundreds of pages of text are devoted to the neurotransmitters mentioned and their receptors. Such effects may be less important than what is not mentioned in much detail: what happens afterward, inside the neuron. Those later second messenger effects are probably more important for the long-term effects of psychotropic agents. Synaptic neurotransmission occurs over minutes to days; second messenger effects over weeks, to months, to years. The first gets matters started; the latter takes them to a conclusion. Both types of pharmacodynamics mechanism deserve attention.

Regarding synaptic neurotransmission, the picture in Figure 2.4 provides the standard description: the axon has synaptic vesicles, carrying neurotransmitters; these are released into the synapse. The axon also has mitochondria with monoamine oxidase, present to degrade excessive neurotransmitters. A reuptake pump on the axon also takes back neurotransmitters released into the synapse. Once released, the neurotransmitters can stimulate autoreceptors on the axon, which have negative feedback effects, reducing the production and release of synaptic vesicles. The dendrite has postsynaptic receptors, which are the endpoint of neurotransmitters, which then bind to and stimulate those receptors. Here the story usually ends.

But what happens after the receptors hug their neurotransmitters? What happens after the happy ending?

As shown in Figure 2.5, a myriad of internal changes happen in the dendrite, involving G-proteins and second messengers. (These effects are most associated with so-called mood stabilizers.) The postsynaptic receptors are typically connected to G-protein complexes. When the neurotransmitters stimulate the postsynaptic receptor, these G-protein complexes are affected: sometimes stimulated, sometimes inhibited. The G-proteins are in turn connected to other proteins inside the dendritic soma, which are stimulated or inhibited by the G-protein. These effects in turn affect other proteins inside the dendritic soma, sending "second" messages (after the "first" message of the neurotransmitter to the postsynaptic receptor), and these proteins in turn

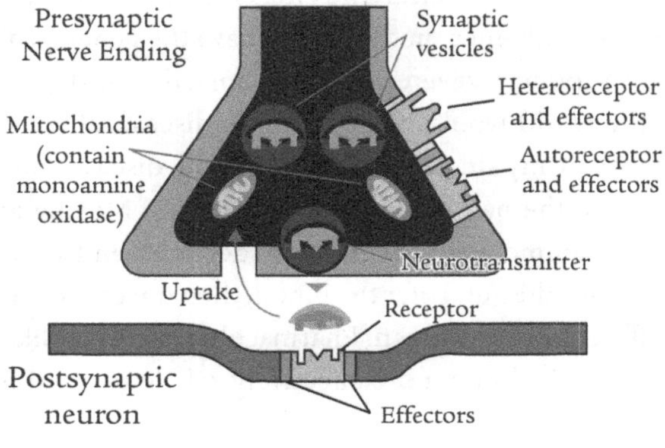

FIGURE 2.4 *The synapse.*

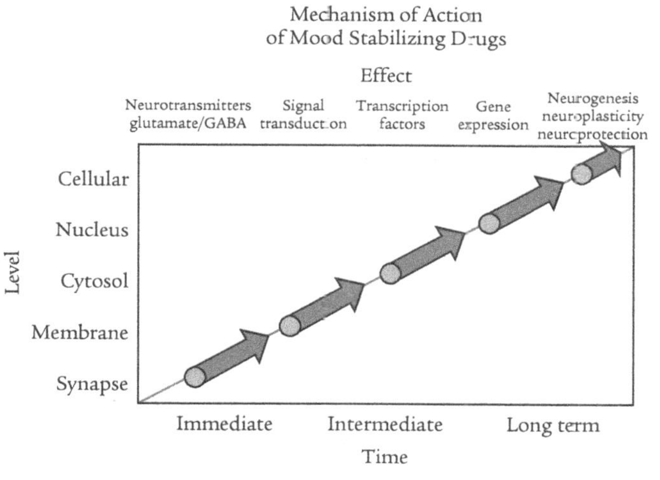

FIGURE 2.5 *After the synapse.*

affect other proteins, which affect other proteins, in a cascade of changes inside the dendrite leading down to the nucleus of the postsynaptic neuron, where genetic transcription is altered.

These genetic changes produce the longer-term consequences desired in neurotransmission. If the goal of the neurotransmission was to stimulate the neuron and tell it to stimulate those it is connected with—say, norepinephrine—then the genetic changes would be to produce more norepinephrine in the synaptic vesicles of that postsynaptic neuron, which, in its axon, would be released and stimulate other neurons at their synapses. And the whole process would be repeated.

It could be that the neuronal message was intended to stimulate the neuron into connecting with other neurons to which it had not yet connected. Then the genetic transcription might produce new sproutings of the axon onto other neurons, making synapses that never existed before. These effects would change, literally, the anatomy of the brain, at a microscopic level. This is what is meant by long-term neuroplastic changes in the brain with psychotropic agents (like lithium).

Metabolism, Excretion, Binding, and the Blood–Brain Barrier

Drugs cannot exert their effects in the brain unless they get there. Pharmacokinetics is about how drugs enter the body, are metabolized and moved around, get to the central nervous system, and are eventually excreted and removed from the body. Pharmacokinetics also involve how drugs affect each other if given at the same time.

The two main organs involved in pharmacokinetics are the liver and the kidney. The liver metabolizes drugs; the kidney excretes them. Much of the work of the liver happens in an enzyme system called the cytochrome P450 system. Some psychotropic drugs, like fluoxetine and paroxetine, block some parts of the P450 system (2D6 and/or 3A4), while other drugs, like carbamazepine and phenytoin, induce the P450 system. Blocking P450 enzymes prevents the metabolism of some drugs, increasing their levels in the body (and thus potentially their toxicity); inducing P450 enzymes enhances the metabolism of some drugs, decreasing their levels in the body (and thus potentially their efficacy).

Once drugs are metabolized in the liver, they pass through the bloodstream to their end-organs and eventually to the kidneys, where they are excreted in the urine. Some drugs, like lithium, bypass liver metabolism and are excreted unchanged by the kidneys. Kidney function is naturally affected by age, with a 1% decline per year in excretion capacity. Thus, a 70-year-old man will excrete 40% less drug than a 30-year-old man; this is one reason why drug doses should decrease with age to avoid toxicity.

Two other important aspects of pharmacokinetics are the BBB and plasma protein binding. The BBB consists of a series of protein pumps at the interface of the dura mater of the brain and spine and surrounding blood vessels. These protein pumps work to keep the internal chemistry of the cerebrospinal fluid (CSF) as stable and consistent as possible. Drugs in the blood can diffuse into the CSF if they are small molecules, but most need to be actively pumped into the brain by protein complexes at the BBB. They may also be actively pumped out of the CSF by the same protein complexes. The BBB can vary depending on the drug (some agents are pumped out more than others), and the patient (some racial/ethnic differences may exist with pumping of medications out of the brain). Perhaps the most clinically relevant fact about the BBB is that it gets more porous with age; older persons will have less active protein pumps and thus more drugs in the blood will enter and remain in the CSF. This can produce more CSF toxicity at standard blood levels (as with lithium; see Chapter 27).

Plasma proteins, namely albumin, are present in the bloodstream and bind some drugs. Drugs that are highly bound to plasma proteins (like valproate) are not available free in the serum so as to diffuse or otherwise cross the BBB. Dosing often needs to exceed plasma-protein binding so that excess drug can freely exist in the serum so as to eventually cross the BBB. Albumin levels are affected by diet (low in malnutrition), and common normal medical processes like pregnancy (where albumin is increased). These changes in plasma protein status can affect the binding of relevant drugs, and thereby increase or decrease the effects of those drugs.

Blood Levels

As shown in Figure 2.6, classic pharmacokinetic studies show that drugs have peak and trough effects. Immediately upon taking a drug, a peak effect occurs, then a degradation process happens as the drug enters the bloodstream and is metabolized or excreted or enters target organs.

The half-life of a drug is defined as when 50% of an initial dose remains in the bloodstream. For most commonly used psychotropic drugs in clinical practice, half-lives vary from 4–12 hours, although some agents can be shorter or longer in their duration of persistence in the bloodstream. Stable blood levels of drugs usually require at least three to five half-lives (hence two to four days for most psychotropic drugs).

Having a stable blood level of a drug is a much-assumed but poorly proven desideratum in clinical practice. Some conditions, like epilepsy, may require stable blood levels for clinical efficacy (i.e., maintenance of a high seizure threshold). Most psychiatric

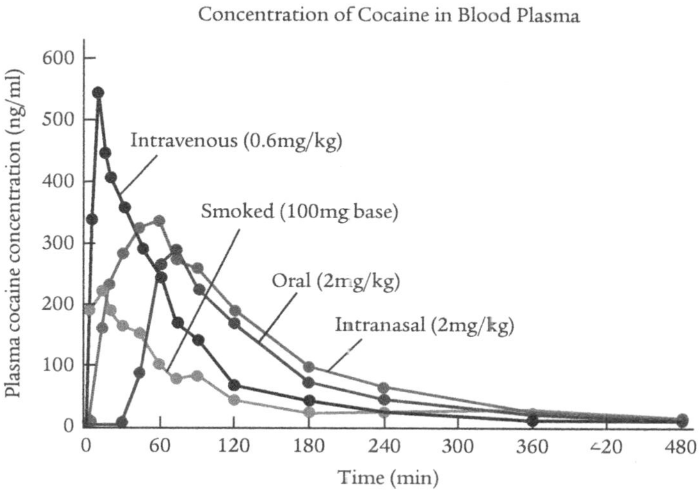

FIGURE 2.6 *Classic pharmacokinetics.* SOURCE: *Adapted from Feldman, Meyer, and Quenzer, Principles of Neuropsychopharmacology, Sinauer Associates 1997.*

conditions do not require stable blood levels because clinical efficacy does not occur on a minute to minute, hour to hour, or even a day to day basis. Psychotropic drugs exert most of their effects postsynaptically, as mentioned, meaning over weeks, to months, to years—not synaptically, over hours to days. Those postsynaptic effects are slow, it bears repeating, because of an extensive second messenger cascade followed by genetic transcription and axonal changes that can even be anatomical. Hence hour to hour fluctuations in blood levels of most psychotropic drugs are likely to be unimportant and irrelevant to their main clinical effects (like alleviating or preventing depressive episodes or psychotic symptoms). An exception may be the use of benzodiazepines for anxiety, where effects are synaptic and immediate, mediated by chloride ion channels; in that use, blood level alterations may be clinically noticeable.

Tolerance and Sensitization

The repeated use of a drug can change its effects. In other words, even drug mechanisms can be affected by pharmacokinetics. Two major types of effects exist: drug mechanisms can decrease in impact, or they can increase. The first is called tolerance, the second sensitization; both can be a problem. With tolerance, repeated administration of a drug leads to less and less benefit; with sensitization, repeated administration leads to excessive effects. With tolerance, drugs stop working; with sensitization, their side effects can increase markedly. An example of tolerance is reduced benefit over time with benzodiazepines for anxiety; an example of sensitization is tardive dyskinesia with repeated dopamine-blocker treatment.

A clarification on tolerance: pharmacological tolerance should be distinguished from clinical tolerance. Pharmacological tolerance means that postsynaptic receptors decrease in number or become less sensitive to the presence of a neurotransmitter.

More drug is needed to have the same effect. Or the effect simply goes away no matter how much drug (or neurotransmitter) is given. This pharmacological process can translate into loss of clinical efficacy. But not all loss of clinical efficacy represents pharmacological tolerance. In other words, clinical and pharmacological tolerance are not identical.

A common example of clinical tolerance happens with recurrent depression and/or mania. Monoamine agonists ("antidepressants") can have short-term benefit, treating an acute mood episode, but they may not have long-term benefit, failing to be effective in maintenance prevention of future mood episodes (see Chapter 6). Thus, if clinicians give monoamine agonists for an acute depressive episode, and then continue the drugs long-term, they frequently observe that the patient improves, and then relapses. This is mistakenly called "tolerance" as if the pharmacological process of postsynaptic receptor desensitization had taken place. Instead, it can simply reflect acute efficacy but lack of maintenance efficacy. The drugs just work acutely, like steroids or antibiotics, but not preventively. The synaptic process may not involve postsynaptic receptor desensitization at all, but simply the fact that monoamine agonism has acute benefits for mood conditions, but has only limited to no long-term prophylaxis benefits.

Dosing Frequency

Generally, frequency of dosing is related to drug half-life. If a drug has a half-life of 12–24 hours, then it can be dosed once daily; if 6–12 hours, twice daily; if less than six hours, thrice daily. As discussed previously, this general rule should be broken, however, if stable blood levels are irrelevant to clinical efficacy, as is the case with most major psychiatric symptoms (excluding anxiety).

As a rule, clinicians should work hard to prescribe psychotropic drugs as infrequently as possible in the course of a day. Once-daily dosing is much preferred to twice; and twice much more than thrice. The main reason has to do with compliance: in classic studies of epilepsy and migraine, once-daily dosing was found to produce about 80% compliance; twice daily, 60% compliance; thrice daily, 52%; and four times daily, 40% compliance. This is the case in persons who are otherwise mentally normal. If one introduces psychiatric illness, which impairs cognition and frequently is associated with poor insight as well as stigma—one can expect much higher noncompliance rates with multiple daily dosing. As a result, in psychiatric conditions, it is to be expected that more than once-daily dosing probably results in noncompliance in at least half, if not the majority, of patients.

No drug works if it isn't taken: therefore, the frequent practice, completely unjustified pharmacologically, of prescribing most psychotropic drugs twice daily or more is a major impediment to the real-world effectiveness of psychotropic drugs. And removing this major impediment is completely within the power of psychiatric clinicians. They should prescribe almost all drugs once daily, unless forced to do otherwise—rather than the reverse. A classic example is lithium, which commonly is prescribed twice or thrice daily despite having a 24-hour half-life. This unnecessary and harmful clinical practice should cease.

GENETICS, ENVIRONMENT, AND PSYCHOPHARMACOLOGY

It is accepted that neurobiology is an important factor in the etiology and pathophysiology of major psychiatric conditions—like schizophrenia and manic-depressive disease, as well as in other psychiatric clinical pictures. The general summary usually provided is that neurobiology represents a diathesis to psychiatric conditions, which is supplemented by environmental stress to produce observed clinical pictures. This mixture of genetics and environment is oversimplified in the minds of most mental health professionals. Most clinicians seem to think the mix is generally 50/50. They then justify the use of combined psychotropic drugs and psychotherapies accordingly. In fact, the mix depends on the illness. In the case of the major psychiatric diseases of schizophrenia and manic-depression, the mix is 80% genetic and 20% environmental factors (based on summary analyses of twin genetic heritability studies). The only physical state more genetic than these diseases is eye color, which is almost completely genetic in twin heritability studies. Physical height is 80% genetic; the environmental component is not very influential, and represents in part statistical "noise."

Hence, schizophrenia and manic-depression are almost completely genetic conditions. Without the genetic susceptibility, the diseases do not happen, despite the most adverse environments. Perhaps this fact has something to do with the fact that psychotropic drugs are essential to the treatment of these diseases—a statement that no scientifically minded mental health professional can deny any longer (despite about a century of such denials until recent decades).

In contrast, personality "disorders" and personality traits are less than 50% genetic, more than 50% environmental; post-traumatic stress reactions are centrally environmental, but also have about 50% genetic components; substance abuse conditions are about 60% genetic and 40% environmental. The more or less "50/50" rule applies to this wide range of psychiatric conditions (excluding schizophrenia and severe mood illnesses, including severe recurrent depression). In these conditions, the notion that psychotropic drugs can be symptomatically helpful may be true, but it should be admitted that psychotropic drugs cannot change environments, and thus generally are insufficient to produce major improvement (unlike the major psychiatric diseases, especially manic-depression).

Our understanding of the role of neurobiology in the etiology and pathogenesis of psychiatric conditions can influence how we use psychotropic drugs. A distinction should be made between diseases of the brain or body—such as conditions that are genetic almost completely, like schizophrenia and bipolar illness—and clinical pictures of psychological impairment that are not caused by diseases of the brain or body, such as some personality states or grief-related sadness.

In the case of diseases, psychotropic drugs are necessary, and often sufficient, not only for symptom improvement but for something akin to a cure: complete removal of all or almost all symptoms forever, as long as the drug is taken. In those cases, psychotropic drugs should be used as much as possible, and long-term.

In the case of non-disease clinical pictures, psychotropic drugs are neither necessary nor sufficient; they can produce short-term symptomatic benefits, but their long-term benefits are limited and often outweighed by their harms. In those conditions, psychotropic drugs should be avoided as much as possible, and used with caution and short-term.

SELECTED REFERENCES

Bienvenu, O., Davidow D. S., Kendler K. S., et al. (2011). Psychiatric "diseases" versus behavioral disorders and degree of genetic influence. *Psychological Medicine, 41*, 33.

Gilman, S., Newman, S. W. (2002). Manter and Gatz's Essentials of Clinical Neuroanatomy and Neurophysiology, 10th Edition. F. A. Davis Company, Philadelphia.

3

Fundamental Psychotropic Drug Structures and Mechanisms

A BASIC KNOWLEDGE OF THE PHARMACOLOGICAL STRUCTURE OF PSYCHOtropic drugs can be helpful, not because one can leap from the visual image of those structures to clinical effects, but because some common clinical misconceptions can be minimized.

A few basic ideas can be stated: Two drugs that are very similar in pharmacological structure can differ wildly in clinical effect. Two drugs that differ markedly in pharmacological structure can exert similar clinical effects. Understanding pharmacological structure is most useful for appreciating classification with similar agents structurally. Clinical conclusions should be based, however, on clinical confirmation or refutation of similarity of effect to other drugs in the same class.

In short, no *a priori* clinical judgments should be made based primarily on pharmacological structure. Structure is a beginning point to understand what drugs do, not the end.

Drugs are often developed by pharmaceutical companies based on variations on the same basic structure: if clinical results are similar, a "me-too" effect ensues, either for efficacy or for side effects. Yet, despite similarities in some clinical outcomes, drugs can have differing effects on other clinical outcomes. The cry of "me too" should not be made cynically.

The rest of this chapter provides basic structure and mechanisms of action of dopamine blockers ("antipsychotics"), monoamine agonists ("antidepressants"), second messenger modifiers ("mood stabilizers"), GABAergic agonists ("anxiolytics"), and other agents.

DOPAMINE BLOCKERS (ANTIPSYCHOTICS)

The original "antipsychotic" was chlorpromazine, the classic agent in the phenothiazine class of drugs (Figure 3.1).

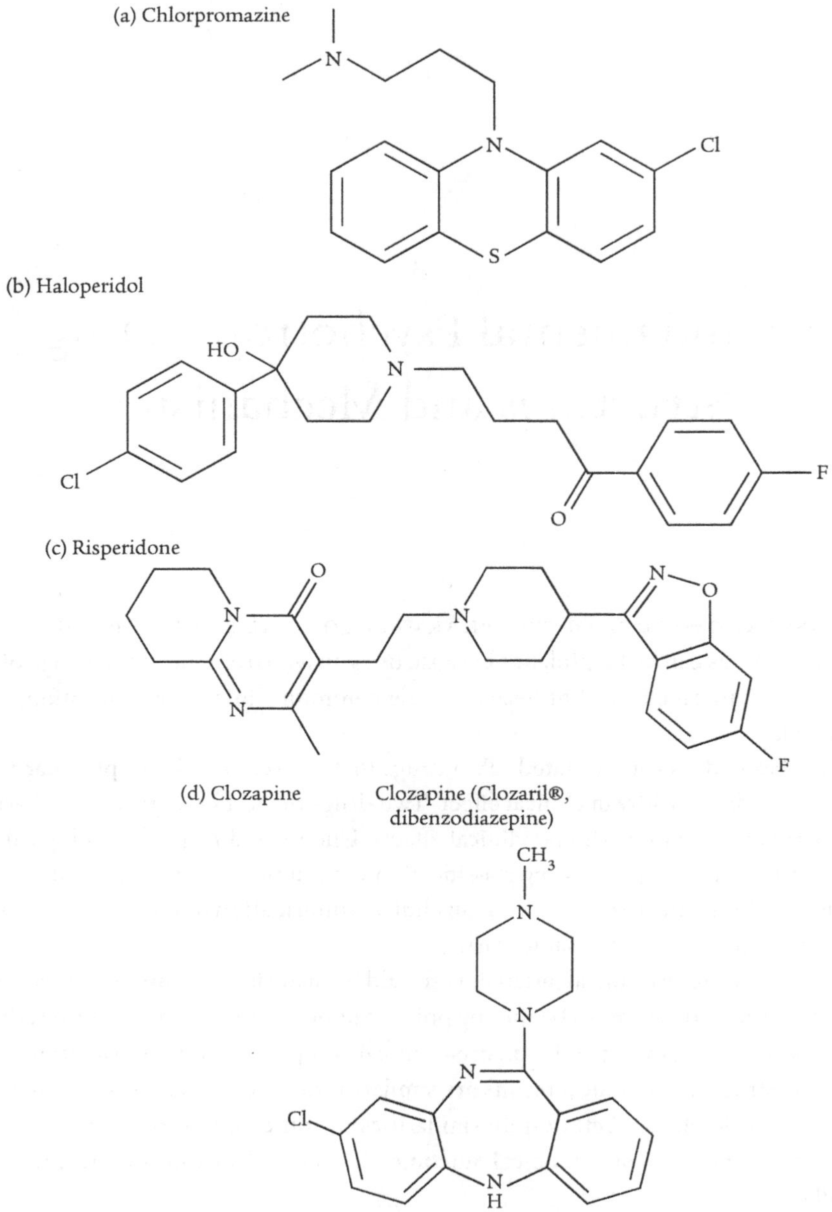

FIGURE 3.1 *Pharmacological structures of dopamine blockers.*

(e) Olanzapine

Olanzapine (zyprexa®, dibenzodiazepine)

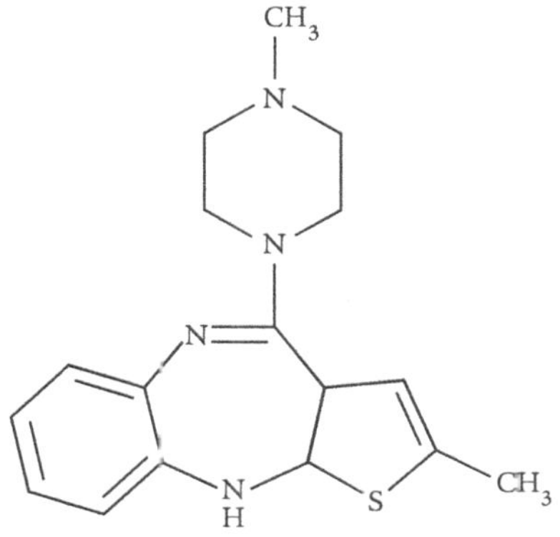

(f) Quetiapine

Quetiapine (Seroquel®, dibenzothiazepine)

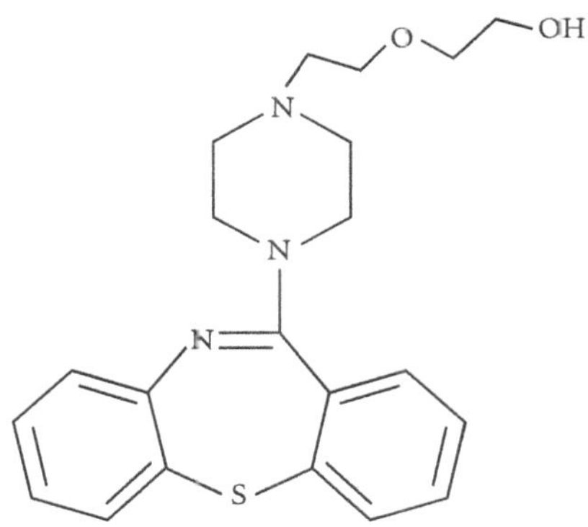

(g) Aripiprazole

Aripiprazole (Abilify®, piperazinylquinolinone)

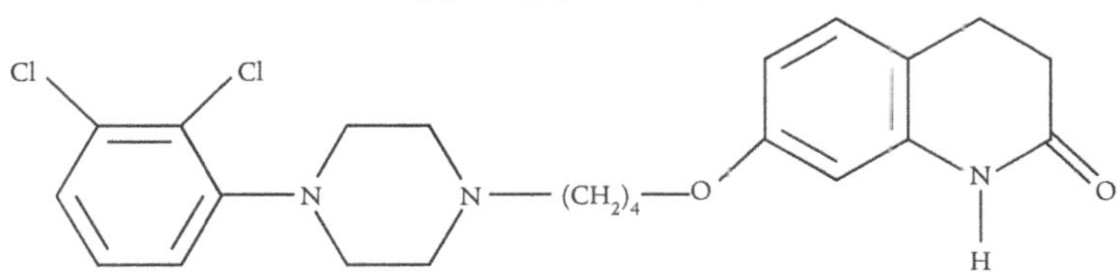

(h) Ziprasidone

Ziprasidone (Geodon®, benzisothiazole)

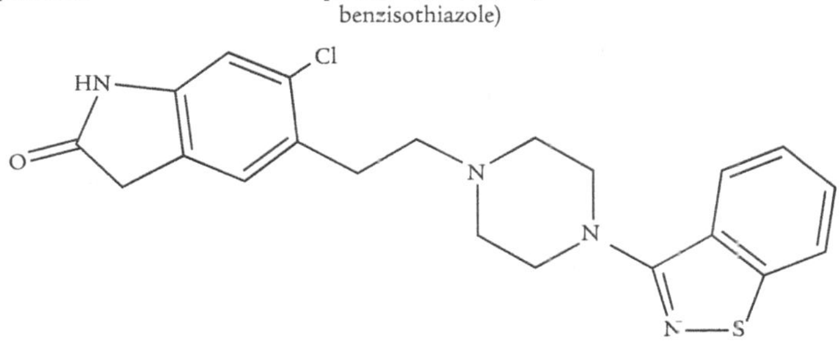

FIGURE 3.1 *Continued*

As seen in Figure 3.1a, chlorpromazine has the classic tricyclic structure: two benzene rings connected by a heterocyclic structure. The center ring is anchored by a nitrogen atom at its top and a sulfur atom at its bottom. Connected at the nitrogen link is a carbohydrate side chain with a terminal amine group. This amine group comes at the end of three carbohydrate links, hence it is called a *tertiary amine group*. Clinical studies find that most tricyclic agents with this tertiary amine group have an extensive series of similar side effects: anticholinergic (dry mouth, cognitive impairment, constipation), antihistaminic (weight gain, sedation), and antiadrenergic (sexual dysfunction, orthostatic hypotension, cognitive impairment) effects.

Chlorpromazine was found to have benefits for psychosis in mania and schizophrenia in the 1950s, in the classic work of the French psychiatrist Jean Delay and his collaborator Pierre Deniker. In the ensuing two decades, multiple other phenothiazines were developed, and demonstrated clinical benefit for psychosis. By the 1970s, haloperidol—an agent in a different pharmacological class, the butyrophenones—was found to be clinically effective for psychosis without most of the tertiary amine side effects associated with chlorpromazine and a number of other phenothiazines. This drug was developed by the Scandinavian psychiatrist and pharmacist Paul Janssen (Figure 3.1b). Structurally, it has absolutely no similarity to phenothiazines. It is a long carbohydrate chain with a benzene ring at each end, and one heterocyclic structure connected to the benzene ring on one end. That ring has a chloride ion; the opposite benzene rink includes a fluoride compound. The remaining carbohydrate chain is simple except for a double-bonded oxygen atom at its center. Chlorpromazine and haloperidol are the iconic traditional dopamine blockers (sometimes called "typical" for reasons that typically are not clear).

In the 1980s and 1990s, Janssen, who had started his own pharmaceutical company, tried to adapt the haloperidol compound to reduce its EPSs and/or enhance its clinical efficacy. He combined the haloperidol molecule with an agent known to block serotonin receptors, ritanserin. The new compound was risperidone (Figure 3.1c). The altered molecule has the recognizable fluoride ion in a benzene ring at one end, but that benzene ring is now connected to a heterocylic structure with an amine double bond, which is connected in turn to another heterocylic structure, followed by a short carbohydrate chain, connected to another benzene ring, and ending finally on another heterocyclic structure. A quite complex molecule, risperidone was similar to haloperidol in its clinical efficacy, but, as hoped for, somewhat lower in its EPSs, especially, in what was a major breakthrough, a markedly lower rate of tardive dyskinesia (a common clinical misconception holds that this is not the case; the definitive clinical evidence will be provided in Chapter 10).

Risperidone was a major breakthrough, and was followed immediately by olanzapine, and then quetiapine, both of which were chemically derived from the structure of clozapine. All these agents provided serotonin receptor blockade along with standard dopamine blockade found with all these agents. These dopamine/serotonin blockers (often called "atypical," a misnomer since it is not clear what was "typical" about the prior agents) are by far the most commonly used current class of dopamine blockers.

As a matter of chronology, clozapine preceded risperidone as the first in this subclass of dopamine blockers (Figure 3.1d). This agent was first marketed in the 1960s and quickly came into clinical use in some countries in Europe. The observation of a number of deaths from agranulocytosis led to its removal from the European market in the 1970s, though, until it was resuscitated in the late 1980s and reintroduced into clinical use with weekly blood tests to identify agranulocytosis at its earliest signs and prevent death by immediately discontinuing the drug. The return of clozapine from perdition paved the way for risperidone and the other dopamine/serotonin blockers, since clozapine was clearly more effective than traditional dopamine blockers. The early 1990s saw the last renaissance of a truly effective drug leading to discharge from mental hospitals of many patients who were not able to be released for years, sometimes decades, using traditional dopamine blockers. Unfortunately, it turned out that no later dopamine/serotonin blocker was, like clozapine, more effective than traditional dopamine blockers. Clozapine remains to this day in its own class, clinically speaking. Unfortunately, besides it agranulocytosis risk, it is clearly the most dangerous dopamine blocker in its many medical risks, especially cardiovascular morbidity and mortality (see Chapter 10).

For our present purposes, the structure of clozapine can be noted in Figure 3.1d. Although classified in the dibenzodiazepine class, clozapine's structure is based on the familiar tricyclic structure at its base, just as is seen with chlorpromazine, the only difference being that clozapine has an amine group in the heterocylic structure connecting the two benzene groups (while chlorpromazine has a sulfur atom in that location). Unlike chlorpromazine, clozapine has a heterocyclic amine side chain (as opposed to a tertiary amine side chain). With these two apparently minor structural differences (an amine group instead of a sulfur atom, and a heterocylic rather than tertiary amine side chain), clozapine is notably more effective than chlorpromazine, causes many fewer EPSs, does not cause tardive dyskinesia at all, and is medically dangerous in multiple ways (agranulocytosis, cardiovascular morality—far more risk on these outcomes than with chlorpromazine). There are some other similarities of side effects (the anticholinergic, antiadrenergic, and antihistaminic effects common to most tricyclic agents), but the example of clozapine versus chlorpromazine provides a key lesson in psychopharmacology: small differences in pharmacological structure can portend major differences in clinical efficacy and/or side effects.

Risperidone was an advance in terms of risks and side effects compared to clozapine: no agranulocytosis existed, and later it became known that its cardiovascular risks were much lower than those of clozapine. Unlike clozapine, though, risperidone was not more effective than traditional dopamine blockers. Figure 3.1e Olanzapine was developed using the structure of clozapine as a template, with the hope of developing a dopamine/serotonin blocker that was both more effective than prior agents, and not as dangerous as clozapine. Olanzapine satisfied the latter but not the former hope: it was safer than clozapine, but, like risperidone, not more effective than haloperidol or other traditional dopamine blockers. Since it was derived from clozapine, it is not surprising to note the classic tricyclic structure at the base of olanzapine, but with a slight alteration: one of the benzene rings was changed to a heterocyclic structure with an sulfur group and only one double bond. The three rings at the base are, in other words, two heterocyclic structures and one benzene group, rather than two benzene groups and one heterocyclic structure, as with the classic tricyclic structure of chlorpromazine and clozapine. Otherwise, olanzapine is just like clozapine, with the same heterocylic amine side chain. Again, a relatively minor change, replacing one benzene group with a heterocyclic sulfur compound, produced major clinical changes: there was no medical risk of agranulocytosis, but there was a major loss of clinical efficacy compared to clozapine.

Next came quetiapine, another attempt to mimic clozapine while removing its medical risks. As seen in Figure 3.1f, there is the same tricyclic structure at its base, with a return to the two benzene rings and a middle heterocyclic structure, like clozapine and unlike olanzapine. The main difference with clozapine is that an extra carbohydrate side chain has been added to the heterocylic amine side chain. Another minor change; still the same result: quetiapine is not as effective as clozapine, and like olanzapine and clozapine, still has notable cardiovascular risks and a range of tricyclic-like side effects (antihistaminic, anticholinergic, antiadrenergic). All three dibenzodiazepines are serotonin blockers, though not as strongly as risperidone; they all have major weight gain as well, more than risperidone, and much more than traditional dopamine blockers, especially haloperidol.

The 21st century began with this list of dopamine blockers. One might consider clozapine and its analogues, olanzapine and quetiapine, along with risperidone, as the first generation of dopamine/serotonin blockers. All these agents were variants on clozapine, or haloperidol combined with ritanserin. In the last 15 years or so, about half a dozen new dopamine/serotonin blockers have been developed that differ pharmacologically in their structure in major ways from their first-generation serotonin/dopamine predecessors. This second generation of dopamine/serotonin blockers began with aripiprazole (Figure 3.1g), quickly followed by ziprasidone (Figure 3.1h). Recently, a number of other agents have come to the market: asenapine, lurasidone, iloperidone, and cariprazine.

Despite technically belonging to different pharmacological classes (aripiprazole is a phenylpiperazine; ziprasidone is a benzisoxazole), these six newer dopamine/serotonin blockers all have a basic structural similarity: they are long carbohydrate chains usually including multiple benzene and heterocylic groups at both ends with a non-cyclic carbohydrate link in the center of the overall molecule. This description is not, in itself, pharmacologically or clinically diagnostic of any outcomes; but it is structurally noteworthy as being markedly different from the tricyclic base structure of most traditional dopamine blockers and first-generation dopamine/serotonin blockers. This overall long complex molecule with multiple benzene and heterocylic rings is more similar, in a general sense, to haloperidol and risperidone than to other drugs with clinical antipsychotic and antimanic effects. Perhaps this general difference may account for some clinical similarities: these drugs all have notable EPSs, but limited-to-no weight gain or other cardiovascular risks. They are not more effective than prior antipsychotic agents, unlike clozapine.

Aripiprazole and ziprasidone stand out with a basic difference compared to other dopamine blockers: they have "antidepressant"-like biochemical mechanisms of monoamine agonism. Aripiprazole is a mild dopamine agonist, providing about 30% receptor stimulation. Thus, even though it is also a strong dopamine receptor blocker—reaching, at higher doses, 90–95% blockade or more—this dopamine blockade is counteracted, in a way, by the 30% receptor stimulation (Figure 3.2).

Hence this agent is not able to fully achieve more than about 70% overall blockade of activity of the dopamine system. A consequence of this inability to achieve full dopamine blockade may be that aripiprazole is not able to have very strong antipsychotic efficacy in severe schizophrenia. In contrast, the partial dopamine agonism of this agent may give it some benefits in treating depressive symptoms more effectively than other dopamine blockers.

The other agent with some monoamine agonism is ziprasidone. This agent has strong serotonin and norepinephrine reuptake blockade effects, equivalent to standard SRIs and TCAs (Figure 3.3).

Thus, taking ziprasidone is like taking a full dopamine blocker along with an SRI or TCA. Again, this monoamine agonism may limit the ability of this agent to have full antipsychotic effects in severe schizophrenia, but at the same time provide some benefits in the treatment of mood symptoms. These monoamine agonistic effects of aripiprazole and ziprasidone may also make these two agents prone to causing mania in some patients.

These mood effects are dose-related. Counterintuitively, these two drugs have more benefits for depression at *lower* doses (and thus more risk of causing mania), while they have more benefits for mania and psychosis at higher doses. For aripiprazole, depression studies found more efficacy at less than 10 mg/d, and less efficacy at higher doses. Above 10 mg/d, dopamine blockade with this agent increases and begins to approximate 90% or greater. For ziprasidone, strong serotonin and norepinephrine reuptake blockade occurs from the lowest dose, but dopamine blockade does not begin to reach high levels (80–90%) until 80 mg/d or greater. Thus, below 80 mg/d, ziprasidone is a strong monoamine agonist with mild to moderate dopamine blockade; this combination may be useful for depressive symptoms, but it also can cause mania.

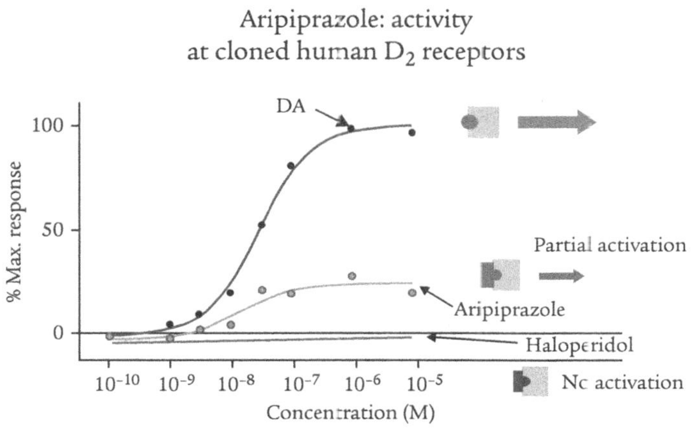

FIGURE 3.2 *Aripiprazole's dopamine agonism.*

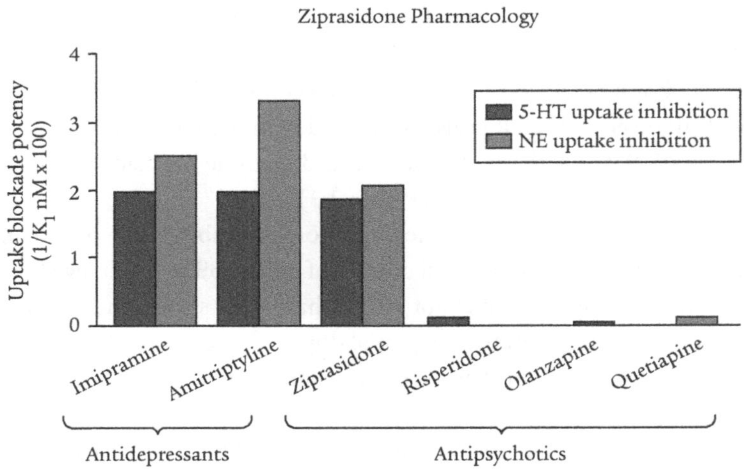

FIGURE 3.3 *Ziprasidone's monoamine reuptake blockade.*

Other new dopamine blockers (lurasidone, iloperidone, cariprazine, asenapine) do not have appreciable monoamine agonistic effects, and thus, compared to aripiprazole and ziprasidone, they may be more effective for severe psychosis in schizophrenia or more effective for mania. They still may have some depression benefits nonetheless, partly through utility for mixed states, as discussed later.

MONOAMINE AGONISTS ("ANTIDEPRESSANTS")

There are four major classes of monoamine agonists, developed mainly for the treatment of depressive conditions, working backwards chronologically: serotonin reuptake inhibitors (SRIs), tricyclic antidepressants (TCAs), monoamine oxidase inhibitors (MAOIs), and amphetamines (dopamine agonists). A fifth category of variable agents that do not fit distinctly into any of these classes has a few recent occupants. Each category of monoamine agonists will be considered, in reverse chronological order.

Serotonin Reuptake Inhibitors

SRIs were initially marketed in the late 1980s in the United States, and exploded in number and usage in the 1990s. The first agent in the United States was fluoxetine (Prozac), and in Europe, citalopram (Celexa). Prozac became a cultural icon, inspiring a number of books extolling either its extreme virtues or equally radical vices. There is no doubt that SRIs radically changed the outpatient treatment of depressive illnesses in the 1990s, not only in the hands of psychiatrists, but in general medicine. The reasons for this massive impact, whose consequences are only now being faced realistically in clinical practice, are numerous and will be addressed in more detail later (Figure 3.4).

These agents were sold as "SSRIs" or "selective" serotonin reuptake inhibitors. This name was a marketing decision by the makers of Prozac, to try to differentiate these agents from TCAs and MAOIs, which increased norepinephrine and/or dopamine activity as well. The idea was that "selectivity" was good, with fewer side effects in particular. In fact,

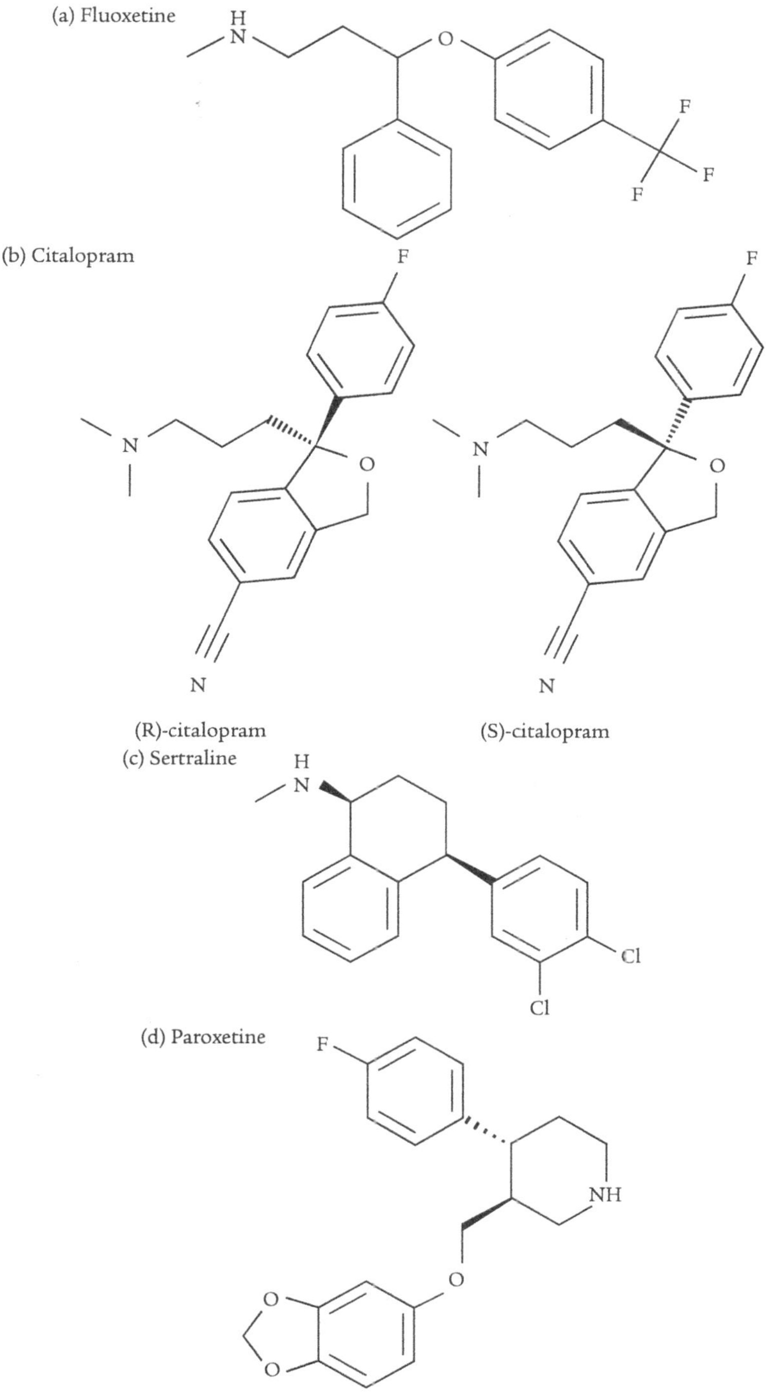

FIGURE 3.4 *Pharmacological structure of main serotonin reuptake inhibitors.*

(e) Venlafaxine

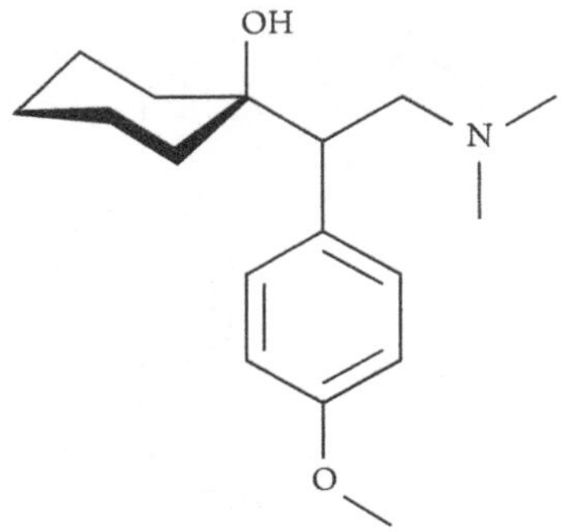

(f) Duloxetine

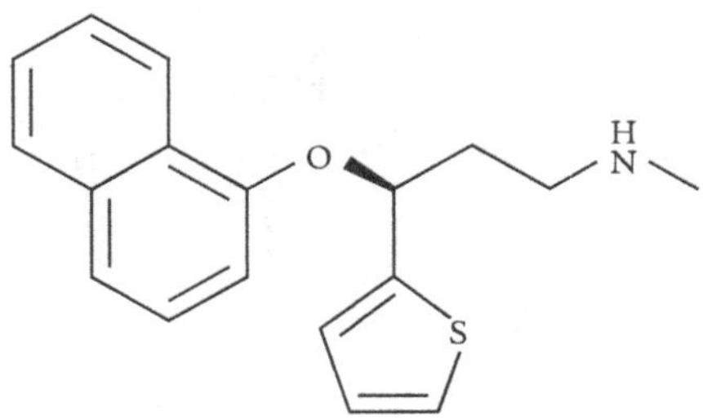

FIGURE 3.4 *Continued*

with the exception of citalopram, this class is not selective, and the acronym "SSRI" is not correct pharmacologically. Hence this text will prefer and use the phrase "SRI," removing the first "S" for "selectivity." This is because most SRIs also affect other monoamines. The SRI agents that also are norepinephrine reuptake inhibitors (NRIs) are fluoxetine, venlafaxine, desvenlafaxine, paroxetine, duloxetine, and vortioxetine. Sertraline is also a dopamine reuptake inhibitor (Figures 3.5, 3.6, 3.7 and 3.8).

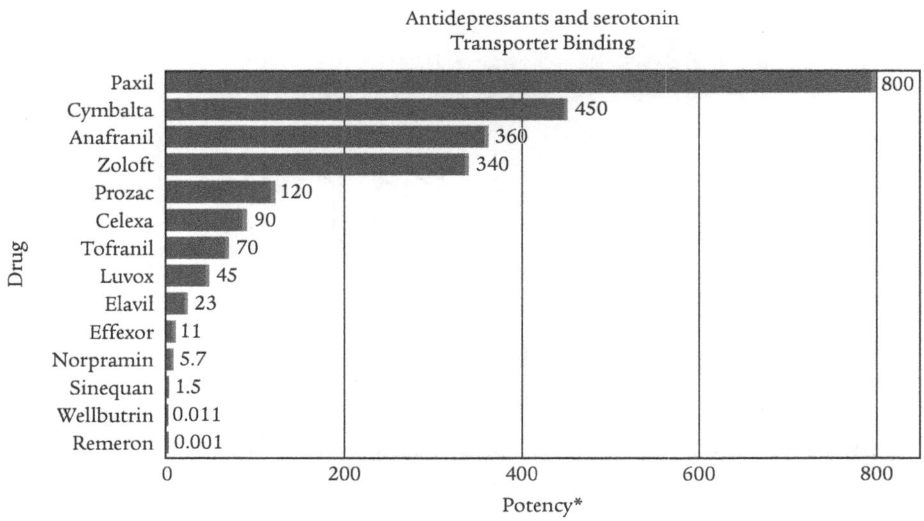

$*10^{-7} \times 1/K_D$, where K_D = equilibrium dissociation constant in molarity

FIGURE 3.5 *Serotonin reuptake inhibition.* SOURCE: *Richelson, E. (2001). Pharmacology of antidepressants. Mayo Clinic Proceedings, 76(5), 511–527. Reprinted with permission from Elsevier.*

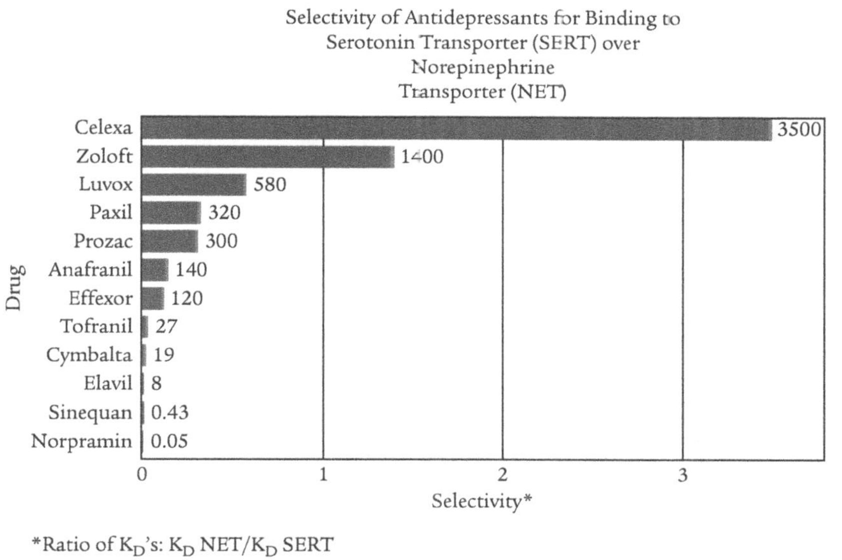

FIGURE 3.6 *Selectivity for serotonin reuptake blockade.* SOURCE: *Richelson, E. (2001). Pharmacology of antidepressants. Mayo Clinic Proceedings, 76(5), 511–527. Reprinted with permission from Elsevier.*

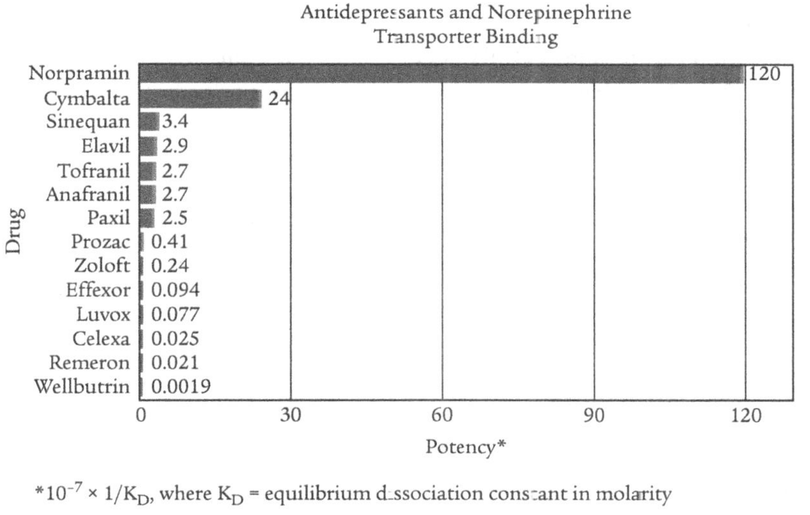

FIGURE 3.7 *Norepinephrine reuptake inhibition.* SOURCE: *Richelson, E. (2001). Pharmacology of antidepressants. Mayo Clinic Proceedings, 76(5), 511–527. Reprinted with permission from Elsevier.*

Trazodone, nefazodone, and vilazodone are SRIs that also block 5HT-2 and 5HT-3 receptors. This effect theoretically increases serotonin neurotransmission down 5HT-1 receptors, which some think would be more specific for depression benefit. Clinically, these agents are seen to cause less sexual dysfunction than standard SRIs. Furthermore, they appear to improve sleep, in contrast to the worsening of sleep patterns caused by most SRIs.

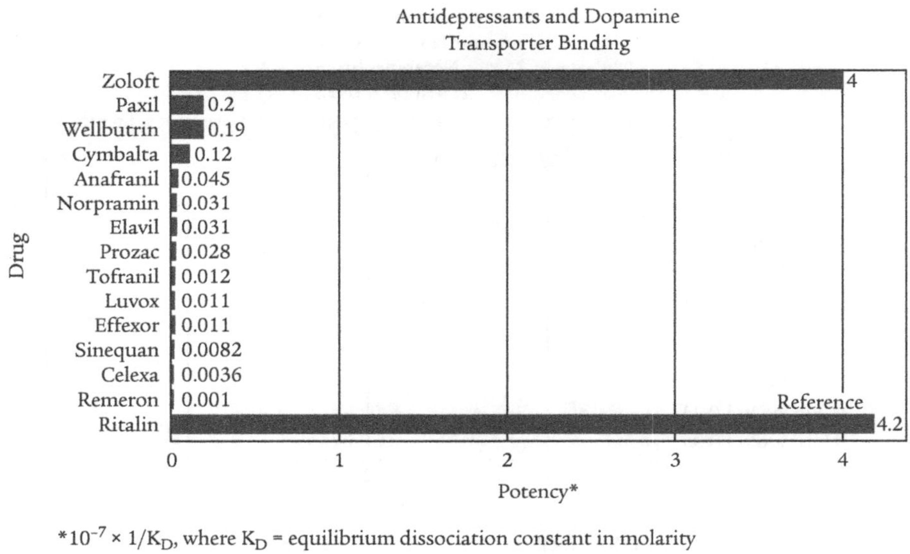

FIGURE 3.8 *Dopamine reuptake blockade.* SOURCE: *Richelson, E. (2001). Pharmacology of antidepressants. Mayo Clinic Proceedings, 76(5), 511–527. Reprinted with permission from Elsevier.*

Only citalopram (and its enantiomer, escitalopram) and trazodone and its variants, are pure SRIs, without any reuptake inhibition of other monoamines.

Still, as mentioned previously, all SRIs affect serotonergic axons that travel in the median forebrain bundle (MFB), which mediates all three major monoamine neurotransmitter projections to limbic and frontal regions. Those projections intermingle and interdigitate, communicating with each other in the MFB, before they reach their ultimate limbic destinations. Hence it is impossible to affect one of the monoamines without affecting the others.

For all these reasons, pharmacologically and anatomically, there is no truly "selective" serotonin reuptake inhibitor, and hence the acronym "SSRI" is a marketing tool that has no valid scientific meaning. Use the acronym "SRI" instead.

Tricyclic Antidepressants

TCAs were developed in the 1950s, with imipramine as the initial medication shown to be effective for endogenous depression by Roland Kuhn and his colleagues in Switzerland (Figure 3.9). Over time, numerous agents were developed and widely used into the 1980s, after which they have been superseded by SRIs and other new agents.

Two basic classes of TCAs exist: tertiary and secondary amines. The tertiary amines are imipramine and amitriptyline; their metabolites are the secondary amines: desipramine and nortriptyline, respectively. The tertiary amines are strong reuptake inhibitors for both serotonin and norepinephrine. The secondary amines are weaker in their serotonin reuptake inhibition, and more selective for norepinephrine reuptake inhibition. Desipramine

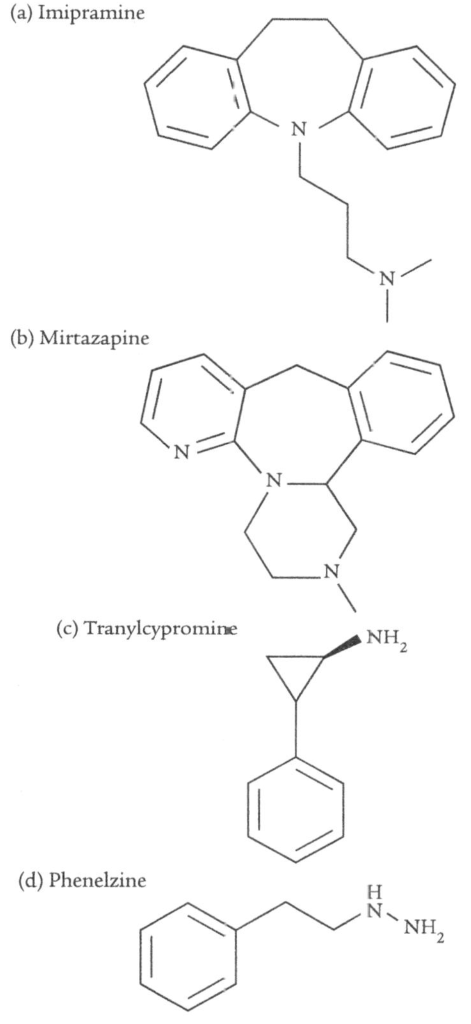

FIGURE 3.9 *Pharmacological structure of representative tricyclic antidepressants and monoamine oxidase inhibitors.*

is a pure selective NRI, the only such agent in psychopharmacology besides atomoxetine (see below).

Besides the agents noted previously, there are numerous other TCAs with few differences, but with some niche uses: Clomipramine, a tertiary amine with serotonin and norepinephrine reuptake inhibition, has been popular for use for obsessive-compulsive disorder (OCD). Molindone is a TCA with dopamine blockade, which was marketed and used for psychotic depression. Doxepin is a tertiary amine TCA with immensely potent antihistamine properties, is markedly sedating, and is used in lower doses for sleep, and in higher doses to alleviate "neurotic excoriations" (skin-picking, dermatological manifestations of anxiety or depression).

Monoamine Oxidase Inhibitors

Along with the TCAs, the MAOIs were introduced in the 1950s, with Nardil (phenelzine) developed by Nathan Kline. Later, Parnate (tranylcypromine) joined it, as did Marplan (isocarboxazid). The MAOIs irreversibly block the function of the enzyme monoamine oxidase, which metabolizes the three monoamines (dopamine, norepinephrine, and serotonin). Hence those monoamines remain in synapses, and their activity is increased markedly.

Because of the major increase in norepinephrine activity in particular, MAOIs can increase blood pressure and produce hypertensive crisis. Furthermore, drug interactions exist with opiate drugs and with other serotonergic drugs, which can produce serotonin syndrome. These potential medically fatal effects—hypertensive crisis and serotonin syndrome—have led to a decline in use of MAOIs, after the development of TCAs and SRIs.

Because of the similarity of tyramine, which is found in some foods, to tyrosine, which is the precursor to norepinephrine, patients treated with MAOIs had to utilize a restricted diet in which tyramine-rich foods were excluded, so as to avoid hypertensive crisis. This diet generally involved avoiding aged cheeses, red wine, and soy sauce in particular, as well as some other foods. The hassle factor of the MAOI diet and medical risks with dietary noncompliance were other factors that limited use of these agents.

In recent years, reversible inhibitors of MAOI (RIMAs) were developed, like moclobemide. This agent was marketed in Europe and Canada but never came to the U.S. market. It was not found to be more effective than other available monoamine agonists. Selegiline was another MAOI that only blocked metabolism of dopamine at low doses. These agents didn't entail the need for the MAOI diet because norepinephrine metabolism was not affected much. Selegiline has been marketed in patch form in recent years for depression (as opposed to pill form for Parkinson's disease); at higher doses (9–12 mg/d in patch form, 20–30 mg/d in pill form), it does block MAO activity related to norepinephrine and serotonin, and thus at those doses, adherence to the MAOI diet is recommended.

Dopamine Agonists (Amphetamines and Other Agents)

Amphetamines are strong reuptake inhibitors of dopamine, and also direct agonists on dopamine receptors (Figure 3.10). There are two basic types of prescribed amphetamines: dextroamphetamine and its variants, and methylphenidate and its variants. The latter agent also has norepinephrine reuptake blockade.

Other dopamine agonists that are not amphetamines in pharmacological structure include modafinil (Provigil) and armodafinil (Nuvigil). These agents have more norepinephrine blockade, but still have similar "stimulant" effects as standard amphetamines.

It is true, but not known commonly, that bupropion (Wellbutrin) is also an amphetamine in its structure, hence its dopamine and norepinephrine agonist effects. It may be less potent in those effects than standard amphetamines (Figure 3.11).

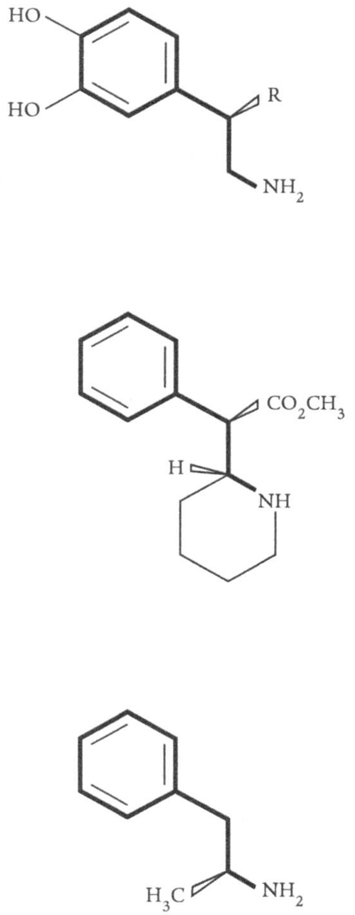

Dopamine; R = H

Norepinephrine; R = OH

(*d*)-R,R-Methylphenidate

(*d*)-S-Amphetamine

FIGURE 3.10 *Amphetamine stimulants.*

Bupropion: An amphetamine

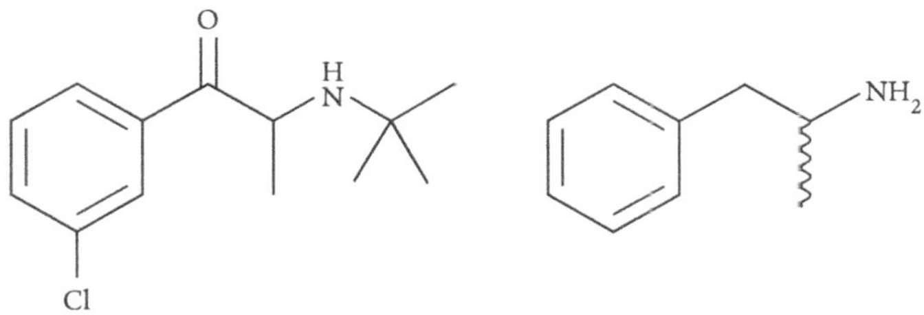

Bupropion

Amphetamine

FIGURE 3.11 *Bupropion.*

Other Monoamine Agonists

Mirtazapine (Remeron) increases norepinephrine activity by blocking a negative feedback loop: the presynaptic alpha-2 receptor, when stimulated by norepinephrine in the synapse, sends messages back into the axon to reduce norepinephrine production (Figure 3.12). Mirtazapine blocks those presynaptic alpha-2 receptors, and thereby increases availability of norepinephrine in the synapse. This agent also directly stimulates serotonin receptors and blocks 5HT-3 receptors, thereby increasing neurotransmission of serotonin by 5HT-1 and 5HT-2 receptors, which are thought to mediate depression symptom benefits. Hence, via these complex effects that do not involve reuptake inhibition, mirtazapine produces the same outcome as multiple SRIs: it is a norepinephrine and serotonin agonist. By blocking the 5-HT3 receptor, mirtazapine

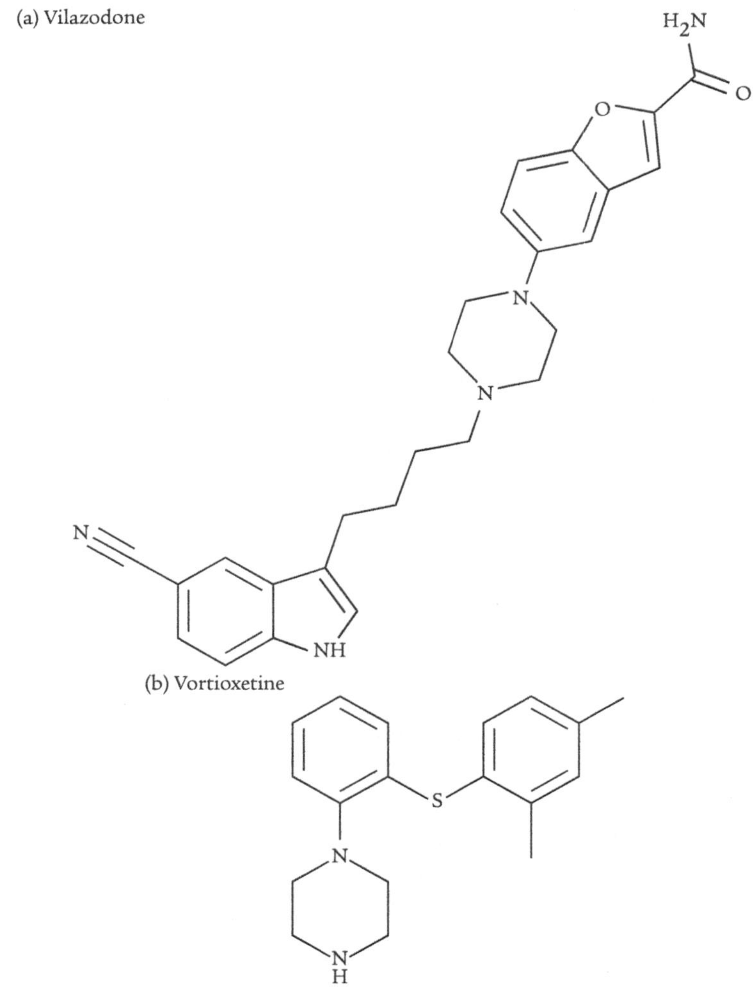

FIGURE 3.12 *Other antidepressants.*

reduces the sexual side effects of SRIs, but this comes at the cost of notable weight gain, unlike most SRIs.

Atomoxetine (Strattera) is a pure NRI, a kind of modern version of desipramine. Like the latter, it is clearly an "antidepressant," but it wasn't marketed as such (despite proven efficacy in clinical trials) by its manufacturer around 2000, when it entered the U.S. market. Desipramine had long been known to be effective in childhood ADHD. Since atomoxetine would join a long list of many "antidepressants," but could be the first specifically marketed non-amphetamine agent for ADHD, its manufacturer opted to obtain an indication for ADHD. It added a twist: rather than being one of many agents for childhood ADHD, the manufacturer obtained FDA approval to be the first agent for "adult" ADHD. What has followed is a major change in research studies supporting the concept of adult ADHD, in contrast to the pre-Strattera era, when most research studies indicated that ADHD did not persist into adulthood. This clinical matter is addressed in more detail in Appendix III.

SECOND MESSENGER MODIFIERS ("MOOD STABILIZERS")

Lithium is the iconic agent in this class. It has multiple second messenger effects that involve signal transduction. This process often is poorly understood by clinicians. The neurotransmitters (like monoamines) are the "first" messengers (Figure 3.13). They communicate between the axon and dendrite by stimulating or blocking postsynaptic receptors. After this first message, communication is further transmitted inside the axon, from the postsynaptic receptor to cyclic adenosine monophosphate (AMP), G-proteins, and then a host of internal proteins inside the axon (such as pyruvate kinase A or C or phosphotidylinositylphosphate, PIP). These molecules (cyclic AMP, G proteins, and internal proteins) are called "second" messengers (Figure 3.14).

Most psychotropic agents are "first" messengers, with synaptic activity. Further changes inside the affected axons are indirect. Lithium, valproate, and carbamazepine bypass the synapse and directly affect these second messengers inside axons. Of these agents, lithium has the most extensive second messenger effects. It stimulates some G-proteins and blocks others; it inhibits pyruvate kinase C and the PIP cascade. It has a range of effects, which end in affecting genes in the nucleus of the axonal neuron. Those genes then change what neurotransmitters they produce, and change their connections with other neurons.

This is a very slow process, but the result is a change in microanatomy of the brain. The connections and projections of the affected neurons are altered over time.

Among its effects, lithium increases activity of neuroprotective proteins, such as brain-derived neurotrophic factor (BDNF), and blocks proteins that cause neuronal death, like bcl-2. With this range of effects, lithium keeps neurons alive longer, and these effects probably are also involved in the increased neuronal connectivity that occurs with lithium.

(a)

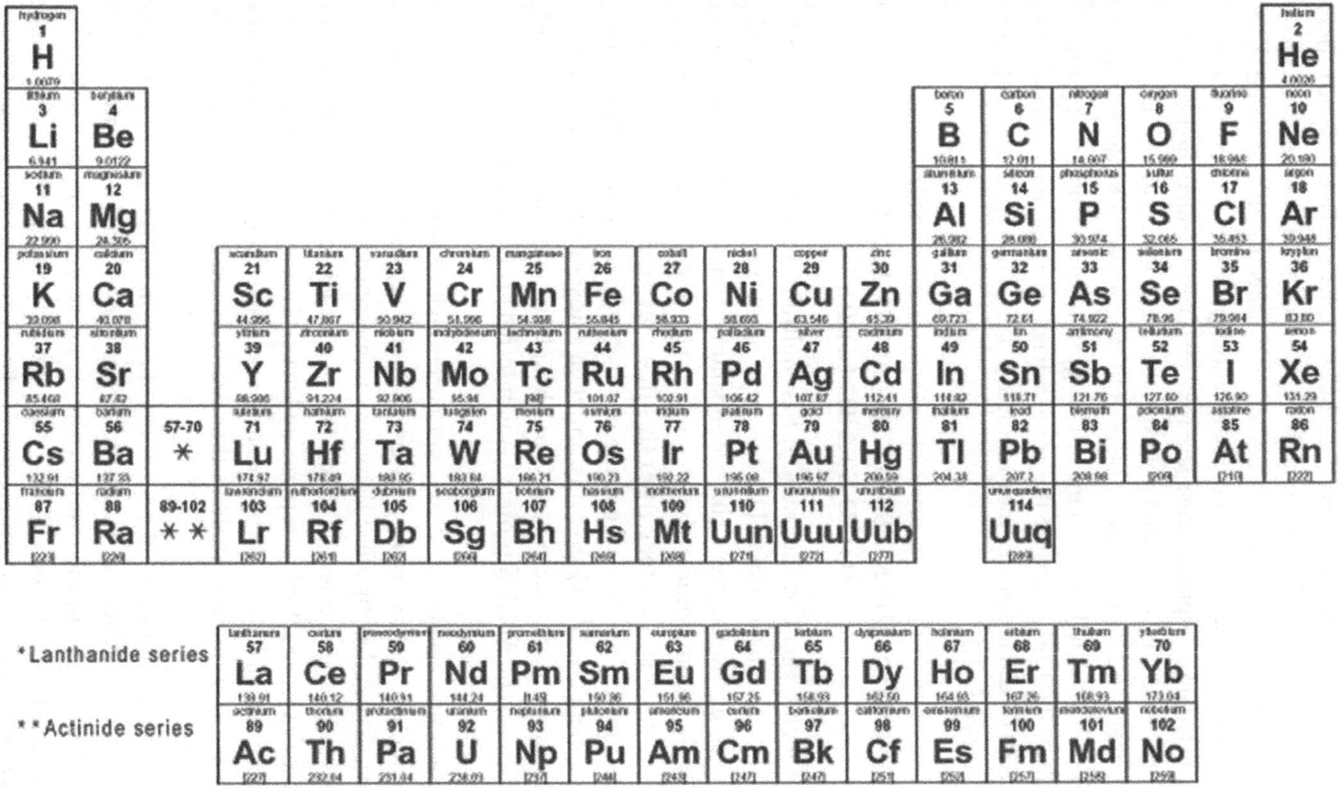

FIGURE 3.13 *a. Lithium*

b. Valproate

c. Carbamazepine

d. Lamotrigine

e. Oxcarbazepine

(b) Valproate

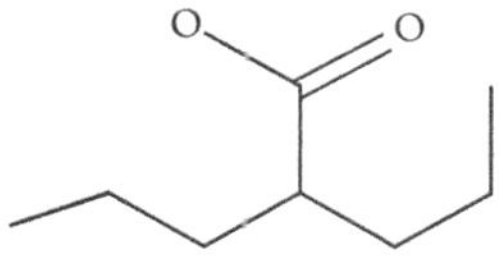

(c) Carbamazepine

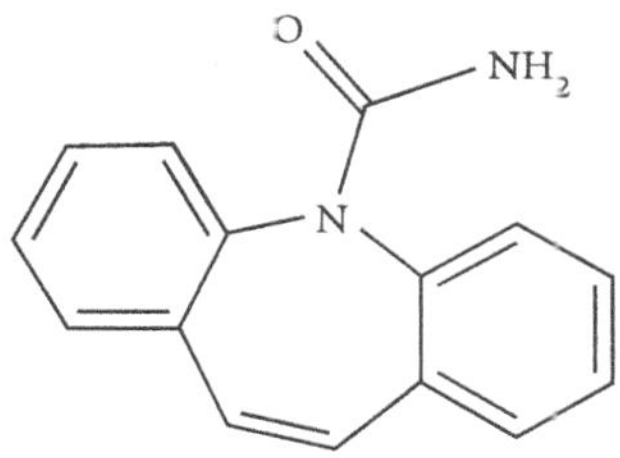

Imipramine

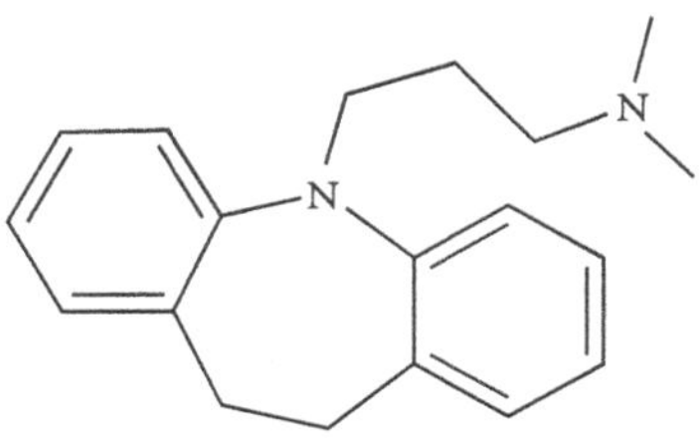

Chlorpromazine

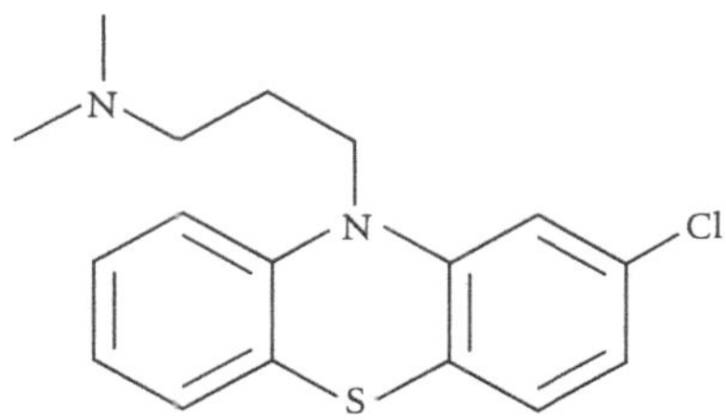

(d) Lamotrigine

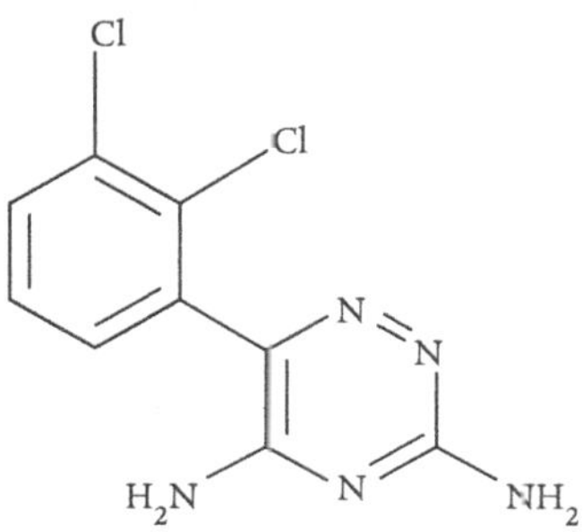

(e)

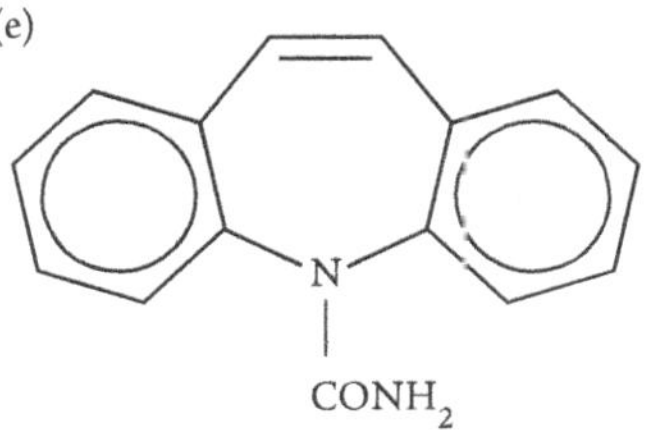

Carbamazepine

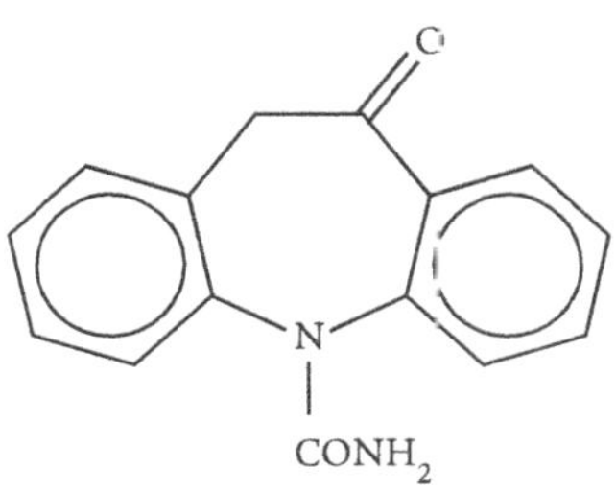

Oxcarbazepine

FIGURE 3.13 *Continued*

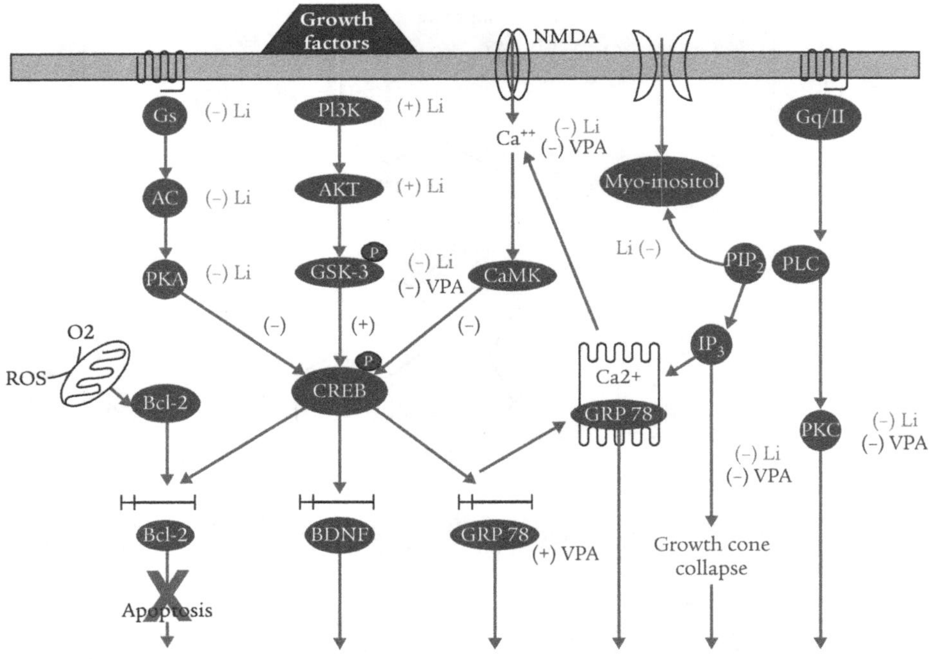

FIGURE 3.14 *Second-messenger effects of lithium and valproate.*

Valproate and carbamazepine are more limited in their second messenger effects. Valproate inhibits pyruvate kinase C activity and affects some other second messengers. Carbamazepine affects cyclic AMP and G-proteins but has few other internal second messenger effects.

These agents can have some mild synaptic effects on neurotransmitters, rather than solely on second messengers. Lithium and valproate mildly stimulate serotonin receptors, and valproate moderately stimulates GABA receptors. But these effects are limited and much less relevant to clinical properties, in most cases, than their second messenger effects.

The only other agent that has benefits like these "mood stabilizers"—that is, in prevention of mood episodes—is lamotrigine. This agent blocks glutamate receptors, and it does not have any known, appreciable, direct second messenger effects. It is an exception to the rule that "mood stabilizers" are second messenger modifiers.

GABAERGIC AGONISTS ("ANXIOLYTICS")

The central class of drugs within this group is the benzodiazepines, agents like diazepam (Valium), lorazepam (Ativan), alprazolam (Xanax), and others (Figure 3.15). These agents stimulate GABA receptors directly, opening chloride channels, which lead to repolarization of neurons. This produces an inhibition of cell transmission.

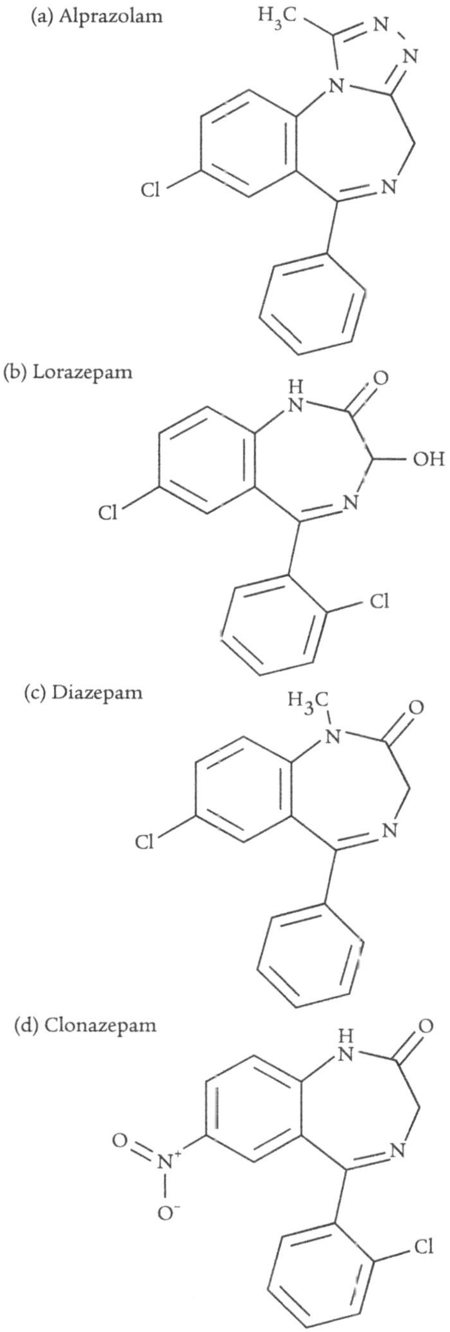

FIGURE 3.15 *Pharmacological structure of benzodiazepines.*

Other sedatives that supposedly are "non-addictive" also are GABAergic: zolpidem (Ambien), zaleplon (Sonata), and eszopiclone (Lunesta) (Figure 3.16). All three agents directly stimulate same GABA-a receptor subunits that are affected by benzodiazepines.

Gabapentin and its metabolite pregabalin stimulate GABA receptors on a different subunit than benzodiazepines (Figure 3.17).

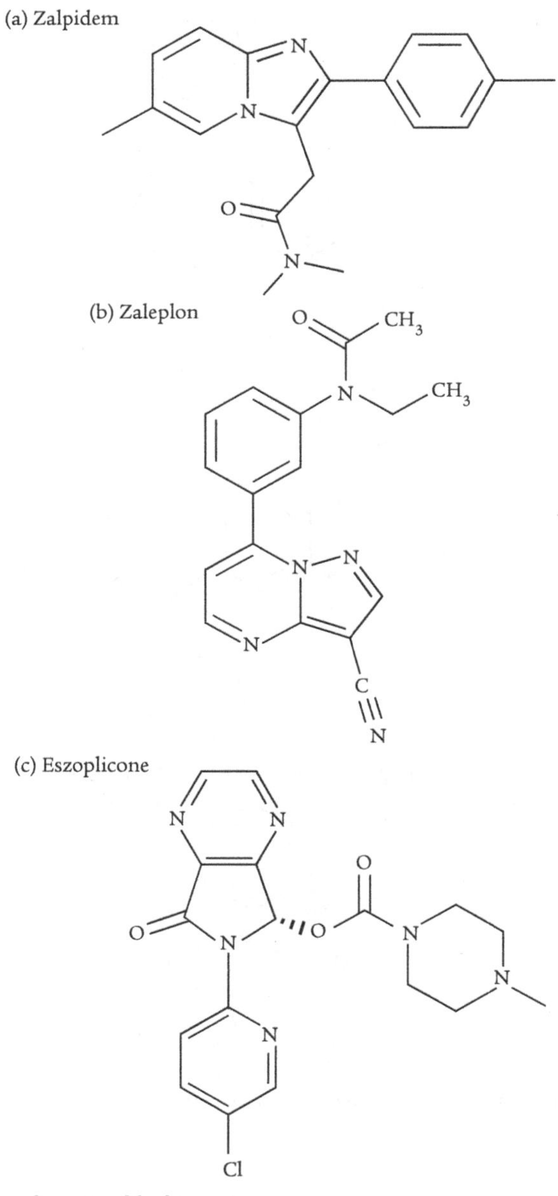

FIGURE 3.16 *Benzodiazepine-like hypnotic agents.*

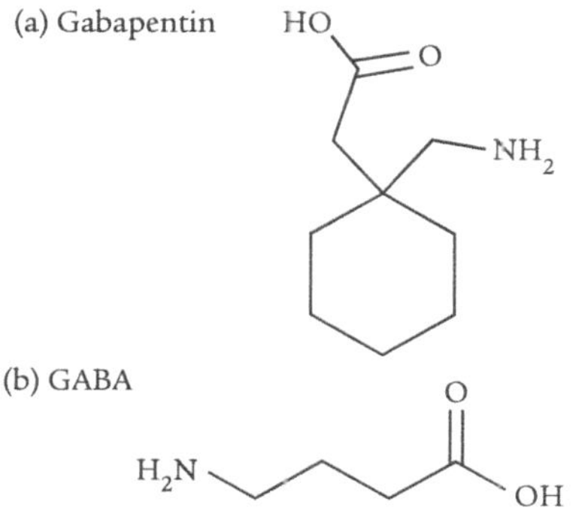

FIGURE 3.17 *GABA and Gabapentin.*

OTHER PSYCHOTROPIC AGENTS

Other miscellaneous agents that have psychotropic properties and are sometimes used in clinical psychopharmacology include the following:

Antihistamines: These agents block histamine receptors, and are used for anxiety and insomnia. They include diphenhydramine (Benadryl) and hydroxyzine (Vistaril).
Melatonin agonists: Ramelteon (Rozerem) is a direct melatonin receptor agonist used for insomnia.
Alpha-adrenergic blockers: Clonidine is a blocker of postsynaptic alpha-1 receptors, used for anxiety and for nightmares.

SELECTED REFERENCES

Brunton, L., et al. (Eds.). (2017). *Goodman and Gilman's The pharmacological basis of therapeutics,* 13th ed. New York: McGraw Hill.

Cusack, B., Nelson, A., Richelson, E. (1994). Binding of antidepressants to human brain receptors: focus on newer generation compounds. Psychopharmacology. 114: 559–565.

Leonard, B. (Ed.). (2004). *Fundamentals of psychopharmacology,* 3rd ed. New York: Wiley & Sons.

SECTION II

Clinical Research Concepts for Psychopharmacology

4

The Limitations of Clinical Experience

Believe none that you hear, and half that you see.

—Edgar Allan Poe

POE'S INSIGHT IS REFLECTED IN AN OLD SAYING IN MEDICINE; THE medical professor tells his students that half of what he will teach them is true, and half is not; he just doesn't know which half. This is the central insight to all clinical practice in medicine, including clinical psychopharmacology.

The most important idea in learning to practice clinical psychopharmacology scientifically, and in understanding clinical research, is the concept of bias. This means systematic error (as opposed to chance, which reflects random error). With systematic error, one makes the same mistake repeatedly because of some inherent problem with observations. "Confounding" is a kind of bias that has to do with factors, of which one often is unaware, that can influence observed results.

As seen in Figure 4.1, the confounding factor is associated with the exposure (the apparent cause) and leads to the result. The real cause is the confounding factor; the apparent cause, which we observe, is just along for the ride. Coffee is associated with cancer, but it doesn't cause cancer, because coffee drinkers are more likely to smoke cigarettes, the actual cause of cancer.

Randomization is the best solution to confounding bias. By randomly assigning people to getting a drug or not, we equalize confounding factors in both groups; the confounding factors then cancel each other out. That is why one can interpret the results straightforwardly: whatever happens can be attributed to the drug. That is also why one can never interpret any non-randomized data straightforwardly: whatever happens could have happened because of many factors, often unmeasured or even unknown.

This bias is why the basic concept of evidence-based medicine is that randomized data are more valid, more accurate and true, than non-randomized data. This includes one's own clinical experiences, the ultimate non-randomized data, as we will discuss.

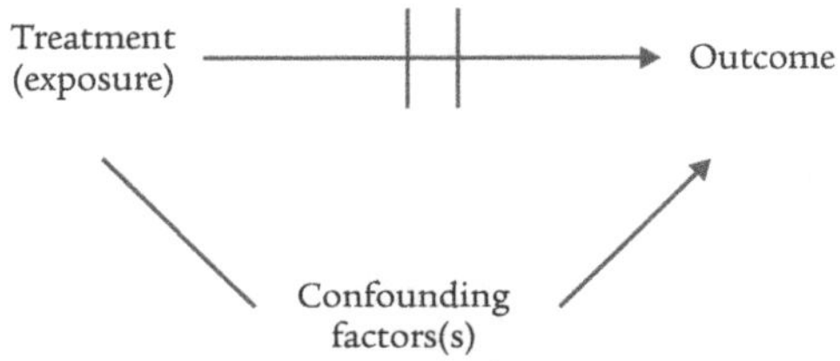

FIGURE 4.1 *The "eternal triangle": Confounding bias in clinical practice.*

In this text, clinical research will be examined to support, reject, revise, inform, and advance clinical experience in the direction of scientific clinical psychopharmacology. The importance of confounding bias in clinical practice takes us to understanding statistics as central to the practice of scientific clinical psychopharmacology. Many clinicians are undereducated or worried about statistics. Elsewhere, the author of this text has provided a book-length exposition of statistics for mental health clinicians. Here, some basic points will be emphasized.

THE "THREE C'S"

The validity of any study involves the sequential assessment of *confounding bias,* followed by *chance,* and then *causation* (the Three C's). Any study needs to pass these three hurdles before accepting its results. Once one accepts that no fact or study result is accepted at face value (because no facts can be observed purely, but rather all are interpreted), then one can turn to statistics to see what kinds of methods we should use to analyze those facts. These three steps are widely accepted and form the core of statistics and epidemiology.

The First C: Confounding Bias

The first step is confounding bias, by which is meant *systematic* error (as opposed to the random error of chance). "Systematic error" means that one makes the same mistake over and over again because of some inherent problem with the observations being made. There are subtypes of bias (selection, confounding, measurement), and they are all important, but what is perhaps the most common and insufficiently appreciated kind of bias is confounding. Confounding has to do with factors of which we are unaware that influence our observed results. It is so central to clinical knowledge that it has been called the "eternal triangle" of clinical research.

This is the lesson of confounding bias: *We cannot believe our eyes.* Or perhaps more accurately, we cannot be sure when our observations are right, and when they are wrong. Sometimes they are one way or the other, but, more often than not, observation is wrong rather than right due to the high prevalence of confounding factors in the world of medical care.

The major confounding factor that results from the behavior of doctors is *confounding by indication* (also called *selection bias*). This is a classic and extremely poorly appreciated source of confusion in medical research.

As a clinician, one is trained to be a non-randomized treater. What this means is that one is taught, through years of supervision and more years of clinical experience, to tailor treatment decisions to each individual patient. One does not treat patients randomly. By practicing non-randomly, one automatically biases all clinical experience. Clinicians think their patients are doing well because of their treatments, whereas they could be doing well because clinicians are tailoring treatments *to those who would do well with them*. In other words, it often is not the treatment effects that one observes, but the treatment effects in specially chosen populations. If one then generalizes from those specific patients to the wider population of patients, one will be mistaken.

The larger topic here is bias, or systematic error; and besides confounding bias, there is one other major source of bias: *measurement bias* (sometimes also called *information bias*). Here the issue is not that the outcomes are due to unanalyzed confounding factors, but rather that the outcomes themselves may be inaccurate. The way the outcomes are measured, or the information that is obtained on which the outcomes are based, is false. Often this can be related to the impact of either the patients' wishes or the doctors' beliefs; thus double-blinding is the usual means of handling measurement bias.

So randomization is the best means of addressing confounding bias, and blinding the means for handling measurement bias. While blinding is important, it is not as important as randomization. Confounding bias is much more prominent and multivaried than measurement bias. Clinicians often focus on blinding as the means of handling bias; this only addresses the minor part of bias. Unless randomization occurs, or regression modeling or other statistical analyses are conducted, the problem of confounding bias will render study results invalid.

The Second C: Chance

If a study is randomized and blinded successfully, or if observational data are appropriately analyzed with regression or other methods, and there still seems to be a relationship between a treatment and an outcome, one can then turn to the question of chance. After randomization, one can assert that any differences seen are probably not due to some hidden bias in observations; now the question is whether they just happened by chance, as random error.

The convention is that a relationship is unlikely to be erroneous if, using mathematical equations designed to measure chance occurrence of associations, it is likely to have occurred 5% of the time, or less frequently, due to chance. This is the famous *p-value*.

The application of these mathematical equations is a simple matter, and thus the assessment of chance is not complex at all. It is much simpler than assessing bias, but it is correspondingly less important. Often what happens is that the first C is ignored, bias is insufficiently examined; and the second C is exaggerated: not just one, or two, but 20 or 50 p-values are thrust upon the reader in the course of an article. The p-value is abused until it becomes useless, or worse, misleading.

The Third C: Causation

Should a study pass the first two hurdles, bias and chance, it still should not be seen as valid unless we assess it in terms of causation. This is an even more complex topic, and a part of statistics where clinicians cannot simply look for a number or a p-value to give them an answer. The problem of causation is this: If x is associated with y, and there is no bias or chance error, still we need to then show that x *causes* y.

This is a problem that has been central to the field of clinical epidemiology for decades. The classic handling of it has been ascribed to the work of the great medical epidemiologist A. Bradford Hill, who was central to the research on tobacco and lung cancer. A major problem with that research was that randomized studies could not be done. This research was observational and liable to bias; Hill and others devised methods to assess bias, but they always had the problem of never being able to completely remove doubt. The cigarette companies, of course, exploited this matter to constantly magnify this doubt and delay the inevitable day when they would be forced to back off on their dangerous business.

With all this observational research, they would argue to Hill and his colleagues, you still cannot prove that cigarettes *cause* lung cancer. And they were right. So Hill set about trying to clarify how one might prove that something causes anything in medical research with human beings. Hill basically pointed out that causation cannot be derived from any one source, but that it could be inferred by an accumulation of evidence from multiple sources. It is not enough to say a study is valid, but one also wants to know if these results are replicated by multiple studies, if they are supported by biological studies in animals on mechanisms of effect, if they follow certain patterns consistent with causation (like a dose–response relationship), and so on. An important feature of establishing causation is to insist on replication. No single study should stand on its own, no matter how well done. Even after crossing the barriers of bias and chance, a study should be replicated and confirmed in other samples and other settings.

In sum, an understanding of clinical psychopharmacology needs to be based on a basic understanding of statistical concepts in clinical research. The three C's are a basic way of getting one's bearings: Confounding bias, chance, and causation—these are the three basic notions that underlie statistics and epidemiology. If clinicians understand these three concepts, then they will be able to believe their eyes more validly.

SELECTED REFERENCES

Abramson, J. H., & Abramson, Z. H. (2001). *Making sense of data*. New York: Oxford University Press.

Ghaemi, S. N. (2009). *A clinician's guide to statistics and epidemiology in mental health*. Cambridge, UK: Cambridge University Press.

5

Evidence-Based Medicine

Pro and Con

With a somewhat ready assumption of cause and effect and, equally, a neglect of the laws of chance, the literature becomes filled with conflicting cries and claims, assertions and counterassertions.

—Austin Bradford Hill

EVIDENCE-BASED MEDICINE (EBM) IS A CONTROVERSIAL TOPIC, WITH BOTH supporters and critics. It is really a simple notion, though, a natural consequence of the main message of the prior chapter, that all clinical experience is distorted by confounding bias. What follows is the most important feature of EBM: the concept of *levels of evidence.*

The originator of the EBM movement, David Sackett, toyed with different names; he initially thought about the phrase "science-based medicine" but opted for the term "evidence" instead. This is unfortunate since "science" tends to engender respect, while "evidence" is vaguer. Proponents of EBM say things like: "That opinion is not evidence-based" or "Those articles are not evidence-based." The folly of this kind of language is evident if we use the term "science" instead: "That opinion is not science-based" or "Those articles are not science-based." Once we use the term "science," it becomes clear that such statements raise the question of what science means. Yet many use the term "evidence" without pausing to think what it means. "Evidence" is contrasted with "opinion," but since "facts" always involve interpretation (which involves opinions or subjective assessments), they are not so distinct.

A better approach to the matter would focus on understanding what kinds of evidence are used, and then to use the best kinds feasible. This is the concept of *levels* of evidence. EBM is *not* about an opposition between having evidence or not having evidence; it is about ranking different kinds of evidence.

LEVELS OF EVIDENCE

The EBM literature has various definitions of specific levels of evidence. Standard EBM texts use letters (A through D). One could also use numbers (I through V). The basic idea is that randomized studies are higher levels of evidence than non-randomized studies, and that the lowest level of evidence consists of case reports, expert opinion, or the consensus of the opinion of clinicians or investigators.

Levels of evidence provide clinicians and researchers with a roadmap that allows consistent and justified comparison of different studies so as to adequately compare and contrast their findings. In psychiatry, the following five levels of evidence have been suggested (Box 5.1), ranked from level I as highest and level V as lowest.

The key feature of levels of evidence to keep in mind is that each level has its own strengths and weaknesses, and as a result, no single level is completely useful or useless. All other things being equal, however, as one moves from level V to level I, increasing rigor and probable validity occurs.

Level V means a case report or a case series (a few case reports strung together), or an expert's opinion, or the consensus of experts, or clinicians' or investigators' opinions (such as in treatment algorithms), or personal clinical experience, or the wisdom of *Great Professors* (like Freud or Kraepelin or Galen). All of this is same level of evidence: the lowest. This does not mean that such evidence is wrong, nor does it mean that it is *not* evidence; it *is* a kind of evidence, just a weak kind. It could turn out that a case report is correct, and a randomized study wrong, but, in general, randomized studies are much more likely to be correct than case reports. We simply cannot know when a case report, or an expert opinion, or a saying of Freud, is right, and when it is wrong. Authority is not the last word.

All of medicine functioned on level V until the introduction of statistics in the 18th and 19th centuries, which opened the way to level IV, the small observational study, which can detect large effects. "Observational" is a synonym for *not randomized*. So level IV is the

BOX 5.1
LEVELS OF EVIDENCE IN PSYCHIATRY

Level I: Double-blind, placebo-controlled randomized trials
Level II: Unblinded randomized trials
Level III: Non-randomized (observational) studies
  IIIa: With control group
  IIIb: Without control group, large (n > 100)
Level IV: Small observational studies (non-randomized, uncontrolled, n < 100)
Level V: Case series (n < 10), Case report (n = 1), Expert opinion

(No permission needed)

same as clinical experience, except that there is some quantification. Patients are counted, and results are reported with numbers in some way. There may or may not be control groups, or other aspects that might improve validity. But the key is simply quantifying the results, as opposed to relying on a simple anecdote or vague generalizations.

If an observational report is conducted in a large number of people, then level III is reached, the large observational study. Usually, such work goes beyond merely quantifying clinical experience, and instead involves planning and organizing a research project. A typical large observational study is the prospective cohort study, the staple of the field of epidemiology, where a group of people are followed over time. Often large observational studies are cross-sectional, like an examination of a national database, or insurance records, for treatment effects of a drug. Observational studies can be retrospective as well, looking back at medical charts to examine past treatments and outcomes.

Levels II and I are the highest levels of evidence due to randomization, which is the best tool to minimize confounding bias. Level II represents open (not double-blind) randomized clinical trials (RCTs), where a placebo is not used; and level I represents double-blind RCTs, where a placebo is often used.

JUDGING BETWEEN CONFLICTING EVIDENCE

The recognition of levels of evidence allows one to have a guiding principle by which to assess a literature. Basic rules are:

1. All other things being equal, a study at a higher level of evidence provides more valid (or powerful) results than one at a lower level.
2. Researchers should base judgments as much as possible on the highest levels of evidence.
3. Levels II and III are often the highest level of evidence attainable for complex conditions, and are to be valued in those circumstances.
4. Higher levels of evidence do not guarantee certainty; any one study can be wrong, thus, look for replicability.
5. Within any level of evidence, studies may conflict based on other methodological issues not captured by the parameters used to provide the general outlines of levels of evidence.

One major advantage of a levels-of-evidence approach to an examination of data is that there is not a huge leap between double-blind, placebo-controlled studies and other, less rigorous levels. In other words, clinicians and some academics sometimes imagine that all studies that are not level I, double-blind RCTs are equivalent in terms of rigor, accuracy, reliability, and information. In reality, there are many intermediate levels of evidence, each with particular strengths as well as limits. Open randomized studies and large observational studies, in particular, can be extremely informative and sometimes as accurate as level I studies. The concept of levels of evidence can also help clinicians who are loath to rely on level I controlled clinical trials, especially if those results contradict their own level V clinical experiences. While the advantages to level V data mainly revolve around hypothesis generation, to devalue higher levels of evidence is unscientific and dangerous.

PRO

In any discussion of statistics and evidence-based medicine, it is important also to address some of the reservations that many clinicians have. A key rationale for EBM is historical: clinical observation, with statistical evaluation, is needed because otherwise the practice of medicine becomes mediocre; before the scientific and statistical methods were developed that are summarized in EBM, clinicians believed in false theories for immense periods of time, and repeatedly made faulty observations. This matter is discussed in more detail in Chapter 16, but here one can briefly state that two basic philosophies of medicine always have conflicted. One is Galenic—the reliance on a theory, often biological, to explain clinical experience. The theory could be the *four humours* or the *three monoamines* or the *ego and the id*; it's the same basic idea. The error is not so much in the content, but in the method of this way of thinking: the focus is on speculation rather than observation. The opposite approach, focused on clinical observation, was held by the Hippocratic school. It was more willing to admit ignorance and to refrain from treatment. From two millennia, most physicians practiced Galenically, based on biological speculation, with the common and frequent use of the gold standard treatment of bleeding.

The core problem behind this history is confounding bias, the limitations of clinical experience, as described before, combined with the influence of authority. Two thousand years of error ended when statistics were introduced to medicine in the 19th century—that is, with EBM. The French physician Pierre Louis disproved bleeding for pneumonia with one of the first small observational studies, showing that more patients died with bleeding than without it.

A century after that study, the biologist Ronald Fisher invented randomization in the 1920s, and the first RCT in medical illness was conducted in 1948. Finally, there was a way to tell what was true in medical treatment, as opposed to being limited by the distortions of confounding bias. RCTs exploded in the 1950s and 1960s, and the EBM movement evolved in the 1970s as a way to make sense of this revolutionary change in medical research. Clinical medicine could be placed on solid scientific ground in a way that was not feasible before the 1950s. Indeed, perhaps the greatest public health advance of our era—the linking of cigarette smoking and cancer (led by the person who conducted the first RCT, A. Bradford Hill)—was both the source and the consequence of EBM methods.

If it is accepted that clinical observation is the core of medicine (rather than theory), and that confounding bias afflicts it, and that randomization is the best solution, then the validity of EBM follows. That is the core of the argument for EBM.

CON

Despite this evidence in favor of EBM, some legitimate critiques can be made. None get at the core rationale for EBM, the reality of confounding bias, but they raise questions about how EBM has evolved and is used today.

A surprising consequence of the popularity of EBM in the last few decades is that it has become a new ideology, almost as Galenic as what it had supplanted. Some academics and researchers hardly ever see or treat patients, but they analyze research studies on a large scale (such as with immense meta-analyses) and then they produce results that are supposed to guide clinical practice. Central to this ideology is the view that unless there are double-blind, randomized, placebo-controlled data, then there is no evidence.

As discussed before, this view is simplistic: there always is evidence; indeed the whole point of EBM is to give us a method to weigh that evidence. Even non-randomized evidence may be correct and useful in the absence of randomized data or given certain constraints; for instance, the link between cigarettes and smoking is completely based on non-randomized evidence but with a great deal of careful statistical analysis to assess confounding factors. If the ivory-tower EBM set the standard, then clinicians should avoid penicillin and support tobacco. (Neither issue has never been studied in RCTs.) This kind of fetishization of RCTs reflects a misunderstanding of science.

In sum, those who oppose EBM ignore the history of medicine. Clinical practice was mostly false and mostly harmful for two millennia, and has begun to change only recently with clinical research, in the Hippocratic tradition of clinical observation, and its statistical correlates in the need for combating confounding bias. On the other hand, ivory-tower EBM is a new way of making mistakes, analyzing numbers alone instead of conducting better clinical research studies. Recovering the Hippocratic heritage of scientifically sound clinical observation—above and beyond biological theory and industrial number-crunching—is the way forward to more effective, scientific, and progressive practice of clinical psychopharmacology.

SELECTED REFERENCES

Ghaemi, S. N. (2009). The case for, and against, evidence-based psychiatry. *Acta Psychiatrica Scandinavica, 119*(4), 249–251.

Hill, A. B. (1962). *Statistical methods in clinical and preventive medicine*. Oxford, UK: Oxford University Press.

6

Maintenance Treatment Designs

"Enriched," But Not Better

IN THIS CHAPTER, THERE WILL BE A DISCUSSION OF THE RESEARCH DESIGN used for maintenance studies in psychiatry. This topic is important because it raises some questions regarding scientific proof of the long-term effectiveness of many commonly used psychotropic drugs, such as dopamine blockers (antipsychotics) and monoamine agonists (antidepressants). This discussion is provided in some detail because the critique described is novel, but it has major implications for decision-making regarding long-term clinical treatment and psychopharmacology.

Although classical RCTs are the gold standard for proof of drug efficacy, the FDA has increasingly allowed a different design, called *randomized discontinuation trials* (RDTs), for indication purposes. These RDTs, called "enriched," are used routinely in psychiatric maintenance trials for FDA registration. The core critique here is of the *concept* of RDTs—that is, their internal validity, not just their external validity or misuse or misinterpretation.

A metaphor may help explain the problem: chocolate and vanilla cake. Do you like chocolate cake? Suppose that a pharmaceutical company decided to market chocolate cake. It wanted an FDA indication for maintenance treatment with chocolate cake. It consulted with the FDA and got approval to design the pivotal research study this way: First, a sample of research subjects would eat chocolate cake and vanilla cake. If they liked vanilla cake only, they would be excluded from further study. If they liked chocolate cake only, they would now be entered into a research study where they would be randomized to continue eating chocolate cake or eat vanilla cake instead.

What do you think the results of the "randomized" clinical trial would show? Have we now proven that chocolate cake is better than vanilla cake? This is how the FDA approves maintenance treatment for antipsychotics for bipolar illness (and also for antidepressants in major depressive disorder).

The key issue in adjudicating the question of whether antipsychotics are mood stabilizers involves how the research studies test that question. The maintenance studies of dopamine blockers all use a similar basic design: they are "enriched" studies, or RDTs. The term "enriched" refers to the fact that the sample is enhanced in such a way that it is more likely to show a treatment effect. Put another way, the sample is preselected for subjects who have already responded to the medication being studied. The problem is that those studies test treatment response samples that are already preselected for treatment response.

This is obviously a tautology, if true. The only way it could be valid is if the kind of treatment response in the maintenance trial was a different response than the acute treatment response. This question is examined in the following discussion.

The basic enriched design of a RDT is as follows: a dopamine blocker, for instance, is given to a group of patients with acute mania; those who don't respond or don't tolerate medication are then excluded; the remaining patients who have responded to the dopamine blocker for acute mania are then entered into the randomized maintenance trial, in which they either stay on the dopamine blocker or come off it (receive placebo). They are followed for up to one year to see if new mood episode relapse occurs. If they relapse quickly on placebo, it is inferred that the dopamine blocker prevented the mood episode from occurring as quickly. The critique here is that most relapses occur within the first few months of the maintenance trial, meaning usually within three months after the dopamine blocker was stopped. These studies aren't really showing benefit for prevention of mood episodes six months to one year or longer after the acute phase, but rather they are showing benefit during and soon after improvement from the acute phase.

All this research design analysis can be translated into clinical experience as follows: Suppose you have an acutely manic patient in hospital. You give that patient a dopamine blocker. The patient improves. You then stop the medication one month later. The patient relapses two months afterward. Have you just proven that this medication is a long-term preventive agent for mood episodes that would happen years into the future?

In other words, patients are preselected for short-term acute efficacy. In the supposed maintenance trial, one is still assessing short-term acute efficacy rather than true long-term prophylaxis. This is the main critique here.

The main response from the supporters of the enriched design is that the maintenance trial is capturing a different phase of illness; namely, new mood episodes occurring outside of the acute phase of treatment. Let's examine if this is correct.

Another way to answer this question can be found in an analysis of enriched maintenance trials of lamotrigine in bipolar illness. The analysis was applied to antipsychotics for their enriched maintenance trials in bipolar illness, because the research design issues were the same. GlaxoSmithKline, the maker of lamotrigine, agreed to give its data to some researchers for analysis after its medication had gone into generic use. Researchers were able to reanalyze their data to address the questions being raised here.

In that analysis, relapse in the maintenance phase was assessed in two ways: (a) Did it occur before or after six months; (b) What was its polarity? One enriched maintenance trial preselected patients who had acutely responded to lamotrigine for a depressive episode, and then they were randomized to either continue or stop it. Another study preselected lamotrigine response for an acute manic episode, and then they were randomized to stay on or come off. Six months or longer was chosen to represent the maintenance phase of relapse, based on natural history research that shows that the untreated average acute manic or depressive episode in bipolar illness lasts about three to six months. Polarity of relapse gave an indication of whether the supposedly new mood episode was indeed different from the acute mood episode. If the polarity of the relapse was the same as the acute episode, and it occurred very quickly after the acute episode was treated, the apparent relapse was likely to reflect the same recent mood episode, rather than representing a completely new mood episode. Indeed, most relapses occurred in less than six months after the maintenance trial began.

Furthermore, all the mood episodes that occurred in the first six months were of the exact same polarity as the acute mood episode that had been used for preselection before the study began. In contrast, almost all the mood episodes that occurred after six months were of the opposite polarity of the original index mood episode before the study began. This finding is consistent with a century of natural history research indicating that mood episodes in bipolar illness cycle from one phase to the other. In other words, mania typically is followed by depression, and depression is followed by mania. If the opposite phase is not prevented, then the next mood episode is not prevented.

The rest of this chapter will examine the science behind the RDT maintenance design in more detail.

RATIONALE FOR THE RDT DESIGN

The enriched RDT design involves the following scenario: To prove long-term maintenance efficacy of a psychiatric drug, patients who enter a double-blind RCT are initially selected, before the study begins, to receive the relevant medication non-randomly for an acute phase of the illness (e.g., an acute depressive or manic episode). Typically, the medication already has been proven effective in RCTs in the acute phases of illness; the question is whether it is effective for maintenance treatment. If a patient responds (e.g., for the acute mood episode), he/she enters the RCT that tests whether he/she will stay well by remaining on that medication, as opposed to having it stopped (whether receiving placebo or active control). Thereby, for patients who respond to a drug in an initial non-randomized phase of acute treatment, enriched RCTs test whether they continue to respond.

Three types of enrichment can be defined:

1. "Practical" enrichment, which produces a more homogeneous sample, thus reducing statistical "noise";
2. "Predictive" enrichment, which produces a more treatment responsive sample, thereby increasing effect size;
3. "Prognostic" enrichment, which produces a sample more likely to have the desired outcome (identifying high-risk subjects who are more likely to have the outcome to be measured).

All three strategies should enhance statistical power, allowing for more efficient, ethical, and cost-effective clinical trials.

The critique here applies mainly to the second type of *predictive* enrichment, which is the most common use of this design strategy in the psychiatric setting. While the other two types of enrichment are likely to be valid, certain types of predictive enrichment are prone to producing scientifically questionable results, and when used as the basis of FDA indication, they could pose public health risks.

INDEPENDENT VERSUS DEPENDENT PREDICTORS

For FDA indication purposes, RDTs appear to be most extensively used in psychiatric illnesses, but published RDT studies also are found in oncology, neurology, and immunology, among other fields. For instance, estrogen-receptor-positive tumors are more responsive to drug treatments that affected that receptor, such as tamoxifen. It thus made sense to design studies in which patients were initially preselected as estrogen receptor positive, and then randomized to receive tamoxifen or placebo. Similarly, a population of patients with high renin status would be expected to be more responsive to an angiotensin-converting enzyme (ACE) inhibitor antihypertensive agent versus placebo.

Such predictors are *independent* of the treatment being studied. For instance, an individual may be estrogen receptor positive or negative; this fact has nothing to do with whether that person receives tamoxifen or not in a randomized trial. In FDA simulation analyses of oncology designs, RDTs have been seen as most valid and efficient when assessing this kind of independent predictor, *viz*. molecular targets that are sensitive to chemotherapeutic agents in a subset of tumors.

Another kind of independently predictive RDT is when the predictor is different from the outcome. A classic example is the important negative Cardiovascular Arrhythmia Suppression Trial (CAST) of drugs proven to acutely suppress paroxysmal ventricular contractions (PVCs). A subsample of subjects who initially responded to such agents with greater than 70% PVC reduction were randomized to continue drug or switch to placebo, with mortality as the primary outcome—a different outcome than the preselected predictor. Surprisingly to some, the anti-arrhythmic agents increased mortality, a negative outcome.

Such independent predictive RDTs can be either positive or negative, and are informative either way. Unfortunately, even in oncology and cardiology, and certainly in psychiatry, predictive biological markers are often unknown, and hence enrichment in RDTs based on independent predictors is not possible.

When independent biological predictors are not known, it has been proposed that the response to treatment by the test drug can be the predictor for enrichment to (further) assess drug treatment response. Therefore, a predictor that is known to be *dependent* on the outcome is used: treatment response is used to identify treatment response. The only way this approach could be non-tautological would be if the specific type of treatment response was different between predictor and outcome; that is, *acute* treatment response (treatment of a *current* episode) as a predictor of *maintenance* treatment response (prevention of future *new* episodes). Posed clinically, this design answers the question "If a patient initially responds to a medication, will that patient continue to respond to that medication in long-term treatment?"

DEPENDENT PREDICTOR AND OUTCOME: ARE THEY THE SAME?

The use of the dependent predictor of acute treatment response to measure the outcome of maintenance treatment response raises a question of validity: Are predictor and outcome the same? If so, this variety of the RDT design would be statistically invalid.

In psychiatric conditions for which RDTs are used, primarily mood illnesses, the underlying illnesses are remitting and relapsing, not chronic. Mood episodes come and go; they tend not to come and stay unchangingly or worsen unremittingly. Chronic constant depression lasting even one year is rare, occurring in less than 10% of unselected mood illness populations. In some of the early RDT proposals in oncology, the context of a progressive chronic disease was taken for granted. RDTs in those studies involved cancers that always worsened, gradually and inexorably. Spontaneous remission was rare. This difference may be a key feature to understanding why RDTs may be being misused in psychiatry.

Most psychiatric studies of maintenance treatment have involved drugs that have been repeatedly proven effective in acute disease states versus placebo, and then they are tested in RDT samples of patients in whom the acute response is confirmed. These studies are invariably positive in the putative maintenance outcome. For instance, an FDA analysis found that all *maintenance* RDTs of antidepressants in MDD over the past 25 years have claimed efficacy (14/14 studies), while only about half (38/74 studies) of acute, classical, non-enriched RCTs of antidepressants for *acute* depression in MDD showed efficacy.

One reason for this outcome may be that the apparent maintenance outcome is merely a reassessment of the acute phase outcome. In other words, the same outcome is being measured twice: once before randomization (when acute non-randomized responders are selected), and again after randomization (when those taken off the acutely effective drug relapse back into the acute phase). The failure to measure a different outcome, prevention of a new episode in the maintenance phase, is suggested by the rapid relapse of most patients in psychiatric RDTs. As discussed before, the natural history of the acute phase of depressive episodes is that they tend to last three to six months in bipolar illness and six to twelve months in unipolar depression. The majority of relapses in RDTs of those conditions occur in the first three to six months after the study begins; that is, after treatment of the acute phase to initial response. Typically, the non-randomized treatment of the enriched acute phase (before the RDT of the purported maintenance phase begins) occurs for about two months (range up to four months). Thus, most relapses are occurring in RDTs just a few months into an acute mood episode, which is still within the natural history of the acute phase of illness. New episodes occurring 6–12 months later are infrequently observed in RDTs, and the drug efficacy is driven mostly by early relapses in the first six months of follow-up; in other words, NOT in the maintenance phase.

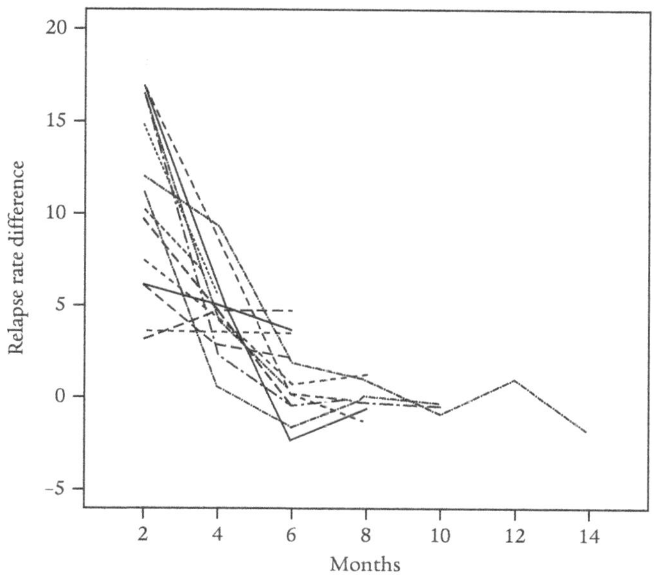

FIGURE 6.1 *Relapse rate differences between drug and placebo arms at each double-blind phase time point in antidepressant maintenance studies*[a]. [a] *Each curve represents a study.* SOURCE: *Borges, S., et al. Review of maintenance trials for major depressive disorder: A 25-year perspective from the US Food and Drug Administration. The Journal of Clinical Psychiatry. 75, 205–214. Copyright 2014, Physicians Postgraduate Press. Reprinted with permission.*

This complete reliance on short-term withdrawal in the first six months, rather than true maintenance prevention of new mood episodes is seen in the FDA analysis of 15 maintenance RDTs of antidepressants in MDD. As seen later, almost all the difference between drug and placebo relapse occurs in the first six months. After six months, there are no differences (Figure 6.1). In other words, psychiatric RDTs are tautologous in what they measure: they preselect patients for acute response; then they measure acute response again (but they label it "maintenance response").

Hence it may not be surprising to note that there are few, if any, studies of a drug that is effective in an acute disease state, which is then given for maintenance treatment in an RDT design, in which the result has been negative. We identified only one potential case in psychiatric studies (a study of electroconvulsive therapy [ECT], a device intervention) out of at least 30 such studies in unipolar and bipolar illness as well as schizophrenia. Since a valid scientific design should be falsifiable, the infrequency of negative studies raises questions about the RDT design's validity.

THE INVERSE ENRICHED DESIGN

One can see how the RDT design can mistakenly suggest drug efficacy rather than spontaneous recovery if RDTs in unipolar depressive illness are examined in what might be called a "reverse" enriched design, where study populations are enriched with placebo responders. Patients treated acutely who respond to *placebo* stay on placebo, or are switched to antidepressant, for the maintenance phase. In seven RDTs with such data available, there is *more* maintenance depressive relapse with antidepressant (42%) treatment versus placebo (25%). Should we conclude that placebo is more effective than antidepressants in maintenance treatment of unipolar depression? If one reverses the terms, in the standard RDT analysis of antidepressant maintenance efficacy in those preselected to respond to antidepressants, antidepressants are more effective than placebo in the maintenance phase. Presumably the reverse enriched RDT design preselects for patients who will do well on placebo, perhaps because they have a more spontaneously recovering illness. However, this may not mean that placebo is inherently more effective than the drug. Similarly, the standard enriched RDT design preselects for patients who will do well on a drug that is effective acutely, at least for some time in the continuation phase of treatment. However, this equally may not mean that drug is inherently more effective than placebo. Which enriched RDT analysis is valid: the one enriched for placebo, or the one enriched for antidepressant? It seems apparent that the RDT analysis cannot adjudicate efficacy in the scenario of a spontaneously recovering illness such as unipolar depression.

A detailed analysis of potential rejoinders to this critique is discussed elsewhere (Ghaemi and Selker, 2017). The main clinical consequences of this critique of enriched RDT maintenance designs in psychiatry follow.

CLINICAL ASSUMPTIONS: ACUTE VERSUS MAINTENANCE RESPONSE

The main clinical claim for the RDT design is that it tests whether a drug that is effective for acute use should be continued or not, and for how long. It is unclear whether the RDT design answers this question any better than a classic RCT.

Clinicians sometimes seem to assume that acute treatment response necessarily implies maintenance response. But counterexamples are common in medicine: indomethacin is an acute treatment for gout but not maintenance, while allopurinol is effective maintenance treatment but is not effective (indeed, counterproductive) for acute use; sumatriptan is an acute treatment for migraine but not maintenance, penicillin can treat acute pneumonia but is poor at maintenance prophylaxis; steroids are much more effective for acute episodes of autoimmune illnesses than for prophylaxis. Lithium and lamotrigine are much more effective in prevention of mood episodes of bipolar illness than in treatment of acute episodes. In a large National Institute of Mental Health (NIMH)-sponsored study, antidepressants were about twice as effective in treating acute depressive episodes as in preventing them. Hence, an equivalence between acute and maintenance efficacy needs to be proven; it cannot be assumed.

GOING BACKWARD ON GENERALIZABILITY

This analysis of the limitations of RDTs, both in validity and efficiency, relates to an increasing appreciation that "efficacy trials" on highly selected participants are less helpful, because of their lack of generalizability and applicability to usual care, than "effectiveness trials." There is a consensus in the clinical trial community that traditional randomized efficacy trials do not provide enough clinically useful information for usual medical practice. RDTs are a step in the opposite direction, with even less generalizable results (and also diminished validity) than usual efficacy trials. Some investigators have even proposed extending the RDT approach from maintenance studies to acute trials in psychiatry. This approach, which has received support from FDA, would appear to head the psychiatric field in the wrong direction, in terms of both validity and generalizability. Hence a reconsideration of RDTs should be undertaken in the context of this general trend, apparently in most of medicine other than psychiatry, towards recognizing a need for less, rather than more, preselection and manipulation of samples in randomized drug trials.

This critique of enriched RDT maintenance designs in psychiatry should be kept in mind in relation to the discussions in Chapter 9 on monoamine agonists (antidepressants) in long-term maintenance prevention of depressive episodes in unipolar depression, and the discussion in Chapter 10 on dopamine blockers in long-term maintenance prevention of mood episodes in bipolar illness. In both cases, some doubt is cast on claims of maintenance efficacy in those settings, and the scientific rationale for that doubt has been provided in this chapter.

SELECTED REFERENCES

Borges, S., et al. (2014). Review of maintenance trials for major depressive disorder: A 25-year perspective from the US Food and Drug Administration. *Journal of Clinical Psychiatry*, *75*, 205–214.

Ghaemi, S. N., & Selker, H. P. (2017). Maintenance trial designs in psychiatry Enriched but not better. *Journal of Clinical and Translational Science*, June; *1*(3), 198–204.

Goodwin, F. K., Whitham, E. A., & Ghaemi, S. N. (2011). Maintenance treatment study designs in bipolar disorder: Do they demonstrate that atypical neuroleptics (antipsychotics) are mood stabilizers? *CNS Drugs*, *25*, 819–827.

7

Negative Studies

The Failure to Know What Isn't Known

There is a type of interaction between human beings which proceeds not from knowledge, or even lack of knowledge, but from failure to know what isn't known.

—John Kenneth Galbraith

THE MEDICAL LITERATURE MEETS GALBRAITH'S DESCRIPTION. SOME things we know, and know that we know. Other things we do not know, and know that we do not know. But perhaps the largest class involves the things we do not know, and do not realize that we do not know. This latter state of affairs is exemplified by the problem of negative studies.

It has become increasingly clear that the medical literature is biased toward positive studies; negative studies are less frequently published. Sometimes this may reflect loss of passion, as disappointed researchers file away their negative results. Sometimes it may be systematic, as pharmaceutical sponsors may actively suppress negative data that would adversely impact their marketplace sales. And journals may also systematically reject negative studies—which will generate fewer readers, fewer citations, and lower impact factors for the journal—more frequently than positive ones.

Negative studies may provide important information. "Negative" does not mean "unimportant," and proving something is ineffective is as important, perhaps more so, than proving it effective. To be a good physician, knowing when not to use which medications, as Pinel famously said, is even more important than knowing when and how to use them. Drugs that are ineffective might be somewhat harmful; almost all drugs are harmful in some way; thus the risk–benefit calculation is always hurtful for an ineffective drug. Furthermore, drugs that are effective are often *not* used, since the ineffective drugs are seen as effective, and thus the truly effective drugs, which sometimes have more side effects, are pushed aside. In short, unpublished negative studies are needed to put positive studies in perspective.

The clearest example in psychiatry is that of antidepressants. The published literature is almost entirely positive, but when unpublished negative studies at the FDA are added, 51% of the actual studies are positive and 49% negative. Had clinicians known for the past two decades that the actual research evidence base had a score of 51 vs. 49, not 90 vs. 10, perhaps they would have been more judicious in their use of antidepressants.

THE CASE OF LAMOTRIGINE

The issue of lamotrigine and its negative studies is more complex because lamotrigine has been proven effective for bipolar illness in some circumstances; namely, maintenance treatment. It was also proven ineffective in other situations (everything else: as explained later in this chapter). The author of this book was a principal investigator in the maintenance studies with lamotrigine in the mid-1990s, and also served on the Lamictal National Advisory Board for its manufacturer, GlaxoSmithKline (GSK). Despite this extended access to the pivotal clinical research trials on this agent, it was a surprise to this author when the existence of numerous negative lamotrigine studies came to light around 2006. In 2004, a paroxetine-related settlement with New York State Attorney General's office forced GSK to post a registry that would include much more information about pretrial and clinical drug study results. Of the nine lamotrigine-related bipolar disorder studies posted on the website, two were positive and published supporting the FDA-approved indication for delay of relapse in the long-term treatment for bipolar disorder patients. A negative study in rapid-cycling bipolar disorder and another in acute bipolar depression were published, but both emphasized positive secondary outcomes as opposed to the negative primary outcomes. Five other negative studies involving rapid-cycling bipolar disorder, acute bipolar depression, and acute mania were unpublished at the time, and some were never published.

Failure to adequately publish these negative studies led to the creation of a clinical impression that lamotrigine is an "antidepressant." This mistaken impression occurred partly because the prophylactic benefits of lamotrigine for depressive episodes were confused with a presumed acute benefit. Partly it was due to the publication of one apparently positive study, and the non-publication of several negative studies. The clinical relevance of the lamotrigine studies is notable: taking the negative outcomes into account, as of now, one might say that this agent is reasonably effective in maintenance treatment of bipolar disorder, particularly in prevention of depression. It is proven ineffective, however, in acute mania, rapid cycling disorder, and acute bipolar depression.

It is worth noting that the FDA has encouraged this state of affairs by viewing negative studies as uninformative, due to the possibility that they were "failed" studies rather than truly negative (i.e., the sample may have simply been unresponsive, or dosing might have been too low, and so on). Thus drugs could have two positive studies and 10 or so negative ones, as did a number of SRIs: for which the FDA not only allowed approval but it did not require that the pharmaceutical industry publish its negative results. The pharmaceutical industry did the minimum necessary; and the FDA set the minimum far below what should have been the acceptable scientific standard. Furthermore, even though the FDA is supposed to allow access to information about all studies of drugs for which it provides an indication, in fact it still does not allow access to raw data from industry-sponsored studies, which are viewed as confidential and proprietary. Rather, the researchers who have attempted to access such studies through the Freedom of Information Act (FOIA) are met with abstracted summary results. While summary results are better than no results, full access to scientific data should be the standard at the FDA.

It is relevant that GSK eventually published some of these data on lamotrigine in combined form in one paper a few years ago, and also a meta-analysis of the combined acute bipolar depression studies. However, these publications were slow in coming, years after the medication had been on the market and had been advertised extensively, without reference to its negative studies. Furthermore, combining multiple papers in one location, and doing so only once, has much less influence than publishing each paper separately when the results are positive, or publishing several papers from the same single positive study, as is common practice. Positive papers also get published in journals with high impact factors and are commonly associated with press releases and related media coverage. As for the meta-analysis, a kind of "statistical alchemy" is performed whereby the overall negative results, although acknowledged, are leavened by the inclusion of a positive subgroup analysis in severe acute bipolar depression. Although this positive subgroup analysis may be valid, it is not emphasized that the effect size is small, and not clinically meaningful. Again, one is faced with the inability to simply state the overall negative outcome as negative. Furthermore, the meta-analysis did not include the other negative studies in acute mania, rapid cycling, or acute unipolar depression. Those studies remain unpublished in any form.

EBM—or, more simply put, the science of medicine—cannot be taken seriously, and is certainly not valid, if the evidence base is only partial. Meta-analyses of large published datasets are not as meaningful as they seem when unpublished data languish elsewhere. Statistical tests for publication bias can only provide some sense of the problem. Clinicians should realize that the published scientific literature provides an overly positive bias towards assuming a greater amount of drug efficacy than is likely to be the case in reality.

SELECTED REFERENCE

Ghaemi, S. N. (2009). The failure to know what isn't known: Negative publication bias with lamotrigine and a glimpse inside peer review. *Evidence Based Mental Health, 12*, 65–68.

8

Side Effects and Generalizability

Beyond *P*-Values

The p-value is a mathematical replacement for sensible thought.

—Alvan Feinstein

ONE OF THE MOST COMMON MISCONCEPTIONS IN CLINICAL RESEARCH IS that "statistical significance" is meaningful in some profound manner. All this phrase means is that the famous "*p*-value" is below 5%. This concept is abused and misunderstood, and bears examination, along with a discussion of effect estimation methods, of confidence intervals (CIs), and numbers needed to treat (NNT), as better methods for clinicians to understand and apply clinical research to practice.

"*P*" stands for probability, and the *p*-value may be defined as follows: *The probability of observing the observed data, assuming that the null hypothesis is true.* The *p*-value is not a real number; it does not reflect a real probability, but rather the likelihood of chance effects *assuming* (but not knowing) that the null condition is true. It is not the probability of an event, but the probability of our *certainty* about an event. Indeed, in this sense, it is a central expression of LaPlace's concept of statistics as quantifying, rather than disclaiming, our ignorance. A *p*-value attempts to quantify our ignorance, rather than establish any reality. Thus, if we use a standard *p*-value cutoff of 0.05 or less as the definition of *statistical significance,* what we are saying is that *we will be rejecting the null hypothesis by mistake 5% of the time or less.*

The key relevance for the *p*-value is not the specific number, but the concept of rareness, the idea that one should examine how likely the play of chance could be, and to interpret one's results more definitively as the likelihood of chance becomes more and more rare.

The term "statistical significance," so widely used in medical research, basically reflects the *p*-value cutoff at which the null hypothesis (NH; i.e., no difference between groups) can be rejected. Unfortunately, the word "significance" has other uses in the English language outside of statistics, hence this shorthand for a statistical result of research is often manipulated for the sometimes less wholesome goals of the human beings who do the research.

The term "statistical significance" (SS) has purely statistical meaning in relation to *p*-values. It has no meaning in any other way. Yet, since the word "significance" in English means, roughly, something that is important, then the words "statistical significance" tend to be interpreted by doctors and clinicians as meaning, if present, that the results are important, and, if absent, that the results are not important. Yet, as discussed in more detail in statistical texts, the results of a study may be falsely positive (and thus the apparently important SS results are in fact not important) or they may be falsely negative (and thus the apparently unimportant SS results are in fact important). Briefly, false positive results occur when too many *p*-values are tested ("multiple comparison"); when repeated over and over, the apparent 5% cutoff (chance results 1 in 20 times) occurs more frequently (if 20 analyses are conducted, one of them will be positive, and give a *p*-value of 0.05, by chance). False negative results happen when the sample size is too small, since *p*-values increase with small samples, and decrease with larger samples. A medium effect size may be statistically significant in 200 patients, but not in 100 patients. The same result will be deemed "real" in the larger study and not real in the smaller one. Hence, a result can be statistically significant but clinically meaningless; or statistically insignificant yet clinically meaningful.

In summary, the concepts of *p*-values and statistical significance, though useful when used appropriately, are based on numerous assumptions that are not themselves based on statistics. In other words, there are some important features of these notions that are arbitrary and open to debate, not simply absolute truths to which we must pledge obedience.

EFFECT ESTIMATION

The effect estimation approach breaks out the factors of effect size and precision (or variability of the data), and provides more information, and in a more clearly presented form, than the hypothesis-testing approach. The main advantage of the effect estimation approach is that it does not require a preexisting hypothesis (such as the null and alternative hypotheses), thus we do not get into all the hazards of false negative and false positive results.

The best way to understand effect estimation, the alternative to hypothesis testing, is to appreciate the classic concept of a 2 x 2 table. There are two groups in such a table: one that had the exposure (or treatment), and one that did not. Then there are two outcomes: yes or no (response or non-response; illness or non-illness).

Using a drug treatment for depression as an example, the effect size can simply be the percentage of responders: number who responded (a + c) ÷ number treated (a + b). Or it can be a relative risk: the likelihood of responding if given treatment would be a/a + b; the likelihood of responding if not given treatment would be c/c + d. So the relative likelihood of responding if given the treatment would be a/a + b ÷ c/c + d. This is often called the "risk ratio" and is abbreviated as RR.

Another measure of relative risk is the odds ratio, abbreviated as OR, which mathematically equals ad/bc. The odds ratio is related to, but not the same as, the risk ratio. Odds are used to estimate probabilities, most commonly in settings of gambling. Probabilities can be said to range from 0% likelihood, to 50-50 (meaning chance likelihood in either direction), to 100% absolute likelihood. Odds are defined as p/1 – p if p is the probability of an event. Thus, if the probability is 50% (or colloquially "50-50"), then the odds are 0.5/ 1 – 0.5 = 1. This is often expressed as "1 to 1." If the probability is absolutely likely, meaning 100%, then the odds are infinite: 1/1 – 1 = 1/0 = infinity. ORs approximate RRs; the only reason to distinguish them is that ORs are mathematically useful in regression models. When you are not using regression models, RRs are more intuitively straightforward.

THE EFFECT SIZE

The effect estimation approach to statistics thus involves using effect sizes, like relative risks, as the main number of interest. The *effect size*, or the actual estimate of effect, is a number; this is whatever the number is: it may be a percentage (e.g., 68% of patients were responders), or an actual number (the mean depression rating scale score was 12.4), or, quite commonly, a relative risk estimate: RRs or ORs.

Many people use the term "effect size" to mean *standardized effect size*, which is a special kind of effect estimate. The standardized effect size, called *Cohen's d*, is the actual effect size described before (such as a mean number) divided by the standard deviation (the measure of variability). It produces a number that ranges from 0–1 or higher, and these numbers have meaning, but not unless one is familiar with the concept. Generally, it is said that an effect size of 0.4 or lower is small; 0.4 to 0.7, medium; and above 0.7, large. Cohen's d is a useful measure of effect because it corrects for the variability of the sample, but it is less interpretable sometimes than the actual unadulterated effect size. For instance, if we report that the mean Hamilton Depression Rating Scale score (usually above 20 for severe depression) was 0.5 (zero being "no symptoms") after treatment, we can know that the effect size is large, without needing to divide it by the standard deviation and get a Cohen's d greater than 1. Nonetheless, Cohen's d is especially useful in research using continuous measures of outcome (like psychiatric rating scales) and is commonly employed in experimental psychology research.

Another important estimate of effect, newer and more relevant to clinical psychiatry, is the *number needed to treat* (NNT) or the *number needed to harm* (NNH). This is a way of trying to give the effect estimate in a clinically meaningful way. Let us suppose that 60% of patients responded to a drug, and 40% to placebo. One way to express the effect size is the risk ratio of 1.5 (60% divided by 40%). Another way of looking at it is that the difference between the two groups is 20% (60–40%). This is called the "absolute risk reduction" (ARR). The NNT is the reciprocal of the ARR, or 1/ARR: in this case, 1/0.20 = 5. Thus, for this kind of 20% difference between drug and placebo, clinically we can conclude that we need to treat five patients with the drug to get benefit in one of them. Again, certain standards are needed. Generally, it is viewed that a NNT of 5 or less is very large, 5–10 is large, 10–20 is moderate, above 20 is small, and above 50 is probably meaningless.

A note of caution: this kind of abstract categorization of the size of the NNT is not exactly accurate. The NNT by itself may not fully capture whether an effect size is large or small. Some authors note, for instance, that the NNT for prevention of heart attack with aspirin is 130; the NNT for cyclosporine prevention of organ rejection is 6.3; and the NNT for effectiveness of psychotherapy (based on one review of the literature) is 3.1. Yet aspirin is widely recommended, cyclosporine is seen as a breakthrough, and psychotherapy is seen as "modest" in benefit. The explanation for these interpretations might be that the "hard" outcome of a heart attack may justify a larger NNT with aspirin, as opposed to the "soft" outcome of feeling better after psychotherapy. Aspirin is also cheap and easy to obtain, while psychotherapy is expensive and time-consuming (similarly, cyclosporine is expensive and associated with many medical risks). NNT provides effect sizes, therefore, which need to be interpreted in the setting of the outcome being prevented and the costs and risks of the treatment being given.

The converse of the NNT is the NNH, which is used when assessing side effects. Similar considerations apply to NNH, and it is calculated in a similarly way as the NNT. Thus, if an antipsychotic drug causes akathisia in 20% of patients versus 5% with placebo, then the ARR is 15% (20–5%), and the NNH is 1/0.15 = 6.7.

THE MEANING OF CONFIDENCE INTERVALS

The rationale for CIs stems from the fact that we are dealing with probabilities in statistics and in all medical research. We observe something: say a 45.9% response rate with drug Y. Is the real value 45.9%; not 45.6%, or 46.3%? How much *confidence* do we have in the number we observe? The concept of CIs is a conceptual construct that helps us appreciate how well our observations have approached reality.

We can, therefore, make the following statements: *Confidence intervals* can be defined as *the range of plausible values* for the effect size. Another way of putting it is that it is *the likelihood that the real value for the variable would be captured in 95% of trials.* Or, alternatively, *if the study was repeated over and over again, the observed results would fall within the confidence intervals 95% of the time.*

The p-value gives a yes or no answer to this question: Are the data highly likely (meaning $p > 0.05$) to have been observed by chance? (Or, alternatively, are we highly likely to mistakenly reject the NH by chance?): yes or no. The CIs give more information: they provide actual effect size (which p-values do not), and (like p-values) they provide an estimate of precision (which p-values do not: how likely are the observed means to differ if we repeat the study?). Since the information provided by a p-value of 0.05 is the same as what is provided by a CI of 95%, there is no need to provide p-values when CIs are used (although researchers routinely do so, perhaps because they think that readers cannot interpret CIs). Or, put another way, CIs provide all the information one finds in p-values, *and more*. Hence, the relevance of the proposal, somewhat serious, that p-values should be abolished altogether in favor of CIs.

SIDE EFFECTS

As a corollary to the need to limit the number of p-values, a common error in assessing the results of a clinical trial or of an observational study is to evaluate side effects across patient groups based on whether or not they differ on p-values (e.g., drug group vs. placebo group). However, most clinical studies are not powered to assess side effects, especially when side effects are infrequent. Significance testing is not appropriate, since the risk of a false negative finding using this technique in isolation is too high.

Side effects should not be interpreted based on *p*-values and significance testing because of the high false negative (type II) error risk. They are not hypotheses to be tested, but simply observations to be reported. The appropriate statistical approach is to report the effect size (e.g., percent) with 95% CIs (the range of expected estimated observations based on repeated studies).

These issues are directly relevant to the question of whether a drug has a risk of causing mania. In the case of lamotrigine, for instance, a review of the pooled clinical trials, which failed to find a difference with placebo, reported no difference. Those studies were not designed to detect such a difference. It may indeed be that lamotrigine is not a higher risk than placebo, but it is concerning that the overall risk of pure manic episodes (1.3%) is four-fold higher than placebo's (0.3%) (RR = 4.14, 95% CI 0.49–35.27): in fact, the sample size required to "statistically" detect (i.e., using "significance hypothesis testing" procedures) this observed difference in pure mania would be achieved with a study comparing two arms of almost 1,500 patients each (at a type II error level of 0.80, with statistical assumptions of no dropouts, perfect compliance, and equal-sized arms).

To give another example, if we accept a spontaneous baseline manic-switch rate of about 5% over two months of observation, and further assume that the minimal "clinically" relevant difference to be detected is a doubling of all events at a 10% rate in the lamotrigine group, the required sample size of a study properly powered to "statistically" detect this "clinically" significant difference should be almost 1,000 overall (assuming no dropouts, perfect compliance, and equal-sized arms). Only with such a sample could we be confident enough that a reported *p*-value greater than 0.05 really reflects a substantial, clinical equivalence of lamotrigine and placebo in causing acute mania. These pooled data involved 693 patients, which is somewhat more than half the needed sample, but even larger samples would be needed due to the statistical assumptions requiring no dropouts, full compliance, and equal sample size in both arms.

The methodological point is that one cannot conclude that there is no difference when studies are not designed to test a hypothesis. This is a "false negative" conclusion, which is a major problem with overuse of *p*-values, especially for side effects in clinical trials.

GENERALIZABILITY

After crossing the hurdles of confounding bias and chance, a reader might conclude that the results of a study are valid. The final step is to assess the scope of these valid results. This is the topic of *generalizability*, which is quite different from *validity*. For generalizability (sometimes called "external validity," as opposed to "internal validity"), one should ask the question, "Given that these results are right, to whom do they apply?" In other words, who was in the sample? More directly, clinicians might want to compare their own patients to those in the sample to determine which of their patients might be affected by what they learned from that study. To some extent, validity is a relative concept: e.g., investigators observe that one group of patients does better than another. But generalizability is an absolute concept: How many patients did better? And who were those patients? One has to search the methods section carefully to answer this question, usually by looking for the "inclusion and exclusion criteria" of a study.

One way in which generalizability is often discussed is by using the term *efficacy* for the results of the samples of patients in clinical trials, and *effectiveness* for the results in larger populations of patients in the real world. If patients have to go through all the hoops of randomization, blinding, placebo, rating scales, and so on, one might expect that only some patients would agree to participate in research studies with all those limitations. Various studies suggest that, for any major psychiatric condition, about 10% of patients with the relevant diagnosis will quality for and agree to participate in available randomized controlled trials (RCTs). The assumption in the world of clinical trials is that the research conducted on this 10% is generalizable to the other 90%. This may or may not be the case: another place where statistics has its limits, and where clinicians should use statistical data with judgment (not simply rejecting nor unthinkingly accepting them).

Figure 8.1 provides a visual example of the problem of generalizability. The faces on the side were combined in a computer simulation to provide the picture in the middle, who is neither male nor female, nor white nor black. This is analogous to RCTs, where the final outcome is an average result for the average patient. But the "average" patient does not exist; only specific individual patients exist. The job of the clinician is to use the general results of RCTs to inform individual decisions. Exceptions are allowed, but not

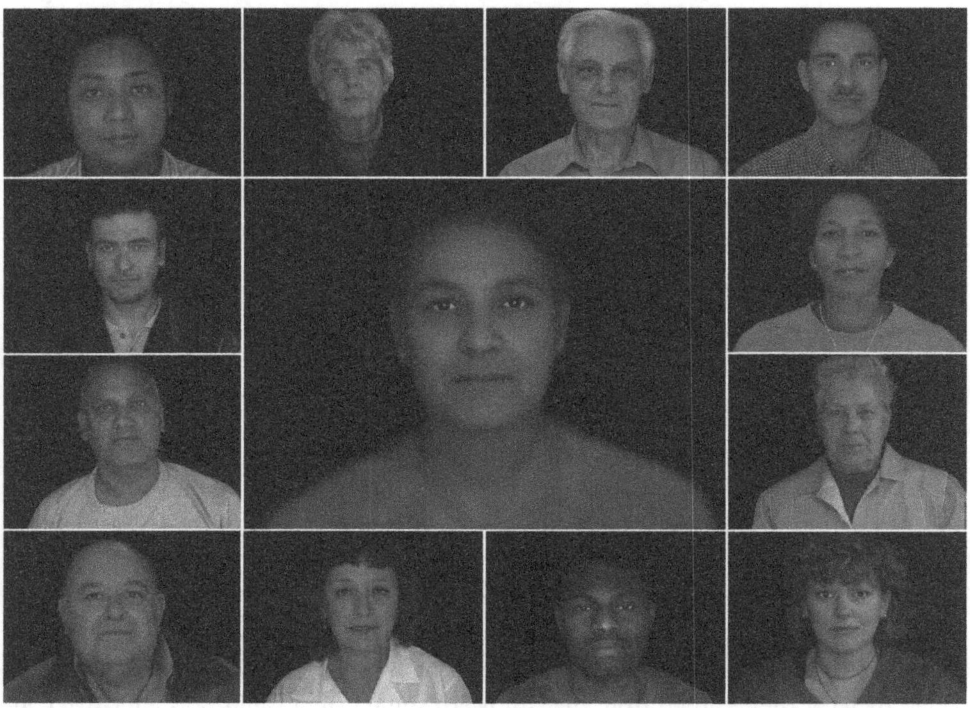

FIGURE 8.1 *Many faces become one face. © Chris Dorley-Brown, Haverbill 2000. Reprinted with permission.*

in the majority of cases. This is where the art of practice has to be added to the science of clinical research.

SELECTED REFERENCES

Feinstein, A. R. (1998). *P*-values and confidence intervals: Two sides of the same unsatisfactory coin. *Journal of Clinical Epidemiology, 51*(4), 355–360.

Ghaemi, S. N. (2009). *A clinician's guide to statistics and epidemiology in mental health.* Cambridge, UK: Cambridge University Press.

Kent, D. M., & Hayward, R. (2007). When averages hide individual differences in clinical trials. *American Scientist, 95*, 60–68.

SELECTED REFERENCES

SECTION III

Clinical Psychopharmacology of Drug Classes

9

Monoamine Agonists ("Antidepressants"), Including Dopamine Agonists ("Stimulants")

MONOAMINE AGONISTS (ANTIDEPRESSANTS) ARE THE MOST WIDELY USED class of psychotropic drugs. There are three major monoamines, and thus three main effects of monoamine agonists: serotonergic, noradrenergic, and dopaminergic. As described in chapter 3, these effects are more often combined than pure.

SEROTONIN AGONISTS

The main serotonin agonists are inhibitors of serotonin reuptake pump. Though they are commonly called selective serotonin reuptake inhibitors (SSRIs), we drop the term "selective" to refer to these agents only as "SRIs." As discussed in Chapter 2, this correction is made because the monoamine system in the brain is interrelated, and thus it is impossible to be purely selective for effects on only one monoamine system (Box 9.1).

If there is an increase in serotonin activity, there will be effects on norepinephrine and/or dopamine activity, via the medial forebrain bundle, which has numerous interdigitations between axons of the different monoamine systems. Even at the level of the synapse, most SRIs are not selective for serotonin, but they can be reuptake inhibitors of other monoamines, as described in chapter 3.

Thus the classic SRI, fluoxetine (Prozac), has as much norepinephrine reuptake blockade as venlafaxine (Effexor), which is marketed as a so-called serotonin/norepinephrine reuptake inhibitor (SNRI). Also, sertraline (Zoloft) has as much dopamine reuptake blockade as the amphetamine methylphenidate, and more than bupropion, which is commonly thought of as a dopamine agonist. The only truly selective serotonin reuptake inhibitor at the level of the synapse is citalopram (Celexa), and its active enantiomer

BOX 9.1
GENERAL TIPS FOR SRI TREATMENT

1. Dose all agents once daily in the morning, with the exception of paroxetine (which can be sedating) and fluoxetine (in the minority of persons who experience sedation).
2. Fluoxetine requires a longer therapeutic trial, but has less serotonin withdrawal.
3. Sertraline works well in weekend drug holidays for sexual dysfunction.
4. Citalopram is the most selective for serotonin reuptake.
5. Sertraline and citalopram have the fewest drug interactions.
6. Paroxetine may have the most anxiolytic effect.
7. Observe carefully for mixed states in misdiagnosed bipolar disorder, as well as akathisia, as potential risk factors for suicidality.

escitalopram (Lexapro). But again, even this effect is not selective at the brain level because of the interconnections of monoamine systems in the median forebrain bundle. Clinical effects of these agents are next discussed in turn.

Efficacy

SRIs have not been proven to be more effective than the tricyclic antidepressants (TCAs); rather, their advantage seems to be improved tolerability and patient acceptability. This is a strong point worth emphasizing. Many clinicians in the United States almost exclusively use SRIs, often going through all medications in this class, occasionally trying some of the newer atypical antidepressants, and rarely or never using TCAs or monoamine oxidase inhibitors (MAOIs). This approach assumes that SRIs have equal or better efficacy than the other agents. In fact, TCAs, MAOIs, and venlafaxine are more effective than SRIs in specific populations, especially hospitalized and melancholic patients.

Safety is an important matter, though, and the popularity of SRIs is not without reason. Sometimes, clinicians confuse pharmacological safety with clinical safety. In other words, since SRIs are not lethal due to direct physiological effects, clinicians act as if they are safe and non-lethal in any clinical circumstance. This is not the case for certain situations, the most important of which are bipolar depression and akathisia. In bipolar depression, SRIs can induce a mixed manic state highly associated with suicide. There is also the possibility that SRI-induced akathisia can also result in suicide. Therefore, the pharmacological safety of SRIs does not imply that clinicians can use them with impunity regardless of the clinical circumstances. The Food and Drug Administration (FDA) published a “black box warning” for such SRI-related suicidality, specifically in relation to children and young adults (below age 25); this important topic is discussed later in this chapter.

Drug Interactions

Differences among SRIs in effects on hepatic metabolic enzymes are also essential to understanding how to use these various medications.

Serotonin Withdrawal Syndrome

It has taken about two decades of use with SRIs for many clinicians to become aware that there is a major problem with these agents that had not been appreciated previously: they have a severe withdrawal syndrome. Previously, the side effects noted here had been the main concern with these agents: sexual dysfunction, gastrointestinal effects, apathy, and the like. It is clear now that these side effects are minimal in the face of the more common and long-term risk of serotonin withdrawal syndrome. This issue is so important that it makes sense for clinicians and patients to ask themselves, before beginning any SRI prescription, as in the decision to go to war, "what is the exit strategy?" How long should patients take the SRI? An endpoint duration should be in mind, as opposed to the common practice of indefinite long-term treatment. These questions should be asked because all SRIs cause serotonin withdrawal syndrome when used, it appears, for about one year or longer.

This condition consists of a range of physical and psychological symptoms, including fatigue, flu-like symptoms, lightning-bolt sensations, paresthesias, headache, marked anxiety, and dysphoric mood. One analogy would be to the experience of a panic attack that never goes away. The constellation of anxious/dysphoric mood with fatigue can make the syndrome seem like a depressive episode, and it is misinterpreted frequently as a depressive relapse, with the conclusion that one "needs" the SRI. This would be analogous to saying that someone needs an opiate when faced with the gastrointestinal pains of opiate withdrawal. This is the problem: one cannot tell whether SRIs are truly effective in maintenance prevention of depressive episodes in that setting, or whether they have produced a withdrawal syndrome phenomenon. The latter is more proven than the former.

An aspect to the withdrawal syndrome is that it can be so painful and extreme that some patients become suicidal, and there is evidence that suicidal ideation and attempts increase during the serotonin withdrawal syndrome. This withdrawal syndrome should not be tolerated by patient or clinician. Efforts should be made to prevent or ameliorate it aggressively. One approach is to avoid the agents that are most likely to cause it. This is one feature in which these agents can differ markedly. It is clear that the worst with venlafaxine, paroxetine, and duloxetine. The mildest serotonin withdrawal syndrome occurs with fluoxetine, which has the longest half-life.

Often, it is necessary to use fluoxetine as cross-tapering agent. It should be used routinely when managing termination of treatment with the three agents described before that have the worst withdrawal syndromes. Usually it is safer to switch patients to fluoxetine, and then taper the latter, rather than trying to taper paroxetine or duloxetine or venlafaxine directly. Clinicians can take a long time to taper off SRIs, especially during a fluoxetine cross-taper. Three to six months is reasonable, or longer, for a gradual taper off SRIs. More rapid taper over one month or so is not necessary, and often leads to severe withdrawal. Abrupt discontinuation is rarely tolerated. If very long-term treatment is expected, then patients should understand that they are making a commitment to indefinite SRI treatment, with notable potential complications of serotonin withdrawal syndrome should they ever need or decide to stop it.

Sexual Dysfunction

Sexual dysfunction is probably the most common side effect of SRIs. Despite low reports in early controlled clinical trials, later experience indicates that about 50% of patients treated for the long term with SRIs develop sexual dysfunction. Dysfunction varies from decreased libido to inability to obtain orgasm, and erectile difficulty. This effect may partly be due to stimulation of 5HT-2 receptors, as agents that block that receptor (like nefazodone and mirtazapine) produce less sexual dysfunction. Weekend "drug holidays," particularly with sertraline as noted later, are sometimes used to minimize this side effect. It is a clinical reality that sexual dysfunction is under-reported if it is not specifically examined by clinicians; patients often will not report sexual side effects due to embarrassment or perhaps due to lack of recognition of those symptoms as medication-related.

This problem is especially common in SRI treatment of depression since many depressed patients experience sexual dysfunction as part of the depressive syndrome, and it may be difficult to recognize further impairment due to the medications. A clinician should be suspicious if most depressive symptoms improve except for sexual function. Again, the clinician needs to consistently query about sexual function to pick up on such lack of improvement.

Other Side Effects

Other side effects common to the entire class are gastrointestinal side effects and disruption of sleep architecture. Gastrointestinal side effects usually involve diarrhea and nausea. It is an often under-recognized fact that there are more serotonin receptors in the enteric nervous system of the gut than in the brain. The gut's enteric nervous system is an independent peripheral nervous system, mostly consisting of serotonergic connections utilizing 5HT-3 receptors. Mirtazapine, a 5HT-3 blocker, produces fewer gastrointestinal side effects. Another way to manage such side effects can be to add ondansetron, a selective 5HT-3 receptor antagonist FDA-indicated to treat chemotherapy-related nausea, to the offending SRI.

The effect of SRIs on sleep architecture (progression from one sleep stage to another) is also common. Sleep stages are highly influenced by serotonergic neurons in the raphe nuclei of the medulla and pons. Progression from one stage of sleep to another is disrupted by SRIs. Clinically, patients experience mid-cycle awakenings in the middle of the night, as well as vivid dreaming. Trazodone regularizes the transitions between sleep stages, resulting in its popularity as an anti-insomnia adjunct in polypharmacy with SRIs. Nefazodone and bupropion also appear to improve sleep architecture. Because of these sleep effects, SRIs should generally be dosed in the morning, with the exception of some persons who experience sedation with paroxetine and occasionally fluoxetine, which should be dosed in the evening in those individuals.

The "Better Than Well" Syndrome

Prozac (fluoxetine) and SRIs have become famous for possibly making people "better than well," the concept introduced by Peter Kramer that such SRIs may alter what used to be called the "melancholic personality," a mixture of dysthymic and anxious chronic symptoms. Such persons seemed to become less anxious and more extroverted with SRIs. This topic has generated much controversy, both as to whether it really occurs, and if so, what it means ethically and clinically. One perspective is that some patients indeed have such responses to SRIs, which are partly changes in personality and partly improvements in depressive syndromes that had been excluded from DSM-III, such as "neurotic depression" (as discussed in Chapter 19). These effects of SRIs should always be distinguished from the common occurrence of misdiagnosed bipolar depression with resultant hypomania or mania.

The Apathy Syndrome

The opposite effect can occur as well. Some individuals with a baseline personality that is low in anxiety and highly extroverted (often hyperthymic) will experience the anxiety-reducing effects of SRIs as restrictive. SRIs appear to induce an apathy syndrome in such persons. This effect is not clearly understood, but it is speculated that SRIs might reduce frontal lobe activity in some patients (although most SRIs increase frontal lobe activity). This effect results in a flattening of affect, sometimes described by patients as an decreased ability to "feel" experiences, or an attenuation of normal fluctuations in mood. In other words, patients may not be able to be appropriately sad when they should be, or appropriately happy when they should be, compared to the manner in which most non-depressed persons would react in those circumstances. This apathy syndrome can be a subtle effect for patients or clinicians to recognize. It can be mistaken as a continuation of depressive anhedonia, or possibly seen as a recurrence of depression. In patients who recover from most of their neurovegetative symptoms except anhedonia, the apathy syndrome should be suspected.

Suicide and Akathisia

An unavoidable topic in relation to the SRIs is the risk of suicide. This issue is most frequently raised in relation to fluoxetine, but this relationship probably reflects the longer availability of fluoxetine relative to other SRIs. Legal cases arguing for an association with suicide have been raised with most SRIs, and the FDA has instituted a black box warning of SRI-induced suicidality in children. This topic is discussed in more detail in Chapter 27, but a brief summary is provided here.

The FDA warning is based on a meta-analysis of multiple randomized clinical trials in children, many of which are unpublished, which demonstrated more than 50% increased relative risk of suicidality (attempts or increased suicidal ideation) in a total sample of about 5,000 children studied. While this is important, indicating a real risk, it should also be borne in mind that the absolute rates of suicidality were about 4% with SRIs versus about 2% with placebo, meaning that this increased risk probably occurs in about 5% or less of treated children. Nonetheless, this fact, as well as the absence of completed suicides in those studies, should not engender false complacency. As with all randomized clinical trials, the subjects who enter are carefully chosen to be low-risk and highly compliant; suicidal ideation of any significance was an exclusion criterion for almost all those studies. If anything, therefore, the FDA meta-analysis underestimates the true risk in the general population of children. Furthermore, there are nuisance side effects, and there are fatal side effects. A 5% risk of nausea is irrelevant, but a 5% risk of death is unacceptable, even if the drug also saves lives (which has not yet been proven with SRIs in relation to preventing suicide).

Thus, the consequence of the FDA ruling should be what the FDA intended and what has in fact happened: prior indiscriminate use of SRIs has been replaced by a greater exercise of clinical judgment, which should have always been the case. The opposite extreme, of never using SRIs, is also inappropriate.

If we now accept that SRI-induced suicidality occurs, the next question is, why? Some critics seem to believe that there is something inherently dangerous about these medications; this claim has not been substantiated. Two other potential causes seem to be, in my view, much more likely, and are also preventable.

First, there is the likelihood of either misdiagnosed bipolar illness, or an early prodrome to later bipolar illness. Some studies of children indicate that up to 50% of depressed children (mean age 12) develop manic or hypomanic episodes in a decade of follow-up. Keeping in mind that the age of onset of bipolar disorder is much earlier than unipolar depression (late teens versus late 20s), clinicians should always have a high index of suspicion for latent bipolar disorder in depressed children. Furthermore, manic episodes in children are usually mixed, and about 60% of mixed states involve increased suicidality, a figure that is even higher than the occurrence of suicidality in pure depression. Statistically, if 50% of apparently depressed children are indeed bipolar, than one would easily expect that 10% of them (or more) would develop manic episodes if given antidepressant monotherapy; these figures could easily explain the 5% suicidality rate observed in the FDA database.

Second, SRIs can cause the extrapyramidal symptoms of akathisia (discussed in more detail in Chapter 10). Akathisia is a very uncomfortable, dysphoric experience, often misinterpreted as agitation or worsening of depression. When unrecognized and untreated, it can increase suicidal ideation, and it seems to have been a factor in a number of the rare cases of fluoxetine-associated suicide. Though probably less common than SRI-induced mania, SRI-related akathisia has been reported to occur in up to 10% of treated individuals.

What should clinicians do? First, carefully rule out bipolar illness, keeping in mind that it cannot be effectively ruled out in children since they may not have yet had their first manic or hypomania episode. In children, therefore, the bipolar spectrum concept, including an emphasis on family history, may be especially relevant (see Chapter 28). In addition, clinicians should warn patients about akathisia and carefully look for this side effect, especially in the first few months of treatment, and should be prepared to either reduce the SRI dose or stop the SRI, or treat with propanolol. Akathisia should never be left to fester: it needs to be terminated as soon as possible.

INDIVIDUAL SRIS

See Table 9.1 for a summary of individual serotonin reuptake inhibitors.

Fluoxetine (Prozac)

The groundbreaking medication in this class was fluoxetine, introduced in the United States in 1989. This agent was quickly followed by sertraline, paroxetine, fluvoxamine, and citalopram, in that order. Fluoxetine was also the first of these agents to become available in generic form (2001), after more than a decade of blockbusting profits. It was not the "best" SRI, but it had the major advantage of being the first on the market. Both clinicians and patients quickly became familiar, and usually comfortable, with this medication. By initiating the change in prescriptions from TCAs to newer antidepressants, fluoxetine also became the symbol of the new generation of "kinder, gentler" psychiatric medications. From a sober medical perspective, however, fluoxetine has some advantages and some disadvantages that do not seem to distinguish it from its SRI compatriots.

TABLE 9.1 Individual Serotonin Reuptake Inhibitors

Drug	Effective dose (mg/d)	Comments
Fluoxetine (Prozac)	20–80	Longest half-life of any antidepressant, requiring longer duration for a therapeutic trial but also producing less serotonin withdrawal; somewhat noradrenergic; marked drug interactions (all cytochromes, esp. 2D6 & 3A4)
Sertraline (Zoloft)	50–200	Dopaminergic; useful in weekend holidays for sexual dysfunction; mild drug interactions
Paroxetine (Paxil)	20–50	Very anxiolytic; moderately anticholinergic; some weight gain; somewhat more serotonin withdrawal; multiple FDA indications; cytochrome 3A4 inhibitor
Citalopram (Celexa)	20–60	Most potent serotonin reuptake inhibition; most selective agent for serotonin; minimal drug interactions; especially useful in the elderly
Fluvoxamine (Luvox)	50–250	Highly potent serotonin reuptake inhibition; indicated for OCD

A unique feature of fluoxetine is that it, and its active metabolite norfluoxetine, have quite long half-lives, the longest, in fact, of any major psychotropic agent. The half-life of fluoxetine is about one day, and of norfluoxetine about three to five days. Thus, on average, it takes four days for a dose of fluoxetine to be 50% eliminated. Since it takes three half-lives to achieve a steady-state blood level, it takes 12 days just to achieve a steady-state level of this agent. All antidepressants require about four to eight weeks' time delay for their pharmacological effects to translate into a clinical antidepressant effect. This delay probably reflects intracellular second messenger and genetic changes. However, this four- to six-week delay occurs after steady state is achieved. For most antidepressants, a steady state blood level is achieved in one or two days. For fluoxetine, the 12-day delay on average means that the clinical effect of the medication may be delayed another one to two weeks. This is why fluoxetine is the only antidepressant that requires a six- to eight-week period for a full therapeutic trial (as opposed to four to six weeks). This fact may be a partial disadvantage: if a patient is not responding to fluoxetine at four weeks of treatment, one cannot change to another medication knowing that a full trial has been given, unless one waits another two weeks. This is not the case with other antidepressants, in which no response at all at four weeks is a sufficient therapeutic trial. On the flip side, a potential advantage to this long half-life is that fluoxetine does not leave the body quickly, and it thus may be less prone to causing serotonin withdrawal syndrome.

Another feature of fluoxetine is that, contrary to what is sometimes assumed, it is not purely selective for serotonin. In fact, fluoxetine also mildly blocks the reuptake of norepinephrine. This effect of fluoxetine is not minor, and it is somewhat similar to the effect of venlafaxine. This feature may possibly account for the "stimulating" effects frequently reported with fluoxetine.

Like all SRIs, fluoxetine can disrupt the sleep architecture. Combined with its potentially stimulating effects, fluoxetine can cause insomnia. Nonetheless, a small subgroup of patients appears to become sedated with it.

Another major effect of fluoxetine is that it is a strong inhibitor of most hepatic cytochrome P450 enzymes, thereby increasing the blood levels and effects of many other medications, including dopamine blockers, TCAs, and some mood stabilizers. Despite its side effect of sometimes causing "stimulation," fluoxetine often has the pharmacological effect of decreased anxiety, as do all SRIs.

Since fluoxetine has been available for the longest amount of time, it has been studied in the largest number of conditions, with reports of efficacy in bulimia nervosa, anorexia nervosa, PTSD, personality disorders, obsessive-compulsive disorder (OCD), and panic disorder. It has efficacy in these conditions, but all SRIs are likely to be useful in similar conditions. Fluoxetine is now FDA-indicated (under a different trade name) for the treatment of "premenstrual syndrome" (late luteal phase dysphoric disorder).

As noted, some clinicians believe that fluoxetine exerts a special beneficial effect on personality. This perspective holds that some depressed and even non-depressed individuals become "better than well" on fluoxetine; that is, not only are they no longer depressed, they also do not return to their premorbid personality. They often become more extroverted and fun-loving, and a patient may feel that her personality on fluoxetine is her "real" self. When reported, this effect seems to be rare, and it seems not to be clearly specific to fluoxetine. It might be explained as an effect on personality, separate from any antidepressant effects of the medication. Some researchers have provided evidence that some aspects of personality, especially what has been called "harm avoidance," may be associated with serotonergic areas of the brain. By increasing serotonin availability, SRIs may alter the personality by making persons less harm-avoidant: that is, less cautious or shy or introverted. As a result, this at one level mysterious effect of fluoxetine may simply be a straightforward effect on the biochemistry of personality. At another level, however, this effect of fluoxetine needs to be balanced with an apparently equal potential for less positive effects on personality, such as the apathy syndrome.

Sertraline (Zoloft)

Sertraline is an SRI with a moderate amount of dopamine reuptake blockade. It has a shorter half-life than fluoxetine, about one day, and causes much less inhibition of hepatic cytochrome P450 enzymes. This does not mean it has no hepatic enzyme effect; especially at higher doses, its effect can be clinically notable. Usually, though, its hepatic effects are mild and do not lead to clinically significant drug interactions.

Sertraline shares with other SRIs a general antianxiety effect, as well as a potentially disruptive sleep effect. It is also FDA-indicated for the treatment of PTSD. While fluoxetine possesses an FDA indication for premenstrual syndrome, sertraline is also useful in this setting, and perhaps more so if an individual prefers to use the SRI for five days before and after the menstrual period, rather than continuously. Such short-term use is effective with all SRIs except fluoxetine (again, due to the latter's long half-life). The short half-life of sertraline may also be useful in the context of drug holidays for sexual dysfunction.

This discontinuation would not work with fluoxetine due to its long half-life, and it might be more difficult with paroxetine or venlafaxine, due to their short half-lives and the consequent risk of serotonin withdrawal syndrome. The weekend drug holiday seems to work well with sertraline, however, which may partly reflect the fact that sertraline's metabolite, desmethylsertraline, has a half-life of about three days. As a result, in weekend drug holidays, sertraline is short-acting enough to leave the body such that sexual function temporarily improves, but not so short-acting that serotonin withdrawal symptoms begin.

A potential disadvantage of sertraline's mild dopaminergic effect may be that in particular susceptible individuals, this biochemical property may lead to increased psychosis. This has been reported in otherwise nonpsychotic individuals, though infrequently.

Paroxetine (Paxil)

Paroxetine is also short-acting, with a half-life of about one day, and perhaps more short-acting than sertraline (since the latter has a metabolite with a long half-life). Paroxetine is more potent than either sertraline or fluoxetine in its serotonin reuptake effect, which means that if a higher degree of serotonin reuptake is needed, then paroxetine may be useful. In other words, even strictly on the issue of serotonin reuptake effect, these

SRIs are not identical. This difference may account for the clinical experience that some patients respond to one SRI and others to another SRI.

Paroxetine also possesses moderate anticholinergic effects. While prominent in vitro, in vivo studies in humans suggest that these anticholinergic effects are not marked and are certainly less severe than with TCAs. In susceptible persons, though, clinically notable anticholinergic effects may occur. These include dry mouth, sedation, constipation, and cognitive side effects.

Most SRIs are weight-neutral, with some persons losing weight and a small number of persons gaining weight. Of the SRIs, paroxetine appears to be the most liable to some amount of weight gain, though not, on the whole, to a severe degree. Some individuals will experience significant weight gain.

Among the SRIs, which all have anti-anxiety effects, paroxetine holds the reputation of having the most consistent anxiolytic effects, and it is FDA-indicated in the treatment of generalized anxiety disorder, panic disorder, and social phobia (social anxiety disorder). Unfortunately, paroxetine's short half-life makes it somewhat more liable to serotonin withdrawal symptoms than other SRIs, which is a major problem.

Paroxetine has minimal effect on the cytochrome P450 2D6 system, unlike fluoxetine, but it is a strong inhibitor of the cytochrome P450 3A4 system, like fluoxetine. In terms of drug interactions, paroxetine has an intermediate effect—not as marked as fluoxetine, but not as mild as sertraline.

Citalopram (Celexa)

Citalopram was used in Europe for a number of years before it was introduced into the United States in 1999. (In Europe it predated fluoxetine.) It is even more potent in its serotonin reuptake blockade effect than paroxetine. It also the most purely serotonergic agent in this class, with almost no other effects on other neurotransmitter systems. It has minimal effect on hepatic enzymes, and a short (but not too short) half-life of about one day. In many ways, then, citalopram (and its enantiomer escitalopram) is the only "SRI" that deserves the label of a *selective* SRI (SSRI).

Overall, it probably has benefits similar to most SRIs as regards anti-anxiety and other effects. Due to its "cleaner" biochemical profile, it has been thought to be helpful in older persons, in whom it is less likely to cause avoidable side effects or drug interactions. Unfortunately, because of its cardiac side effects, it is not preferable for use in older persons.

Citalopram is associated with cardiac arrhythmias at doses above 40 mg/d, and thus should not be prescribed above that dose, and it probably should be avoided in persons with cardiac arrhythmias. There should also be caution in its use in persons with cardiovascular diseases that may increase the risk of arrhythmias. It is not effective in bipolar depression, having been disproven in a large placebo-controlled trial in bipolar depression (see Chapter 19).

Escitalopram (Lexapro) is the active enantiomer of citalopram; except for the ability to get the same effect of citalopram at lower doses, claims to better tolerability than citalopram have not been clinically confirmed.

Fluvoxamine (Luvox)

Fluvoxamine is FDA-indicated for OCD, but it probably has benefits for depression and anxiety similar to other SRIs'. Like paroxetine and citalopram, it is potent in its serotonin reuptake blockade. It has few other biochemical effects, and no other real advantage over other SRIs. It is a strong inhibitor of the cytochrome P450 3A4 system, perhaps even more than paroxetine, and thus has some disadvantages in terms of drug interactions.

Venlafaxine (Effexor)

This agent is sold as a serotonin-norepinephrine reuptake inhibitor (SNRI), but it hardly has any more noradrenergic effects than fluoxetine, or even paroxetine at higher doses. It is about 30 times more potent for serotonin versus norepinephrine reuptake blockade. Thus venlafaxine is just another SRI with some noradrenergic effects. The norepinephrine reuptake blockade is higher with venlafaxine at higher doses, especially 150 mg/d or more.

It is typically dosed at 150–300 mg/d, given once daily at night. At 75 mg/d, it is a pure SRI with anxiety symptom benefits, and is FDA-indicated for generalized anxiety at that dose. Its average dose in studies of major depressive disorder (MDD) is about 225 mg/d. The maximum approved dose is 375 mg/d.

It has few drug interactions and does not interact with the cytochrome P450 system extensively. It has a brief half-life of about five hours, even with the extended-release formulation, which leads to very severe serotonin withdrawal syndrome. Its active metabolite, O-desmethylvenlafaxine, has a somewhat longer half-life of nine hours. The extended release has a half-life of about 15 hours. In all cases, serotonin withdrawal syndrome tends to be severe.

Unfortunately, venlafaxine raises the blood pressure and has cardiovascular risks of sudden cardiac death. These harmful cardiovascular effects were underplayed by the manufacturer for years and have not been well appreciated by the clinical community. In 2004, the United Kingdom regulatory body responded to the evidence for cardiac arrhythmia leading to death with overdose of venlafaxine by restricting its use to persons without cardiovascular disease. A great deal of pushback from the manufacturer and from clinicians led to a revision of the U.K. restriction to contraindication in persons with uncontrolled hypertension or past cardiac arrhythmias. No such restrictions have been implemented by the FDA in the United States. Nonetheless, it is clear that venlafaxine is the riskiest SRI for persons with cardiovascular disease.

It also is not appreciated that venlafaxine has about double the risk of causing mania in persons with bipolar depression, compared to other SRIs or bupropion. Thus venlafaxine should also be avoided in bipolar depression.

It has been argued that venlafaxine is more effective than other SRIs in refractory clinical depression. There is some evidence to this effect, especially in hospitalized depression. Some of the published meta-analyses of this topic were limited by not including unpublished studies that demonstrated inefficacy with venlafaxine. Thus, the extent to which it may be more effective than other monoamine agonists is questionable.

Desvenlafaxine (Pristiq)

The active metabolite of the agent desmethylvenlafaxine (Pristiq) also has been patented as a stand-alone agent, dosed up to 50 mg/d, given once daily at night. Higher doses have been studied but not proven more effective for MDD. The mechanisms and risks and benefits of this agent do not appear to differ notably from venlafaxine's. It is somewhat more noradrenergic than the parent compound, but is still ten times more potent as an SRI as it is in norepinephrine reuptake inhibition.

Duloxetine (Cymbalta)

This agent is more of a true SNRI than venlafaxine, since it is notably more potent in its norepinephrine reuptake blockade, but it is still primarily an SRI, similar to desvenlafaxine in this regard (about tenfold more potent for serotonin than for norepinephrine reuptake blockade). It is dosed 20–60 mg/d, given once daily at night. The maximum approved dose is 120 mg/d, but doses above 60 mg/d have not been shown to be more effective. It is FDA-indicated for MDD, generalized anxiety disorder (GAD), fibromyalgia, chronic musculoskeletal pain, and diabetic peripheral neuropathy. Physical pain symptoms were studied with this agent in its depression trials, and pain benefits were shown, leading to FDA indications. It is likely that other monoamine agonists, especially those with noradrenergic effects, also will have pain benefits, but most of them were not studied on this matter systematically. Duloxetine has a half-life of about 12 hours, and very severe serotonin withdrawal syndrome.

Given the previous discussion, Table 9.1 summarizes overall general tips on the use of SRIs in clinical practice.

DOPAMINE AGONISTS: BUPROPION AND "STIMULANTS"/AMPHETAMINES

Bupropion (Wellbutrin)

This agent predated fluoxetine, reaching the U.S. market in the late 1980s as one of the first modern antidepressants after the TCAs. Unlike the latter, bupropion (Wellbutrin) was seen as being safe, without risk of fatal overdose due to cardiac arrhythmias, unlike TCAs. Unfortunately, this agent was soon faced with fluoxetine (Prozac), which was marketed aggressively as better than bupropion due to a small seizure risk found with the latter. Also, Prozac had a good marketing story to tell: it was a "selective" SRI, unlike TCAs, which were nonselective serotonin and norepinephrine reuptake inhibitors. It is known now that this is not true, and that both Prozac and TCAs are serotonin and norepinephrine reuptake inhibitors, but it was a good story. And it was true that Prozac was safe in overdose, unlike TCAs.

But the makers of bupropion did not have a story to tell, because they did not know how their drug worked. And for many clinicians, its mechanism remains a mystery. All that is known is that this agent has mild dopamine agonism effects, and perhaps mild

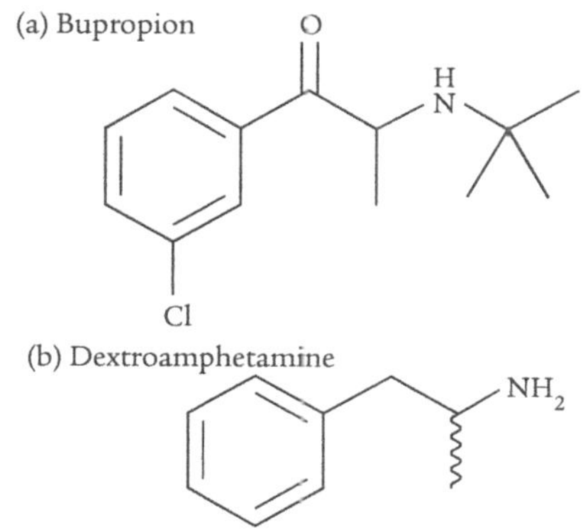

FIGURE 9.1 *a. Bupropion b. Dextroamphetamine*

norepinephrine agonism effects; but these effects are often seen as too mild as to explain its robust antidepressant properties.

A solution can be found to this dilemma once one observes the chemical structure of bupropion and compares it to dextroamphetamine. Then it becomes clear that bupropion is a variant on amphetamine. Upon drawing this conclusion, it makes sense that this agent has mild dopaminergic and noradrenergic effects, is "stimulating," causes weight loss, enhances sexual drive, causes insomnia, worsens anxiety, and has been shown to be effective in attention deficit disorder (ADD) in children—all classic amphetamine effects (Figure 9.1).

A slow-release formulation (Wellbutrin SR) reduces the risk of seizures from 0.4% to 0.1%, making it similar to SRIs on that risk. This preferred formulation comes in 100 mg capsules, with a standard dose of 200–400 mg/d for depressive episodes. Higher doses produce higher seizure risk. Other slow-release formulations (XL) exist so that one pill daily can be provided for a 300 mg/d dose. Bupropion has been shown to have low to no risk of causing mania at these standard doses or lower, but it has been shown also to be ineffective in treating depression in bipolar illness. It is often used by clinicians for its amphetamine-like properties of weight loss and sexual enhancement, and often added to SRIs to counteract the sexual side effects of the latter. As noted, it can cause insomnia and anxiety as side effects, and it can have benefits for improving attention, as in ADD, as do all amphetamines.

Amphetamines

Although now used for ADD, this class of medications was the first class of antidepressants, introduced for that use in the 1930s and remaining the prime class of antidepressant treatments for 40 years. These agents are all variants on one of two basic structures: methylphenidate and dextroamphetamine. The methylphenidate variants are the standard compound (Ritalin), Focalin, and Concerta. The dextroamphetamine variants are the standard compound (Dexedrine), Adderall, and vyvanse, among others (Table 1.7).

These agents are all dopamine agonists with direct stimulation of dopamine receptors. Some also stimulate norepinephrine receptors. Their typical side effects are insomnia, anxiety, and jitteriness, and they can cause mania in bipolar illness. Their main medical risks are cardiac arrhythmias and neurotoxicity in animals.

They also produce weight loss and increase sexual libido in all persons, effects often used to enhance one's appearance or sexual function. They also improve attention in all persons, not only in ADD, which has led to their use for performance enhancement in sports as well as in academic or white-collar work circumstances.

Their neurotoxicity often is underappreciated. This is a consistent finding in animal studies, particularly in rodents. These studies find that animals exposed to methylphenidate or other amphetamines will develop hippocampal atrophy and show increased excitotoxicity of neurons. They also have harmful behaviors such as increased anxiety and depression in animal models. Human research is small and inconclusive, neither clearly supporting nor refuting these animal data.

Cardiotoxicity also is important, especially in adults, who have more cardiac risk factors than children. Some research finds almost a doubling of the risk of sudden cardiac death due to ventricular arrhythmias with methylphenidate. When analyzed to calculate an absolute frequency of risk, it was about 1:1000. If true, this risk is a concern with the increasing use of these agents for presumed adult ADD.

OTHER NEW MONOAMINE AGONISTS

Several new monoamine agonists have entered the market in the last few years. In general, none of these agents are shown to be any more effective than the standard agents described here, nor do they have appreciably fewer side effects. They are used often in patients who have failed to improve with the standard agents, but there is no efficacy proven in refractory depressed patients.

Vilazodone

This agent is the child of trazodone, an SRI with 5HT1a receptor partial agonism, which limits sexual dysfunction. Like its precursor nefazodone, this derivative of the trazodone parent compound is less sedating in doses that are effective in depression. Its effects on sleep have not been studied yet, but may be beneficial, as with trazodone. Although it has less sexual dysfunction than other SRIs, it will have other side effects similar to those in agents in that class.

Vortioxetine

This agent is an SRI with 5HT1A agonism (complete, not partial), similar to trazodone and vilazodone but with somewhat higher serotonergic potency. Although these effects are unknown in their relevance, this agent also blocks 5HT3 and 5HT7 receptors.

Its manufacturer has tried to market it in a way that would distinguish it from other SRIs by calling it a serotonin "modulator." This is a marketing gimmick, as vilazodone and trazodone long have had the same mechanism. Furthermore, mirtazapine also is a partial serotonin reuptake agonist and a blocker of 5HT2 receptors, along with noradrenergic effects. Hence there is nothing truly unique about the mix of monoamine receptor blockade and partial agonism and blockade of other serotonin receptors.

This agent has a very long half-life of 66 hours, which should minimize serotonin withdrawal. It is dosed 10–20 mg/d for the acute phase of MDD.

One randomized study found that it improved cognition in persons during depressive episodes, even when depressive symptoms had not improved notably. Thus, there is some thought that it may enhance cognition in addition to mood symptoms.

Levomilnacipran

This agent is an SNRI with much more norepinephrine reuptake blockade than venlafaxine or duloxetine. It is FDA-indicated for the acute phase of MDD, in the 40–120 mg/d dose range. It is an enantiomer of milnacipran, which has been used in Europe for many years for depression. In the United States, the latter agent is FDA-indicated for fibromyalgia. Being highly noradrenergic, it appears to increase blood pressure, which may limit its use in persons with risk factors for cardiovascular disease. It may be useful in depression related to chronic pain in particular.

Agomelatine (Not in the U.S. but in Canada and Europe)

This medication is a melatonin receptor agonist and blocker of serotonin 5HT2C receptors, approved for use for MDD in Canada and Europe, but not in the United States. It is the only agent used for depression that is not a monoamine agonist, although its serotonin blockade mechanism may be relevant to its possible depressive symptom benefits. Because of its lack of monoamine effects, it has the advantage of not having typical side effects such as sexual dysfunction or serotonin withdrawal syndrome. However, there is considerable debate regarding its efficacy. Since it was being studied in phase III randomized trials to come to the U.S. market, but the company owning its rights decided not to bring it to the market, it is fair to conclude that those studies probably did not show that it was effective over placebo in MDD. In fact, in the international literature, it is effective in 6 of 10 randomized trials of MDD. This frequency of efficacy may seem questionable, but it is similar to other standard monoamine agonists (as discussed in Chapter 19).

Ketamine

This agent has received a great deal of attention. Ketamine is studied and given mainly intravascularly (IV), which makes its clinical use complex. Nonetheless, ketamine clinics exist to provide this medication IV. Available research has claimed that it provides rapid antidepressant effect, within hours, and lasting one week after a single dose, as opposed to having effects within weeks to a month or more with standard oral antidepressants. This effect also is claimed to occur in persons who have not responded to standard antidepressants, although randomized data are few, limited in sample size, and completely dependent on retrospective recall to claim treatment resistance. Efficacy in bipolar depression also has been reported in small, short, randomized trials. Ketamine is a medication used mainly in anesthesia, or used as a recreational drug of abuse. It certainly causes a "high"; the view that its rapid antidepressant effect is something other than a drug "high" is based on reported benefit for a range of depressive symptoms. Nonetheless, as with all drugs of abuse, its rapid immediate effects correlate with a rapid loss of effect; hence the need for repeated treatment over time. Whether this "maintenance" treatment is effective is questionable, since it has not been studied in randomized clinical trials.

In animal studies, ketamine is neurotoxic at standard doses used in human recreational drug abuse, but it is reported not to be neurotoxic at the low doses used in psychiatric drug treatment of depression. Its possibly harmful effects on the human brain have not been studied in randomized trials.

A nasal version of this agent, esketamine, has been studied in phase III randomized trials and has been fast-tracked by the FDA for approval. If used, it will have a similar profile to standard ketamine, including biological evidence of neurotoxicity, although with the more convenient intranasal, as opposed to intravenous, route of administration. Further discussion of ketamine is provided in Chapter 19.

SELECTED REFERENCE

Richelson, E. (2001). Pharmacology of antidepressants. *Mayo Clinic Proceedings, 76*(5), 511–527.

10

Dopamine Blockers ("Antipsychotics")

Dopamine blockers are agents used to treat psychotic symptoms such as delusions and hallucinations. These medications have been developed mostly for use in schizophrenia, but they always have been found to be effective in acute mania as well. For the latter reason, they have been used in bipolar illness also. Several of these agents have been proven effective in the depressive phase of bipolar illness, not just the manic phase. Furthermore, some of them have been shown to be effective in the depressive phase of unipolar mood illness.

Outside of these uses based on randomized trials and registration indications, this class of medication has been used off-label for decades for agitation and aggression in general. The most common scenarios for this latter usage include emergency room–based control of intoxicated persons, hospital-based treatment of delirium in medically ill persons, agitation in the context of dementia, and agitation/aggression in a range of neuropsychiatric syndromes (traumatic brain injury, mental retardation, epilepsy, Parkinson's disease). In addition, they commonly have been used in low doses to manage self-injury in borderline personality and/or agitation in post-traumatic stress disorder (PTSD).

This chapter will review common side effects and risks with the class as a whole, and then the specific pharmacology and clinical effects of each agent.

PHARMACOLOGY

Common class terms are "typical" versus "atypical," or "conventional" versus "modern," or "first-generation" versus "second-generation" agents. The claim is that the "typical" or conventional dopamine blockers were pure dopamine blockers, whereas the "atypical" or modern agents also are serotonin blockers. Sometimes this phrasing is shortened to "the atypicals." Yet, the majority of agents in common use today, now about ten of them, are serotonin/dopamine blockers; hence the term "atypical" loses its meaning when the standard agents are now of that variety. The term "modern" is less meaningful as well, now that we are into the third decade of existence of the newer agents.

As proposed earlier in this book, the phrase "dopamine blocker" better captures all these agents, with the understanding that they also have other effects, with most of the newer generation of agents also being serotonin blockers. Some of the older generation also were serotonin blockers, so that distinction is not neat. In this book, the phrase "dopamine blockers" will be used for all these agents, and non-technical adjectives will be used to refer to earlier versus later generations of these medications.

MECHANISMS OF ACTION

It is thought that dopamine blockers generally need to block about 80–90% of D2 receptors, or more, to produce an antipsychotic effect. Most of the newer generation of dopamine blockers also block almost all (>90%) serotonin-2 (5HT2) receptors. It has been argued that the newer dopamine blockers possess greater selectivity for dopamine receptor blockade in the limbic regions of the brain (which subserve mood and thought) rather than the nigrostriatal areas (which produce extrapyramidal side effects [EPS]). This claim has been found in some animal studies, but its verification in human studies is limited.

It's important to note that despite these beliefs, two important dopamine blockers appear to produce antipsychotic effect with limited dopamine blockade. Clozapine and quetiapine only block about 20–40% of dopamine receptors, at any dose.

A GENERAL CLASSIFICATION

A common way of classifying traditional dopamine blockers has been to divide them into high, mid, and low-potency classes based on D2 blockade (Table 10.1). The same approach can be taken to the newer dopamine blockers based on D2 and 5HT2 blockade, as seen in the table. Clozapine and quetiapine are low-potency atypical dopamine blocker agents because they do not block over 90% of 5T2 receptors (more in the 40–80% range), and they do not block D2 dopamine receptors at higher than 40% levels, even at higher doses. Furthermore, like their traditional counterparts, these agents block multiple other receptor systems, with anticholinergic, antihistaminic, and antiadrenergic effects. Olanzapine is a mid-potency agent because it blocks over 90% of 5HT2 receptors at all doses, it produces dose-related increased D2 blockade reaching over 80% at 20 mg/d, and it has anticholinergic, antihistaminic, and antiadrenergic effects. Risperidone and ziprasidone are high-potency agents because they block over 90% of serotonin receptors, they produce dose-related D2 blockade that exceeds 80–90% at high doses, and they have few other receptor effects. As with traditional dopamine blockers, potency differences among newer dopamine blockers influence side effects. Lower-potency agents have fewer Parkinsonian effects, more anticholinergic effects, and more weight gain; higher-potency agents possess more Parkinsonian effects and less weight gain; with mid-potency agents midway on all accounts. However, with newer agents, some other differences apply due to the added effect of serotonin blockade, which may predispose to weight gain. Due to the complex influences of serotonin and histamine blockade on weight gain, olanzapine

TABLE 10.1 Classification of Traditional and Second Generation Neuroleptics Based on Potency

	Low potency	Mid potency	High potency
Traditional dopamine blockers	Chlorpromazine (Thorazine) Thioridazine (Mellaril)	Perphenazine (Trilafon) Trifluoperazine (Stelazine)	Haloperidol (Haldol) Fluphenazine (Prolixin)
	Less D2 potency Less Parkinsonian EPS Multiple receptor blockade effects	**Intermediate on all counts**	More D2 potency More Parkinsonian EPS Few other receptor blockade effects
Second-generation dopamine blockers	Clozapine (Clozaril) Quetiapine (Seroquel)	Olanzapine (Zyprexa) Asenapine (Saphris)	Risperidone (Risperdal) Ziprasidone (Geodon) Aripiprazole (Abilify) Iloperidone (Fanapt) Lurasidone (Latuda) Cariprazine (Vraylar)
	Less D2 potency Less 5HT2 potency Fewer Parkinsonian EPS Multiple receptor blockade effects More weight gain	Intermediate, with exception of weight gain for olanzapine	More dose-related D2 potency More Parkinsonian EPS Few other receptor blockade effects Less weight gain

Note: Akathisia and TD do not differ in general between potency groups, for either traditional or second generation neuroleptic classes.

causes more weight gain than quetiapine, which has more than risperidone. As with traditional dopamine blockers, risk of tardive dyskinesia (TD) and akathisia does not seem to differ significantly between potency groups.

Note that most of the newest dopamine blockers tend to be high-potency agents. This is the case because these agents are developed on purpose with the goal of not causing metabolic syndrome and weight gain, as appears to happen mainly with the low-potency dopamine blockers (clozapine and quetiapine) and with olanzapine.

DOPAMINE BLOCKER CLASS SIDE EFFECTS

The main shared class side effects of these medications involve EPS. Some agents, but not all, also can have cardiovascular/diabetes harms ("metabolic syndrome"). These two major types of side effects are now considered in turn.

Extrapyramidal Symptoms (EPS)

EPS are defined as Parkinsonian tremor, rigidity, akathisia, dystonia, and TD. Most clinicians appear to identify EPS with Parkinsonian tremor and rigidity, and they will often include TD as part of EPS. This definition omits akathisia, described further later, which can be seen as the most important type of EPS, as it is associated with suicidality, is easily confused with other conditions, and is most highly associated with noncompliance.

The risk of developing EPS has been shown to increase when D2 receptor occupancy reaches between 70% and 80%. Additionally, some studies suggest that the occupancy of 5-HT2a receptors may mitigate EPS induced by high rates of D2 occupancy. Clozapine and quetiapine have the lowest D2 occupancy rates at therapeutic doses, and appear to be associated with less EPS. Moreover, EPS rates with both clozapine and quetiapine do not appear to be dose-dependent. In contrast, risperidone and olanzapine have higher striatal D2 occupancy rates and are associated with more EPS. Although, both drugs have high 5-HT2a affinities, at higher doses they appear to induce a greater risk for EPS. These findings are consistent with animal models that support the positive relationship between D2 occupancy, EPS, and therapeutic effect.

Acute Dystonias

Dystonic reactions (acute muscle spasms, usually of the head or neck) occur shortly after initiation of drug treatment; 50% occur within 48 hours, 95% within 96 hours. Risk factors include family history of dystonia, prior dystonic reactions, recent history of cocaine or alcohol use, young age, and male gender. Acute dystonic reactions occur with modern dopamine blockers, though probably less often than with traditional dopamine blockers.

Parkinsonism

Medication-induced Parkinsonism is characterized by rigidity, resting tremor, masked faces, generalized slowing of movements, and cogwheel rigidity. Mental abnormalities associated with Parkinsonism include emotional blunting, apathy, anhedonia, and social withdrawal. Modern dopamine blockers repeatedly have demonstrated lower rates of Parkinsonism than typical neuroleptics. Absolute rates are not minimal, however. For instance, in one RCT, EPS emerged in 55% of patients with haloperidol, but were also noted in 26% with olanzapine. Other randomized evidence suggests similar rates with risperidone, but lower rates with quetiapine (in the 5–10% range). Clozapine also appears to have low Parkinsonism rates.

Clinicians sometimes assume that risperidone should have more Parkinsonism than olanzapine, due to presumed higher D2 binding affinity with risperidone. But both agents in fact have similar D2 blockade binding affinity, especially at higher doses. If there is lower Parkinsonism with olanzapine compared to risperidone, it might be due to the anticholinergic, instead of D2, effects of olanzapine. Empirical head-to-head studies have not demonstrated lower Parkinsonism with olanzapine compared to risperidone, though some suggestion of this can be found in a few available studies. In one observational report, the Parkinsonism rate with olanzapine was 1/20 (5%) versus 4/25 (16%) with risperidone. In another long-term comparison of 29 patients, Parkinsonism rates were the same.

Akathisia: The Most Important EPS

About one-half of EPS represent akathisia. If akathisia is missed, one-half of the cases of EPS will be misinterpreted as other conditions. Conservative estimates indicate that about 25% of patients treated with traditional dopamine blockers develop akathisia. About half of the cases of akathisia are delayed, not occurring until after the first month of treatment, but most cases occur within three months. (There are rare cases of extremely delayed and chronic, or "tardive," akathisia.)

Akathisia has subjective and objective components. Subjectively, it consists of an intense feeling of dysphoria and extreme anxiety, as occurs with panic attacks. Objectively, it is associated with observed physical restlessness and an inability to sit still. This restlessness is not necessarily consistent, but it can be intermittent, occurring for a few hours in a day or less. Hence akathisia cannot be ruled out based on lack of observed physical restlessness during an office visit. Clinicians often ask patients whether they feel like they need to "jump out of their skin." In my experience, if positive, this symptom is almost pathognomonic of akathisia; but its absence does not rule out akathisia.

Based on these characteristics, akathisia is frequently confused with other conditions. The most common misdiagnosis is vaguely observed "agitation." Frequently, such agitation is simply ascribed to the offending medication, but this vague description gives no guidance to a clinician about how to manage it. The same issue holds for the more vague term "activation," which I often hear in relation to atypical dopamine blockers as well as SRIs like fluoxetine. Especially with SRIs, many of these cases of "activation" or "agitation" are cases of akathisia. Another common misdiagnosis is mania; this mistake is linked to the "agitation" problem. Sometimes clinicians will observe agitation in a patient with bipolar disorder, and conclude that it represents mania (rather than systematically assessing mania criteria). It is my hunch that many purported cases of "mania" related to atypical dopamine blocker use really represent undiagnosed akathisia. Lastly, such agitation can be misinterpreted as worsening psychosis in patients with schizophrenia.

One of the leaders in research on akathisia in the 1970s and 1980s, Theodore Van Putten, conducted a number of studies that indicated that up to 10% of patients with schizophrenia experienced worsening psychosis driven by akathisia. In those patients, the distinction from psychosis unrelated to akathisia was crucial, since in the case of akathisia-related apparent psychosis, the symptoms improved with lowered antipsychotic dosing, whereas in other cases of psychosis, the appropriate treatment would have been to increase the antipsychotic dose.

Besides the fact that akathisia represents one-half of the cases of EPS, it is important to diagnose this side effect because it is associated with noncompliance and suicidality. Many patients appear to tolerate a mild degree of Parkinsonian tremor or rigidity, but even mild akathisia is highly disagreeable, and patients need immediate relief. This usually requires reduction in dosing of the dopamine blocker, or, where reduced dosing leads to less efficacy, the addition of a beta-blocker like propanolol. Unfortunately, propranolol has a very short half-life of four hours, thus it is difficult to dose it frequently enough to prevent breakthrough akathisia. It is recommended to use slow-release preparations of this agent; in the United States, recently a generic formulation has become available, propranolol extended-release (ER), given in doses of 60 mg, 80 mg, or 120 mg tablets. It should be given at night, since it can be sedating, beginning with 60 mg at night of the ER formulation, increasing as need to 80 mg at night, then 120 mg at night and if needed, up to 240 mg at night. It is important to check a baseline pulse, and to follow the pulse as one increases the dose, not increasing the dose beyond a minimal pulse of 50 beats/minute.

There are no clearly informative studies comparing different kinds of beta-blockers in the treatment of akathisia. Cardioselective agents, such as atenolol, are helpful at times and have the advantage of not crossing the blood–brain barrier, unlike propanolol. Sometimes clinicians will avoid propanolol due to reported risks of depression or sedation related to its central nervous system (CNS) activity. Meta-analyses indicate that the relative risk of depression with propanolol is quite low, and patients with bipolar disorder rarely appear to develop depressive symptoms in relation to propanolol. Propanolol also has the advantage of providing some direct CNS anxiolytic relief for the subjective experience of akathisia. Other general risks with beta-blockers can sometimes limit their use, such as the risk of elevation of cholesterol in long-term use, sexual dysfunction (impotence) in men, and a relative contraindication in patients with severe diabetes or asthma.

Consequently, akathisia can sometimes be sufficient reason to change the dopamine blocker medication, when lowered dosing or the addition of beta-blockers are either ineffective or not indicated. In any case, akathisia should never be allowed to fester; this side effect calls for immediate and quick relief.

Sometimes akathisia can lead to suicidality. On occasion, this is how the side effect presents: the patient reports feeling more suicidal, without reporting the classic features of motor restlessness. When suicidality occurs or increases rapidly upon dopamine blocker treatment, clinicians should immediately think about akathisia and stop the dopamine blocker, asking questions later. The dose later can be reduced, or given with propranolol ER. It is important to warn patients about this potential side effect, and to say that if they become more suicidal, they should stop the medication and then call their clinician, not vice versa.

This process sometimes involves a lack of recognition on the part of patients that their intense dysphoria, anxiety, and restlessness may be a side effect; these symptoms are more frequently attributed to their depressive or manic syndromes, leading to demoralization, and they sometimes see suicide as the only viable form of relief. This process may have been related to a number of the cases of fluoxetine-related suicide that have been published. Again, clinicians need to educate their patients about the nature of akathisia, and when it is suspected, all efforts should be made to resolve akathisia as soon as possible so as to reduce the suicide risk.

Differential EPS Risks of Newer Dopamine Blockers

It is important to emphasize that all dopamine blockers cause EPS. The difference with traditional dopamine blockers is that newer agents may cause fewer EPS, not that the newer agents do not cause any EPS. Clinicians often see reports of clinical trials where EPS rates with newer dopamine blockers are described as equal to traditional agents'; this does not mean that there are no EPS with those agents. Clinical trial patients are "clean," lacking medical and other psychiatric comorbidities that may increase EPS rates, leading to lowered rates in their cases. Such side effects are often more accurately obtained in the "uncontrolled" environment of real-world clinical experience ("naturalistic" studies). A good example of this is the case of sexual dysfunction with SRIs, which were initially denied in clinical trials but became obviously common in clinical practice. Consequently, to summarize the relationship of newer dopamine blockers to EPS, Parkinsonian side effects may be lower with the less potent dopamine blockers, but akathisia rates differ less in the different potency classes.

Community-based studies on risperidone similarly report more EPS than previously expected. In one study, EPS prevalence with risperidone (49%) was similar to that with haloperidol (48%). In another, 50% of elderly patients with dementia demonstrated moderate Parkinsonism with risperidone. Two other reports on small samples, one with schizophrenia and another in bipolar disorder, found an akathisia prevalence of 14%.

One study that compared extrapyramidal symptoms in patients treated with clozapine (n = 19), risperidone (n = 9), and typical dopamine blockers (n = 22) found the prevalence of akathisia to be 10.5% with clozapine, 11.1% with risperidone, and 22.7% with typical dopamine blocker agents. Parkinsonian symptoms were reported to be 0% with clozapine, 11.1% with risperidone, and 31.8% with typical dopamine blockers.

Low-binding affinity drugs, like clozapine and quetiapine, have the reputation of causing minimal EPS, yet a blind review using the Extrapyramidal Rating Scale (ERS) found akathisia to be present in 39% of clozapine-treated patients (n = 23) compared with 45% of patients treated with typical neuroleptic agents (n = 29), with comparable severity of akathisia based on the ERS in both groups. Similar findings were reported in another blind review of 151 patients with schizophrenia participating in a multicenter study, in which akathisia was as common with clozapine as with chlorpromazine, while Parkinsonism was less common with clozapine.

RCTs repeatedly report akathisia rates with olanzapine, for example, in the 14–16% range, which again, though lower than with haloperidol (35–52%), is still not insubstantial. New randomized data with aripiprazole also report an akathisia rate of 10% versus 18% with haloperidol.

In summary, akathisia rates tend to run in the 10–20% range with newer generation dopamine blockers, and while they appear somewhat lower than traditional comparators, they remain a major problem.

Pimavanserin

It should be noted that the previous observations held until the introduction of pimavanserin as a treatment for delusions or hallucinations associated with Parkinson's disease. This agent is the only potential medication that has antipsychotic effects that is not a dopamine blocker. It is discussed further later, but it should be noted that this medication is the exception to the rule that some dopamine blockade is needed for the basic antipsychotic effects that are central to this class of medications, and it does not cause the EPS and other dopamine blockade-related side effects discussed here.

Tardive Dyskinesia (TD)

It commonly is believed that the risk of TD worsens with time, that TD is irreversible, that acute EPS predict increased risk for later TD, and that all dopamine blockers have been shown to cause it. However, schizophrenia is associated with a spontaneous TD rate in healthy young adults of about 0.5% per year. This contrasts with the normal population and patients with affective disorders, who do not have any notable incidence of spontaneous TD below age 60. After age 60, however, in the non-psychiatrically ill general population, there is a spontaneous incidence of TD that approximates about 0.5% per year. These spontaneous rates probably reflect abnormalities in the extrapyramidal neuronal tracts of the brain. Hence, there is a TD risk throughout life in schizophrenia, possibly due to abnormal brain structures in that condition in those areas, and there is a TD risk occurring in late life in the general population, presumably due to gradual degeneration of brain function in susceptible persons in those areas. Consequently, TD occurs unrelated to dopamine blocker medications. When interested in the risks related to those medications, one must be careful not to attribute spontaneous TD to dopamine blockers.

Probably the most carefully conducted long-term study of TD with traditional dopamine blockers was conducted at Yale. In that study, 398 patients with psychotic disorders (mostly schizophrenia) were followed prospectively with TD rating scales every three months for eight years (1985–1993). An average TD incidence of about 5% per year was noted, but the important finding, which conflicts with accepted opinion, was that almost 20% of patients developed TD in the first three years of treatment. After the first three years, the TD rate seemed to plateau at a rate of about 1% per year. It is important to remember that the spontaneous TD rate in schizophrenia is about 0.5% per year. Thus, the added risk due to dopamine blockers is about 0.5% per year after the first three years of treatment. The earlier TD literature seems to suggest overall TD rates of about 40–50% after about 20 years of dopamine blocker treatment. The myth is that this risk is linear (see Figure 10.1); the Yale study shows that the risk is asymptotic, with half the TD

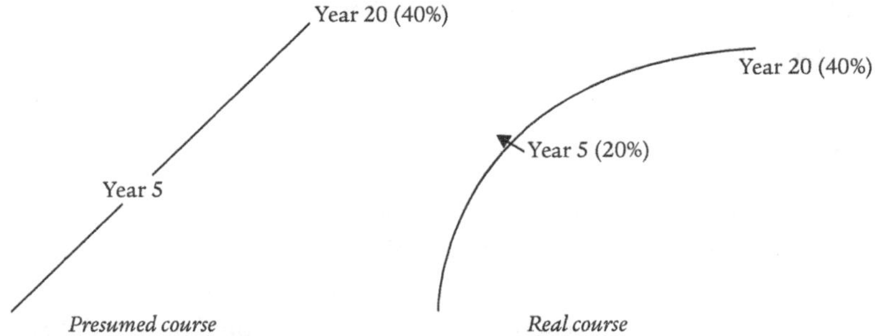

FIGURE 10.1 *Real versus presumed courses of TD.*

occurring in the first few years of treatment, and the other half occurring very gradually over the following two decades.

In other words, as the Yale study investigators note, in contrast to accepted wisdom, TD risk is highest early in treatment, in the first few years of new treatment with dopamine blockers in a person never previously treated with those agents. If a person has taken a dopamine blocker for 19 years, they are not very likely to develop TD in year 20. After the first few years of treatment, those who have not developed TD represent a relatively TD-resistant cohort of patients. Such patients are much less at risk for TD than someone who has never taken dopamine blockers before and is newly being prescribed them. Thus, there is no indication to stop a dopamine blocker due to fear of future TD in someone who has taken it for longer than 5–10 years without developing TD.

It is also important to bear in mind, in relation to the previous figures, another myth, which is the idea that TD is inherently irreversible. In fact, TD is temporary in about one-half of cases, with complete resolution over one year if dopamine blockers are stopped. The problem in some diseases like schizophrenia is that dopamine blockers cannot be stopped, thus TD persists. The continuation of TD is an ongoing drug effect in many people, not an underlying irreversible biological change. Thus, in non-schizophrenia uses, if TD occurs, all efforts should be made to stop and avoid future use of dopamine blockers. With this approach, at least half, if not most, cases of TD will improve over time.

The findings of the Yale study have generally been confirmed by a number of other prospective studies of TD, with the added proviso that the risk of TD in the elderly (above age 60 for the purposes of research) patients with schizophrenia is even higher. In the first year of treatment with a traditional dopamine blocker, the risk of TD has been shown to be 25–38%, and after only two years, about 34–66% in various studies. Hence, the elderly patient has about as much TD risk in one year as occurs in five years in a young adult.

These points directly bear on our ability to know whether dopamine blockers possess much risk of TD. Clinicians sometimes think that we do not have enough experience with dopamine blockers to understand their TD risk. This view assumes that we need 10–20 years of follow-up to be able to make such assessments. However, based on the data provided here with traditional dopamine blockers, three to five years of data should provide evidence on the highest-risk period, and we do have such data with most atypical dopamine blockers. For risperidone, double-blind, controlled data on its use in the first year of treatment in clinical trial conditions ($n = 3{,}298$) indicates a TD incidence of 0.6% versus 2.7% with haloperidol. With olanzapine, in clinical trials of 1,714 patients with schizophrenia, schizoaffective disorder, or schizophreniform disorder treated for up to 2.6 years with either olanzapine or haloperidol in a double-blind fashion, the one-year risk of TD was 0.52% with olanzapine versus 7.45% with haloperidol ($p = 0.002$). The risk ratio was 11.86 (95% CI = 2.30, 61.14); thus the risk of TD is almost 12 times higher with haloperidol than with olanzapine. The rates with risperidone and olanzapine were equal to the spontaneous rate in schizophrenia. One would expect rates in the 5–10% range as seen with the haloperidol control if atypical dopamine blockers were as risky as traditional agents in the first year of treatment. The first year of treatment is the highest-risk period for TD. Risk of TD with risperidone has also been studied in the high-risk elderly population with schizophrenia, with a TD rate of about 5% with risperidone at nine months of treatment versus about 30% with haloperidol (total $n = 122$).

It should be noted that, in the Clinical Antipsychotic Trials of Intervention Effectiveness (CATIE) study, patients who had preexisting TD were excluded from assignment to treatment with perphenazine, thus TD risk comparisons could not be made between earlier and newer dopamine blockers in that study.

Dopamine Blocker–Induced Mania

Controversy existed in the mid-1990s about whether dopamine blockers could cause mania. Most of that speculation has been put to rest with the clear efficacy of these agents in treating mania. However, current clinical experience suggests that perhaps some of the newer agents, like ziprasidone and aripiprazole, may in fact cause mania in some cases. These agents have antidepressant-like biochemical mechanisms that may put them at higher risk of such effects in a subgroup of patients.

DOSING FOR MOOD VERSUS PSYCHOSIS

Two decades of experience with second-generation dopamine blockers support the general conclusion that these agents should be dosed in bipolar illness at about half the dose used in schizophrenia. This lower dose may reflect increased side effects in bipolar disorder (particularly EPS) and/or increased efficacy at lower dose (where the profile of maximal serotonin blockade and moderate anti-dopamine effect is most evident). Hence, with risperidone, 2–4 mg/d is usually sufficient; with olanzapine, 5–15 mg/d; with quetiapine and clozapine, 100–200 mg/d; with ziprasidone, 20–80 mg/d; with asenapine, 2.5–10 mg/d; and with lurasidone, 20–60 mg/d.

METABOLIC SYNDROME

A clinical definition of metabolic syndrome could be given as the triad of diabetes, hypertension, and hypercholesterolemia, with associated abdominal obesity and dyslipidemia. Differing definitions exist, however; another common definition of metabolic syndrome is any three of the following: central obesity (waist circumference), hypertriglyceridemia, low high-density lipoprotein (HDL) cholesterol, hypertension, and elevated fasting plasma glucose. The underlying pathophysiology of the metabolic syndrome is thought to be hyperinsulinemia and insulin resistance. Persons with schizophrenia are more likely than the general population to develop metabolic diseases such as hyperlipidemia and type 2 diabetes. Relevant risk factors include poor diet, inadequate physical exercise, unhealthy lifestyles, and lack of financial, medical, and social resources.

The agents most associated with this outcome are clozapine, olanzapine, and quetiapine, but not risperidone, ziprasidone, aripiprazole, or any of the other newer agents. In fact, now it can be said that the majority of second-generation dopamine blockers do *not* cause metabolic syndrome. Nonetheless, the FDA has put a black box warning on all drugs in this class for potential risk of diabetes and lipid abnormalities. The guidelines of the American Diabetes Association (ADA) to prevent and manage metabolic risks with dopamine blockers include fasting glucose, lipid profiles, and blood pressure measurement three months after treatment, and then yearly, along with more frequent weight measurements. It is important to note that the risk of metabolic syndrome is independent of weight gain, although obviously if there is weight gain, there will also be an even higher risk of metabolic syndrome.

Modern dopamine blockers differ in other side effects besides EPS, weight gain, and metabolic syndrome. Clozapine has a serious risk of seizures and agranulocytosis, requiring weekly or biweekly blood monitoring. Risperidone is associated with prolactin elevation; while this effect is common at the laboratory level, clinically associated side effects are infrequent (5–10% of patients; mainly galactorrhea, amenorrhea, or sexual dysfunction). This effect is most relevant to postmenopausal or dysmenorrheic women, where prolactin elevation is associated with increased risk of osteoporosis. Ziprasidone is associated with prolongation of the QT interval on the electrocardiogram (EKG) to a greater extent than other atypical dopamine blockers, though less so than some traditional dopamine blockers. The newest atypical dopamine blocker, paliperidone, which is an active metabolite of risperidone, also appears to have some risk of QT prolongation. In cases where cardiac history is present, baseline EKGs may be prudent.

Weight Gain

Nearly one-half of adults in the United States currently meet criteria for being overweight (body mass index [BMI] 25 to 29.9) or obese (BMI > 30). Obesity is a known risk factor for hypertension, elevated triglycerides, insulin resistance, and diabetes mellitus. As adiposity increases, particularly excess abdominal fat, so does the occurrence of metabolic abnormalities. In the Framingham Offspring Study cohort, small increments of weight gain led to significantly increased occurrence of type 2 diabetes. Even modest increases in BMI (>1.0) show a positive linear correlation with increased mortality from cardiovascular disease.

Head-to-head comparison studies indicate that clozapine appears to induce the greatest weight increase among atypical antipsychotics, followed by olanzapine and quetiapine, respectively. One meta-analysis of short-term clinical trials (mostly about one month in duration) reported the most mean weight gain with clozapine at 4.45 kg, followed by olanzapine at 4.15 kg, risperidone at 2.10 kg, and ziprasidone at 0.04 kg. (Quetiapine was not included in that analysis due to insufficient data.)

Follow-up studies have provided more data on the extent of the problem. In one RCT of one year or greater clozapine use, 58% of patients gained at least 10% of their baseline weight. Calculations derived from the Framingham Heart Study suggest that treatment with clozapine may reduce 416 deaths due to suicide in a population of 100,000 schizophrenic patients. However, further calculations also reveal that approximately 492 deaths due to cardiovascular disease associated with weight gain are likely to occur in the same population.

Also, BMI increases of almost 10% and weight gain in excess of 10 kg have been observed after one year of olanzapine treatment at commonly prescribed doses. Furthermore, a review of four studies (about 3,000 patients) indicated that patients treated with olanzapine experienced a mean increase of 11.8 kg at high doses (12.5–17.5 mg/d) and 3 kg at lower doses. Overall, 40.5% of olanzapine patients gained more than 7% of baseline weight. Risperidone also is associated with weight gain in their major clinical trials compared to placebo, though less severe in magnitude than clozapine, olanzapine, or quetiapine.

An important methodological point is that some studies of olanzapine and quetiapine report no weight gain in one-year follow up. However, in these studies, the majority of patients dropped out of follow-up (often due to weight gain) before one year, and thus were not included in the survival curve at end point. Thus, these survival curves are interpreted invalidly when it is claimed that weight gain "plateaus" after one year.

Dyslipidemia

One comparative RCT designed to address dyslipidemia with dopamine blockers was a prospective, randomized, double-blind 14-week trial of clozapine, olanzapine, risperidone, and haloperidol in hospitalized patients (n = 157) with schizophrenia or schizoaffective disorder. At eight weeks, cholesterol levels rose for clozapine (14.7 ± 30.5 mg/dl) and olanzapine (12.3 ± 28.1 mg/dl), but not haloperidol or risperidone (–4.9 ± 17.7 and 4.2 ± 29.7 mg/dl, respectively). At 14 weeks, in completers, the increases with clozapine and olanzapine were even greater (16.3 ± 39.6 and 20.1 ± 26.8 mg/dl, respectively), haloperidol remained unchanged (–4.4 ± 25.2 mg/dl), and risperidone was somewhat higher, but judgment is precluded by the small subsample (n = 14) and the wide standard deviation of risperidone at this time point (9.2 ± 36.7 mg/dl). Thus, there was dyslipidemia with clozapine and olanzapine, not with haloperidol, and probably not with risperidone.

Most observational studies do not pay adequate attention to confounding variables, thus reported conclusions vary markedly. In a study of clozapine (n = 117), triglyceride levels rose from 184.6 mg/dl to 273.4 mg/dl in men, and from 164.9 mg/dl to 223.3 mg/dl in women, adjusted for age, weight, gender, daily antipsychotic dose, and concurrent medications. Similar results were found in another study comparing clozapine with typical neuroleptics, corrected for age and gender.

A large case control study in the United Kingdom (n = 9,226) similarly found a fivefold higher odds ratio of dyslipidemia with olanzapine compared to no treatment, and a threefold higher rate with olanzapine compared to typical antipsychotic treatment. No such associations were found with risperidone.

In a non-randomized study in which 36 non-obese patients on clozapine, olanzapine, or risperidone were matched for BMI, fasting total cholesterol levels were higher with clozapine (155.6 ± 31.2 mg/dl) and olanzapine (182.6 ± 62.5 mg/dl) than risperidone (129.1 ± 26.7 mg/dl; p = 0.05). HDL was somewhat higher with risperidone, and low-density lipoprotein (LDL) somewhat lower, but these differences were not as marked as the overall total difference. Triglyceride levels were notably higher with clozapine (193.5 ± 145.4 mg/dl) and olanzapine (205.9 ± 147.1 mg/dl) than risperidone

(73.6 ± 17.4 mg/dl; $p = 0.07$). RCTs for quetiapine indicate a 17% increase in triglycerides along with an 11% increase in total cholesterol levels versus placebo. RCT data with ziprasidone and aripiprazole and newer agents do not find evidence of dyslipidemia.

Diabetes Mellitus

In schizophrenia, the risk of developing type 2 diabetes is two to three times greater than in the general population; in fact, the lifetime prevalence of type 2 diabetes is estimated to be at least 15% among patients with schizophrenia. A study of 345 hospitalized patients with bipolar disorder found the prevalence of diabetes to be 9.9%. Cigarette smoking, poor diet, physical inactivity, and obesity are more common among patients with schizophrenia than the general population, and all of these factors are known to increase the risk of type 2 diabetes. Several documented cases of insulin and glucose resistance were noted by physicians prior to the introduction of neuroleptics. In addition, some studies have found that the prevalence of type 2 diabetes, impaired glucose tolerance, and insulin resistance are more common in schizophrenic patients not receiving antipsychotic treatment than in those on such drugs.

While these features of schizophrenia may account for some cases of type 2 diabetes within the population, a growing body of literature implicates the use of modern dopamine blockers, specifically a 9% increase in type 2 diabetes versus conventional antipsychotic agents. One study of schizophrenic patients treated with clozapine, olanzapine, risperidone, or a typical antipsychotic found that glucose and insulin levels were increased, independent of increased adiposity, only in patients treated with modern dopamine blockers versus no-treatment control group.

At one level, case reports provide a first line of evidence regarding the risk of diabetes mellitus with atypical antipsychotics. A study pooling the results from the U.S. FDA MedWatch surveillance system and other published case reports identified modern dopamine blockers associated new-onset diabetes in 242 clozapine-treated patients, 225 olanzapine-treated patients, and 78 risperidone-treated patients. Furthermore, the development of metabolic acidosis or ketosis was cited in 80 clozapine patients, 100 olanzapine patients, and 26 risperidone patients. Deaths were also found to be associated with 25 clozapine, 25 olanzapine, and 4 risperidone-treated patients during hyperglycemic episodes. Another study analyzed 45 case reports of new-onset diabetes and diabetic ketoacidosis and found 20 were associated with clozapine, 19 with olanzapine, 3 with quetiapine, and 3 with risperidone. 42% of those with new diabetes mellitus presented as diabetic ketoacidosis, and 50% had no weight gain. Fifty-nine percent experienced glucose abnormalities within three months of treatment, and 84% did so by six months.

One randomized comparative study designed to assess impaired glucose tolerance involved 157 patients who were randomized to clozapine, olanzapine, risperidone, or haloperidol treatment, and 101 patients provided blood samples. In the first eight weeks of treatment, fasting glucose level rose 17.1 ± 29.6 mg/dl for clozapine, and 8.4 ± 17.7 mg/dl for haloperidol, but was unchanged for olanzapine or risperidone (1.9 ± 16.9 and −1.3 ± 14.9 mg/dl, respectively). At 14 weeks, in a completer analysis, only olanzapine demonstrated elevation in plasma glucose level (14.3 ± 25.5 mg/dl). Thus, this study, which is the best-designed clinical study to assess this issue, found evidence of increased risk of diabetes, at least in the short term, with clozapine and olanzapine, but not risperidone.

In a non-randomized study in which 36 non-obese patients on clozapine, olanzapine, or risperidone were matched for BMI, fasting plasma glucose level was higher with clozapine (97.8 ± 7.8 mg/dl) and olanzapine (95.3 ± 13.8 mg/dl) than risperidone (88.9 ± 5.5 mg/dl; $p = 0.09$). Fasting serum insulin was also higher with clozapine (11.1 ± 8.1 mg/dl) and olanzapine (10.6 ± 8.8 mg/dl) than risperidone (4.3 ± 3.2 mg/dl; p = 0.05). Insulin sensitivity index was lower with clozapine (3.2 ± 4.1 mg/dl) and olanzapine (4.5 ± 2.7 mg/dl) than risperidone (0.9 ± 0.5 mg/dl; $p < 0.001$). This study has the advantage of using more sensitive measures of glucose metabolism than simply fasting glucose levels.

Laboratory studies also tend to support these clinical studies. They generally find that clozapine, olanzapine, and quetiapine, but not other modern dopamine blockers, are associated with marked increases in plasma glucose, plasma insulin levels, and insulin resistance following oral and intravenous glucose tolerance tests. RCT data with risperidone, ziprasidone, aripiprazole and newer dopamine blockers do not find evidence of diabetes mellitus.

CLINICAL RECOMMENDATIONS

The literature reviewed here clearly shows the strongest association of metabolic syndrome with clozapine, olanzapine, and quetiapine compared to the other agents. Furthermore, due to the direct effects of these agents on insulin resistance, independent of weight gain, one must assess these changes in all individuals. Also, due to the risk of diabetic ketoacidosis, early attention to blood glucose levels is necessary. Ongoing monitoring of lipid profiles is also important. This monitoring makes sense for all of these agents given the limitations of the current literature, but special attention should be paid to clozapine, olanzapine, and quetiapine, with less risk with other agents.

Specific Dopamine Blocker Agents

After the above discussion of the class as a whole, the rest of this chapter will examine specific agents.

Traditional Low-Potency Dopamine Blockers

The first antipsychotics agents were phenothiazines, and they came to be known as "low-potency" agents because it took higher doses of them to produce 90% or more dopamine blockade. Besides this common feature, these agents tended to have many other neurotransmitter effects beyond their core dopamine effects. They tended to block acetylcholine muscarinic, histamine-1, and norepinephrine alpha-1 receptors. Thus, besides being antidopaminergic, these agents were anticholinergic, antihistaminic, and antiadrenergic. In short, they were "dirty" (in contrast to the later "clean" agent, haloperidol, which was purely antidopaminergic).

The first agent in the antipsychotic class was chlorpromazine (Thorazine), discovered in the early 1950s and first published as effective by a classic paper from the University of Paris chairman Jean Delay, and his colleague Pierre Deniker. Chlorpromazine was later followed by thioridazine (Mellaril) and other agents. The chemical structure of these agents was tricyclic, with two benzene rings connected by a heterocylic chain. In this basic tricyclic structure, chlorpromazine was similar to the first modern antidepressant, imipramine (Elavil), which was discovered similarly in the mid-1950s. It was a matter of some speculation why agents with such chemical similarity should differ so markedly in clinical effect. One treated mania; the other caused it. One treated delusions; the other caused them. One treated depression; the other didn't.

The standard dose needed to reach antipsychotic effect was about 300 mg/d with these agents. One might oversimplify and divide by 10 to identify the standard dosing of each drug class: 300 mg/d for low-potency agents like chlorpromazine, in contrast to about 30 mg/d with mid-potency agents like perphenazine, and 3 mg/d with high-potency agents like haloperidol.

Despite their "low" potency, it is a common mistake to believe that these agents have less EPS or TD risk than higher-potency agents. All traditional antipsychotic agents were used at doses that led to about 90% or higher D2 dopamine receptor blockade. It didn't matter that the doses need to reach that level of dopamine blockade differed by drug class; the result was the same: almost all dopamine receptors would be blocked. EPS would follow similarly between potency groupings. Furthermore, regarding TD, long-term studies found no lower rates of TD with low-potency versus high-potency dopamine blockers.

The impression of lower EPS, especially Parkinsonism, with low-potency agents probably had to do with their inherent anticholinergic effects, which would reduce Parkinsonian symptoms. However, anticholinergic effects do not reduce the risk of akathisia appreciably, and they have no impact at all in the prevention of TD.

It is notable that the dirty multi-receptor blocking effects of low-potency agents produce an overall sedating effect, above and beyond the anti-agitation effects of dopamine blockade. Thus, low-potency agents became popular as "major tranquilizers"; that is, as strong sedatives, especially in the highly agitated emergency room or hospitalized psychotic patient. This strong sedating effect was often the endpoint of treatment, not necessarily any reduction in delusions or hallucinations. Sometimes this sedating effect could be achieved with low doses of chlorpromazine, especially if given intramuscularly. In that setting, where 90% dopamine blockade wasn't needed or sought, EPS could be limited with these agents.

Traditional Mid-Potency Dopamine Blockers

These agents are in the middle in their dopamine potency as well as in their multiple neurotransmitter effects. They do not have a large range of dosing, thus one can reach 90% dopamine blockade relatively easily. Yet there is enough of a range that very low doses can be given for low dopamine blockade. They have moderate anticholinergic, antihistaminic, and antiadrenergic effects, not as much as with low-potency agents, but not as minimally as with high-potency agents. In many patients, these lowered multi-receptor effects are such that no observable side effects occur. In patients who are sensitive to these non-dopaminergic effects, though, these mid-potency agents can still be intolerable.

One utility of a mid-potency agent is that one can begin with it as an initial strategy, a "hedge," to see if the patient is more prone to antidopaminergic EPS or to the other neurotransmitter (anticholinergic/antihistaminic/antiadrenergic) effects. Clinicians would begin with the mid-potency agent, and then move up to the high-potency agents if too many anticholinergic/antihistaminic/antiadrenergic side effects occurred. They would move down to the low-potency agents if too many antidopaminergic EPS occurred. If patients did well instead, they remained on the mid-potency agent.

The classic drug in this class is perphenazine (Trilafon); it became a popular initial agent of choice in the 1980s and 1990s. Another alternative was trifluoperazine (Stelazine). A third was thiothixene (Navane).

Traditional High-Potency Dopamine Blockers

The classic high-potency dopamine blocker, and the first in its class, was haloperidol (Haldol). It differed from the initial phenothiazines in its chemical structure and pharmacological class; it was a butyrophenone, and it did not have a tricyclic structure. These major differences led to important clinical changes. Haloperidol was a pure dopamine blocker, and it did almost nothing else: no anticholinergic, antihistaminic, or antiadrenergic effects at all. Hence it wasn't "sedating" in the traditional sense of the term, but, because of its anti-dopamine effects, it reduced agitation, both in psychosis and in other settings like delirium. "Vitamin H" became a popular injectable intramuscular or intravenous agent in emergency rooms and psychiatry wards. Despite all the progress with other agents, it remains widely used for agitation.

Haloperidol was invented by a pharmacist and psychiatrist, Dr. Paul Janssen, in Belgium, who would found the pharmaceutical company bearing his name. In the early 1960s, Dr. Frank J. Ayd, Jr., an American psychiatrist and one of the leading founders of clinical psychopharmacology in the United States, flew to Belgium to learn about this new drug that was supposed to have so many fewer side effects than chlorpromazine. He flew back with the first haloperidol pills that would be given to American patients, tucked safely in a vial in his wife's purse.

By the 1970s, haloperidol had eclipsed chlorpromazine as the most commonly prescribed antipsychotic. It was so popular, and its side effects so low, that there seemed to be no limit to its dosing. Although later studies would establish its full efficacy at no more than 5–10 mg/d, it commonly was used orally at doses of up to 40–60 mg/d. Eventually, cases of neuroleptic malignant syndrome, acute dystonic reactions, and severe akathisia began to accumulate, as did longer-term severe TD outcomes. It became clear that clinicians were succumbing to the First Fallacy of Psychopharmacology: "more is better." Since haloperidol wasn't sedating, they kept giving more until the patient became "calmer," which often reflected pure rigidity.

THE NEUROLEPTIC THRESHOLD

In the 1980s, a great deal of controversy and research ensued, with the eventual establishment of the "neuroleptic threshold," the dose of haloperidol at which 90% or more of dopamine receptors were blocked. New neuroimaging methods established that this classic threshold for antipsychotic efficacy, which also corresponded to the onset of and higher risk for EPS, was visible clinically by the detection of "cogwheel rigidity." The examiner would place his finger or thumb on the patient's pronated biceps tendon, at its insertion into the fossa of the elbow. With his other hand, the examiner would move the patients arm up and down slowly, keeping the elbow anchored to the arm of a chair. When moving the arm downward, the sensation of resistance, which would start and stop and start again, like a cogwheel, would establish the presence of this EPS. At the first dose that produces that clinical sign, the neuroleptic threshold, or 90% dopamine blockade, was reached. It was found that this point was reached with about 4 mg/d of haloperidol. Higher doses, like 10 mg/d, 20 mg/d, or 40 mg/d, only took dopamine blockade from 90% to 95% to 97% to 99%, minor biological changes that produced no appreciable clinical benefit, and only increased the risk of more consistent and more severe EPS. For a few years, some controversy ensued, until the whole fuss was rendered moot by the introduction of a new generation of dopamine blockers, beginning with clozapine, which were characterized by lower EPS than the traditional agents of prior decades.

THE INTRODUCTION OF "ATYPICAL" ANTIPSYCHOTICS

The modern use of clozapine began to happen in the mid-to-late 1980s, and it immediately became clear that this agent was different in kind from prior antipsychotics. In fact, clozapine was not a new agent, but had been introduced in the 1960s, and was seen as another "me, too" low-potency traditional neuroleptic. It fell out of favor quickly, though, because of deaths due to agranulocytosis, and was withdrawn from the market in the 1970s. By the mid-1980s, as it became clear that all of the traditional dopamine blockers suffered from severe and unavoidable EPS, and as the haloperidol dosing controversy raged, some researchers turned back to clozapine because of its reported low EPS rates. They noted that it was not a pure dopamine blocker, but also a serotonin blocker. It was brought back to the market and a randomized study proved that it was more effective than chlorpromazine in treatment-resistant schizophrenia, the first time one antipsychotic was proven more effective than another in schizophrenia (and still the only time this has been proven). Interest rose, and Dr. Paul Janssen's team in Belgium tweaked their haloperidol molecule, adding an agent that was a serotonin blocker to produce a new compound, risperidone, marketed in the United States in 1994. This new agent had notably lower EPS than haloperidol. Then Janssen's competitor Eli Lilly tweaked the clozapine molecule, producing an agent that did not cause agranulocytosis, olanzapine, marketed in the United States in 1996. And the modern generation of dopamine/serotonin blockers was off to the races.

Modern Low-Potency Dopamine Blockers

Clozapine, as noted, was the first modern dopamine blocker. Like chlorpromazine, it is a low-potency agent in that it has multiple other receptor-blocking effects: it is markedly anticholinergic, antihistaminic, and antiadrenergic. These receptor effects translate to its many major side effects: marked constipation, weight gain, and sedation. Unlike chlorpromazine, the low-potency nature of clozapine's dosing is not that it takes a lot to eventually reach 90% or more dopamine receptor blockade, as with chlorpromazine. Rather, with clozapine, no matter how high the dose, one never gets anywhere near 90% dopamine receptor blockade. Instead, dopamine receptor blockade never seems to rise above 30–40%, which is reached at about 300–400 mg/d and plateaus thereafter.

This is the mystery of clozapine. It clearly is the most effective antipsychotic, but it is one of few (along with quetiapine and nuplazid) that doesn't have potent dopamine receptor blockade.

Why, then, is clozapine so effective? It isn't that clozapine also has serotonin blockade, for so do other modern dopamine blockers that are no more effective in treatment-resistant schizophrenia than other agents (unlike clozapine). It isn't that clozapine is a "dirty" drug because it affects many other receptors, because so do multiple other traditional and modern agents. The only thing unique about clozapine is that its low dopamine receptor blockade involved D1 and D2 receptors, which are the usual receptors involved in animal and human studies of psychosis. Dopamine is a weak blocker of those receptors. But it is a strong blocker of the D4 receptor, which had never been seen as being important. Given this sole unique effect of clozapine, specific pure D4 blockers were developed by the pharmaceutical industry, but they were ineffective for schizophrenia. The mystery remains unsolved.

Importantly, clozapine causes agranulocytosis, which can be fatal, in almost 1% of treated persons (0.8% is the exact cited figure). Reversible neutropenia is more common, and occurs in about 2% of patients. The severity of the agranulocytosis led to restrictions in the United States such that weekly blood-count monitoring was required for clozapine. The frequency of this monitoring has now been reduced to monthly after six months of treatment, since the observed risk seems highest in the first six months after final dosage is reached.

Unlike traditional low-potency dopamine blockers, clozapine is not a phenothiazine in its pharmacological structure. Rather, it is a dibenzodiazepine. This structure was used to develop olanzapine, as discussed later. The other relevance of the benzodiazepine structure may involve similar risks and benefits with that class of anxiolytic agent. This structure could explain some of clozapine's efficacy for anxiety and agitation, and perhaps reflect some risk of withdrawal syndrome, as is occasionally experienced by patients. There is no known evidence of addiction and tolerance with clozapine.

The other major low-potency modern dopamine blocker is quetiapine (Seroquel). It is a dibenzothiazepine, and thus is related pharmacologically to the dibenzodiazepines clozapine and olanzapine (the difference being a single sulfur atom). Thus, it makes pharmacological sense that these three dopamine blockers all have the same major medical harm of metabolic syndrome.

Like clozapine and olanzapine, quetiapine has many multi-receptor effects, being antihistaminic, antiadrenergic, and anticholinergic; thus it has the same range of nuisance side effects associated with those receptor blockade profiles: sedation, weight gain, hypotension, cognitive impairment, and constipation. Like clozapine, quetiapine is a weak dopamine inhibitor, never reaching about 30% D-2 receptor blockade, despite whatever dose is used above 300 mg/d. It is a weak serotonin-2 receptor blocker as well, never getting to 80–90% blockade, unlike most other modern dopamine/serotonin blockers in this class.

A popular theory to explain quetiapine's efficacy despite its low dopamine blockade is the fast dissociation hypothesis. This idea is that quetiapine in fact does block 90% of dopamine receptors or more, but it does so briefly, dissociating rapidly from the receptor, so that when it is measured using standard methods, only about 30% remains at the receptor. This observation has been supported using positron emission tomography (PET) imaging in humans. The speculation is that quetiapine has a kind of tweaking of the dopamine receptors, blocking them briefly enough to get an antipsychotic effect, but not so long so that longer-term EPS occur. This speculation may or may not be true. Critics note that "fast dissociation" may be simply a synonym for "weak blockade."

In any case, the low long-term dopamine blockade seen with this agent may be a biological rationale for the clinical observation in practice that quetiapine is not, unlike clozapine, notably effective in the most severe cases of delusions/hallucinations, as in severe schizophrenia or schizoaffective illness. Because of its limited antipsychotic potency, many clinicians have shifted to using this agent at lower doses for a range of non-psychotic uses.

It has strong antihistamine blockade effects, which are well known in classic over-the-counter (OTC) drugs like diphenhydramine (Benadryl) to be useful for sedative purposes to treat insomnia and also as mild anxiolytic agents. Thus, clinicians often use quetiapine in low doses (25–100 mg/d) for sleep or for anxiety. This usage should not be surprising, since the same usage was common before the newer generation of dopamine blockers was developed. In the 1980s and earlier, the traditional dopamine blocker equivalent of quetiapine was probably thioridazine (Mellaril), an agent with a wide dose range for which lower doses in the 25–100 mg/d range were used for sedation and anxiety. At those low doses, thioridazine had limited dopamine blockade, and thus low EPS. The same holds true for quetiapine, which has lower akathisia rates than other dopamine blockers, according to the CATIE study, even at standard doses. EPS are rare with it at very low doses. Some clinicians are concerned that low doses may still predispose patients to other harms, such as TD and metabolic syndrome. TD is extremely rare in this class in patients not previously exposed to traditional dopamine blockers, with only a single such case reported with quetiapine in the published literature (and in that case, with mild symptoms). It is not clear if metabolic syndrome is dose-related, but it is likely that at least to some extent this is the case; long-term cardiovascular and diabetes harms probably are mitigated at lower doses, though not absent.

The maker of quetiapine has studied it extensively for non-schizophrenia and non-mania uses, and has sought many other FDA indications. Pharmaceutical industry–sponsored studies showed in randomized trials that quetiapine at 75 mg/d was more effective than placebo for generalized anxiety disorder, but the FDA did not grant an indication for this use. Pharmaceutical industry–funded randomized trials also were showed benefit for acute bipolar depression, as well as an adjunct to SRIs for the acute depressive episodes in MDD, and an FDA indication was granted for the latter use.

Modern Mid-Potency Dopamine Blockers

As noted, olanzapine is a dibenzodiazepine, which its manufacturer, Eli Lilly, tried to market as clozapine without agranulocytosis. It turns out that olanzapine certainly does not cause agranulocytosis, but it does have other major risks, similar to clozapine, which were unknown when this agent was first introduced to the U.S. market in the mid-1990s, namely, metabolic syndrome and a wide range of cardiovascular and diabetes harms, as explained previously. Furthermore, olanzapine shares the whole range of low-potency multi-receptor side effects: it is very anticholinergic, antihistaminic, and antiadrenergic. Hence, unlike most other mid-potency agents, it has low-potency–like harms of marked constipation and cognitive impairment, weight gain, and sedation.

Despite sharing most of these harms with clozapine, olanzapine did not inherit the treatment-efficacy benefit of clozapine. In other words, though it has been studied repeatedly for this effect, olanzapine is *not* more effective than other dopamine blockers for psychotic symptoms, whether in schizophrenia or other conditions.

Hence, except for the important improvement of not causing agranulocytosis, olanzapine was not an improvement on clozapine, but in fact a retrogression on efficacy, and just as bad for a wide range of other medical and nuisance harms. Nonetheless, since it had little competition in the mid-1990s, and was well marketed, olanzapine quickly rose in usage in the United States and became the leading antipsychotic used into the 2000s. This wide usage spread in particular in non-schizophrenia indications, especially bipolar illness, where olanzapine was studied extensively, and received important FDA indications that allowed for extensive marketing.

Besides olanzapine, other mid-potency modern dopamine blockers are aripiprazole, brexpiprazole, cariprazine ziprasidone, and lurasidone. All these agents are potent dopamine and serotonin blockers, and have no metabolic syndrome harm (with usually no or limited weight gain as well), but each has certain unique qualities.

Aripiprazole (Abilify) is a partial dopamine agonist, stimulating about 30% of D2 receptors. Thus, despite greater than 90% dopamine blockade, the simultaneous stimulation of about 30% of dopamine receptors does not allow for full dopamine blockade. Again, with the exception of clozapine, there is a clinical correlation between limited antipsychotic efficacy and incomplete dopamine blockade. Thus, clinical studies confirm that aripiprazole is not very effective in the most severe psychotic states. Yet this partial dopamine agonism could confer some benefits in terms of depressive symptom improvement, which is supported by the efficacy of this agent, leading to FDA indication, in adjunctive treatment of the acute depressive episode of MDD. It also has a mania FDA indication, but not for bipolar depression, partly because of a research design mistake. This agent is

FDA-indicated for maintenance treatment of bipolar illness, although it did not prevent depressive episodes.

Brexpiprazole (Rexulti) is a newer agent, similar pharmacologically to aripiprazole, with greater dopamine agonism, up to 70% stimulation of dopamine receptors, combined with the usual high amount of dopamine blockade. Its manufacturer only sought indication from the FDA in the United States for adjunctive treatment of the acute depressive episode for MDD, which was granted. Its potential efficacy in bipolar illness or schizophrenia is unknown. It is the first dopamine blocker that was brought to the market for a non-schizophrenia indication.

Cariprazine (Vraylar) also is a partial dopamine receptor agonist, more for D3 than for D2 receptors, though any potential clinical efficacy benefits of its D3 effects are unclear and speculative. It has proven efficacy and FDA indications for schizophrenia and mania, but not for any depressive conditions yet.

Ziprasidone is a potent dopamine blocker, reaching 90% or greater blockade by about 80 mg/d. It has structural similarities to risperidone. It also is a strong serotonin and norepinephrine reuptake inhibitor, similar in potency in some data to standard SRIs and TCAs. With this profile, one would expect potent benefits for depressive episodes and perhaps some harm for mania or psychosis, which can be worsened with monoamine agonists. Indeed clinical studies and experience again indicate that ziprasidone is not a strong antipsychotic for severe psychotic states of schizophrenia. It is proven effective and FDA-indicated for schizophrenia and mania, though. In studies of acute bipolar depression, it was not more effective than placebo, but in a randomized study of the depressive mixed state, it was effective. It has not been studied in unipolar depression. Thus, its biochemical profile may indeed be confirmed with at least some efficacy in some kinds of depressive states. It just has been studied by its manufacturer less thoroughly than other agents like quetiapine or aripiprazole. It clearly has no metabolic syndrome harm and in the CATIE study was the most beneficial dopamine blocker on cardiovascular and diabetes risk effects. However, it has the highest risk of cardiac arrhythmias of almost all modern dopamine blockers (with the exception of iloperidone). This is seen with a prolongation effect on the QTc interval of about 11 milliseconds.

Lurasidone is a partial serotonin receptor agonist, along with its strong dopamine and serotonin receptor blockade effects. This monoamine agonist effect could confer some benefit for depressive symptoms, and its manufacturer brought this agent to the U.S. market from the beginning with efficacy shown and FDA indications received for schizophrenia and for acute bipolar depression. The manufacturer did not study or seek indication for mania, which leaves open the question of the extent of its anti-manic efficacy. It has randomized data showing efficacy in acute mixed episodes of MDD, as defined in DSM-5 as "MDD with mixed features," but the FDA declined to give an indication for this treatment. It also has randomized data showing benefit in maintenance prevention of bipolar mood episodes. As with maintenance data for all dopamine blockers, there is a concern about the validity of the "enriched" research design used for those studies (see Chapter 6).

Modern High-Potency Dopamine Blockers

There are four modern high-potency dopamine blockers: risperidone, paliperidone, iloperidone, and asenapine. Risperidone was the first modern second-generation dopamine/serotonin blocker. It was developed by Janssen Pharmaceuticals as an evolution of haloperidol. That pure dopamine blocker was combined with a pure serotonin blocker, ritanserin, which had shown some antipsychotic potency. The result was risperidone, the first new strong dopamine-plus-serotonin blocker. The drug was created in 1984 and reached the U.S. market a decade later in 1994. By then, clozapine had been rediscovered, after some studies in the late 1980s, and its serotonin blockade was noted. But clozapine was a weak dopamine blocker and a weak serotonin blocker, as noted before. So it remained uncertain whether it truly was effective because of this combination effect. Risperidone answered that question, showing good efficacy for psychosis as well as lowered EPS, compared to haloperidol, in its randomized clinical trials. The introduction of risperidone led to a rapid shift in treatment from the traditional dopamine blockers to the modern agents, since the weekly blood testing and agranulocytosis risks of clozapine no longer were impediments. In addition, unlike the low-potency agent clozapine, the high-potency agent risperidone did not have most of the multi-receptor blockade effects of clozapine, and thus did not cause marked sedation, constipation, cognitive impairment, and weight gain. Risperidone did cause some weight gain, but much less than clozapine. Risperidone has antiadrenergic effects, though, which can lead to orthostatic hypotension, and in some patients, cognitive impairment. Later, when metabolic syndrome harms were identified with clozapine and olanzapine, it was found that risperidone did not cause these harms; that is, it does not have direct anti-insulin effects and thus doesn't increase the risk of diabetes, nor does it cause hypertension, nor worsen most lipid profiles. Risperidone does have an effect of hypertriglyceridemia, though. Like haloperidol, its parent compound, risperidone also increases prolactin levels, which can lead in some cases to clinical symptoms, such as galactorrhea.

When first introduced, risperidone was dosed rapidly as follows: 1 mg twice daily for three days, then 2 mg twice daily for three days, then 3 mg twice daily. This dosing is much too rapid for most patients, and was introduced in its early days when risperidone was being used for severe acute psychotic exacerbations in schizophrenia. Now that it is used broadly in other conditions, this rapid dosing is unnecessary and harmful, often leading to severe akathisia. The manufacturer never incurred the expense to return to the FDA to change initial dosing labeling, however; thus many clinicians continue to give risperidone in this rapid high dosing unnecessarily.

As a rule of thumb, all dopamine blockers initially developed for schizophrenia can be reduced in dosage by half when given for other conditions, like bipolar illness or depression. Thus, the dosing of risperidone for schizophrenia tends to be 4–6 mg/d, but in bipolar illness, it usually is sufficient to give 2–4 mg/d for mania, and often less for depressive symptoms or maintenance treatment.

Risperidone has a half-life of 20 hours, and thus need only be dosed once daily at night, not twice daily as is common practice.

Paliperidone (Invega) is 9-hydroxy-risperidone, the active metabolite of risperidone. It has similar efficacy and similar side effects, though its dosing is somewhat different, about 6–12 mg/d.

Both risperidone and paliperidone are available in long-acting intramuscular injectable formulations that can be helpful in patients who are non-adherent to treatment, especially in schizophrenia and severe bipolar illness. The risperidone formulation is Risperidone Consta, given once monthly, and the paliperidone formulation is Invega Sustenna, given once every two weeks.

Iloperidone (Fanapt) is structurally similar to risperidone, and has a similar profile of potent dopamine and serotonin blockade, as well as alpha-1 adrenergic blockade. It is FDA-indicated for schizophrenia only, without reported studies in mood conditions. It has no metabolic syndrome effects, including, unlike risperidone, no increased occurrence of hypertriglyceridemia. Like ziprasidone, it has a prolongation effect on the QTc interval of about 11 milliseconds, which would increase cardiac arrhythmia risks.

Asenapine (Saphris) differs structurally from the other high-potency agents, and it also differs in its clinical effects. It is a potent dopamine and serotonin blocker, and has some serotonin receptor agonist effects, like lurasidone. It is a highly sedating agent, and in this respect is most similar to quetiapine among modern dopamine blockers. Yet, unlike quetiapine, it does not cause metabolic syndrome harms; thus, for sedating purposes, it may be a safer alternative. It needs to be taken sublingually, which for some persons produces a distasteful effect, although an attempt has been made to formulate it with flavors that will make it more palatable. It is FDA-indicated in mania and schizophrenia, but has not been studied extensively in mood conditions, although its partial serotonin agonism might suggest potentially utility for depressive symptoms.

A Non–Dopamine Blocking Antipsychotic Agent

Recently, a new antipsychotic has been developed that is not a dopamine blocker at all, but rather a serotonin blocker. Pimavanserin (Nuplazid) is now FDA-indicated for delusions and hallucinations in Parkinson's disease. It is marketed as a serotonin "inverse agonist," which to me, sounds simply like serotonin blockade.

In fact, the classic serotonin antagonist, ritanserin, also was effective mildly to moderately in psychotic symptoms, like pimavanserin. The chemical structures of the two agents share some similarities (Figure 10.2).

Ritanserin was shown to be effective to a moderate degree when added to standard dopamine blockers in schizophrenia studies of the 1980s. Janssen Pharmaceuticals decided to combine it with haloperidol to create a new molecule, risperidone, rather than try to marked ritanserin as a separate add-on treatment for psychosis. Now, 30 years later, pimavanserin has been marketed on its own for mild to moderate psychosis in Parkinson's disease, and initial research in schizophrenia has shown moderate benefit when it is added to dopamine blockers, like risperidone. In this regard, it seems similar to its progenitor, ritanserin. Whether pimavanserin will prove to have stand-alone benefit for psychotic symptoms outside of Parkinson's disease (as in schizophrenia or mania) remains to be seen. It is possible it might have some use in non-psychotic affective illness, such as

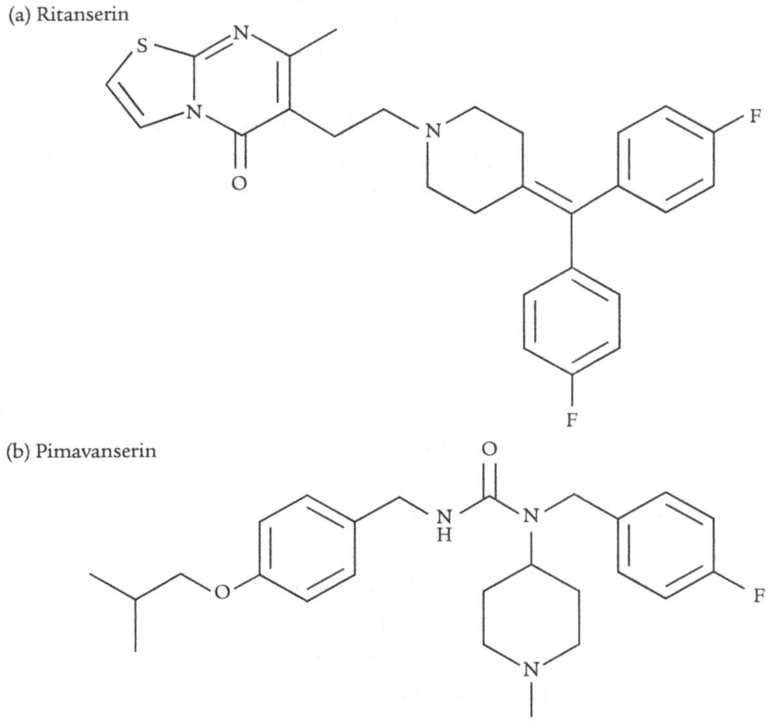

FIGURE 10.2 *a. Ritanserin*
b. Pimavanserin

manic or depressive episodes, but those studies have not been conducted yet either. In Parkinson's disease, this agent has the obvious benefit that, if it works, it does not cause or worsen Parkinsonian and EPS.

DOSING

Dopamine blockers should be dosed differently for different indications. As noted, a rule of thumb is that these agents should be dosed half as much in affective illness as in schizophrenia. The dosing for schizophrenia or severe delusions/hallucinations in schizoaffective illness tends to be higher than for non-psychotic uses, such as non-psychotic depressive episodes in unipolar or bipolar illness. The treatment of severe mania, whether psychotic or not, tends to be high-dose, as in schizophrenia or schizoaffective illness, but in mild to moderate mania, lower doses, akin to those used in unipolar or bipolar depression, tend to be sufficient.

Some specific nuances of dosing apply to a number of individual agents based on their unique pharmacological profiles. These include the following considerations.

Risperidone has strong alpha-2 antagonist effects. Alpha-2 receptors are presynaptic receptors that are part of a negative feedback loop for norepinephrine neurotransmission. Norepinephrine in the synapse stimulates post-synaptic alpha-1 receptors, which has an excitatory effect, depolarizing the axon and stimulating the next neuron. But norepinephrine in the synapse also stimulates presynaptic alpha-2 receptors, which are on the dendrite, and that then signal the neuron, which has released norepinephrine, to stop producing and releasing norepinephrine into the synapse. Thus, blocking alpha-2 receptors should allow more norepinephrine to be released into and remain in the synapse, which would then have an excitatory effect on the axon of the next neuron. This mechanism is similar to one of the properties of mirtazapine: by increasing norepinephrine activity, depression symptom benefit is expected. In the case of risperidone, this potential benefit has not translated robustly in clinical studies of acute depressive episodes in bipolar illness, though some benefit is seen in those studies.

Quetiapine and olanzapine are said to have mild noradrenergic effects in frontal cortex, based on animal studies conducted by their manufacturers. Confirmation of these reported effects in humans has not been published. The relevance of this purported mechanism to depression clinical benefits is unknown.

Aripiprazole and brexpiprazole are D1 and D2 agonists, more for the latter than the former (about 70% dopamine agonism versus about 30% in animal studies). Cariprazine also is a partial dopamine agonist, though more for D3 than for D2 receptors.

Ziprasidone is an SRI, similar in potency to other agents like fluoxetine in animal studies. It also is an NRI, similar in potency to other agents such as imipramine in animal studies. Thus, ziprasidone has potent monoamine agonist properties, which would suggest benefits for depressive symptoms. Though it was ineffective in two randomized trials of bipolar depression, it was effective in a study of the depressive mixed state. A number of cases of mania induction with this agent are consistent with its monoamine agonist effects.

Lurasidone is a partial serotonin receptor agonist, as is asenapine. These effects would predict benefit for depressive symptoms.

INJECTABLES

Injectable formulations come in two varieties, immediate emergency agents and long-acting agents. These agents are given intramuscularly in all cases, except for haloperidol, which has an intravenous form also.

Immediate emergency injectable agents exist for multiple traditional dopamine blockers, such as chlorpromazine and haloperidol. Among modern agents, such acute short-acting injectable forms exist for olanzapine and ziprasidone. The latter agent is well tolerated in the elderly, though attention should be given to QTc risks.

Long-acting depot formulations exist for multiple traditional dopamine blockers, such as haloperidol decanoate and fluphenazine (Prolixin) decanoate. These are given in monthly intramuscular injections. Among modern agents, such long-acting depot formulations exist for risperidone (Consta), paliperidone (Sustenna), and aripiprazole (Maintena). Risperidone Consta and aripiprazole Maintena are given once monthly intramuscularly, while paliperidone Sustenna is given every two weeks.

Intravenous haloperidol can be given for short-acting effects for immediate control of emergency agitation in the hospital, typically in the setting of delirium. When given intravenously, haloperidol does not go through first-pass metabolism in the liver. Some clinicians think this may be the reason why very high doses of haloperidol (over 10–20 mg/d, and in some reports up to 80–100 mg/d) can be tolerated intravenously, whereas they would be much too sedating or cause severe extrapyramidal effects (especially rigidity or dystonia) in oral or intramuscular administration. Very high intravenous haloperidol has a notable risk of QTc prolongation, though, and concern exists regarding cardiac arrhythmia induction with such usage.

SELECTED REFERENCES

Morgenstern, H., & Glazer, W. M. (1993). Identifying risk factors for tardive dyskinesia among long-term outpatients maintained with neuroleptic medications. Results of the Yale Tardive Dyskinesia Study. *Archives of General Psychiatry, 50*, 723–733.

Shirzadi, A. A., & Ghaemi, S. N. (2006). Side effects of atypical antipsychotics: Extrapyramidal symptoms and the metabolic syndrome. *Harvard Review of Psychiatry, 14*, 152–164.

11

Second-Messenger Modifiers ("Mood Stabilizers")

THE STANDARD MOOD STABILIZERS EACH HAVE STRENGTHS AND weaknesses. Lithium is still the gold standard, most proven agent; no other drug has been clearly shown to be more effective than lithium. Furthermore, lithium is the only psychotropic agent shown to prolong life, by preventing completed suicide and decreasing cardiovascular mortality; no other psychotropic agent, including antidepressants, have been shown to have those benefits. Also, lithium has long-term cognitive benefits, preventing neuronal death and reducing long-term cognitive impairment in bipolar illness. These clinical benefits are explained further later in this chapter.

LITHIUM

Lithium is the classic second messenger modifier.

Mechanisms of Action

Lithium is a naturally occurring cation. The standard lithium formulation is lithium carbonate. Other lithium formulations include lithium citrate, which can be better tolerated than the carbonate compound in the setting of severe nausea, and slow-release preparations, such as lithium carbonate extended-release (ER). Other formulations include an over-the-counter (OTC) version, lithium orotate.

For many years, the mechanism of action of lithium was unknown. Lithium has mildly pro-serotonergic effects, but it does not significantly affect other major neurotransmitters (like dopamine or norepinephrine). Research in recent decades has shown that the main effects of lithium do not occur at the synapse with neurotransmitters, but post-synaptically, at the level of G-proteins and other second messengers (such as phosphatidylinositol phosphate: PIP). It is these cellular effects that probably mediate lithium's clinical utility.

Specifically, lithium inhibits the alpha unit of G-proteins, especially those connected to beta-adrenergic receptors via cyclic adenosine monophosphate (cAMP). By blocking the G-protein transmission of messages from these noradrenergic receptors, lithium may interfere with the neuronal activity that occurs with mania. Similar effects on G-proteins linked to other neurotransmitters may produce lithium's antidepressant effects. Furthermore, lithium inhibits PIP function when PIP is excessively active, but lithium has no effect when PIP is normally active. Lithium inhibits protein kinase C (PKC), a central protein involved in the second-messenger cascade of neurons. Lithium augments the activity of brain-derived neurotrophic factor (BDNF), and blocks the activity of bCL2, an apotopic agent; these actions subserve lithium's effects on keeping neurons alive longer. Thus, by its complex second-messenger functions, lithium may essentially be reestablishing intracellular homeostasis and enhancing neuronal viability, growing or preserving connections to other neurons that may involve larger neural circuits subserving mood, accounting for its mood episode benefits.

Lithium Levels

The usual dosage of lithium carbonate is around 900 mg/d (range 600–1200 mg/d). It often is given two or three times daily, but it should be given in a one-time dose since its mean half-life is about 24 hours. It is dosed to a serum therapeutic range of 0.6–1.0, and somewhat lower in the elderly (0.4–0.6). A typical level for acute and maintenance treatment is 0.8 (0.4 in the elderly). Maintenance studies suggest similar results in the 0.6–0.8 range. No studies show more benefit above 0.8, thus higher levels should be avoided, certainly above 1.0. There is no clinical efficacy rationale for such higher levels, and the risk of toxicity increases as one gets closer to the borderline-toxic range of 1.2–1.5, with minimal side effects of tremor, nausea, diarrhea, and ataxia. Levels from 1.5–2.0 are associated with a higher risk of seizures. Above 2.0, acute renal failure can occur, and dialysis may be warranted. Above 2.5, coma and death can occur, and dialysis is indicated. In the elderly, these signs of toxicity can occur at half the levels. A special warning is appropriate for the elderly depressed patient who experiences diminished appetite: decreased fluid intake will raise lithium levels to toxic ranges quickly. If renal failure is produced, lithium levels rise exponentially, greatly increasing the risk of death. Thus, dialysis is essential in such cases.

Lithium is not metabolized in the liver and is excreted unchanged by the kidney. Thus, its only drug interactions involve other medications that can affect its renal excretion.

Dosing Titration

Like most medications, lithium should be dosed to clinical efficacy, not blood level. This is a common clinical error. A lithium level is not "subtherapeutic" if the patient is responding to it clinically. The levels described before are established mainly in studies of the acute manic episode, and to some extent in prophylaxis studies of future mood episodes. Those studies usually are conducted in type I bipolar illness. Those levels may differ in type II illness, or the acute depressive episode, or for other uses of lithium, such as in affective temperaments of cyclothymia or hyperthymia.

In general, a very slow titration of lithium is wise, because it limits side effects and allows for efficacy at lower doses than are commonly used. An exception for this titration is that if someone is markedly symptomatic with severe depression and/or mania, and the clinician has other reasons to believe they will tolerate lithium (such as past use without side effects): in that case, a more rapid titration to standard levels is reasonable. Outside of those circumstances, a slower titration such as the following may be suggested.

Begin lithium 300 mg nightly at bedtime (qHS) for 2–3 weeks; if insufficiently effective, increase to 450 mg qHS for 2–3 weeks; if insufficiently effective, increase to 600 mg qHS for 3–4 weeks; if tolerated but insufficiently effective increase, to a full dose of 900 mg qHS and check a level with a goal of 0.8 at that dose. If the patient begins to improve at lower doses, leave lithium at the lowest effective dose and check the lithium level only for documentation.

Dosing Frequency

Lithium should only be dosed once daily since it has a half-life of 24 hours. The common practice of dosing lithium multiple times daily is based on habit without any general rationale. In some cases, if lithium is dosed all at once, a patient may experience some sedation or cognitive impairment. In such cases, more than once-daily dosing may be necessary. Dosing lithium at night minimizes such side effects. Another option is to use slow-release lithium (like generic lithium carbonate ER or various trade alternatives, such as Eskalith), which minimizes the peak blood-level side effects. Slow-release formulations may also lead to somewhat less impairment of urinary concentration capacity. If gastrointestinal effects predominate, the liquid lithium citrate formulation may be best tolerated.

Laboratory Tests

It is advisable to check thyroid and kidney function tests upon beginning lithium, and again about three months later, and then every 6–12 months in maintenance treatment. When checking thyroid function, it is useful to obtain free T4 levels in addition to TSH due to potential subclinical hypothyroidism in which free T4 levels are low or low-normal while TSH levels can be normal.

Side Effects

Lithium can have many side effects, and it has the medical risks of possible long-term renal impairment and hypothyroidism. Most of those side effects can be managed or treated, or in the worst cases, if intolerable, lithium can be discontinued. It is important to note that with slow titration, most patients are able to tolerate lithium reasonably well.

As with all side effects, it is useful to divide risks into two major groups: nuisance and medically serious harms. Two other specific risks with lithium include toxicity and teratogenicity.

Nuisance Side Effects

Nuisance side effects occur at therapeutic levels or lower, are often related to non-compliance, and are experienced as troublesome. These include sedation, cognitive difficulties like poor concentration and memory, a sense of decreased creativity, dry mouth, hand tremor, increased appetite, weight gain, increased fluid intake (polydipsia), increased urination (polyuria), nausea, diarrhea, psoriasis, and acne. Polydipsia and polyuria persist in about 25% of patients during maintenance treatment with lithium. When severe, this increased urination may represent nephrogenic diabetes insipidus, a condition stemming from lithium's inhibition of the kidney's sensitivity to the pituitary's antidiuretic hormone (ADH, or vasopressin).

Some of these side effects are treatable: sedation and cognitive effects may improve with the controlled-release formulation; dry mouth can be minimized by use of sugar-free candy; increased appetite and weight gain can be responsive to carbohydrate restriction (since lithium has a mild insulin-like effect) and exercise; nausea and diarrhea may respond to the citrate formulation; hand tremor may improve with the use of propanolol; and polydipsia/polyuria can improve with the use of thiazide diuretics, like the hydrochlorothiazide/triamterene combination. Since thiazide diuretics increase lithium levels, lithium doses should be decreased by about 50% in co-administration, and levels followed. It should be noted that because of lithium's mild insulin-like effect, the insulin regimen of diabetic patients receiving lithium may also need to be altered. Frequently, despite these measures, individuals are unable to tolerate lithium solely due to these nuisance side effects, which are the main source of lithium non-compliance.

Medically Serious Side Effects

Medically serious side effects (excluding toxicity) fall into three sub-categories: thyroid abnormalities, chronic renal insufficiency, and cardiac effects.

THYROID ABNORMALITIES

Lithium's thyroid effects can occur early in treatment, but often appear after years of use as well. Lithium has a direct, reversible antithyroid effect, thus it can lead to hypothyroidism (usually in about 5% of patients). It inhibits the thyroid gland's sensitivity thyroid-stimulating hormone (TSH). High TSH levels on laboratory tests indicate a need to either discontinue lithium or supplement it with thyroid hormone replacement. Either T4 or T3 formulations can be used, alone or in combination; the most common practice is to use T4 (l-thyroxine), since it is metabolized in the body to T3 naturally.

KIDNEY EFFECTS

Lithium's kidney effect is more long-term, occurring in 1–5% of persons after 10–20 years of chronic therapy. Unlike the acute, direct inhibition of renal concentrating ability (including diabetes insipidus), this long-term effect of lithium is often irreversible and may involve renal glomerular function, resulting in a mild azotemia in most cases (mildly elevated creatinine levels). Lithium appears to reduce glomerular filtration rate, usually slightly. In rare instances, it can lead to severe chronic renal insufficiency and nephrotic syndrome, with glomerular pathologies of varying types. In the setting of new azotemia, the clinician needs to consider switching from lithium to another agent, although sometimes lithium can safely be continued, as long as future kidney function tests do not worsen beyond mild abnormalities.

Prospective studies show that there are two main risk factors for chronic renal insufficiency with lithium: acute lithium toxicity, and multiple daily dosing. Acute toxicity kills nephrons and decreases the long-term renal reserve that declines with aging. Keeping lithium levels normal but not high-normal minimizes risk of inadvertent toxicity, especially due to dehydration in older persons. Thus, the proven lithium level is 0.8–1.0; higher levels are not needed and should be avoided. Low lithium levels are sometimes effective when combined with standard therapeutic levels or doses of other mood stabilizers (like Depakote or Tegretol or Lamictal), thus one can diminish lithium exposure while maintaining some benefit at least with such combination treatment. Multiple daily dosing leads to higher consistent blood levels of lithium to which the kidney is exposed. As noted, lithium has a half-life of 24 hours, and it only needs to be dosed once daily. By reducing the mean lithium concentration in the blood after the initial peak with a one-time dose, the kidney is given a breather. Thus, less lithium is seen by the kidney. By also using a slow-release preparation, one smooths off the peak and keeps the kidney from exposure to brief but high lithium levels. Thus once-daily dosing of slow-release lithium at night will minimize long-term kidney impairment. The kidney risks are a central reason why lithium should be dosed almost always once daily, not multiple times per day.

CARDIAC EFFECTS

Lithium's cardiac effects mainly consist of some decrease in cardiac conduction efficiency, which can result in sick sinus syndrome. Lithium can produce blockade of the sinoatrial node, premature ventricular beats, and atrioventricular blockade. If lithium use is essential in a patient with these effects, a cardiac pacemaker may be necessary. Otherwise, the use of a different mood stabilizer may be indicated.

It is noteworthy that lithium mildly increases free calcium levels, possibly by stimulating direct release of parathyroid hormone from the pituitary gland, but this effect has little clinical significance, and hypercalcemia is not a serious problem. Lithium can also produce a mild leukocytosis, although this as well is without clinical sequelae.

Early reports based on retrospective data found that lithium was associated with increased levels of congenital cardiac malformations in children of mothers treated during pregnancy. Specifically, Ebstein's anomaly, a malformation of the tricuspid valve, was associated with lithium use in the first trimester of pregnancy. Recent prospective studies report lower risks than in the past. However, cardiac malformations, specifically Ebstein's anomaly, are still generally thought to be a risk with lithium use during pregnancy. These risks are probably lower than the risks of neural tube defects associated with the use of anticonvulsant mood stabilizers, like divalproex and carbamazepine, in pregnancy. Thus, in the severely ill manic patient who requires treatment, lithium use, with or without high-potency conventional antipsychotics, may at times be necessary, ideally after the first trimester of pregnancy.

Clinical Benefits

Lithium is quite effective in pure mania (i.e., euphoric mood), but less effective than the anticonvulsants in mixed (depressive, dysphoric) mania. It is by far the agent most well proven in the prevention of mood episodes, of both depression and mania, in bipolar disorder. A number of common misconceptions need to be addressed. First, it is often held that anticonvulsants are more effective than lithium in treatment of rapid cycling; yet head-to-head studies indicate that both carbamazepine and divalproex are similar to lithium in that difficult-to-treat population. Furthermore, lamotrigine has been twice shown to be equivalent to placebo in patients with rapid cycling. Second, it is commonly thought that lamotrigine is more effective than lithium in prevention of bipolar depressive episodes. Yet those studies only included patients who initially responded to lamotrigine, and thus they were not fairly designed to compare lamotrigine and lithium. Thirdly and similarly, one study compared olanzapine to lithium in patients who initially responded to olanzapine for acute mania, with the observation of better prevention of mania with olanzapine than with lithium; again, that study is biased in favor of olanzapine due to its "enrichment" design, and thus does not allow for a meaningful claim of superiority over lithium. Fourth, recent FDA indications for maintenance treatment with some antipsychotics (olanzapine and aripiprazole) are based on only one placebo-controlled randomized study with each drug. In the case of lamotrigine, two such randomized maintenance studies exist. In all those cases, the studies were solely conducted by their corporate sponsors. In contrast, lithium maintenance studies have been conducted over five decades by numerous independent research groups, and number in the thirties (though many of them are relatively small). Hence, the amount of evidence supporting lithium's efficacy far exceeds those other agents'.

In both treatment of acute bipolar depression and prevention of bipolar depressive episodes, antidepressants (both tricyclic agents and SRIs) have repeatedly been shown to be no better than lithium, and sometimes worse. Furthermore, in refractory unipolar depression, lithium is the most proven effective adjunctive treatment in randomized studies, though it is worth keeping in mind that most of these studies were conducted in the pre-DSM-IV era and thus probably included patients with bipolar II disorder.

Lithium is the psychotropic agent best proven to reduce mortality in any psychiatric illness, with evidence of reduction in death from suicide as well as from cardiovascular disease. Recently, evidence is also emerging that lithium has neuroprotective effects, by promoting various neurotrophic factors, which may lead to protection from long-term cognitive impairment as a result of the deleterious physiological effects of repeated mood episodes.

Dementia Prevention

There is also another important use of lithium to consider: there is a two- to threefold increased risk of dementia in persons with severe mood disorders; we think this risk has to do with the excitotoxic effects of steroid activity, which is increased with depression and mania. Since severe anxiety is also associated with increased endogenous steroid activity, there may be some reason for long-term concern in such cases, as well of increased risk of dementia. Mood illnesses are often associated with cognitive symptoms, which may improve when mood is controlled, or there may be some cognitive symptoms left over. Either way, it is worth considering a possible alternative, based on the extensive evidence that lithium has neuroprotective and neurotrophic effects, far more consistently and clearly than any other psychotropic drug. These effects are present in some animal studies at any dose of lithium, raising the possibility of benefits even with low-dose lithium, which would be especially useful due to side effects and risks in the elderly. Lithium-treated mood disorder patients do not have increased risk of dementia, unlike other mood disorder patients. The specific efficacy of lithium for this purpose has been studied in a few prospective randomized studies, mostly with promising results. If confirmed, these initial findings could suggest the addition of very low-dose lithium, such as 150 mg every other day, for potential long-term cognitive benefits (if lithium is not otherwise being used in the treatment regimen at higher standard doses for mood benefits).

Clinical Limitations

It has been demonstrated that lithium response is lower in patients with rapid-cycling, psychotic features, or substance abuse (compared to not having those states). However, those clinical pictures are generally treatment-refractory, and, contrary to common opinion, anticonvulsants have not been shown to be more effective than lithium in those states. The only condition in which anticonvulsants have clearly been shown to be more effective than lithium is the mixed episode.

Lithium Withdrawal Syndrome

It is important to recognize that lithium should not be abruptly discontinued (except in a medically dangerous case of acute lithium toxicity). If it is stopped suddenly, there is a 50% risk of sudden mania within one month, as well as some evidence of a marked increased short-term risk of suicide. If tapered over two weeks or longer, those risks appear to subside. Thus, lithium should generally be tapered at that speed; often a reduction of 300 mg per week is sufficient.

Clinical Nuances

Despite the previous discussion, psychiatrists often are hesitant to prescribe lithium. Older psychiatrists may have had bad experiences in the past, when, in the absence of viable alternatives, lithium was often dosed at higher blood levels than currently proven in the search for better response (often leading to toxicity). Younger psychiatrists are simply unfamiliar with how to use it.

Dr. Frederick Goodwin, former head of the National Institute of Mental Health (NIMH) and a key lithium research in the 1960s and 1970s, once expressed the view that "If you can't use lithium, or won't use lithium, get out of the business of treating bipolar disorder." Another way of thinking about the many benefits of lithium, which exceed its harms, is the following: "All other things being equal, for the average person with bipolar illness, one need not find reasons to prescribe lithium; one needs reasons *not* to prescribe lithium."

Some clinicians worry that patients might overdose on lithium, but since it is proven to prevent suicide, this risk is uncommon. In other words, patients are less likely to overdose on lithium than not, because lithium reduces the desire to overdose.

Sometimes the doctor is willing, but the patient is not. Often this reluctance has to do with the fact that lithium has long been associated with the diagnosis of manic-depressive illness, and thus may carry more stigma than newer drugs. In other cases, patients may have taken lithium in the past, often in the hospital, with many side effects. The latter scenario often involves high blood levels of lithium combined with polypharmacy with antipsychotics or other agents. Patients may not have side effects with lithium alone, especially if it is titrated very gradually.

In the case of stigma, it is worth noting that the choice of medication does not increase or decrease the severity of an illness. If one describes the benefits of lithium, especially for mortality and cognition, patients tend to be more open to it. Finally, for those patients especially attracted to natural treatments, like herbal medications, due to their being found in nature and not synthetic, it is worth noting that lithium is a mineral found in rocks, a natural resource that is part of the table of chemical elements.

VALPROATE

Mechanisms of Action

Like most antiepileptic agents, valproate blocks sodium channels, but this effect is not thought to be relevant to its psychotropic mechanism. Valproate also has moderate GABAergic and mild serotonergic effects, which may provide some anti-anxiety benefit, but probably are not prominent components of its mood effect. It is likely that valproate, like lithium, provides mood-stabilizing effects mainly through second-messenger mechanisms. Recent research has found that valproate, like lithium, is a potent inhibitor of PKC, an essential ingredient in the second-messenger cascades of many monoamine neuronal systems.

Dosing

Valproate, also known in generic form as valproic acid, is marketed in the United States as divalproex sodium (Depakote). Divalproex appears to possess a somewhat longer half-life and somewhat milder gastrointestinal side effects than valproic acid. The half-life of valproate is usually greater than 12 hours. Partly due to many active metabolites with long half-lives, it generally can be dosed once daily, which also assists compliance. Multiple daily dosing has been advocated in the epilepsy clinical trials so as to keep blood levels as stable as possible. While this effect may be relevant to epilepsy, it is less relevant to the long-term effects of valproate, which as explained before, involve second-messenger changes that occur over months or longer. An extended-release formulation (Depakote ER) has been developed but is not needed for once-daily dosing.

The usual dosage of valproate is about 750–1500 mg/d (range 500–2000 mg/d). It is dosed to a serum therapeutic range of 50–120 ng/dl. In the outpatient setting, I begin with 250 mg at night, then increase by 250 mg/d intervals every five to seven days until either it is intolerable or therapeutic range doses are achieved. In the inpatient setting, it is effective to begin with 500 mg at night, increase by 250–500 mg/d intervals every one or two days. A standard level for acute and maintenance treatment is in the 60–90 mg range. In the definitive clinical trials for acute mania, the mean level was in the 90s. It should be remembered that those trials were monotherapy trials (valproate vs. lithium vs. placebo). If valproate is being used with a neuroleptic, somewhat lower levels may be effective, but levels below 60–70 mg are probably insufficient for acute mania. In maintenance treatment, similar levels seem effective, though in my experience, levels in the 90s or higher are not frequently necessary. In patients with bipolar type II disorder or cyclothymia, some evidence exists that low valproate levels may be sufficient, such as 30–60 ng/dl. Some clinicians have the impression that higher levels may worsen depressive symptoms (especially in bipolar II disorder), but this clinical belief has been contradicted by randomized data that demonstrate efficacy with divalproex for bipolar depression at standard levels (around 80 mg). Nonetheless, combined with lower side effects at lower levels and a common reluctance to take mood stabilizers on the part of patients with bipolar II disorder, such low levels should be offered as a treatment option to those patients.

One of the major advantages of valproate is its decreased toxicity and large therapeutic index. The difference between a therapeutic level and a toxic level is much larger than with lithium. When levels exceed 100 or 120 ng/dl, toxicity symptoms are not as severe with valproate as with lithium and are usually associated with severe nausea, sedation, and perhaps dizziness, but not usually serious medical conditions.

Side Effects

Overall, valproate is not limited in its side effects, but, carefully titrated, it is often well tolerated. Some of valproate's side effects appear to be, based on clinical experience and available studies, similar in kind and severity to lithium's. These include weight gain, sedation, cognitive impairment, nausea, diarrhea, and tremor. These side effects are generally dose-related, and can respond to lowered serum valproate levels if clinically appropriate. Valproate-induced nausea or weight gain can also respond to supplementation with histamine-2 (H2) blockers, such as over-the-counter ranitidine. Valproate also can cause hair loss, which may be treatable with supplemental zinc plus selenium used at higher-than-recommended daily allowance amounts.

Medical Risks

Medically serious side effects consist mainly of hepatic failure and pancreatitis. Other medical effects, which generally are not potentially lethal, include thrombocytopenia, mild anticoagulation, and possible endocrine abnormalities in women with associated polycystic ovarian syndrome.

Valproate's hepatic effects are usually the most commonly discussed. In reality, potentially lethal hepatic risks are extremely rare in adults. A recent review of mortality due to hepatitis with valproate found only one reported case in an adult receiving valproate monotherapy, and that patient was 19 years old. Most cases also involved polypharmacy with multiple antiepileptics. Valproate can cause non-dangerous elevations of liver function tests (LFTs) in many more persons, but it is important to realize that abnormal LFTs are relatively common and unrelated to the rare and sudden cases of severe hepatitis. If LFT scores are less than two- to threefold increased, some clinicians even continue valproate and simply follow the LFT results. Especially if valproate is uniquely effective for a patient, then mildly elevated but stable LFTs are not a reason for immediate discontinuation of valproate. In most cases, though, abnormal LFTs continue to rise, and then discontinuation of valproate is prudent.

A key medical risk is acute pancreatitis, which is unpredictable and can occur at any age. In adults, pancreatitis poses at least as serious a risk as hepatitis. Since there is no way to predict this occurrence, any valproate-treated patient who experiences new abdominal pain should be quickly examined by a physician. If there is any uncertainty, valproate should be held, and amylase and lipase levels drawn. If abdominal pain is severe, immediate recourse to an emergency room visit is indicated.

Clinicians sometimes worry about thrombocytopenia—excessively, in my view, as reduced platelet levels rarely fall below 50,000, and even more rarely into the dangerous level of less than 20,000. Thrombocytopenia is usually mild and stable. This effect would only be of concern in patients with other risks for bleeding. Similarly, the anticoagulant effects of valproate, mediated by clotting factors, are mild and usually clinically limited. Again, patients at risk of even minimal effects, such as those with past cerebral bleeding, should be carefully followed.

Despite causing weight gain, valproate does not seem to lead to increased risk of metabolic syndrome. Indeed, it seems to do the reverse, with evidence in recent randomized data with the ER formulation of decreased total cholesterol levels with valproate compared to placebo. Also, in patients with schizophrenia given antipsychotics like olanzapine, which increase lipid levels, co-administration with valproate led to normalization of lipid levels.

There is an association between valproate and polycystic ovarian syndrome (PCOS), occurring in 10% of valproate-treated women with bipolar illness versus about 1% of lithium-treated women. PCOS is a condition of elevated concentrations of androgenic hormones in women, with associated cysts on ovaries and increased infertility. Since valproate causes weight gain, it has been suggested that PCOS may really be a secondary effect of the weight gain, rather than a direct effect of valproate. If so, one would expect PCOS to occur as frequently with other anticonvulsants or mood stabilizers, like lithium, that cause weight gain; yet data from the Systematic Treatment Enhancement Program for Bipolar Disorder (STEP-BD) study show that this does not appear to be the case. Other in vivo animal studies also seem to find a direct effect of valproate on increasing androgen activity, unrelated to weight gain.

Despite valproate's association with PCOS, clinicians need not avoid valproate in general due to this reason. In persons with other risk factors, such as those with amenorrhea, infertility, and weight gain, the possibility of PCOS should be considered as one factor among many in deciding among mood stabilizers.

Teratogenicity

Valproate is associated with neural tube defects, as is carbamazepine, and this effect is more frequent than lithium-related teratogenic effects. Some neurologists continue valproate during pregnancy in some patients with epilepsy, but most psychiatric specialists recommend that it be avoided during pregnancy in patients with bipolar disorder.

It has also been shown that fetuses exposed to valproate appear to have slower neurobehavioral development in childhood and lower IQ in middle childhood. Thus valproate appears to have somewhat harmful cognitive effects in children exposed to it in pregnancy.

In women who are not stable, or highly non-compliant, or sexually unreliable, despite valproate usage, then it probably should be deemphasized compared to other agents with fewer pregnancy risks, like lithium, lamotrigine, or antipsychotics. However, valproate should not be avoided in general simply because many persons with bipolar disorder experience sexual impulsivity or are non-compliant when they are symptomatic.

Drug Interactions

Valproate is a mild inhibitor of the cytochrome P450 2D6 system, though this effect probably does not lead to much in the way of clinical drug interactions. On the other hand, valproate is very tightly bound to plasma proteins, and thus can lead to drug interactions with other agents that are highly protein-bound. The most prominent example is in combination with lamotrigine, where blood levels of the latter are markedly elevated in the presence of valproate, leading to a higher rash risk. There are case examples of pedal edema with valproate plus atypical neuroleptics, which may be related to plasma protein binding. Valproate is also a mild inhibitor of certain clotting factors, which can lead to increased bleeding risk with aspirin or other anticoagulants.

Clinical Effectiveness

Acute Mania

Valproate is quite effective in mania, equally so whether in pure or mixed episodes (unlike lithium, which is half as effective in mixed as in purely manic episodes). Valproate also has the advantage of more rapid onset of action than lithium, with benefit notable in one week or so, compared to two weeks or longer with lithium. Valproate can also be loaded orally, at 20 mg/kg/day, and with that dosing, benefit has been reported within days of initiating treatment. Valproate loading has also been shown to be similar in speed and amount of antimanic effect to haloperidol. Valproate loading is especially useful in severe non-psychotic hospitalized manic episodes; in psychotic manic episodes, or extremely agitated and potentially dangerous manic patients, combination treatment with neuroleptic agents makes sense.

Prophylaxis

Frequently, clinicians assume that if a drug is "approved" for mania, then it is a "mood stabilizer." This is an important and confusing issue. If one identifies mood stabilizer usage with prophylactic efficacy, some would argue that by this definition, valproate and carbamazepine are not mood stabilizers, partly because they do not have FDA indications for maintenance treatment. This criticism is questionable, however.

Two major concepts need to be understood regarding the only placebo-controlled maintenance prophylaxis study of valproate in bipolar illness (a one-year randomized comparison with lithium and placebo). First, both lithium and valproate were the same as placebo due to a high placebo-response rate, probably reflecting the exclusion of severely ill patients by researchers due to ethical concerns about placebo use. Since lithium is proven effective, one cannot conclude, therefore, that the study showed valproate to be ineffective, but rather that the study could not have shown that anything was effective, given the nature of the sample. Second, the study utilized the most difficult design with which to demonstrate efficacy: a non-enriched design. In this approach, patients are allowed into the study as long as they are well (euthymic), no matter what previous medications they might have taken to get well. It is an underappreciated fact that in a secondary analysis limited to those who initially responded to valproate, valproate was more effective than lithium and placebo. This latter design, called "enriched," in fact became the standard approach in future lamotrigine and antipsychotic trials. In other words, if one compares the studies using the same research design, valproate shows the same efficacy as lamotrigine or antipsychotics. (The reason the FDA did not give an indication for valproate was that its analysis that showed efficacy was not the *a priori* primary outcome for which the study had been designed.)

Acute Depression

Many clinicians assume that valproate is not effective in the treatment of acute bipolar depression. There is some clinical lore that valproate may be "depressogenic."

In fact, multiple randomized studies show notable benefit with valproate for acute bipolar depression over placebo. When combined in meta-analysis, valproate is shown to be effective. While still limited, this evidence of benefit is much stronger than lamotrigine's, which has been repeatedly proven ineffective in acute bipolar depression.

Special Populations

Valproate is often preferable to lithium in older persons due to lithium's low therapeutic index. Valproate may be preferable also in adolescents who are non-compliant with lithium. Small studies suggest that valproate can improve substance abuse as well as bipolar illness in patients with comorbid conditions. Valproate provides notable anxiolytic benefit, probably due to direct GABAergic effects. Since valproate is proven effective for migraine, it is an especially useful treatment in patients with bipolar disorder and migraine.

CARBAMAZEPINE (TEGRETOL)

Carbamazepine's spectrum of efficacy is similar to valproate, with the exception that it has perhaps more studies supporting efficacy in prophylaxis and acute bipolar depression. Some long-term studies report less preventive benefit with carbamazepine than with lithium, however. Also, in one randomized long-term study, carbamazepine also did not reduce mortality from suicide, unlike lithium-treated patients in the same study. The main limitations to greater use of carbamazepine have to do with its drug interactions.

Formulations, Mechanisms, Dosing, and Pharmacokinetics

Carbamazepine is available in generic form, in standard trade formulation (Tegretol), and in a generic extended release form, carbamazepine ER, as well trade ER forms (Tegretol XR or Equetro/Carbatrol). Standard carbamazepine has a half-life of about six hours, thus requiring at least twice-daily dosing (unlike valproate and lithium), even with the ER formulation. In the outpatient setting, dosing titration can begin with 200 mg at night, or 300 mg at night with the ER formulation, and then increase to 300 mg twice daily (BID) in one week (or 200 mg every morning [qAM] + 400 mg qHS over two weeks). The psychotropic mechanism of action of carbamazepine is unclear. Unlike valproate and lithium, it does not appear to affect many second-messenger systems (like PKC), but it does affect the second-messenger cAMP. Carbamazepine usually requires doses around 600 mg/d (range 400–800 mg/d) in BID dosing for an effective serum level of about 8 (range 4–12). This serum level is most relevant for acute mania.

Drug Interactions

Perhaps the most important pharmacological effect of carbamazepine is its strong induction of the hepatic cytochrome P450 enzyme system. Hence, carbamazepine reduces efficacy or blood levels of many other medications. This effect is a major problem in treating patients with other medical conditions, such as the elderly. It also can be a problem in treating bipolar illness, since many patients are treated with multiple psychotropic medications.

Carbamazepine's 9,10-epoxide metabolite can be neurotoxic (producing delirium or confusion), and may be produced in greater amount in combination treatment with valproate. Consequently, the valproate-carbamazepine, though safely used in many patients, should be avoided on a routine basis. Another drug interaction of importance is that with lamotrigine. Here the problem is that carbamazepine reduces lamotrigine levels, due to the induction of the hepatic cytochrome p450 enzyme system. Also, there is additive risk of rash, including potentially serious dermatological reactions.

Side Effects

Carbamazepine has important nuisance side effects as well as serious medical risks. Among its associated side effects, which are dose-related, are sedation, double vision (diplopia), ataxia, and dizziness. As an important advantage, carbamazepine does not cause appreciable weight gain in most patients, unlike lithium and valproate.

The slow-release preparations, like carbamazepine ER, have fewer nuisance side effects than generic carbamazepine does. Patients rarely tolerate generic carbamazepine, but they tolerate the ER formulation quite well.

Medical Risks

Carbamazepine is associated with liver function test abnormalities, like valproate, and occasionally, hepatic failure. It is also associated with rare agranulocytosis (1 in 575,000 cases), and rare Stevens-Johnson syndrome (1 in 10,000 cases). Benign reversible leukopenia can also occur, as can hyponatremia (with associated seizure risk). Non-serious rash is also common.

Clinical Uses

Carbamazepine is an under-appreciated drug. Its lack of weight gain should put it at the fore of mood stabilizer options in groups concerned about weight, such as young women. Since lamotrigine is less effective in the long term for manic episode prevention than for depression, and since it is acutely ineffective for mixed or manic symptoms, carbamazepine would seem to have an important niche in the young woman with predominantly mixed episode symptoms, or with a history of more severe mania than depression.

Carbamazepine is most useful in such younger individuals who do not have many medical morbidities and are not taking other medications, thus obviating the drug interaction complications. Furthermore, if a patient with bipolar illness does not respond well to carbamazepine in monotherapy, or in combination with lithium, it may be wise to avoid continuing combinations with antipsychotics or anticonvulsants, due to the undercutting effect of carbamazepine's hepatic enzyme induction on the blood levels of those other agents. In randomized trials of risperidone or olanzapine added to mood stabilizers, the combination with carbamazepine was no better than placebo, although combinations of risperidone or olanzapine with lithium or valproate were better than placebo. In such settings of polypharmacy, carbamazepine is usually best left out of the mix (Table 11.1).

TABLE 11.1 Standard Anticonvulsants

Drug	Effective dose (mg/d)	Side effects	Comments
Valproate (Divalproex, Depakote, Depakote ER)	750–1500	Gastrointestinal (nausea or diarrhea), sedation, cognitive impairment, weight gain, hair loss, tremor, elevated liver function tests, acute pancreatitis, thrombocytopenia, mild anticoagulation, possible PCOS	Reasonably well tolerated, elevated LFTs, risk of pancreatitis, broadly effective, probable PCOS
Carbamazepine ER (Tegretol, Tegretol XR, Carbatrol, Equetro)	400–800	Nausea, diplopia, dizziness, ataxia, sedation, reversible leukopenia, non-serious rash, agranulocytosis, Stevens-Johnson Syndrome, elevated liver function tests, hyponatremia	Multiple nuisance and medically risky side effects, no weight gain

LAMOTRIGINE

Even though lamotrigine is not a second-messenger modifier, but rather a glutamate blocker, it will be included in this chapter since it is so often compared to the second-messenger modifiers. As is well known, lamotrigine tends to be classified among the novel anticonvulsants, including gabapentin, topiramate, oxcarbazepine, zonisamide, levetiracetam, and felbamate. In this long list, the only agent that has been proven effective in prevention of mood episodes in bipolar illness, i.e., a "mood stabilizer," is lamotrigine. General characteristics of novel anticonvulsants that differentiate them from standard anticonvulsants and lithium are that they do not cause weight gain (some can cause weight loss), they mainly produce anticonvulsant effects by either inhibiting glutamate or enhancing GABAergic function (unlike standard anticonvulsants, which mainly block sodium channels), they generally do not cause cognitive side effects (except topiramate), and they do not require or have therapeutic blood levels. In general, these agents are better tolerated than standard mood stabilizers, but, with the exception of lamotrigine, they are also less effective. Despite wishful thinking, they have generally been proven ineffective in acute mania and thus are likely to have no role in bipolar type I disorder as stand-alone mood stabilizers. This lack of efficacy in type I mania does not rule out benefit in type II bipolar disorder, but no randomized data exist in the latter population. These agents may have adjunctive benefits for non-mood uses, such as anxiety or weight, when used with proven mood stabilizers. Other than lamotrigine, the other novel anticonvulsants that are not effective for mood illness will be discussed in other sections later, which correspond to their main biological mechanisms.

Pharmacological Properties

Lamotrigine's biochemical effect involves inhibiting the presynaptic release of excitatory amino acid neurotransmitters such as glutamate and aspartate. It is metabolized by the liver and is moderately (over 50%) protein-bound. Its half-life is 25 hours, which allows for simple once-daily dosing. Some patients find it to be slightly stimulating. Divalproex competes with lamotrigine for hepatic glucuronidation, inhibiting lamotrigine's metabolism and increasing its half-life to 60 hours, while carbamazepine, phenytoin, and primidone enhance its metabolism, decreasing the half-life to 15 hours. When used with valproate, the dose of lamotrigine should be halved due to its markedly longer half-life. Dosing for bipolar illness is discussed in detail later, but efficacy has been shown in the 50–200 mg/d range, though the maximal dose for other purposes can go up to 500 mg/d. It should *not* be dosed more quickly than 25 mg/d due to serious rash risk (see further discussion, next section).

It is not wise to dose lamotrigine above 200 mg/d, mainly because there is no evidence of more benefit at higher doses (400 mg/d was similar to 200 mg/d in one study of prophylaxis). Furthermore, the risk of rash is highest as long as one is increasing the dose, so the higher one goes, the longer the period of risk. Lastly, cognitive side effects are more frequent at doses above 200 mg/d.

Side Effects and Rash

Most side effects with lamotrigine are rare and mild. These include headache, tremor, somnolence, and dizziness; in clinical trials, only 2% of bipolar disorder patients discontinued lamotrigine due to adverse events. However, about 10–20% of patients develop a common but non-serious rash. It is recommended that discontinuation of lamotrigine should occur when rash arises, due to the risk of progression to the rare, but potentially fatal, Stevens-Johnson syndrome. Stevens-Johnson syndrome is a serious rash with which patients can experience symptoms equivalent to a severe burn. Patients die due to bacterial superinfection; those who survive can be disfigured. While obviously severe, Stevens-Johnson syndrome is rare, and seems most associated with rapid titration of lamotrigine. In the early 1990s, when lamotrigine was first studied in large-scale clinical trials, Stevens-Johnson syndrome was observed in 1/1,000 adult patients and 4/1,000 children and adolescents. These rates were observed with relatively rapid titration of the medication. When titration was reduced to the current recommendation of 25 mg/week, the incidence of Stevens-Johnson syndrome fell from about 1/1,000 cases to about 1/ 6,000 cases. Combined therapy with valproate and lamotrigine increases the non-serious rash rate, and potentially the serious risk of rash.

The most conservative approach would be to dose lamotrigine by 25 mg every two weeks, as opposed to every week, in the average patient, and by 12.5 mg every two weeks in any patient in whom other risk factors for rash are present. Thus, achieving a target dose of 100–200 mg per day may take one to three months. This slow titration is justifiable if one keeps in mind that lamotrigine is effective for prevention of future mood episodes, not to treat the current acute depressive episode.

The most important risk factor for rash, besides speed of titration, is other drug allergies, particularly antibiotics. Data on file with the manufacturer indicate that the risk of rash with lamotrigine increases four- to fivefold in persons who have antibiotic allergies. Other risk factors, suggesting immunological reactivity, are asthma, autoimmune disorders, hay fever, allergic rhinitis, and food allergies. In the case of autoimmune syndromes, harmful reactions to lamotrigine can involve a range of immune system–mediated effects: not just rash, but also outcomes like aseptic meningitis.

In such patients, it is best to avoid lamotrigine, or automatically institute a 12.5 mg/two-week titration. Patients' fears can be allayed by pointing out the marked lowering of risk of serious rash with a slow titration. Also, the serious rash risk appears to be highest in the first months of treatment. Once patients are taking a stable dose of lamotrigine for long-term prophylaxis, they no longer appear to possess significant risk of serious rash.

In sum, lamotrigine is effective for maintenance treatment, but not for acute efficacy, with few nuisance side effects. However, it has potential for a serious rash risk, which can be lessened by a slow titration. The non-serious rash variant occurs in 10–20% of patients. Clinicians should avoid simply prescribing lamotrigine without much thought given to the small but real risk of fatality. Patients also need to be cautioned explicitly and carefully, to never increase lamotrigine dosing on their own. Sometimes patients are used to other drugs (like amphetamines), which have immediate dose-related effects; they need to be educated that altering lamotrigine dosing is unwise and sometimes dangerous.

Efficacy

After legal action against its manufacturer for a different agent, it became clear that negative studies on lamotrigine were not published, or were slowly released, so as to create an overly positive image of its efficacy. Under court order, for a brief period, its manufacturer posted those negative data on its website, where the following evidence was present:

1. Lamotrigine was effective in 2/2 studies in prevention of mood episodes in bipolar disorder.
2. It was ineffective in 2/2 studies of acute mania.
3. It was ineffective in 3/3 studies of acute unipolar major depression.
4. It was ineffective in 4/4 studies of acute bipolar depression.
5. It was ineffective in 2/2 studies of rapid cycling.

Almost all of those studies were either not published or were only published in partial form as summary results combined with other studies. A few studies were published as positive, based on secondary analyses, despite negative primary outcomes. What this means is that the drug was the same as placebo in its main analysis, though sometimes later analyses suggested some benefits in a particular subgroup. The latter subgroup benefits were not replicated in follow-up studies, however (e.g., possible benefit in a type II rapid-cycling subgroup in one study was not found in another study).

Overall, although lamotrigine is a useful drug and very helpful to many patients, the glossing over of negative data, combined with the effects of marketing its real positive benefits, resulted in clinicians' forming an overly favorable impression of the extent of efficacy of this drug. Despite its maintenance-preventive benefits, the data strongly indicate that it does not have acute mood benefits and that it does not improve rapid-cycling bipolar illness. Some would argue otherwise, suggesting for instance that its acute mood benefits are hard to demonstrate in two-month studies of acute depression due to its slow titration; that may be the case, but it still is true that it has not been proven effective for acute depression (or mania or rapid cycling).

Turning to its maintenance efficacy, lamotrigine seems to have preventive benefits, more so for depression than for mania prevention. While this is the case based on its two maintenance studies, there is often the misconception that those same studies prove that lamotrigine is more effective than lithium in prevention of depression (and vice versa: lithium better prevented mania than lamotrigine). This may or may not be the case, since those studies were "enriched": they only included patients who had initially responded to lamotrigine *before* they entered the randomized maintenance study. Thus, it was not a fair comparison with lithium (to do so, half of the enrolled patients would have needed to be chosen based on initially responding to lithium before the study). One can say that, in lamotrigine responders for acute mood symptoms, lamotrigine is more effective than lithium in prevention of depression. However, one cannot say, *in general*, that lamotrigine is more effective than lithium in prevention of depression. In contrast, the fact that lithium was more effective in mania prevention, despite the initial preselection of patients as lamotrigine responders, *does* demonstrate that lithium is clearly more effective in prevention of mania.

The simple interpretation of those data led to the marketing of lamotrigine as a mood stabilizer "from below" (more antidepressant than antimanic), in contrast to lithium as a mood stabilizer "from above" (more antimanic than antidepressant). Given the potential invalidity of the enriched design, as discussed in Chapter 6, these marketing phrases would seem to be questionable. It has not been proven, in valid non-enriched designs, that lamotrigine is more effective than lithium in prevention of depression.

In summary, numerous negative studies are now available that indicate that the spectrum of lamotrigine's efficacy is overstated. Besides its maintenance benefits, it is otherwise an ineffective agent for acute mood episodes (whether mania or depression) and rapid-cycling bipolar illness.

Medicolegal Concerns

Legal claims regarding Stevens-Johnson Syndrome (SJS) with lamotrigine have occurred, entailing some important forensic aspects to its use. The usual issues are inadequate warning regarding the risk of SJS, too rapid dosing, or inappropriate indication of lamotrigine. First, with any patient given lamotrigine, the clinician should document: "warned regarding SJS." Further detail can also be provided, such as warning regarding the risk of disfigurement, not only death, and spelling out of the dosing titration. Second, patients should clearly be warned to never increase the dose on their own, and clinicians should not dose the drug faster than 25 mg/week. It is true that FDA dosing instructions allow more rapid titration (25 mg/d for two weeks, then 50 mg/d for two weeks, then 100 mg/d for one month, then 200 mg/d), but this dosing titration was developed for epilepsy, and is unnecessarily fast for the long-term prevention of mood episodes in bipolar disorder. Jumping from 100 to 200 mg/d overnight is risky. In contrast, one cannot be faulted for dosing lamotrigine too slowly, since it has no acute efficacy. Third, lamotrigine has only one proven indication: the prevention of mood episodes in bipolar I disorder. It is not indicated or proven in type II bipolar disorder, or acute major depression in that setting, for instance. Clinicians should not turn to lamotrigine as their first-line drug for type II bipolar depression, since it has not been shown effective in that setting, and since it has real medical risks. If SJS should occur, that kind of indication would increase a clinician's legal risk. If lamotrigine is used, discussion of other standard mood stabilizers should occur and be documented, and the rationale for use of lamotrigine should be given.

SELECTED REFERENCES

Ghaemi, S. N. (2009). The failure to know what isn't known: Negative publication bias with lamotrigine and a glimpse inside peer review. *Evidence-Based Mental Health, 12*, 65–68.

Mauer, S., et al. (2014). Standard and trace-dose lithium: A systematic review of dementia prevention and other behavioral benefits. *Australia & New Zealand Journal of Psychiatry, 48*(9), 809–818.

12

GABAergic Agonists ("Anxiolytics")

BENZODIAZEPINES

Mechanisms

Benzodiazepines are the classic group of medications that have primarily anti-anxiety effects. Mechanistically, they are GABAergic agonists. In this effect, they stimulate activity at the GABA-a receptor. This receptor has two alpha subunits that are bound by gamma amino-butyric acid (GABA) itself, two beta subunits to which barbiturates bind, and one gamma subunit to which benzodiazepines bind. The GABA receptor is connected to a chloride ion channel. When stimulated, the chloride ion activity leads to repolarization of the neuronal membrane, producing decreased neurotransmission. GABA receptors are distributed throughout the neocortex and have a generally inhibitory effect on brain activity. All benzodiazepines have the same basic mechanism of activity. Their differences involved their pharmacokinetics; namely, their half-life and speed of onset. They also differ in potency of effect, with 1 mg of clonazepam being equivalent to about 4 mg of lorazepam, which is equivalent to about 20 mg of diazepam.

Thirteen different benzodiazepine agents are available on the U.S. market. Most were introduced beginning in the 1950s, thus they have been available in practice for decades. These agents are all available generically. As shown in Table 12.1, prototypical agents can be selected that differ in pharmacokinetics.

If one wanted to use the medication that had quick onset of action and short half-life, with the least sedation, then alprazolam could be chosen. If the opposite was needed, a slow-acting agent with a long half-life and more sedation, then clonazepam could be chosen. An intermediate effect would be found with lorazepam. Diazepam is another long-term option, with a long half-life, but a rapid onset. Regarding addictiveness potential, it has generally been thought that the agent with the slowest onset of action and the longest half-life would have the least addictiveness potential, which is why clonazepam has been seen as safest in that regard. However, clonazepam is the most potent benzodiazepine by milligram dosing; thus it, too, can be addictive in susceptible persons.

TABLE 12.1 Pharmacokinetics of Benzodiazepines

Benzodiazepines: 13 agents

Drug	T 1/2	Speed of onset	Dose equivalence	Daily dose (mg/d)	Other
Alprazolam (Xanax)	Short (6–12 h)	Very short (30 minutes)	0.5	0.5–3.0	Most addictive
Lorazepam (Ativan)	Medium (10–20 h)	Short (1 h)	1.0	0.5–3.0	Good as needed
Clonazepam (Klonopin)	Long (20–50 h)	Long (1–4 h)	0.25	0.5–3.0	Least addictive but most potent and most sedating
Diazepam (Valium)	Long (20–100 h)	Short (1 h)	5.0	5–20	Addictive

Efficacy

These medications are mainly effective in acute, short-term, symptomatic improvement of anxiety, and for symptomatic improvement of insomnia. They are not proven effective in long-term treatment of anxiety conditions, nor are they FDA-indicated for such long-term treatment. Despite absence of proof for long-term benefit, these agents are widely used in the general population long-term. It has been estimated that about 2.5% of the U.S. population takes benzodiazepines, and the frequency is higher in older age. In France, 7.5% of the general population takes benzodiazepines, with the frequency rising to above 14% in individuals aged 65 or older. Thirty percent of women in Spain above age 65 take benzodiazepines. The FDA discourages their use beyond six months. Specific language in FDA labeling of lorazepam is as follows: "In general, benzodiazepines should be prescribed for short periods only (e.g., 2 to 4 weeks). Extension of the treatment should not take place without reevaluation of the need for continued therapy. Continuous long term use of product is not recommended." Of the available agents, only alprazolam and diazepam have formal FDA indications for anxiety diagnoses. Lorazepam and clonazepam are mainly FDA-indicated for seizure conditions.

In generalized anxiety disorder (GAD), a meta-analysis of 23 randomized clinical trials was conducted, with 2,336 subjects. Comparisons were made between diazepam, lorazepam, alprazolam, and placebo. An overall relative risk of 0.78 was observed, with confidence intervals touching the null value of one (0.62, 1.00). In other words, these medications have a mild benefit with reduction of anxiety symptoms in this setting by 22%, but the range of benefits seen in these studies could be as little as nothing. No studies were found that had a duration longer than six months.

In insomnia, a meta-analysis of 24 studies including 2,417 subjects above age 60 found a number needed to treat (NNT) of 13, which indicates a small effect size. The correlation of benefit for sleep quality was also very small (r = 0.13). Total sleep time increased by a mean of only 25 minutes. The number needed to harm (NNH) for adverse effects was 6, which is a moderate effect size, with cognitive side effects being over four times more common with benzodiazepines than placebo (RR 4.76, 95% CI 1.47, 15.5). In other words, when comparing amount of benefit with amount of harm, the use of these agents for insomnia in older persons seems questionable.

It is important to note that the use of benzodiazepines for insomnia involves only an immediate sedating effect, not any deeper improvement of sleep itself. In fact, benzodiazepines impair sleep architecture, producing increased alpha and beta activity, and decreased K complexes and delta activity. They also produce decreased non-REM (rapid eye movement) stage 3 and 4 sleep, as well as REM sleep. Stage 3 and 4 non-REM sleep is generally called "slow-wave sleep." By decreasing slow-wave sleep, benzodiazepines impair the restorative benefits of sleep. Thus, even if one sleeps somewhat longer with these agents, one may wake up feeling tired, or without as many of the physiological benefits of sleep as would normally occur.

Side Effects

The main side effects are drowsiness, imbalance, and impaired reflexes. Sedation is highest with clonazepam, lowest with alprazolam, and intermediate with lorazepam. All side effects are dose-related, worsening at higher doses. Ataxia or imbalance can lead to a risk of falls in older persons especially, which is a serious medical risk. Impaired reflexes influence the ability for fine motor activity and/or rapid response. Hence these agents shouldn't be taken just before driving a motor vehicle or any other machine.

Cognitive impairment can occur, especially at higher doses, with long-term use, and in older persons. Clonazepam may be the worst for cognition, especially long-term. Some studies report an association between benzodiazepines and increased long-term risk of dementia, but other studies do not find this association, and animal studies have found that benzodiazepines appear to be neuroprotective, keeping neurons alive longer and helping with recovery in animal stroke models. Thus, cognitive impairment with these agents is more likely to be an immediate effect, and one that is reversible if the agents are stopped.

Drug Interactions

Most benzodiazepines are metabolized by the hepatic cytochrome P450 system via the 1A2 enzyme. Other medications that affect that enzyme can influence benzodiazepine levels. For instance, paroxetine is an inhibitor of the 1A2 enzyme, and thus would increase benzodiazepine levels, producing either more side effects or a need for lower doses.

Since benzodiazepines have a similar GABAergic mechanism to alcohol's, the use of both together can produce excessive GABAergic effects, with the side effects previously noted: ataxia, sedation, poor reflexes. Since there is some respiratory depression in the medulla with these GABAergic effects, at high doses and combined with alcohol, as in overdose, such respiratory depression can be fatal.

Addictiveness

There has been a great degree of controversy for decades regarding the addictiveness potential of benzodiazepines. There was little doubt that addiction happens with these medications, both in animal studies and in humans. Yet the concept of addictiveness varies from very mild effects with some agents, such as coffee, to very powerful effects with other agents, such as heroin or cocaine. Benzodiazepines appear to have risks that are between those extremes. In polysubstance abuse, benzodiazepines are the primary drug of abuse in 32% of subjects. If substance abusers are prescribed benzodiazepines, 15% will eventually abuse them, versus 6% of controls not prescribed benzodiazepines. There is a much lower rate of benzodiazepine abuse in the non–substance-abusing population, in some surveys approximating 1% or less. Thus, in general, it can be said that benzodiazepine addiction is highly unlikely in individuals who do not have past substance abuse. In those with past substance abuse, the risk is probably in the range of 15–30%.

Regarding tolerance, it has been shown in animal studies that benzodiazepine effects in rats decreased with the same dose over time. Tolerance is disputed in human studies, but there are very few randomized trials long-term, and none lasting longer than about six months.

There is a well-known benzodiazepine withdrawal syndrome consisting of anxiety, restlessness, insomnia, dizziness, nausea, headaches, and, in the worst-case scenario, seizures. This withdrawal syndrome is more common with agents with shorter half-lives, like alprazolam, and less common with agents with longer half-lives such as diazepam and clonazepam. It is much more likely if medications are abruptly discontinued, after having been taken continuously for a long period of time, such as months to years.

A range of hypnotics has been marketed as "non-addictive" alternatives to benzodiazepines for insomnia. These agents, described next, are not "non-addictive" as claimed in an absolute sense, but rather may be somewhat less potent than benzodiazepines in their GABAergic effects.

ZOLPIDEM (AMBIEN)

This medication has an onset of action in 15–30 minutes and a half-life of two to three hours. Its mechanism is binding to the GABA-a receptor, to the gamma subunit, just like benzodiazepines. Its dose range is 5–10 mg per day, and it has been marketed at a maximum dose of 10 mg per day. The reason for this maximum dosing has to do with being able to market as "non-addictive." To assess addictiveness potential, the FDA requires a standard research design, where these medications are compared to a known addictive benzodiazepine, like diazepam, and to placebo. These agents are given to former drug abusers, who, in a blinded fashion, report their subjective "high" experience with the agents at varying doses.

In that type of addiction study, 40 mg per day of zolpidem was equivalent to 20 mg per day of diazepam in terms of the subjective experience of high feelings in former drug abusers. Ten milligrams per day of zolpidem was equivalent to placebo. Hence the manufacturer only sought FDA indication up to 10 mg per day so that zolpidem could be marketed as non-addictive. Nonetheless, because of its addictiveness at higher doses, it was labeled by the FDA as a Schedule IV controlled substance.

ESZOPLICONE (LUNESTA)

Eszoplicone is an active isomer of zopiclone, which is an anti-anxiety hypnotic agent widely used in Europe. This medication is another GABA-a agonist. It has a rapid onset of action of one hour and a half-life of six hours, and is typically dosed at 1–3 mg daily. In addictiveness potential studies, 6–12 mg of eszoplicone produced a subjective high experience in former drug abusers similar to 20 mg per day of diazepam. One milligram per day of eszoplicone was equivalent to placebo. Hence eszoplicone was marketed, at doses up to 3 mg per day, as non-addictive, but FDA required that it be classed as a Schedule IV controlled substance.

ZALEPLON (SONATA)

Zaleplon has the same mechanism as zolpidem and eszoplicone; namely, activation of the GABA-a receptor. Its dose range is 5–20 mg per day, and it has an onset of action of 15–30 minutes and a half-life of only one hour. FDA labeling indicates that testing in former drug abusers found that 25–50 mg per day of zaleplon had abuse potential similar to benzodiazepines'. Again, it was marketed at lower doses to allow for claims of non-addictiveness, yet the FDA has classed it is a Schedule IV controlled substance.

Efficacy

The efficacy of most non-benzodiazepine GABAergic agents does not appear to be greater than the efficacy of the benzodiazepines themselves. With eszoplicone, for instance, randomized clinical trials found that treated patients fell asleep about 15 minutes earlier than placebo and slept about 37 minutes longer overall. At the end of such randomized trials, eszoplicone-treated patients still met insomnia criteria.: In other words, the effect size of benefit with these agents for insomnia is small.

GABAPENTIN (NEURONTIN)

Mechanism, Dosing, Pharmacokinetics

Gabapentin is a synthetic analog of GABA, and thus has anxiolytic effects as do all GABAergic agents. It has a wide dose range, depending on its use. The smallest capsule size is 100 mg/d, which can be too sedating for those sensitive to it. Typical doses are 300 mg capsules, given multiple times daily, with a usual dose of around 900 mg/d for anxiety. The range usually is from 600 mg/d to 1500 mg/d in such use. Higher doses can be given if needed, and are used often for neuropathic pain and/or epilepsy, up to 4000 mg/d. Gabapentin is eliminated primarily by the kidneys; it does not induce hepatic enzyme metabolism, nor does it have any known drug–drug interactions. The half-life of gabapentin is six hours, requiring twice- or thrice-daily dosing.

Efficacy

Multiple randomized clinical trials now demonstrate that gabapentin is ineffective for acute mania, and is equivalent to placebo. Yet there is a misconception among many clinicians that this agent is a "mood stabilizer." In fact, it is not an antimanic agent, and was never proven effective for any kind of depressive state. Rather, it has been shown to be effective for anxiety symptoms, such as panic attacks or social anxiety, in randomized clinical trials. Its sedating effects probably can help insomnia.

It is FDA-indicated for epilepsy and for post-herpetic neuralgia. Besides its anticonvulsant effects, it has anti-pain effects, for which it is used frequently in chronic pain syndromes. There are some data that it may help with cocaine and alcohol withdrawal syndrome and possibly help reduce relapse into cocaine and/or alcohol abuse.

Gabapentin was shown in randomized trials to reduce menopause-related symptoms of hot flashes and discomfort, but the amount of change over placebo was small, leading to FDA refusal of indication for that use.

Its active metabolite, pregabalin (Lyrica), has been marketed for chronic pain and studied in anxiety disorders, where there is benefit; its use in mood disorders has been assiduously avoided by the manufacturer, but it probably has a similar profile to gabapentin's. Unlike gabapentin, it is FDA-indicated for fibromyalgia and diabetic neuropathy.

As long as it is clear that this agent is not effective for depression or manic symptoms directly, it may have some use in mood conditions for concomitant anxiety/insomnia and/or pain symptoms.

Side Effects

The most frequently reported adverse events related to gabapentin include somnolence, dizziness, and ataxia. Such side effects generally are moderate and transient. This is its main benefit: it is a safe and generally tolerable drug. There are no known long-term risks, and no known direct harm by overdose. It is not carcinogenic or teratogenic in animal studies.

SELECTED REFERENCE

Schmitz, A. (2016). Benzodiazepine use, misuse, and abuse: A review. *Mental Health Clinician, 6*, 120–126.

13

Other Agents (Glutamate Antagonists, Antihistamines, Melatonin Agonists, and Others)

IN ADDITION TO THE MAJOR PSYCHOTROPIC DRUG CLASSES, THERE IS A MIScellaneous group with varied mechanisms, such as glutamate antagonists, antihistamines, melatonin agonists, and others. These agents have a range of clinical uses, but most are used symptomatically to produce sedation or reduce anxiety or for other symptoms. In this chapter, these agents are reviewed.

GLUTAMATE ANTAGONISTS

Topiramate (Topamax)

This anticonvulsant has been proven ineffective for acute mania in five placebo-controlled studies. This means it is not effective in bipolar illness as a "mood stabilizer" as a primary agent. Topiramate functions by increasing the inhibitory action of GABA in the brain and also by blocking the effect of glutamate. It may also inhibit carbonic anhydrase and block sodium channels. Only about 15% is bound to human plasma proteins; 70% is excreted unmetabolized in the urine.

It has clear weight loss effects, but whether it has any mood effects of any significance is unclear. As noted, it clearly does not improve manic symptoms. It has no known anxiolytic effects. Any benefit for depressive symptoms is mild if present at all.

Topiramate dosing typically is around 100–200 mg/d, with 50 mg/d being a minimally effective dose for either weight loss or possible mood effects. Below 100 mg/d it is generally ineffective; above 200 mg/d, it is frequently associated with excessive side effects, often cognitive.

There are no known drug–drug interactions with lithium, carbamazepine, or divalproex sodium, but its use with other carbonic anhydrase–inhibiting agents may increase the risk for renal-stone formation, a side effect that occurs in 1.5% of patients. Other side effects include somnolence, dizziness, and ataxia, but these side effects are usually mild and transient.

The most troublesome side effect of topiramate is cognitive impairment, which is common, usually consisting of word-finding difficulty, difficulty with attention, or short-term memory impairment. In some cases these effects are mild, in other cases more severe. This effect is dose related, and is very common above 200 mg/d.

Regarding weight loss, some studies report an average of 10–20 lb. weight loss in patients with bipolar illness. Weight loss occurs in about one-half of patients in psychiatric studies, and is also dose-related, with higher prevalence above 100 mg/d.

The weight benefits of topiramate may be relevant in patients who respond to other psychotropic drugs with weight gain, like some dopamine blockers or valproate. In that setting, the addition of topiramate might assist with weight while not worsening the overall psychiatric illness. This use should not be confused with any benefit for psychiatric symptoms, which appear to be minimal to none. Such weight benefit should be balanced against the common cognitive impairment with this agent.

Oxcarbazepine (Trileptal)

Oxcarbazepine is another anticonvulsant commonly used in affective illness. Like topiramate and gabapentin, oxcarbazepine also is ineffective in bipolar illness, and its use should be avoided due to lack of efficacy. Clinicians often are inclined to use this agent instead of carbamazepine, from which it is derived in its chemical structure. As seen in Figure 3.13e, it differs from carbamazepine only in a hydroxy atom. However, this small change produces major differences in clinical effects, both for side effects and in efficacy.

Regarding side effects, unlike carbamazepine, oxcarbazepine has no drug interactions, no known drug levels, and little to no apparent risk of agranulocytosis. These benefits attract clinicians. It also is more sedating than carbamazepine, and has a notable hyponatremia rate of 2.5%, which is more than with carbamazepine, and can lead to seizures. Regarding efficacy, it either is proven ineffective for acute mania or not shown to be effective, unlike carbamazepine. It also is shown not to be effective for prophylaxis of mood episodes in bipolar illness, in contrast to much more proven efficacy with carbamazepine. Clinicians accept the difference in side effects, but seem to assume that there should be no differences in efficacy.

Although basically ineffective in psychiatric uses, the common dose range of oxcarbazepine appears to be about 600–1500 mg/d, with about 900–1200 mg/d being the most-used dose for psychiatric purposes. It is dosed twice daily, due to a half-life of about eight hours.

OTHER ANTICONVULSANTS: ZONISAMIDE, LEVETIRACETAM, TIAGABINE, FELBAMATE

Clinicians and researchers have been excited about prior and current other novel anticonvulsants, most of which have either anti-glutamate or pro-GABA effects. None has proven effective for affective illness or for any important psychiatric use, except perhaps for some mild anxiolytic effects for the GABAergic agents.

Specific agents have been vigabatrin, tiagabine (Gabitril), gabapentin (Neurontin), and pregabalin (Lyrica), among the GABAergic agents, and felbamate (Felbatol), zonisamide (Zonegran), and levetiracetam (Keppra) among the likely anti-glutamate agents. Gabapentin and pregabalin have been discussed previously. Vigabatrin had a very potent effect in refractory epilepsy, working in difficult cases where many other anticonvulsants had failed. Unfortunately, it was taken off the U.S. market in the 1990s on the basis of neurotoxicity in animals. Felbamate elicited interest among some psychiatric researchers but was removed from the U.S. market as well in the 1990s for agranulocytosis. Tiagabine was not found to have much effect clinically except for mild symptomatic anxiolytic effects.

Zonisamide was found to have notable weight loss, but no clear mood or other psychotropic benefits. It may be an alternative to topiramate, with similar benefits (weight loss) and similar limitations (no notable mood or other psychiatric benefits), and with the added benefit of not having as much cognitive impairment as topiramate. Zonisamide has a very long half-life of almost three days (over 60 hours), and potential overlap of risk of rash in persons with sulfa allergies.

Levetiracetam has no drug interactions, a wide dosage range (like gabapentin), and some notable efficacy in epilepsy. However, it has no proven or apparent psychiatric benefits (Tables 13.1 and 13.2).

TABLE 13.1 Novel Anticonvulsants and Psychiatric Effects

Drug	Typical or effective dose (mg/d)	Comments
Lamotrigine (Lamictal)	50–200	Only proven effective agent for mood conditions. Benefit is only in long-term prophylaxis, not acutely. Potentially fatal skin rash risk.
Gabapentin (Neurontin) and pregabalin (Lyrica)	600–1800 (gabapentin) 150–450 (pregabalin)	Well tolerated, no drug interactions, sedation occurs; not effective for mood conditions, effective for anxiety and pain.
Topiramate (Topamax)	100–200 mg/d	Causes weight loss and cognitive impairment; not effective for mood or other psychiatric conditions.
Oxcarbazepine (Trileptal)	900–1200 mg/d	No efficacy for mood or other psychiatric illness. Fewer side effects than carbamazepine. Sedating, 2% hyponatremia risk.

TABLE 13.2 Other Novel Anticonvulsants

Drug	Epilepsy dose (mg/d)	Comments
Felbamate (Felbatol)	1200 (TID)	Aplastic anemia risk, restricted to epilepsy
Tiagabine (Gabitril)	32–56 (BID)	Not effective for mood, may be anxiolytic
Levetiracetam (Keppra)	1000–2000 (BID)	Appears well tolerated, no psychiatric benefits
Zonisamide (Zonegran)	200–600 (qHS)	Causes weight loss like topiramate but with less cognitive impairment. Sedating, renal stones (2–4%), contraindicated if patient sulfa-allergic, 48–72-hour half-life

KETAMINE

There has been a great deal of interest in recent years in ketamine as a novel treatment for depression. This interest has been sparked by the possibility that a new antidepressant mechanism may have been discovered with this agent. Also, it has been claimed that this medication may be especially effective in treatment-refractory depression. Lastly, its effects are rapid, occurring within hours and lasting up to a week, which is much more rapid than the traditional antidepressant onset of effect. This rapid effect may help with suicidality in particular. Ketamine has been used primarily as an anesthetic intravenously, and thus most research to date has been of the intravenous formulation. It has been shown in small randomized clinical trials to be more effective than placebo for the acute depressive episode in both bipolar and unipolar depression. These studies tend to be of a few weeks duration or up to two months at the longest, and there are no long-term data showing or testing any preventive benefit for future depressive episodes. This increasing clinical interest in ketamine led to study of its intranasal formulation, esketamine, which is being evaluated for receiving FDA indication for treatment-refractory MDD.

The mechanism of action of ketamine involves antagonism of N-methyl-D-aspartate (NMDA) receptors, meaning decreased glutamate activity. However, ketamine has a wide range of effects, and its glutamatergic effects are complicated, with some investigators suggesting that use of low doses of ketamine may actually increase glutamate activity by stimulation of glutamatergic α-amino-3-hydroxy-5-methyl-4-isoxazolepropionic acid (AMPA) receptors.

It is well known that ketamine is neurotoxic in animal studies, in both rats and primates. This neurotoxicity varies somewhat based on dose and duration given, as well as the age of the animal. Nonetheless, different types of studies demonstrate neuronal cell toxicity in various ways with ketamine. It has been argued that the very low doses used in treatment of depression may not be neurotoxic. There is no evidence one way or the other about its long-term safety.

Ketamine also is a well-known drug of abuse, used as "Ecstasy," or "XTC," which causes hallucinations and dissociative states. Its proponents argue that at the very low doses proposed for depression, it will not have abuse liability. Again, there are no studies of high quality that have tested this claim.

In summary, the efficacy and safety of ketamine for depressive uses rests almost entirely on the claim that at very low doses, it is much safer than at the doses used for other purposes or in abuse. It cannot be claimed that this is simply a safe drug, but that it is an unsafe drug that is safer at lower doses. Regarding efficacy, the excitement about its use in treatment-resistant depression has led many to believe that it simply is a more effective antidepressant than other agents. The fact that it is clearly a drug of abuse and that its effects are immediate is more consistent with subjective elation as occurs with almost all drug abuse. The long-term continuation of such benefits is more impressive for depressive symptoms, but it is not shown that this medication has long-term benefits beyond a few weeks. The general view of this text is the treatment-refractory depression is more a problem of diagnosis than of treatment. In other words, the problem is not that the monoamine agonist drug classes are not sufficiently effective for MDD. The problem is that MDD is a scientifically questionable concept that is very heterogeneous and includes many different depressive subtypes, and probably is not biologically specific enough to respond effectively to monoamine agonists. This problem will persist with any such agents. The belief and hope with ketamine is that a glutamatergic mechanism will somehow be much more effective than monoamine agonism. This hope has not been demonstrated with agents that have glutamatergic mechanisms in other psychiatric conditions, such as lamotrigine for bipolar illness or topiramate for affective illness. Hence there is room for skepticism, and reason to emphasize the importance of better diagnosis and more accurate clinical phenotyping, rather than simply trying to find more and more drugs for scientifically questionable clinical phenotypes.

ANTIHISTAMINES

Antihistamine agents typically are seen as having anxiolytic and sedating properties. The classic agent is diphenhydramine (Benadryl), which is sold in the United States over the counter in 25 mg doses. At about 50–100 mg at night, it is sedating and can be used for sleep (or at lower doses in some persons). It has mild anxiolytic effects. Hydroxyzine (vistaril) is more sedating and has somewhat stronger anxiolytic effects, and requires a prescription in the United States. Typical dosing for such uses is 50–100 mg/d, although lower doses may be sufficient in some persons. These agents are H1-histamine receptor blockers. Other antihistamines that affect the H2 receptor or other histamine receptors do not have these sedating and/or anxiolytic properties. A number of other older H1 blockers also exist, though they are uncommonly used.

Clinicians like to use antihistamines for anxiety effects, especially in as-needed use, in place of benzodiazepines in persons with current or recent substance abuse. There is no prominent addiction or withdrawal or tolerance with antihistamines. However, some substance addicts will replace other options with antihistamines, and appear to abuse these agents.

Their anxiolytic effects are much milder than benzodiazepines'. Their sedating effects can be mild, but are dose-related and can be rather notable at higher doses.

MELATONIN AGONISTS

Melatonin is a hormone produced by the pineal gland in response to light triggers. It has been known to be part of the physiology of circadian rhythms, and has been studied both for insomnia and for jet lag. It has been shown to be beneficial in some studies for both purposes. Typical doses are 1–5 mg/d, with a range up to 10 mg/d.

Its benefits may be limited by denaturation in the stomach, so specific agonists of melatonin receptors in the brain have been developed. Of these, the only one to come to the U.S. market is ramelteon (Rozerem), which is FDA-indicated for insomnia. It is ten times more potent than melatonin. A direct agonist of the MT1 and MT2 melatonin receptors, its effects appear to be mild. It has a short half-life of about two hours. It is given in 8 mg tablets, with no greater benefit at a higher dose than one pill daily. It has no known serious side effects.

Another melatonin receptor agonist that is used for depression instead of insomnia is agomelatine. Like ramelteon, it is a MT1 and MT2 agonist, but it also is a serotonin 5-HT2c receptor antagonist. This agent is marketed in Europe and Canada, but not in the United States, and has been shown to have benefit for depressive episodes in MDD. Its overall benefit has not been shown to be any greater than that of other agents used for MDD. It is given in doses of 25–50 mg at night. It seems to be well tolerated, with limited side effects.

SELECTED REFERENCE

Stefan, H. I., & Feuerstein, T. J. (2007). Novel anticonvulsant drugs. *Pharmacology & Therapeutics*, *113*(1), 165–183.

14

Drug Class Summaries and Dosing Guidelines

SECOND-MESSENGER MODIFIERS ("MOOD STABILIZERS")

This textbook defines a "mood stabilizer" as a drug that prevents mania and depressive episodes in bipolar disorder. The four drugs that have reasonable evidence that they can do this are lithium, Depakote, carbamazepine, and Lamictal. *Atypical antipsychotics are not mood stabilizers,* despite the FDA maintenance indications which they received, for the reasons given in Chapter 6 on the invalidity of the enriched, randomized, discontinuation maintenance design. Thus, all patients with bipolar illness should receive one of those four mood stabilizers, and dopamine blockers should be used as adjuncts, but not by themselves.

The standard mood stabilizers each have strengths and weaknesses. Lithium is still the gold standard, the most proven agent; no other drug has been clearly shown to be more effective than lithium. Furthermore, lithium is the only psychotropic agent shown to prolong life, by preventing completed suicide and decreasing cardiovascular mortality; no other psychotropic agents, including antidepressants, have been shown to have those benefits. Also, lithium has long-term cognitive benefits, preventing neuronal death and reducing long-term cognitive impairment in bipolar disorder. It obviously can have many side effects, and it has the medical risks of a small risk of long-term renal impairment and treatable hypothyroidism. Most of those side effects can be managed or treated, or in the worst case, if they are intolerable, lithium can be discontinued. But most patients are able to tolerate it reasonably well.

Prospective studies show that there are two main risk factors for chronic renal insufficiency with lithium: acute lithium toxicity and multiple daily dosing. Acute toxicity kills nephrons and decreases the long-term renal reserve that declines with aging. Keeping lithium levels normal but not high-normal minimizes risk of inadvertent toxicity, especially due to dehydration in older persons. Thus, the proven lithium level is

0.8–1.0; higher levels are not needed and should be avoided. Low lithium levels are sometimes effective when combined with standard therapeutic levels or doses of other mood stabilizers (like Depakote or Tegretol or Lamictal), thus one can diminish lithium exposure while maintaining some benefit, at least with such combination treatment. Multiple daily dosing leads to higher consistent blood levels of lithium to which the kidney is exposed. Lithium has a half-life of 24 hours, so it only needs to be dosed once daily. By reducing the mean lithium concentration in the blood after the initial peak with a one-time dose, the kidney is given a breather. And thus, less lithium is seen by the kidney. By also using a slow-release preparation, one smooths off the peak and keeps the kidney from exposure to brief but high lithium levels. Thus once-daily dosing of slow-release lithium at night will minimize long-term kidney impairment.

Lithium should be dosed once daily most of the time. The generic lithium carbonate ER formulation, all dosed at night, is preferred; once-daily dosing is associated with less long-term renal impairment, as well as enhanced compliance. It generally should be dosed to a target blood level of 0.8 (range 0.6–1.0). Creatinine and thyroid stimulating hormone (TSH) should also be followed. In the case of bipolar disorder type II, lower levels may be effective (0.4–0.6) and are better tolerated. If not effective, the higher levels can be used.

A very slow titration of lithium is wise, because it limits side effects and allows for efficacy at lower doses than commonly used. An exception for this titration is that if someone is markedly symptomatic now with severe depression and/or mania, and the clinician has other reasons to believe they will tolerate lithium (such as past use without side effects), then a more rapid titration to standard levels is reasonable. Outside of those circumstances, though, a slower titration such as the following also is reasonable.

Begin lithium 300 mg qHS for two to three weeks; if insufficiently effective, increase to 450 mg qHS for two to three weeks; if insufficiently effective, increase to 600 mg qHS for three to four weeks; if tolerated but insufficiently effective, increase to a full dose of 900 mg qHS and check a level with a goal of 0.8 at that dose. If the patient begins to improve at lower doses, leave lithium at the lowest effective dose and check level only for documentation.

There is also another important use of lithium to consider: there is a two- to three-fold increased risk of dementia in persons with severe mood disorders; we think this risk has to do with the excitotoxic effects of steroid activity, which is increased with depression and mania. Since severe anxiety is also associated with increased endogenous steroid activity, there may be some reason for long-term concern in such a patient's case, as well as increased risk of dementia. Mood illnesses are often associated with cognitive symptoms, which may improve when mood is controlled, or there may be some cognitive symptoms left over. Either way, it is worth considering a possible alternative, based on the extensive evidence that lithium has neuroprotective and neurotrophic effects, far more consistently and clearly than any other psychotropic drug. These effects are present in some animal studies at any dose of lithium, raising the possibility of benefits even with low-dose lithium, which would be especially useful due to side effects and risks in the elderly. Lithium-treated mood disorder patients do not have increased risk of dementia, unlike other mood disorder patients. The specific efficacy of lithium for this purpose has not been studied sufficiently in prospective randomized studies. In the meantime, clinicians need to make a decision for many of our patients in their 50s to 70s now or in the near future to prevent long-term dementia. The suggestion here is to add very low-dose lithium, such as 150 mg every other day, not specifically for mood benefits, but for potential long-term cognitive benefits. (This is relevant if lithium is not otherwise being used in the treatment regimen at higher standard doses for mood benefits.)

Valproate has more weight gain than lithium, but it does not have harmful lipid effects, unlike olanzapine. It has some anxiolytic properties and also have been shown to have benefit in prevention of depressive episodes in bipolar disorder. It is especially effective for the mixed state. Valproate should be dosed once daily at night most of the time. The titration is divalproex 250 mg qHS x 1 week, then 500 mg qHS x 1 week, then 750 mg qHS, then check a blood level. It generally should be dosed to a target blood level of 75 (range 60–90), usually achieved with doses of 750–1500 mg/d. LFTs, platelets, and amylase should also be followed. In the case of bipolar disorder type II, lower levels may be effective (30–50) and are better tolerated. If not effective, the higher levels can be used.

Carbamazepine has similar benefits to valproate's, but it has the added benefit of no weight gain. It has the problem of drug interactions if concomitant antipsychotics in particular are needed. It combines well with lithium and is best used in young persons who don't need much polypharmacy. It has more medical complications than valproate (need to follow complete blood count, CBC, and LFTs). Due to a 1:10,000 risk of Stevens Johnson syndrome (SJS), I prefer not to combine it with lamotrigine.

There is a slow-release carbamazepine, carbamazepine ER, which is much preferred to standard generic carbamazepine, due to many fewer nuisance side effects, such as diplopia and ataxia. This notably enhanced tolerability of carbamazepine ER leads to much better adherence than with generic carbamazepine. Just as generic valproic acid has many more side effects than divalproex, and thus the latter is given, similarly, generic carbamazepine should almost never be given in favor of the much better-tolerated, and now generic, carbamazepine ER formulation. Another benefit of the latter agent is that it comes in 300 mg capsules, not only 200 mg as in the case of standard generic carbamazepine, and thus can be titrated quickly to a therapeutic dose with one pill twice daily (or even all at night if preferred).

The titration is carbamazepine ER 300 mg qHS x 1 week, then 300 mg BID. It generally should be dosed to a target blood level of 8 (range 4–12). LFTs and CBC should also be followed.

Lamotrigine clearly has no acute mood episode efficacy of any kind, whether for acute depression, mania, or mixed states. It also has been shown to be ineffective in two studies of rapid cycling. It is only effective, but importantly so, in long-term prophylaxis, and there, more for depressive than manic episode prophylaxis (though it was better than placebo in mania prevention in the pooled analysis of its clinical trials). However, lamotrigine also has a risk of a 1:1000 reported rate of SJS. Using a slow titration, this risk may be lowered to less than 1:5000.

The view of this textbook is that lamotrigine should be dosed as slowly as possible in general, thus I recommend 25 mg/d for two weeks, then 50 mg/d for two weeks, then 75 mg/d for two weeks, then 100 mg/d. Then wait at that level for months before considering further increases.

Furthermore, a common mistake is to dose Lamictal above 200 mg/d. Instead, it has been proven in the randomized trials of bipolar illness that higher doses up to 400 mg/d are not more effective; they only produce more side effects of anxiety and cognitive impairment and increased risk of rash. Thus doses higher than 200 mg/d are not needed and should not be used in bipolar illness.

One can give lamotrigine in the morning, not at night, since it can be stimulating in most people, and thus impair sleep. If someone gets sedated, it can be given at night, but sedation is uncommon.

Here is a key point: *If antibiotic or other drug rash allergies are present, the risk of rash with lamotrigine is doubled, and the risk of SJS also appears to increase.* So in those cases, either do not use it, or delay its use until other agents have failed, and then at half the titration rate of 12.5 mg every two weeks. If the patient has evidence of immune system hyperactivity as well, like seasonal allergies and asthma, or especially if autoimmune syndromes have occurred, then lamotrigine is probably best avoided.

DOPAMINE BLOCKERS

Clozapine, olanzapine, and quetiapine all are the major agents that cause weight gain and metabolic syndrome, increasing the risk for diabetes and cardiovascular disease. These agents should especially be avoided in middle-aged and older persons.

If quetiapine is used, a common mistake is to dose it lower than the effective dose range shown effective for bipolar depression or mania, which is 200–400 mg/d. The extended release (XR) formulation has less sedation.

Excluding these agents, other dopamine blockers are risperidone, ziprasidone, aripiprazole, and the newer agents. Among these, risperidone is typically dosed 2–4 mg qHS and has more evidence of efficacy for mania than depression.

For bipolar depression, the other agents are shown more effective, with amount of evidence in decreasing order for lurasidone (Latuda), aripiprazole (Abilify), and then ziprasidone (Geodon). None of these agents cause weight gain or metabolic syndrome, but they all have the important risk of akathisia, which can also be associated with suicidality. If akathisia occurs and is severe and/or associated with suicidality, these agents should be stopped immediately. If it is less severe, their doses can be decreased, and/or propranolol ER 60–120 mg qHS can be added.

A very slow titration and overall lower dosing for bipolar depression is needed with these agents so as to minimize akathisia. The dose titrations that follow are recommended in non-schizophrenic indications.

Begin aripiprazole 2 mg qHS for two to three weeks; if insufficiently effective, increase to 5 mg qHS for two to three weeks; if insufficiently effective, increase to 7.5 mg qHS for three to four weeks; with maximum of 10 mg qHS.

Begin lurasidone 20 mg qHS for two to three weeks; if insufficiently effective, increase to 40 mg qHS for two to three weeks; if insufficiently effective, increase to 60 mg qHS, which is the maximum dose.

Begin ziprasidone 20 mg qHS for two to three weeks; if insufficiently effective, increase to 40 mg qHS for two to three weeks; if insufficiently effective, increase to 60 mg qHS for two to three weeks or longer; 80 mg/d is the maximum dose recommended by this text.

Important points to note are that doses higher than the amounts just mentioned are not more effective for bipolar depression; in fact, for aripiprazole, doses higher than 10 mg/d were *less* effective for bipolar depression than doses below 10 mg/d.

Other relevant points for these agents: Ziprasidone biochemically has strong serotonin reuptake blockade, which may suggest an appreciable antidepressant effect. Aripiprazole is a mild dopamine agonist, which can be good for depression, or bad in some cases for mania. Lurasidone is proven effective in bipolar depression and mixed depression, and has maintenance data.

Other new agents are: Asenapine (Saphris), which is sedating, but less so than quetiapine, and is proven effective in mania, but not proven in bipolar depression. Typical dose is 2.5–10 mg qHS in my experience; above that, the dose is too sedating. Iloperidone (Fanapt) is similar to the other agents, except it also seems to have some norepinephrine stimulating effects. It should be dosed low in bipolar illness, in my experience, in the 1–6 mg/d range, beginning at 0.5 mg/d.

Two newer dopamine blockers are cariprazine and brexpiprazole. Both are, like aripiprazole, partial dopamine agonists, in addition to blocking D2 receptors. Both are FDA-indicated for schizophrenia, and cariprazine is FDA-indicated in mania, while brexpiprazole is FDA-indicated in adjunctive treatment of major depressive disorder. Dosing is 1.5–6 mg/d for cariprazine, and 1–4 mg/d for brexpiprazole.

ELECTROCONVULSIVE THERAPY (ECT), TRANSCRANIAL MAGNETIC STIMULATION (TMS), AND KETAMINE

ECT is always an option for short-term treatment if severe suicidality is present. Its benefits are only short-term, with long-term treatment proven to be no more effective than psychotropic medications. The same short-term limited benefit applies for transcranial magnetic stimulation (TMS) and ketamine.

MONOAMINE AGONISTS (ANTIDEPRESSANTS/ STIMULANTS)

When choosing among SRIs, it is commonly said that all agents are equal, thus decision-making can be individualized by the preferences of clinicians and patients. Some overall considerations that are raised often include whether or not the agents have drug interactions, as occurs by the inhibition of cytochrome P450 enzymes by fluoxetine and paroxetine, or whether the medications examined have side effects that are worse than other comparators, such as increased weight gain with paroxetine. Given such considerations, many clinicians tend to begin with sertraline or citalopram or escitalopram, since these medications have the fewest drug interactions and the cleanest pharmacological profile. Recently it has been found that citalopram and its metabolite have some increased risk of cardiac arrhythmias, at least at higher doses, which might argue for a preference for other agents. Venlafaxine tends to have more side effects than other SRIs, and it has cardiovascular risks in middle and older age. Viewed from the perspective of the issues raised here, all other things being equal, it would seem that sertraline might have the lowest overall side-effect profile so as to support its use as an initial agent in this class. It might be followed by low-dose citalopram, and then other agents.

An important feature to consider when choosing among SRIs, which has only begun to receive attention in recent years, is the problem of serotonin withdrawal syndrome. This is one feature in which these agents can differ markedly. It is clear that it is worst with venlafaxine, paroxetine, and duloxetine. The least serotonin withdrawal syndrome occurs with fluoxetine, which has the longest half-life. This matter is important, especially if SRIs are prescribed with the view to long-term usage. If these medications are continued for longer than one year, then patients are being committed to long-term treatment, since discontinuation after that time is likely to be associated with serotonin withdrawal syndrome. For this reason, in long-term treatment, it would be rational to avoid the agents that have the worst search on withdrawal syndrome. In such settings, then, fluoxetine might be the preferred agent. It is important to have a discussion with patients about an exit strategy when giving SRIs. There should be a timeframe in which these drugs are expected to be used and then stopped. When developing such a timeframe, the problem of serotonin withdrawal syndrome should be an important factor in deciding among these agents. If very long-term treatment is expected, then patients should also be notified of such treatment expectations, and decision-making among these medications should take into account the long-term setting of treatment. For instance, in a middle-aged or older patient, long-term treatment with paroxetine or fluoxetine could become complicated by drug interactions with medications often used for other common medical conditions.

The dosing of these agents could be as follows. Fluoxetine is a very interesting medication since it has a long half-life of one to two weeks, or longer for its active metabolite. Thus, it need not be given daily, but it can be given if needed once or twice weekly. Begin with 10 mg per day, or every other day, or twice weekly, or once weekly, depending on the preference of the patient or the condition being treated. In young children, fluoxetine 10 mg once or twice weekly can be sufficient to treat moderate anxiety and/or depressive symptoms. The dose can be increased in 10 mg increments to be in the 20–40 mg range overall as needed in adults, with a maximum of 80 mg/d.

Sertraline can be started at 25 mg per day, and increased in 25 mg increments to a usual dose range of 50–100 mg/d, with a maximum of 200 mg/d.

Paroxetine can be started at 10 mg per day, and increased in 10 mg increments to a usual dose range of 10–30 mg per day, with a maximum of 60 mg/d. At 30 mg/d or above, serotonin reuptake blockade is augmented by norepinephrine reuptake blockade. At lower doses, this agent is more of a pure serotonin blocker.

Venlafaxine can be started at 37.5 mg per day, and increased in 37.5 or 75 mg/d increments to a usual dose range of 75–150 mg per day, with a maximum of 225 mg/d. It usually is given in the XR formulation. At low doses, it is a pure serotonin blocker, and at 150 mg per day or higher, there is more norepinephrine reuptake blockade.

Citalopram can be started at 10 mg per day, and increased in 10 mg increments to the usual dose range of 20–40 mg/d. Higher doses are associated with increased risk of cardiac arrhythmia. Escitalopram is more potent at a lower dose, and can be started at 5 mg per day, with the usual dose range of 10–20 mg/d.

Duloxetine can be started at 30 mg per day, with dose increases as needed by 30 mg increments, to a usual dose range of 30–60 mg/d, with a maximum of 120 mg per day.

Other monoamine agonists include mirtazapine and bupropion.. Mirtazapine can be started at 15 mg/d, with increases in 15 mg increments to maximum of 60 mg/d and a usual dose of 15–45 mg/d. Bupropion is usually given in the slow-release (SR) formulation, beginning with 100 mg/d, increasing in 100 mg increments to the usual dose range of 200–300 mg/d, with the maximum dose of 400 mg/d. It can also be given in extended release (XL) or other formulations.

GABAERGIC AGONISTS (BENZODIAZEPINES)

There are many specific benzodiazepines, with some variations and availability in different countries. It is generally useful to become familiar with and prescribe one agent that has a rapid onset and fast half-life for short-term use, and another agent that has a medium-range onset of action and half-life, and a third agent that has a slow onset of action and a long half-life. In the United States, the medications that fit these parameters are alprazolam, lorazepam, and clonazepam, respectively. The choice of agent depends on the purpose of treatment. For as-needed treatment, the rapid onset of action and short half-life of alprazolam and the similarly quick effects of lorazepam are helpful. For regular dosing, alprazolam is the least useful due to its short half-life, and clonazepam is the most useful, but lorazepam can also be effectively used. Sedation is highest with clonazepam, followed by lorazepam, followed by alprazolam. Clinicians can move from one agent to another, depending on whether sedation is a problem, limiting dosage increase with the medication. For instance, if a patient has sedation with lorazepam at 0.5 mg/d, it would be reasonable to switch to alprazolam. The use of clonazepam in such patients probably would not be tolerated.

Typical dosing is as follows: alprazolam can begin at 0.25 mg/d, increased in 0.25 or 0.5 mg/d increments to usual dose of 0.5 to 1 mg/d. Lorazepam can begin at 0.5 mg/d, with an increase by 0.5 mg increments to usual dose of 0.5–1 mg/d. Clonazepam can begin at 0.5 mg/d with an increase by 0.5 mg increments to usual dose of 0.5–1 mg/d. There is no definitive maximum dose of these agents, and many clinicians prescribed them up to 3 mg/d or higher. The preference in this textbook is that these medications should not be dosed higher than 2–4 mg/d if at all feasible. Higher doses probably reflect other underlying causes of anxiety symptoms that need more direct attention.

As is well known, these medications are associated with possible risk of addiction, as well as consistent tolerance and withdrawal syndromes. The short-acting agents have the worst withdrawal syndromes, and clonazepam has the least harmful withdrawal syndrome. In all cases, though, the medications need to be tapered slowly. Missed doses should be avoided, and refill should be provided sufficiently such that multiple days are not missed if the medications are taken regularly, because of the risk of withdrawal-related seizures.

These medications can be dangerous in overdose, especially if combined with alcohol, and thus attention should be given to prescribing frequent refills with smaller pill counts, as opposed to large pill counts and infrequent refills.

Other agents can be used, like diazepam or temazepam and others, with doses as provided in standard FDA dosing guidelines. Most patients can be managed for most uses, however, with the three major agents described previously.

15

Index of Selected Commonly Used Drugs with Brief Summaries

AMBIEN (ZOLPIDEM)—ADDICTIVE, IF DOSED HIGH ENOUGH

Typical dose: 5–10 mg/d
Biological mechanism: GABA-receptor agonism
Typical side effects: Sedation, nightmares
Medically important side effects: None
Clinically proven efficacy: FDA indication for insomnia

Biological Mechanism

Zolpidem is a GABA-a receptor agonist, the same gamma-1 subunit of GABA that is affected by benzodiazepines.

Clinical Efficacy

Zolpidem is FDA-indicated for insomnia. It has been shown to increase overall sleep time by about 30 minutes on average. It doesn't improve the stages of sleep, but like benzodiazepines, it doesn't worsen sleep stage patterns, such as reducing restorative deep stages 3 and 4.

Many medications used for sleep actually worsen sleep cycles. They tend to sedate people, helping them fall asleep in the beginning of the night. But since they worsen sleep cycle phases, they don't improve sleep stages in the end. The most important part of sleep involves the deep sleep stages 3 and 4. With more sleep in these stages, it's found that immune system function improves, neurons are repaired, and, upon awakening, there is a sense of well-being, with enhanced cognition and energy. It should be noted that these important deep sleep stages aren't improved with zolpidem, although it doesn't worsen them.

Addiction Risk

The standard way of assessing addiction risk is to give such agents to humans with substance abuse histories, and to compare the subjective effects to known addictive agents, like diazepam, and to do so in a double-blind placebo-controlled fashion. With this design, 40 mg/d of zolpidem was experienced as giving a "high" similar to 20 mg/d of diazepam, and more than placebo. But at lower doses of 10 mg/d, zolpidem produced a high similar to placebo. This is why the manufacturer sought FDA indication at a maximum of 10 mg/d so that the drug could be marketed as "non-addictive." In fact, the drug is proven addictive, only less so at the lower doses. Nonetheless, the FDA agreed to allow non-addictive marketing language at the lower dosage range.

Dosing

For the reason just stated, the company sought and received FDA indication for the dose range of 5–10 mg/d. It has a half-life of only two to three hours, which is why its benefits are only for helping patients fall asleep, as opposed to staying asleep. Its onset of effect is rapid, in 15–30 minutes.

Side Effects

The main side effects of zolpidem are sedation and loss of coordination. Nightmares can occur.

Bottom Line

- Zolpidem has minimal benefit for sleep.
- It doesn't worsen or improve deep sleep stages.
- It's an addictive GABAergic agonist, though less so at lower doses.

ASENAPINE (SAPHRIS)—A NEW SEDATING DOPAMINE BLOCKER WITHOUT METABOLIC HARMS

Typical dose: 5–20 mg/d (range)
Biological mechanism: Dopamine and serotonin receptor blockade
Typical side effects: EPS, sedation, bad taste
Less common but important side effects: Weight gain
Medically important side effects: None known

Clinically proven efficacy: Acute mania, schizophrenia

Biological Mechanism

Asenapine is a dopamine blocker with potent D2-receptor blockade, along with strong antiadrenergic effects. The D2 blockade is dose-dependent, such that at 10–20 mg/d, over 90% of D2 receptors are blocked. This level of D2 blockade produces extrapyramidal symptoms (EPS) such as akathisia, which appears to be the main clinical problem with this agent, as with the entire dopamine blocker class.

Like all modern dopamine blockers, it also has serotonin-2-receptor blockade, but it seems to have little to no weight gain. Asenapine does not have apparent anti-insulin effects, and thus it does not appear to cause or worsen the metabolic syndrome of diabetes, hypertension, and hyperlipidemia.

It has moderate anti-alpha adrenergic effects, like risperidone. This effect may be a mechanism for notable sedation with asenapine. Clinically, this sedation is not as extensive as quetiapine, but it is more than other agents. Some patients cannot tolerate this medication due to over-sedation, but for other patients, this effect can help insomnia, and it can be a sedating alternative to quetiapine, without the weight gain and metabolic harms of the latter.

Other Features

It is given sublingually. Despite flavoring attempts, it can be distasteful.

Clinical Efficacy

Asenapine has been shown to be effective for manic episodes and for schizophrenia. It does not have data or FDA indications for bipolar depression or MDD. However, in its mania studies, asenapine improved depressive symptoms in subjects with mixed manic episodes.

Dosing

Doses of 5–10 mg/d are effective for moderate mood states, with higher doses need for severe mania and schizophrenia.

Bottom Line

- Asenapine is proven effective for acute mania and schizophrenia.
- It is a good sedating alternative to other dopamine blockers.
- It has minimal weight gain and no apparent risk of metabolic syndrome or worsening diabetes or cardiovascular risks.
- Akathisia remains an important risk, to be managed by keeping the dose as low as feasible and/or using propranolol.

ATOMOXETINE (STRATTERA)—AN ANTIDEPRESSANT MASQUERADING AS A "STIMULANT"

Typical dose: 40–80 mg/d (range: 10–100 mg/d)
Biological mechanism: Norepinephrine reuptake inhibitor (NRI)
Typical side effects: Anxiety, insomnia
Less common but important side effects: None
Medically important side effects: None
Clinically proven efficacy: Treatment of major depressive episodes and ADD

This medication is an NRI, initially developed as an antidepressant. It was brought to the market as the first drug for adult ADD, rather than one of the last for depression. It differs notably from other "stimulants," though, in its mechanism and risks.

Clinical Efficacy and Inefficacy

In early clinical trials, this agent was found to be effective in major depressive episodes. It was noted that it shared its basic mechanism of pure norepinephrine effects with desipramine, which had been proven effective in childhood ADD. Eli Lilly, the company that was developing atomoxetine, made an economic decision to shift to ADD rather than major depressive disorder (MDD), but even in ADD, there were multiple other agents, mostly amphetamines, that were FDA-indicated in children. However, no agents were FDA-indicated in adults for ADD. Indeed, the whole concept of adult ADD was not used much, and it was not part of DSM-IV. After obtaining academic support, Eli Lilly convinced the FDA to provide the first indication for ADD in adults. The latter designation was then added to DSM-5.

Biological Mechanism

Atomoxetine blocks reuptake of norepinephrine at the synapse. Unlike other "stimulants," it does not have direct or indirect agonism of dopamine activity.

Side Effects and Dosing

The main side effect of this agent, as with the other purely noradrenergic drug, desipramine, is anxiety and feeling agitated or overstimulated. Desipramine, which is a TCA, was also associated with cardiac arrhythmias, but this has not been the case with atomoxetine.

The clinical trials with atomoxetine showed some cases of increased suicidal thoughts with this agent, versus no cases with placebo, which led to an FDA black-box warning in 2005.

Bottom Line

- Atomoxetine is an antidepressant masquerading as a "stimulant" for adult ADD.
- It is an NRI, like desipramine, which tends to cause anxiety.

BENZODIAZEPINES—A LITTLE ADDICTIVE, VERY EFFECTIVE SHORT-TERM BUT NOT LONG-TERM

Three typical agents: Short onset (<30 minutes)/short half-life (6–12 hours)—alprazolam; medium onset (30 minutes)/medium half-life (12–18 hours)—lorazepam; long onset (>30 minutes)/long half-life (30–40 hours)—clonazepam

Typical agents' effective dose: 0.5–2 mg/d for all three agents. Note: Clonazepam is more potent per mg than other agents. Maximum preferable recommended dose is 4 mg/d of any agent

Biological mechanism: GABA agonism

Typical side effects: Sedation, incoordination, poor memory

Less common but important side effects: Withdrawal seizures

Clinically proven efficacy: Acute panic attacks

Questionable efficacy: Long-term management of anxiety

Benzodiazepines were the source of major controversy, and major drug company profits, in the 1980s. Now they are all generic, and as past controversies have subsided, clinicians seem to have settled into two basic camps: one group thinks these drugs are very addictive, and rarely prescribes them; another group thinks addiction concerns are way overblown, and prescribes them commonly. There is a third view: they are addictive, but not in most people. It's useful to provide numbers for addiction concerns. About 15% of persons with severe mental illness (schizophrenia or severe bipolar illness) who are prescribed benzodiazepines eventually become addicted to them. This isn't a small number, but it is a minority. Rates should be even lower in milder anxiety/depressive conditions. Thus, one perspective is that these agents can be given to persons with mild anxiety/depressive conditions, who do not have current or past substance abuse, but they should be avoided in those with more severe psychiatric conditions with past substance abuse. Addiction is highly unlikely in the former, and possible in the latter.

Clinical Efficacy and Inefficacy

Once the addiction question is settled, the main issue is efficacy. These are basically symptomatic drugs that reduce anxiety symptoms immediately, in all persons, normal and sick; that is why they can be addictive. Like amphetamines and other addictive medications, everyone who takes them "gets better"; this doesn't mean that any disease has been treated. As discussed previously re the different kinds of anxiety, the main question is when and how much of these agents should be used for anxiety symptoms. When severe anxiety is caused by another disease, which is the most common case, then the mood disease, for instance, should be the focus, not reducing anxiety symptoms with benzodiazepines. Of course, like Tylenol for fever, these agents can be used temporarily to make patients more comfortable. But the focus should remain on treating the mood disease that is causing the anxiety symptoms. In other types of anxiety, like personality traits, existential anxiety, or neurotic depression, benzodiazepines can have a symptomatic role, but again, as with opiates or nonsteroidal anti-inflammatory drugs (NSAIDs) for pain, clinicians should be aware that the treatment is purely symptomatic and not a long-term solution. The benzodiazepines should be used short-term and at as low a dose at possible, and preferably as needed rather than in a standing dose. This doesn't mean that some persons may not need a standing dose and long-term treatment, but the clinical concepts of anxiety described before, and the scientific literature on benzodiazepine efficacy, do not support such constant and long-term use for these agents. The longest outcome study in a randomized clinical trial for any benzodiazepine (clonazepam) is about six months. FDA language is clear about benzodiazepines: they should be used mainly short-term. In this case, the scientific evidence seems to support the FDA language. Yet it's commonplace for benzodiazepines to be used long-term with little question. It would be preferable if most patients were treated short-term. Of course, tolerance, with reduced response over time, also occurs.

Biological Mechanism

These agents are GABA agonists that work by directly opening chloride channels. This effect is immediate, as is the clinical effect.

Specific Agents

There are over a dozen agents in this class, mostly differing in pharmacokinetics: speed of onset and half-life. Three representative agents that differ in pharmacokinetics are: clonazepam (slow onset, long half-life), lorazepam (medium onset, medium half-life), alprazolam (fast onset, short half-life). One approach would be to begin with lorazepam for most uses, especially intermittent as-needed use. Alprazolam is somewhat more addictive due to its very rapid onset and offset, and clonazepam is usually too slow for as-needed use. Clonazepam can be given for long-term standing use, but as noted, it is preferable to limit long-term benzodiazepine treatment, both on questionable efficacy and addiction grounds. Note that clonazepam has a half-life of two to three days, so *twice-daily and thrice-daily dosing doesn't make biological sense*, and may reflect placebo effects and pill-taking dependence.

Side Effects

Sedation is the most common side effect of the class, along with cognitive impairment (clonazepam being worst for both). Incoordination can be risky (e.g., automobile driving), and ataxia can occur. Withdrawal symptoms include risk of seizures.

Bottom Line

- Since most anxiety treatment is symptomatic, and not reflective of an anxiety disease, these agents are best used short-term as needed.

- Long-term efficacy of benzodiazepines is questionable and isn't established in randomized clinical trials.
- Of the three prototypical agents, lorazepam is most preferable, followed by clonazepam.
- Alprazolam is more addictive than the others and should be avoided generally.
- Side effects include sedation and incoordination.

BREXPIPRAZOLE (REXULTI)—MORE DOPAMINE AGONISM

Biological Mechanism

Brexpiprazole is a dopamine blocker, but it also has dopamine agonism. Its basic mechanism is similar to aripiprazole's. The difference is a matter of potency. As usual, the D2 blockade is dose-dependent, such that eventually, over 90% of D2 receptors are blocked. This level of D2 blockade produces EPS such as akathisia, which may remain the main clinical problem with this agent, as with the entire dopamine blocker class.

The dopamine agonism of this agent is somewhat less than occurs with aripiprazole. In animal studies, there was 43% agonism for brexpiprazole compared to 61% for aripiprazole. The relevance of this distinction may be that brexpiprazole may have less of some of the dopamine stimulation effects that are seen with aripiprazole, which may be observed clinically in terms of mania induction or possibly reduced antipsychotic potency.

Like aripiprazole and other new antipsychotics, brexpiprazole does not appear to cause or worsen the metabolic syndrome of diabetes, hypertension, and hyperlipidemia.

Clinical Efficacy

Unlike most other antipsychotics, brexpiprazole was not initially indicated for the classic antipsychotic indications of schizophrenia and mania. Instead, it was developed to be indicated by the FDA indications for schizophrenia and for MDD as an adjunct to SRIs. It has not yet been studied for mania or bipolar depression.

Dosing

Doses of 2–4 mg/d are proven effective for the preceding indications.

Bottom Line

- Brexpiprazole is proven effective for schizophrenia and as an adjunct for MDD. It has somewhat less dopamine agonism than aripiprazole.
- Brexpiprazole has minimal weight gain and no apparent risk of metabolic syndrome or worsening diabetes or cardiovascular risks. Akathisia remains a potential important risk.

BUPROPION (WELLBUTRIN)—A MILD AMPHETAMINE

Typical effective dose: 100–300 mg/d (SR formulation, maximum 400 mg/d)
Biological mechanism: Mild dopamine/norepinephrine agonism
Typical side effects: Anxiety, insomnia
Less common but important side effects: Mania, seizures
Clinically proven efficacy: Mild/moderate unipolar depressive episodes
Clinically proven inefficacy: Bipolar depression
Other proven uses: Weight loss, sexual dysfunction, smoking cessation

This drug has been with us over 25 years now, yet it is still misunderstood. Bupropion was introduced to the U.S. market in 1988, before fluoxetine (Prozac). It was the first of the new generation of post–tricyclic antidepressants (TCAs); instead of becoming the blockbuster that would be Prozac, it had some bad luck. A few cases of seizures occurred in patients hospitalized at McLean Hospital near Boston, and the makers of Prozac used those cases to beat bupropion into submission. Clinicians turned to the new post-TCA agents mainly for safety reasons, not having to worry about overdose toxicity or cardiac arrhythmias. Prozac opened the way for the antidepressant era as other SRIs (serotonin reuptake inhibitors) quickly followed in the early 1990s. For a number of years, clinicians didn't realize that SRIs produced sexual dysfunction, and by the time they found out, the use of SRIs had already become well established. Two decades later, after all these agents became generic and the pharmaceutical marketing wars had ended, clinicians looked at these agents more objectively, and bupropion made a comeback. More is known now about its benefits: no sexual dysfunction (in fact, it enhances sexual drive); weight loss; and reduction of seizure risk with the slow-release formulation (Wellbutrin SR, which is now generic in the U.S.; the seizure rate is 0.1% with Wellbutrin SR, which is equivalent to SRIs, as opposed to 0.4% with immediate-release bupropion.) Some studies also find low manic switch rates.

Yet many clinicians don't realize is what bupropion is. If asked about its mechanisms, they will say it has mild dopamine agonism (also mild norepinephrine agonism). But how does it produce its mild dopamine/norepinephrine agonism? This mystery shouldn't have persisted for two decades. The solution to the saga of bupropion is: It's just another amphetamine, as is visible in its chemical structure. So it should be no surprise that it enhances libido and leads to weight loss.

Clinical Efficacy and Inefficacy

Clinicians should realize that bupropion has been proven ineffective in bipolar depression, in contrast to unipolar depression (major depressive disorder). In bipolar depression, bupropion was equivalent to placebo, when added to standard mood stabilizers (G. Sachs et al. [2007], *New England Journal of Medicine, 356,* 1711–1722). In other words, it did not improve depression at all. Many researchers emphasize the fact that bupropion did not cause mania more than placebo in that study either, but this is not a justification to use a drug that provides no clinical benefits for depressive symptoms in bipolar illness. Furthermore, although the medium doses used there did not cause more mania than placebo, this does not mean that bupropion will never cause mania. In fact, like all antidepressants, it can cause mania at a high enough dose. In some who are sensitive to it, bupropion will cause mania even at low doses.

Biological Mechanism

Its mild dopamine agonism, it should be noted, is less than occurs with sertraline. This may be why bupropion has avoided being labeled a controlled substance. Yet the drug is still a street drug of value, often ground up and snorted for its addictive properties.

Bottom Line

- Bupropion is a mild amphetamine.
- It is not effective in bipolar depression.
- It does not seem effective in severe depression of any kind.
- Its many benefits are amphetamine-like, and it is abused by some persons.

CARBAMAZEPINE—A NEGLECTED SECOND-MESSENGER MODIFIER WITHOUT WEIGHT GAIN

Typical dose: 400–800 mg/d
Biological mechanism: Cyclic AMP (cAMP) blockade
Typical side effects: Diplopia, imbalance
Medically important side effects: Agranulocytosis, SJS
Clinically proven efficacy: FDA indication for acute mania

Biological Mechanism

Carbamazepine probably exerts its psychotropic effects by blockade of cAMP transmission. It shares this kind of second-messenger type of effect with lithium and divalproex, but not with other anticonvulsants that are not effective psychiatrically. Its anticonvulsant effects occur through the standard mechanism of blockade of sodium channels, which has no psychotropic influence.

Clinical Efficacy

Carbamazepine is FDA-indicated for acute mania and epilepsies. It also has a number of randomized trials for maintenance treatment of bipolar illness showing similar efficacy to lithium.

Dosing

The standard dose is about 600 mg/d, with a blood level of around 8, range being 4–12. The level is not associated with efficacy strongly, and thus it is a general guide only. The half-life is about 12–17 hours in long-term treatment, thus twice-daily dosing has been standard practice. Given that blood level stability is relevant to seizures but not to mood episodes, once-daily dosing at night can be considered also.

Side Effects

Nuisance side effects are diplopia, ataxia, paresthesias, and cognitive impairment. These side effects are reduced markedly with the generic slow release formulation, carbamazepine ER. It is highly preferable that the slow-release formulation be used, otherwise unnecessary side effects will lead to discontinuation.

Medically important side effects are very rare, with (probably less than 1:10,000) risk of agranulocytosis and SJS, and more common non-serious rash.

Importantly, this agent has no weight gain, and it is a better alternative to lamotrigine for that purpose in persons who have notable manic episodes or symptoms (for which lamotrigine is minimally effective, if at all). Other potential side effects include hyponatremia (with risk of seizures) and hepatitis (liver function tests should be monitored).

Bottom Line

- Carbamazepine has no weight gain and is effective in mania.
- The generic ER formulation is highly tolerated, and much preferable to standard generic use.
- It works in mixed depressive states.
- It has no metabolic harm or weight gain, but it can cause cardiac arrhythmia.

CLOZAPINE (CLOZARIL)—MORE EFFECTIVE IN REFRACTORY PSYCHOSIS, MOST METABOLIC EFFECTS

Typical dose: 300–600 mg/d
Biological mechanism: Mild dopamine/serotonin blocker
Typical side effects: Weight gain, sedation, constipation, impaired cognition
Medically important side effects: Cardiovascular disease and diabetes
Clinically proven efficacy: FDA indication for schizophrenia

Biological Mechanism

Clozapine has mild blockade of dopamine and serotonin receptors. This effect is mild, much less than with other antipsychotics. It has no other effects that are known to be associated with clinical efficacy for psychosis. It has many other mechanisms that produce side effects: it is highly anticholinergic, antiadrenergic, and antihistaminic.

Clinical Efficacy

Clozapine is FDA-indicated for schizophrenia. It is the only antipsychotic proven more effective than other antipsychotics for refractory psychosis. It also has FDA-approved language for prevention of suicide attempts, based on a single randomized clinical trial. It did not prevent completed suicides in that trial better than its comparator, olanzapine. It is used for mania and bipolar illness, but it has no randomized trials for affective conditions.

Dosing

The standard dose is about 300–600 mg/d, with lower doses used for depressive episodes in bipolar illness, down to 200 mg/d. Doses below 100 mg/d probably have no clinical efficacy. Above 300–400 mg/d, clozapine reduces the seizure threshold, which may be related to its efficacy and to risk of seizures.

Side Effects

Nuisance side effects involve sedation, constipation, impaired cognition, and weight gain. Clozapine has major anti-insulin receptor effects, which cause cardiac harm and markedly increase the risk of diabetes. In some early studies, mortality was about 1% per year, from cardiac events. Diabetes rates were 30–50% in a decade. These medical harms occurred in schizophrenic patients in their mid-30s. At older ages, and with more cardiac risk factors, the risks are likely to be higher. Clozapine causes marked increase in cholesterol. Clozapine also has a notable seizure risk at medium to higher doses. It causes agranulocytosis in about 0.8% of patients, leading to the need for weekly complete blood count (CBC) checks, later reduced to biweekly or monthly.

Bottom Line

- Clozapine is the most effective available antipsychotic agent.
- The biological mechanism of its strong clinical efficacy is unknown.
- It is also the most harmful available antipsychotic, with major cardiovascular and diabetes harms, along with seizure risk and notable agranulocytosis risk.

DUETETRABENAZINE (AUSTEDO)—THE FIRST TARDIVE DYSKINESIA (TD) TREATMENT

Typical dose: 24 mg/d
Biological mechanism: Monoamine transport inhibitor

Typical side effects: Insomnia
Less common but important side effects: None
Medically important side effects: TD prolongation
Clinically proven efficacy: Treatment of Huntington's chorea and mild TD

Clinical Efficacy

This agent is an agent that had been used for Huntington's chorea and now is FDA-indicated for treatment of TD. It is the first agent proven effective for treatment of TD. In two randomized clinical trials, typical doses of this medication led to about 3-point mean improvement in the Abnormal Involuntary Movements Scale (AIMS) , compared to about 1.5 points with placebo. This benefit was significant statistically, though somewhat small in magnitude. Patients in these trials included both schizophrenia as well as affective illness. The mean baseline AIMS score was about 10, which indicates mild severity of TD. In one study, 24 mg/d was more effective than 12 mg/d, but 36 mg/d was no more effective than 24 mg/d. In a second study, with flexible dosing, the mean final dose used was 38.3 mg/d.

Biological Mechanism

This agent is an inhibitor of the axonal monoamine transporter, by which it reduces the availability of all monoamines (dopamine, serotonin, norepinephrine) in the synapse.

Side Effects and Dosing

Dosing is recommended to start at 6 mg twice daily, with a maximum of 48 mg/d. A standard proven effective dose is 24 mg/d. In the TD trials, its most common side effect was insomnia. Its serious side effects include QT prolongation. It has a black box warning of increased risk of depression and suicidality when given for Huntington's chorea, but not for TD. Its half-life is about 10 hours, leading to the current recommendation of twice-daily dosing.

Bottom Line

- This agent is a new treatment for TD.
- Its TD benefit appears to be small in magnitude, but its risks also appear to be small.

DULOXETINE (CYMBALTA)—SOUPED-UP PROZAC

Typical dose: 20–60 mg/d
Biological mechanism: Serotonin/norepinephrine reuptake blockade
Typical side effects: Sexual dysfunction

Medically important side effects: Severe serotonin withdrawal syndrome
Clinically proven efficacy: FDA indications for MDD, GAD, fibromyalgia, diabetic neuropathy, chronic pain

Biological Mechanism

Duloxetine is similar to fluoxetine, from which it is derived, having serotonin and norepinephrine reuptake blockade. Both agents share the same mechanism; the only difference is in potency. While fluoxetine has mild norepinephrine reuptake inhibition and strong serotonin reuptake inhibition (and thus has more SRI than NRI effects), duloxetine has moderate norepinephrine reuptake inhibition and strong serotonin reuptake inhibition. They are thus more similar than different, and duloxetine still is primarily an SRI (not an "NRI," contrary to its marketing).

Clinical Efficacy

Duloxetine is FDA-indicated for acute depressive episodes in MDD. It also has FDA indications for generalized anxiety disorder, fibromyalgia, chronic pain, and diabetic neuropathy. It has been shown to help pain in depression and tends to be used by clinicians for pain syndromes. It has never been shown to be more effective than any other monoamine agonist (antidepressant) for depressive episodes.

Dosing

The standard dose is about 20–60 mg/d, with a maximum of 120 mg/d, given once daily at night. For MDD, doses above 60 mg/d have not been shown to be more effective. The half-life is about 12 hours.

Side Effects

Nuisance side effects of duloxetine involve sexual dysfunction, diarrhea, and apathy, as with all SRIs. Medically important side effects are uncommon, though, as with all SRIs, there is some risk of osteoporosis and gastrointestinal bleeding (due to inhibition of blood clotting).

The main problem with this agent is that it has a very severe serotonin withdrawal syndrome. This syndrome tends to happen after about one year of constant use. Since this agent is used long-term in many persons for chronic pain, the serious withdrawal syndrome means that if clinicians give this medication long-term, they are committing patients to indefinite treatment, as it will be very difficult to ever come off it. If needed, direct taper is almost impossible. In that case, cross-taper with fluoxetine is the best option.

Bottom Line

- Duloxetine is an SRI with somewhat stronger norepinephrine reuptake blockade than its cousin, fluoxetine.
- It is effective in pain syndromes, like fibromyalgia.
- It has typical SRI side effects, like sexual dysfunction.
- It has terrible serotonin withdrawal syndrome, complicating long-term treatment.

FLUOXETINE (PROZAC)—ONCE-WEEKLY DOSING, IDEAL FOR CROSS-TAPER OFF OTHER SRIS

Typical dose: 20–40 mg/d
Biological mechanism: Serotonin and norepinephrine reuptake inhibition
Typical side effects: Sexual dysfunction, akathisia
Medically important side effects: Suicidality
Clinically proven efficacy: FDA indication for MDD, OCD, panic, bulimia

Biological Mechanism

Fluoxetine is the classic SRI, the first marketed in the United States, in the late 1980s. It is not a "selective" SRI, contrary to popular marketing, but instead has notable norepinephrine reuptake inhibition, similar in potency to medium-dose venlafaxine.

Clinical Efficacy

Fluoxetine is FDA-indicated for acute and maintenance treatment of MDD, bulimia nervosa, OCD, and panic disorder. Combined with olanzapine, it is FDA-indicated for acute depressive episodes in bipolar illness, and for treatment-resistant depression.

Besides these mood effects, fluoxetine and all SRIs have direct and immediate anxiolytic effects, especially at low doses. Patients with anxiety symptoms feel "better," but this effect can be misinterpreted as depression benefit. It may underlie the "better than well" phenomenon.

Dosing

The standard dose is 20–40 mg/d, with a maximum of 80 mg/d. The half-life is very long, being four to six days for fluoxetine, and 16 days for its active metabolite norfluoxetine. Given this very long half-life, it only needs to be dosed once weekly, and a trade Prozac Weekly formulation is proven effective in MDD at 90 mg/weekly.

Side Effects

Nuisance side effects are nausea, diarrhea, apathy syndrome, and sexual dysfunction. Medically risky side effects include akathisia, which can lead to suicidality, which has been shown repeatedly to occur with fluoxetine, especially in children and young adults. As with all antidepressants, mania occurs with fluoxetine, though less when given with dopamine blockers.

Serotonin withdrawal syndrome occurs after stopping this agent after long-term use, but it is less severe than with other SRIs. In fact, fluoxetine is useful as a cross-tapering agent to allow for taper off other SRIs with less serotonin withdrawal syndrome.

Bottom Line

- Fluoxetine is not a pure SRI but has noradrenergic effects.
- It is a powerful immediate anxiolytic, more so than an antidepressant.
- The half-life for its active metabolite is two weeks. It need only be dosed once weekly.
- It causes akathisia and suicidality in young adults and children.
- It is useful as a cross-tapering agent with other SRIs for serotonin withdrawal syndrome.

GABAPENTIN—AN ANXIOLYTIC, NOT A "MOOD STABILIZER"

Typical dose: 300–900 mg/d (range 100–2000)
Biological mechanism: GABA agonist
Typical side effects: Sedation, nausea
Less common but important side effects: None
Medically important side effects: None
Clinically proven efficacy: Treatment of anxiety, alcohol/cocaine withdrawal, diabetic neuropathy, epilepsy

Gabapentin is a medication that has many uses, especially for anxiety and insomnia, but it is frequently misused as if it were a mood stabilizer that could be used by itself in bipolar illness. It's important to know when to use it and also to realize that it is not a "mood stabilizer."

Clinical Efficacy and Inefficacy

Gabapentin was first FDA-indicated for epilepsy. Very quickly, it began to be used for many non-indicated (off-label) purposes. Some of this use outside of epilepsy was based on a certain amount of clinical wisdom, with the observation that gabapentin was effective for anxiety and pain. These anxiety and pain symptoms often occurred in the context of depression, however, and this led to the misinterpretation by many clinicians (including authors of this text) that this medication might be effective for mood illnesses per se.

The company that marketed this medication in the 1990s then began to market those uses to clinicians, which is outside of federal regulations. This led to a backlash from the FDA and those who are critical of the pharmaceutical industry. In the last decade, the opposite scenario evolved. Critics began to claim that gabapentin was useless for anything except epilepsy. The truth is somewhere in between. Gabapentin is experiencing something of a renaissance. It's being used for anxiety, insomnia, menopausal symptoms, chronic pain syndrome, and once again for mood and bipolar illness.

These uses could be potentially valid, but not as a primary mood stabilizer in bipolar illness. Gabapentin was studied about a decade ago in multiple studies of acute mania, and it was proven to be equivalent to placebo. It has never been proven to be effective for bipolar depression or in prophylaxis of mood episodes. It should not be used in place of lithium, valproate, or lamotrigine. Nevertheless, it is useful for anxiety, whether symptomatically or as part of a larger anxiety illness. It's sedating and probably helpful for insomnia in some persons, although it has not been carefully studied in that condition. It's very well proven for pain syndromes and also beneficial for persons with substance abuse who may have anxiety-related self-medication.

Biological Mechanism

Gabapentin stimulates a receptor subunit of GABA, which probably produces its anxiety benefits.

Side Effects and Dosing

The main benefit of this medication is that it has very few side effects, and none that are known to be medically important or harmful long-term. Its main nuisance side effects are nausea and sedation. Dosing has a very broad range, which can be good in terms of being able to reduce the dose greatly to a point that is tolerable for most people. Sensitive individuals usually begin at 100 mg nightly, but for the average patient, 300 mg is a standard starting dose. For anxiety, pain, and insomnia, the typical final dose will be about 300–900 mg nightly. PL recommends giving all the medication at night, even though it has a short half-life of about four hours. This short half-life may be relevant for anxiety, in which case multiple-daily dosing may be needed. If given for other purposes, a single evening dose may be sufficient.

Bottom Line

- Gabapentin is a versatile medication, which can be helpful for anxiety and insomnia.
- It is proven ineffective for mania and should *not* be given as a "mood stabilizer."

LAMOTRIGINE—INEFFECTIVE ACUTELY IN ANY FORM, BUT GOOD FOR PROPHYLAXIS

Typical dose: 50–200 mg/d
Biological mechanism: Glutamate antagonist
Typical side effects: Rash
Less common but important side effects: Anxiety
Medically important side effects: SJS
Clinically proven efficacy: Prevention of mood episodes in bipolar illness

Lamotrigine is an anticonvulsant that has turned about to be the latest, newest, proven effective "mood stabilizer," by which this text means an agent that prevents mood episodes in bipolar illness. The studies that proved lamotrigine's efficacy were conducted over 15 years ago, and now the agent is available as a generic drug.

Clinical Efficacy and Inefficacy

In the late 1990s, when its manufacturer was preparing its studies of lamotrigine, it had an ambitious agenda: multiple randomized clinical trials (RCTs) were conducted for acute mania, acute bipolar depression, and even acute unipolar depression. Along with two studies in rapid-cycling bipolar illness, it added up to about a dozen randomized clinical trials.

In all cases, lamotrigine failed. It was completely ineffective. It was not better than placebo. Luckily for its manufacturer, two RCTs were conducted in maintenance prevention of mood episodes in bipolar illness. In both cases, lamotrigine worked. It was effective. In other words, the drug was proven not to work in any acute mood state, manic or depressive. But it was proven to work in prevention of mood episodes, both manic and depressive.

Why would lamotrigine prevent future mood episodes, but not improve current ones? This seems like a major paradox for many clinicians because they can't get out of the mindset of treating acute symptoms. The thought always has been that if a drug works short-term, it'll work long-term—the Second Fallacy of Psychopharmacology: "What gets you well, keeps you well."

This common clinical belief was disproven by lamotrigine. It doesn't get you well, but it keeps you well. Take lamotrigine when you're well to stay well, not when you're sick to get better. Since these ideas aren't well known, there is a common clinical misconception that lamotrigine is effective for acute depression, whether in bipolar or unipolar illness. When patients have depressive symptoms, clinicians sometimes increase the dose of lamotrigine as if it will improve depressive symptoms within weeks or months.

Multiple RCTs show that lamotrigine will not help current depressive (or manic) symptoms that way. These misconceptions about lamotrigine's acute efficacy were left uncorrected by its manufacturer, which didn't publish the many negative RCTs. After a legal verdict against the parent drug company for a different medication (paroxetine), a court order required the company to publish all its negative data on a website. For a brief period, those data were publicly available on the Internet, from which the author of this text downloaded the results and published them separately. Without that legal intervention, the results never might have been known, due to patent law protection.

Regarding the maintenance studies themselves, another misconception needs correction: it is sometimes thought that lamotrigine only prevents depression, not mania. In fact, in the combined two maintenance RCTs, lamotrigine was more effective in preventing mania than placebo; it did have mania prevention benefit. It just had more benefit in prevention of depression than mania.

Biological Mechanism

Lamotrigine is a novel anticonvulsant, which raises the seizure threshold via glutamate antagonism. Glutamate is an excitatory neurotransmitter distributed throughout the brain. Whether this mechanism is relevant to this agent's mood effects is unknown.

Side Effects and Dosing

The main concern about lamotrigine is rash. Non-serious rash happens in about 5–10% of persons; serious rash usually involves SJS, which is potentially fatal. SJS occurs in about 1/5000 adults given lamotrigine, and in about 1/1000 children or adolescents. These rates assume the standard slow titration of lamotrigine. This text recommends a slower titration than the FDA language, developed originally for epilepsy. The recommendation here is 25 mg/d increased every two weeks in 25 mg increments—no faster. Risk factors for rash and SJS are rapid titration, other drug allergies (such as antibiotics), and autoimmune conditions (like lupus). Of these risk factors, drug allergies and autoimmune illnesses are relevant. Rash risk is higher with drug allergies, and in those cases, lamotrigine shouldn't be used as a first-line agent, and if used, the dosing titration should be even slower (such as 12.5 mg every two weeks). If autoimmune illnesses are present, this text recommends that lamotrigine not be used at all. A number of cases exist of serious medical harm in autoimmune illness, with immunological reactions such as SJS and aseptic meningitis.

The dose range proven effective in RCTs of bipolar illness was 50–200 mg/d. A 400 mg/d dose was studied and was found to be no more effective than 200 mg/d. A common error is to increase the lamotrigine dose to 300 mg/d or 400 mg/d, without realizing that these higher doses aren't more effective for bipolar illness. These higher doses only cause more side effects, particularly anxiety and cognitive impairment.

Bottom Line

- Lamotrigine is effective for prevention of mood episodes in bipolar illness, but not for acute depressive symptom benefit.
- There's no further mood efficacy above 200 mg/d, only more anxiety and cognitive side effects.

LITHIUM—MORE BENEFITS, AND FEWER HARMS, THAN OFTEN ASSUMED

Typical effective dose: 600–900 mg/d. Levels 0.6–1.0
Biological mechanism: G protein and second-messenger effects
Typical side effects: Polyuria, thirst, diarrhea, tremor
Less common but important side effects: Acne, psoriasis, cognitive effects, weight gain
Medically important side effects: Hypothyroidism, renal impairment
Clinically proven efficacy: Acute mania and depression, prevention of mania and depression
Questionable efficacy: Acute mixed episodes
Other proven uses: Suicide prevention

Lithium is one of the first modern psychotropic drugs, discovered for mania in 1949 by John Cade in Australia. It was the first psychotropic drug proven effective in an RCT, in 1952. Yet it's been consistently undervalued by clinicians and patients.

Clinical Efficacy and Inefficacy

In the 1980s, drug makers for anticonvulsants (like valproate) claimed that most patients with bipolar illness didn't respond to lithium. These predictors of negative response were factors like rapid-cycling, substance abuse, mixed states, and psychosis. Now we know that these features predict poor response to all mood stabilizers, including anticonvulsants, not just lithium. Further studies in the last two decades often used lithium as a comparator arm, in studies designed to show benefit for agents like lamotrigine or antipsychotics. Those studies generally found that lithium was as effective, or more, than new putative mood stabilizers. This conclusion isn't appreciated, judging by some claims made by some drug companies. For instance, it's claimed that lamotrigine was more effective than lithium in dementia prevention. But (as reviewed on the PL website) those studies were designed to preselect only lamotrigine responders to enter them; hence they weren't a fair comparison to lithium.

In short, after half a century, lithium remains the best proven, and overall most effective, mood stabilizer, for prevention of both depressive and manic episodes.

Biological Mechanism

For decades, the profession had no clue how lithium worked, because it had few synaptic effects on neurotransmitters. In the last few decades, it's become clear lithium has multiple effects inside neurons, on G-proteins and second messengers. Those effects are extensive, and include many neuroplastic effects that keep neurons alive longer. They probably produce many of lithium's long-term benefits, in prevention of mood episodes and perhaps in anti-suicide and anti-dementia effects.

Side Effects and Dosing

Polyuria is lithium's most common side effect. Cognitive side effects can occur short-term, even though it produces cognitive benefits long-term through its neuroprotective effects. Its medical side effects are known, but the risk of chronic renal insufficiency is about 1% at 20 years . This risk can be decreased by once-daily dosing, as opposed to multiple-daily dosing, and by avoiding acute lithium toxicity (which kills kidney cells). This is why this text strongly recommends not giving levels higher than 1.0, so as to avoid borderline toxicity either by error or by dehydration. Furthermore, levels of 0.6–0.8 are shown equivalent in efficacy to 0.8–1.0 in type I bipolar illness. Thus, there is no need for "high therapeutic" levels. Thyroid effects occur more quickly but are reversible with thyroid hormone supplementation. Weight gain is a common concern, but it's less with lithium than with valproate or other commonly used antipsychotics like olanzapine or quetiapine.

Bottom Line

- Lithium is the most effective mood stabilizer, including for depression and mania prevention.
- Lithium affects second messengers, a unique mechanism providing long-term benefits.
- Levels above 1.0 aren't needed for efficacy.
- Long-term kidney effects are 1% at 20 years.
- Lithium should be prescribed only once daily to minimize long-term renal harm.

LURASIDONE (LATUDA)—A NEW DOPAMINE BLOCKER FOR BIPOLAR DEPRESSION

Typical dose: 20–60 mg/d (range 20–120 mg/d)
Biological mechanism: Dopamine-receptor blockade
Typical side effects: Akathisia, Parkinsonism
Medically important side effects: Suicidality
Clinically proven efficacy: FDA indications for acute bipolar depression, schizophrenia

Biological Mechanism

Lurasidone is a dopamine D2-receptor blocker without other major neurotransmitter effects. Like other new dopamine blockers, it does not cause or worsen metabolic syndrome or have appreciable weight gain.

Clinical Efficacy

Lurasidone is somewhat unusual in that it was never studied and proven for acute mania, as is the case with almost all other dopamine blockers. Instead, after its initial proof of efficacy in schizophrenia, it was studied and proven effective in acute bipolar depression. Those are its two FDA indications.

Further research has been conducted in maintenance treatment of bipolar illness for prevention of mood episodes as well as for MDD with mixed features (MDD-MF). Those latter uses have not been given FDA indications yet, though. A maintenance indication may come in the future, but it appears that the MDD-MF indication will not occur, apparently because this new DSM-5 indication has not been seen by FDA reviewers as worthy of specific drug treatment indication yet. For what it is worth, though, using that DSM-5-defined term, lurasidone was more effective than placebo for mixed features in a randomized trial.

Dosing

In schizophrenia, doses are in the 40–120 mg/d range. In bipolar depression, doses higher than 60 mg/d were proven to be no more effective than doses in the 20–60 mg/d range.

Side Effects

The main side effects are EPS, especially akathisia, but also Parkinsonism. Unlike earlier modern dopamine blockers, this agent does not cause or worsen glucose or lipid profiles. It does not have appreciable weight gain, at least in initial clinical trials.

Akathisia is dose-related, thus the preceding dosing guidelines should be kept in mind. Sometimes akathisia produces suicidal thoughts, which can be how it presents, as opposed to obvious motor restlessness.

Bottom Line

- Lurasidone is effective in schizophrenia and bipolar depression, but not proven in mania.
- It also is likely to be effective in mixed states.

METHLYPHENIDATE, AND ITS VARIANTS—EFFECTIVE IN EVERYONE, BUT NEUROTOXIC

Typical dose: 10–60 mg/d
Variants: Focalin, dex-methylphenidate; Concerta, methylphenidate ER
Biological mechanism: Dopaminergic and noradrenergic agonist
Typical side effects: Insomnia, anxiety, jitteriness
Less common but important side effects: Mania

Medically important side effects: Ventricular arrhythmia, neurotoxicity
Clinically proven efficacy: Treatment of ADD and non-bipolar depressive episodes

The most widely used amphetamine agent is methylphenidate. In fact, all prescribed amphetamines are variants of either methylphenidate or dextroamphetamine.

Clinical Efficacy and Inefficacy

Methylphenidate and its variants have been shown to be effective in ADD, as well as in major depressive episodes. They also produce weight loss and increase sexual libido. They have been found to cause mania and/or worsen bipolar illness.

"Benefit" in ADD for attention is not surprising, since methylphenidate has been shown to be effective in normal individuals to improve attention. In other words, since some inattention is normal, methylphenidate "works" in everyone, and its efficacy is not indicative of presence of an illness.

Biological Mechanism

This agent is a dopamine reuptake inhibitor and directly stimulates dopamine and norepinephrine receptors. Thus, it increases both dopamine and norepinephrine activity.

For some reason, there is a common misconception that methylphenidate is not an amphetamine. It clearly is an amphetamine, based on both its pharmacological structure and its biological effects. It has the same basic structure as dextroamphetamine and dopamine. It also has the same basic biological effect of dopamine agonism as is the case with dextroamphetamine. The only difference is that it also has noradrenergic effects. But this additional effect doesn't remove or cancel out its basic dopaminergic effect, which is part and parcel of its basic amphetamine structure.

Neurotoxicity

Many animal studies have shown that methylphenidate is harmful to neurons, causing atrophy. This has been shown over and over again in many rodent studies. The question often raised is whether this effect occurs in humans. The short answer is that it hasn't been studied in any way that can answer the question. A few small studies exist in adolescents, none of which are followed more than a few years, and all in non-randomized observational settings. Those studies mostly report no cortical atrophy, although some analyses do indicate more atrophy. In any case, because of confounding bias, those studies cannot answer the question. We would need randomized neuroimaging studies, which have never been conducted. Another factor is that animal studies indicate that the most harm occurs if methylphenidate is given early in childhood and continued into adulthood. There has never been even a non-randomized observational study of neuroimaging in human adults who have been exposed to amphetamines in childhood continuously into adulthood.

Side Effects and Dosing

Besides neurotoxicity in animals, methylphenidate is known to have cardiotoxicity, specifically cardiac arrhythmias. This risk may be lower in children than in adults. In adults, a recent analysis found that there was almost a doubling of risk of sudden cardiac death due to ventricular arrhythmias with methylphenidate. The authors tried to explain this result away given the observational setting, and the presence of confounding factors should prevent definitive judgments pro or con. Nonetheless, these are the best data we now possess, and they do indicate some risk as far as we can accept those data. Absolute frequency of risk appears to be about 1:1000. In other words, if these results are correct, methylphenidate can cause sudden cardiac death in one in 1,000 adults. Other studies do not find evidence of such risk, so that at present one cannot be definitive.

In summary, it is not the case that this medication is proven safe in children and adults, as is commonly repeated by some experts.

Bottom Line

- Methylphenidate is an amphetamine.
- It is effective for attention in everyone, not just persons with ADD.
- It is proven neurotoxic in animals, and human studies do not prove or disprove that risk.
- It is possibly cardiotoxic in adults, with 1:1000 risk.
- It is not proven safe in children and adults such that one can prescribe it without any concerns.

OLANZAPINE (ZYPREXA)—SOME BENEFITS, MANY HARMS

Typical dose: 5–20 mg/d
Biological mechanism: Dopamine and serotonin-receptor blockade, anti-insulin effects
Typical side effects: Marked weight gain, EPS, sedation, constipation
Less common but important side effects: Metabolic syndrome
Medically important side effects: Metabolic syndrome
Clinically proven efficacy: Acute mania, schizophrenia

Biological Mechanism

Olanzapine is a dopamine blocker with potent D2-receptor blockade, along with strong anticholinergic effects. The D2 blockade is dose-dependent, such that at 10–20 mg/d, over 90% of D2 receptors are blocked. This level of D2 blockade produces EPS such as Parkinsonian tremor and rigidity, and akathisia. The Parkinsonian effects are somewhat mitigated by this agent's anticholinergic properties, but the latter cause their own side effects, especially cognitive impairment, sedation, and constipation.

Like all modern dopamine blockers, it also has serotonin-2-receptor blockade, which probably produces weight gain. Olanzapine also has strong anti-insulin effects, which produces the dire metabolic syndrome of diabetes, hypertension, and hyperlipidemia, along with marked weight gain and abdominal girth.

Other Features

Olanzapine causes notable abnormalities in liver function tests (LFTs), more so than divalproex, and it can cause death by acute diabetic ketoacidosis.

Clinical Efficacy

Olanzapine has been shown to be effective for manic episodes and for schizophrenia, and also has an FDA indication for maintenance treatment of bipolar illness. It has been proven ineffective in the acute major depressive episode in both bipolar depression and MDD. However, when combined with fluoxetine (olanzapine-fluoxetine combination, Symbyax), it has been proven effective for the acute bipolar depressive episode.

In the CATIE study, it was shown to be very effective for schizophrenia, but it also had more side effects and was less safe than other antipsychotics.

Dosing

Doses of 5–10 mg/d are effective for moderate mood states, with higher doses needed for severe mania and schizophrenia.

Bottom Line

- Olanzapine is very effective for acute mania and schizophrenia.
- It is much less safe than most other dopamine blockers.
- Its other utility, such as in maintenance treatment in bipolar illness, is questionable, given possible invalidity of the "enriched" design, as discussed in chapter 6.

OXCARBAZEPINE—INEFFECTIVE, UNLIKE CARBAMAZEPINE

Typical dose: 600–1200 mg/d
Biological mechanism: Unknown
Typical side effects: Sedation
Less common but important side effects: Rash
Medically important side effects: Hyponatremia
Clinically proven efficacy: None (in psychiatry)

Oxcarbazepine is an anticonvulsant, but its use for psychiatric conditions is mostly for mood states (Figure 15.1). Yet it appears that carbamazepine is effective for mood

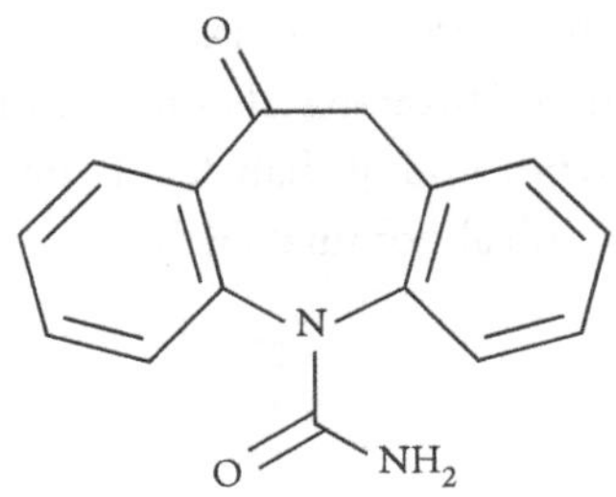

FIGURE 15.1 *Oxcarbazepine.*

illnesses, but not oxcarbazepine (Figure 15.2). The reason for this difference is the same as why chlorpromazine is effective for schizophrenia, but imipramine is not. Small differences in chemical structure can produce large differences in efficacy. The difference between carbamazepine and oxcarbazepine is one carbonyl bond (C=O).

Similarly, the difference between imipramine (a TCA) and chlorpromazine (Thorazine, an antipsychotic) is one chlorine bond and one sulfate bond (Figure 15.3). One is an antipsychotic that works for mania, but doesn't appear to work for depression (chlorpromazine); the other is an antidepressant that causes mania and doesn't work for schizophrenia (imipramine). A chemical bond or two can make a huge difference. This doesn't mean that similarity of chemical structure is irrelevant; sometimes it can imply similar clinical effects, whether for efficacy or for side effects. For instance, chlorpromazine and imipramine share many similar side effects (anticholinergic effects of dry mouth and constipation, and antihistamine effects of sedation and weight gain). But their clinical effects are quite different. Similarly oxcarbazepine and carbamazepine share some side effects (like hyponatremia) but have important differences (e.g., no drug interactions with oxcarbazepine). So one can't assume their clinical effects are similar.

Clinical Efficacy and Inefficacy

What does the clinical research show about the efficacy of oxcarbazepine in psychiatric conditions? Most of the research is in mood illness. In acute mania randomized trials, some studies indicate similar efficacy to haloperidol, but without placebo controls, so we can't infer efficacy, since mania resolves by itself spontaneously within weeks to months. There are no randomized trials in acute bipolar depression.

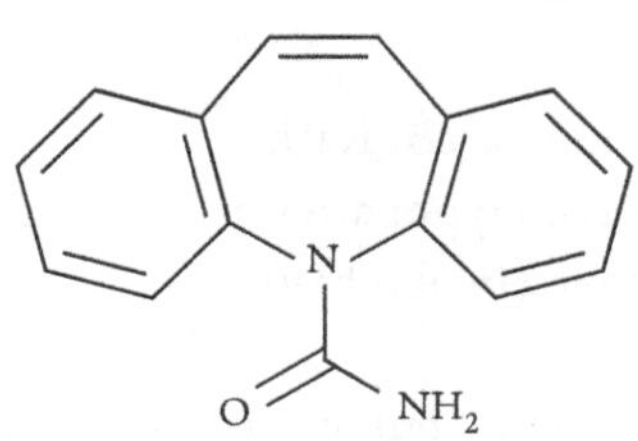

FIGURE 15.2 *Carbamazepine.*

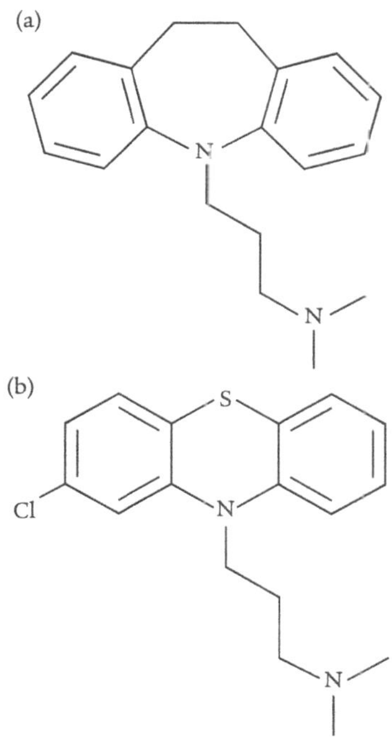

FIGURE 15.3 *a. Imipramine*
b. Chlorpromazine

Observational reports suggest some benefit, but they are contradicted by randomized data. Two maintenance RCTs found no benefit over placebo. More evidence that oxcarbazepine is ineffective overall involves studies of its active metabolite, licarbazepine, which never came to the market, presumably due to negative trials in mania. This inefficacy was proven again by two randomized clinical trials of an enantiomer of licarbazepine (eslicarbazepine), which found again that the agent was equivalent to placebo for acute mania.

In summary, oxcarbazepine and/or its active metabolite or enantiomers have been proven ineffective in acute mania and in maintenance prophylaxis of bipolar illness. It's never been proven effective in any randomized trial of an acute depressive episode.

Biological Mechanism

Like most anticonvulsants, oxcarbazepine raises the seizure threshold via sodium channel blockade. Any biological effects that are relevant to mood are unknown.

Side Effects and Dosing

This agent doesn't have drug interactions, unlike carbamazepine, and thus it can be combined with other agents, such as dopamine blockers or monoamine agonists (antidepressants). It also has less risk of rash or leukopenia. It has more sedation than carbamazepine, however, and it has one potentially serious medical risk that can lead to seizures; namely, a 2% risk of hyponatremia. As with carbamazepine, there's no weight gain. Clinicians should exercise caution in use of this agent in persons with eating disorders, who often wish to take medications without weight gain. Frequently, such persons will drink water excessively as a way of maintaining weight loss. This over-drinking of water, when combined with oxcarbazepine, can lead to dangerous hyponatremia. If sodium levels fall below 120, seizures can occur.

Bottom Line

- Oxcarbazepine probably is ineffective in any psychiatric use.
- If one wants carbamazepine-like effects, one should use carbamazepine.

PAROXETINE (PAXIL)—THE LOWEST RISK OF MANIA IN BIPOLAR DEPRESSION, BUT INEFFECTIVE

Typical dose: 10–80 mg/d (range)
Biological mechanism: Serotonin and norepinephrine inhibition
Typical side effects: Sexual dysfunction, sedation
Less common but important side effects: Weight gain
Medically important side effects: None
Clinically proven efficacy: Treatment of acute depressive episodes in MDD, treatment of OCD

Biological Mechanism

Paroxetine is an SRI that, at low doses, is highly selective for serotonin, but at higher doses, also inhibits norepinephrine reuptake. In general, it's often thought that norepinephrine reuptake leads to increased induction of mania. Thus, the observation of low acute mania induction with paroxetine may be due to its selectivity for serotonin at lower doses. However, the flip side is that at higher doses, paroxetine probably does not have a low risk of acute mania induction.

This agent also has anticholinergic effects, which have been associated with sedation; some patients also report weight gain.

Clinical Efficacy

Paroxetine has been shown to be effective for depressive episodes in MDD, but it has been shown to be ineffective in bipolar depression. It also has efficacy for, and is FDA-indicated in, OCD, and is probably effective for a range of anxiety symptoms.

Dosing

Paroxetine produces pure serotonin reuptake inhibition at 10–20 mg/d, whereas norepinephrine reuptake inhibition begins to increase at higher doses, and is definitely present with 40 mg/d or more. Low doses, less than 20 mg/d, are less likely to be associated with causing mania. Higher doses, like 40–80 mg/d, tend to be used for OCD.

Other Features

When stopped, paroxetine possesses a severe serotonin withdrawal syndrome, though it has a relatively long half-life of 21 hours. Given this long half-life, it need not be dosed more than once daily, and frequently it is best to give it at night due to sedation.

Bottom Line

- Paroxetine is a pure SRI at very low doses.
- It is an NRI at higher doses.
- At low doses, it is less likely to cause mania, but it is ineffective for acute bipolar depression.
- It has a severe serotonin withdrawal syndrome.

PIMAVANSERIN (NUPLAZID)—THE FIRST NON-DOPAMINE BLOCKER ANTIPSYCHOTIC

Biological Mechanism

Pimavanserin is the first proven antipsychotic that does not cause dopamine blockade. A number of prior putative antipsychotics, which were not dopamine blockers, had been studied over the years; most of those agents were pure serotonin blockers. When studied in clinical trials, though, those agents didn't work. This agent appears to be the first to have proven some clinical efficacy, in this case for psychotic symptoms in Parkinson's disease. The purported mechanism of pimavanserin is "inverse agonism" of the serotonin 1A receptor. This mechanism is thought to result in complete blockade of serotonin activity at that receptor, as opposed to other prior serotonin blockers, which still allowed a small amount of activity at that receptor. Whether this mechanism truly explains the antipsychotic efficacy of this agent remains to be seen.

Clinical Efficacy

For now, this medication is only FDA-indicated for psychosis in Parkinson's disease. However, a randomized trial in schizophrenia has shown efficacy over placebo. We'll need to see if that efficacy is replicated and then followed by FDA indication. If this occurs, this would be a major shift in treatment of severe psychosis in schizophrenia, as well as possibly for mania or bipolar illness, since this agent would be the first non-dopamine blocker that would be effective for classic psychosis.

Dosing and Other Features

The effective dose is 34 mg/d for Parkinson's psychosis, with pill sizes of 17 mg per pill. This agent has a very long half-life of 2 1/2 days. Thus it would take one to two weeks to achieve a steady state, if not longer, in older persons with Parkinson's disease. This feature of this medication should be kept in mind.

Side Effects

The main observed side effect in the clinical trials in Parkinson's disease was peripheral edema. There was no weight gain or metabolic syndrome.

Bottom Line

- Pimavanserin is a pure serotonin blocker that is proven effective for psychosis in Parkinson's disease. It does not cause EPS.
- Pimavanserin has a very long half-life of two to three days.

PROPANOLOL ER—JACK-OF-ALL-TRADES

Typical dose: 60–120 mg/d
Biological mechanism: Centrally acting beta-blocker
Typical side effects: Sedation
Less common but important side effects: Fainting
Medically important side effects: Bradycardia
Clinically proven efficacy: Treatment of akathisia, anxiety, PTSD, tremor, migraine; antihypertensive

Propranolol is the first of the beta-blocker class of medications used mainly for hypertension. It has many potential psychotropic uses as well, including for PTSD.

Clinical Efficacy and Inefficacy

Focusing on psychotropic uses, some studies have found that if beta-blockers are given in the emergency room setting soon after an acute trauma, later PTSD symptoms may be lessened. If given later, beta-blockers can reduce anxiety and physiological symptoms of PTSD. Most beta blockers affect the peripheral nervous system, reducing the sympathetic drive, thereby decreasing arousal and anxiety. Propranolol also enters the central nervous system, and thus can reduce anxiety directly through effects on the brain.

A specific kind of severe anxiety for which propranolol appears to be helpful is akathisia—marked psychomotor restlessness that occurs as a side effect of dopamine blocking medications. This agent also helps tremor, such as can be induced by lithium or valproate. In older persons, especially those with medical illnesses, beta-blockers have some risk of causing depression.

Biological Mechanism

Propranolol causes central and peripheral blockade of beta-receptors on noradrenergic neuronal synapses.

Side Effects and Dosing

The use of the generic slow-release version of this agent, propranolol ER, is recommended strongly, since the standard generic agent has a very short half-life of only one to four hours and thus needs to be dosed multiple times daily, which is not practical for most persons. Furthermore, the ER formulation can be given at night, so that sedating effects help sleep and do not cause problems in the daytime. Other side effects besides sedation are potential fainting or dizziness from excessive blood pressure reduction or from bradycardia. This agent reduces the heart rate, so bradycardia is the main concern. Resting pulse should be assessed before using this medication, and it should not be prescribed if baseline pulse is 60 beats/minute or lower. Dosing should start at 60 mg at night, then increased to 80 mg at night, and further increased if needed as long as the pulse stays around or above 60 beats per minute. Attention should be paid to some risk of masking diabetic ketoacidosis symptoms and/or worsening of obstructive pulmonary disease. Hence, in diabetes and obstructive lung disease, these agents should be avoided or used with caution.

Bottom Line

- Propranolol ER is a versatile medication, which can be helpful for anxiety.
- Its use in akathisia is important to allow for effective use of dopamine blockers.

QUETIAPINE (SEROQUEL)—SEDATING, WITH LOW EPS

Typical effective dose: 50–150 mg/d for anxiety or insomnia, 200–300 mg/d for bipolar depression, 300–400 mg/d for mania, 300–800 mg/d for psychosis/schizophrenia

Biological mechanism: Mild dopamine blockade

Typical side effects: Sedation, weight gain, metabolic syndrome/cardiovascular harms, diabetes, akathisia

Less common but important side effects: Orthostatic hypotension
Clinically proven efficacy: Acute bipolar depression, acute mania, schizophrenia
Questionable efficacy: Unipolar depression, anxiety, maintenance prevention of bipolar mood episodes

Clinicians of a certain age will remember thioridazine (Mellaril). At low doses, it helped sleep and reduced anxiety; at higher doses where it helped psychosis or mania, it knocked people out. But at least it wasn't a benzodiazepine, and it didn't have as serious EPS as other neuroleptic agents, especially at low doses. So clinicians loved it. And so did many patients.

Quetiapine is the Mellaril of the 21st century. Unlike thioridazine, it has very minimal risk of TD, so it has proved a natural replacement for a drug that clinicians can give to patients for that inevitable request: "Doctor, please give me something to help me sleep" (or in another variant, "to help me be less anxious"). Benzodiazepines are the class of medication for those uses, of course, but their potential dependence limits their use in some people. Hence the never-ending search for the holy grail of the benzodiazepine-like drug that doesn't cause addiction. Hence quetiapine.

Clinical Efficacy and Inefficacy

The popularity of quetiapine isn't about schizophrenia, although this medication is listed among antipsychotics. It has been used most extensively for bipolar depression, and also was studied for generalized anxiety disorder and MDD, and some benefit reportedly was seen at low doses (<200 mg/d), but FDA reviewers were reluctant to give FDA indication for monotherapy for those uses, given concerns about medical harms from widespread use in the primary care setting. It does have FDA indication now as an adjunct to SRIs for MDD, however. Efficacy in acute mania has been shown in standard studies. Efficacy in maintenance prevention of bipolar illness has been shown using randomized discontinuation trial designs, which may have questionable validity (see Chapter 6).

Biological Mechanism

Although it's called an "antipsychotic," quetiapine is different from other treatments for psychosis in that it never reaches, at any dose, more than mild amounts of dopamine blockade. From about 400 mg/d to 800 mg/d, there is a plateau of about 30–40% D2-receptor blockade, nowhere near the 80–90% D2 blockade obtained with all other antipsychotics except clozapine.

Side Effects

Sometimes, similarity of chemical structure entails similar side effects. Quetiapine's basic chemical structure is similar to those of clozapine and olanzapine. All three have notable antihistamine, anticholinergic, and antiadrenergic effects, all of which add up to marked sedation. Importantly, all share the major harm of metabolic syndrome: increasing susceptibility to hypertension, diabetes, and hyperlipidemia. All these are major cardiovascular risk factors. Apart from these direct physiological effects (decreasing insulin sensitivity), quetiapine *also* causes weight gain, which further worsens these cardiovascular risk factors. Regarding neuroleptic effects, quetiapine can cause akathisia, although apparently less frequently than other dopamine blockers (based on the CATIE study); it doesn't cause much Parkinsonism because its inherent anticholinergic effects reduce Parkinsonian symptoms; TD is rare.

Bottom Line

- Quetiapine is a mild dopamine blocker.
- It is effective in bipolar depression, mania, and schizophrenia; sedation effects may be interpreted as mood and psychosis benefits.
- Long-term efficacy in bipolar illness can be questioned based on study design questions.
- Benefits for anxiety/insomnia/agitation are probably related to antihistamine/antiadrenergic/anticholinergic effects.
- It causes metabolic syndrome, worsens cardiovascular risks, and has notable weight gain.

RISPERIDONE—THE CLASSIC MODERN DOPAMINE BLOCKER

Typical dose: 2–4 mg/d
Biological mechanism: Dopamine/serotonin-receptor antagonist
Typical side effects: Akathisia, Parkinsonism
Less common but important side effects: Rigidity, dystonia
Medically important side effects: Potential stroke in elderly
Clinically proven efficacy: Treatment of schizophrenia and acute mania

Clinical Efficacy

Risperidone is FDA-indicated for schizophrenia and mania. Risperidone can be thought of as haloperidol with somewhat less EPS. Like its parent compound, it is very effective for manic symptoms and for acute psychotic symptoms. Hence it is useful in severe acute exacerbations of schizophrenia or mania. For bipolar depression, it has been studied less, but it appears to have less benefit than do some other dopamine blockers. It also has not been as well studied for long-term prevention of mood episodes in bipolar illness, although it probably is effective, especially as adjunct to standard mood stabilizers.

Biological Mechanism

Risperidone is a dopamine and serotonin blocker. It was the first of the modern class of such agents, developed as a combination of haloperidol (pure dopamine blocker) and ritanserin (pure serotonin blocker). It was created in the 1980s by Dr. Paul Janssen, who had previously created haloperidol in the 1960s.

Side Effects and Dosing

EPS are its major side effects, mainly akathisia but also Parkinsonism, and sometimes rigidity and dystonia. It has some weight gain, but much less than olanzapine or quetiapine, yet it is not weight-neutral. It can increase triglycerides, but does not cause the metabolic syndrome (i.e., does not cause diabetes or hypertension or worsen other lipid profiles). It has few medically serious side effects, although an association with stroke in the elderly has been reported, with an FDA black-box warning. It has a wide dose range, from 0.5 mg/d to 6 mg/d, and is typically effective for mania or schizophrenia at 2–4 mg/d, with higher doses needed in severe cases. It can be effective at very low doses of 0.5–2.0 mg/d in older persons or for mild manic symptoms. Its half-life is 20 hours and only needs to be dosed once daily.

Bottom Line

- Risperidone is a classic effective dopamine-blocking agent for psychosis and mania.
- Its main limitation, which it shares with all dopamine blockers, is EPS, like akathisia.
- It has some weight gain but does not cause metabolic syndrome.
- Its wide dose range allows for benefit with very low doses in some settings.

SELEGELINE PATCH (EM-SAM)—NOT MORE EFFECTIVE THAN OTHER ANTIDEPRESSANTS

Typical dose: 6–12 mg/d
Biological mechanism: monoamine oxidase-B (MAO-B) inhibition
Typical side effects: Anxiety, insomnia
Less common but important side effects: None
Medically important side effects: Hypertensive crisis at high doses (>12 mg/d)
Clinically proven efficacy: Treatment of acute depressive episodes in MDD

Biological Mechanism

Selegiline is a selective monoamine oxidase-B (MAO-B) inhibitor. In contrast, classic monoamine oxidase inhibitors (MAOIs) block both the A and B enzymes. MAO-A metabolizes serotonin and norepinephrine; MAO-B metabolizes dopamine. By blocking the B enzyme, selegiline is a purely dopaminergic drug. In contrast, classic MAOIs (like phenelzine or tranylcypromine) are also noradrenergic and serotonergic. These differences in neurotransmitter effects may help explain why selegiline should not be seen as a simple MAOI, similar in effect to other agents in this class, and also why selegiline should not be assumed to be as effective as other MAOIs.

MAO-A blockade is associated with greater clinical benefit, but, since norepinephrine activity is robustly increased, it is associated with a risk of hypertensive crisis if a person eats food rich in tyramine. Tyramine is converted to tyrosine and then norepinephrine; in the setting of irreversible MAO-A inhibition, the massive presence of norepinephrine leads to very high blood pressure, which can produce a stroke and be fatal.

Hence the dilemma of MAOIs: If they work robustly, they're dangerous. If they're not dangerous, they don't work robustly. This is the fallacy with selegiline: It is marketed as a "safe" MAOI, but this is because it is not a very effective MAOI.

Clinical Efficacy

As is well known, an extensive literature shows that classic MAOIs, like phenelzine and tranylcypromine, are more effective than other antidepressants, like TCAs or SRIs. Many clinicians assume this greater efficacy extends to selegiline. This is not the case. No clinical trials have ever proven that selegiline is more effective than other antidepressants. Since selegiline does not increase norepinephrine or serotonin activity, unlike other MAOIs, it makes sense that it may not have similar clinical effects.

Dosing

The diminished efficacy of selegiline relative to other MAOIs is more relevant to the patch form of this medication, as opposed to the oral pill. FDA indication for MDD exists for the patch, but not the pill, mainly because the pill is generic; thus, the pharmaceutical industry was able to obtain profits by producing and studying a patch formulation. Biologically, the patch is a selective MAO-B inhibitor at 6–12 mg/d, but at higher doses, it blocks MAO-A. This is good if you want more antidepressant effect, but it is bad if you want to avoid the restrictive diet needed with classic MAOIs to prevent hypertensive crisis.

MAO-A inhibition begins at 9 mg/d but increases markedly above 12 mg/d, hence the pharmaceutical company's decision to cut off dosing at 12 mg/d. FDA recommendations are that MAOI dietary restrictions begin at 9 mg/d in any case based on the theoretical concern of MAO-A inhibition, although clinical harm through tyramine dietary exposure has not been reported extensively at that dose.

If the oral pill is used, the FDA-approved dose for Parkinson's disease is 5–10 mg/d. At that dose the drug is a selective MAO-B inhibitor, and no dietary restrictions are needed. At 15 mg/d, dietary restrictions often are recommended, and at 20–30 mg/d, some clinical studies find efficacy for acute depressive episodes, although such use of the oral pill would be off-label. At such doses, MAO-A inhibition occurs, and dietary restrictions should be instituted. Some experts thinks that selegiline may have less risk of hypertensive crisis, even at higher doses that inhibit MAO-A, than other MAOIs, but this clinical hypothesis has been neither proven nor disproven.

Bottom Line

- Selegiline is a mild dopaminergic agent.
- It is a selective MAO-B inhibitor, which is good for avoiding dietary restrictions, but bad for clinical efficacy.
- MAO-A inhibition is required for extensive antidepressant effects.
- Selegiline is not as effective as other MAOIs.
- It is not more effective than other antidepressants.

SERTRALINE (ZOLOFT)—DOPAMINERGIC, BELIEVED TO BE SAFE IN HEART DISEASE, BUT PERHAPS NOT

Typical dose: 50–100 mg/d (range 25–200 mg/d)
Biological mechanism: Dopamine and serotonin reuptake inhibition
Typical side effects: Sexual dysfunction, diarrhea
Medically important side effects: None known
Clinically proven efficacy: FDA indications for MDD, OCD, panic disorder, PTSD, social anxiety, premenstrual dysphoric disorder

Biological Mechanism

Sertraline is a classic SRI, well-known to most clinicians. It's easy to dose and has a wide range of uses.

What few know is that it isn't a pure SRI. It has notable dopamine reuptake inhibition. In some animal studies, its dopamine reuptake blockade is similar to methylphenidate's. It's hard to know whether this mechanism has important clinical effects in humans, though. One would expect weight loss and enhanced sexual function with such dopaminergic effects, yet these clinical outcomes don't tend to occur in humans.

Sertraline is the best-studied antidepressant in persons with heart disease, and it's the most proven, safest agent in the setting of cardiovascular diseases. The Sertraline Against Depression and Heart Disease in Congestive Heart Failure (SADHART) study didn't find that sertraline improved cardiac outcomes, though some analyses suggest some such benefits. But at least, it was commonly argued, it can be stated that it doesn't worsen cardiac outcomes and has no known cardiac risks. (The same cannot be said of many other antidepressants, such as bupropion, which has an amphetamine-related structure and can cause cardiac arrhythmias; or venlafaxine, which has some association with increased risk of sudden cardiac death, which is also the case with methylphenidate.) Further analysis of the SADHART data indicated elevated stroke risk and a small increase in overall cardiovascular mortality (see Chapter 32). Hence presumed cardiac safety may be questionable.

Clinical Efficacy

It often isn't appreciated that the randomized trial literature of sertraline in MDD, conducted in the 1990s, was almost entirely outpatient, not conducted in hospitalized patients. Thus, there is no appreciable scientific evidence that sertraline is effective in hospitalized or severe depression.

It has few drug interactions and can be used without much concern about liver interactions, unlike some other SRIs.

Dosing

At low doses (25–50 mg/d), sertraline is more purely serotonergic and has anxiolytic effects. Its mean effective dose in the MDD studies was about 75 mg/d (with a range of 50–100 mg/d). Though it can be dosed higher, it hasn't been proven to be more effective for MDD above 100 mg/d than below that dose.

Bottom Line

- Sertraline is a versatile agent, but not proven effective in severe depression.
- It has dopaminergic mechanisms, but clinical implications are unclear.
- It is believed to be the safest antidepressant in persons with cardiovascular disease, but this common belief may not be correct.

TRAZODONE—THE PERFECT INSOMNIA DRUG?

Biological Mechanism

Trazodone is an SRI with partial serotonin-receptor 1 (5HT1a-receptor) agonism.

Clinical Efficacy

Trazodone is FDA-indicated for MDD, not insomnia. It was developed originally in the late 1980s as one of the first SRI antidepressants. It was found to have little to no sexual dysfunction, but it was too sedating at antidepressant doses. This weakness became its strength, as it began to be used ubiquitously as an add-on treatment for insomnia, which was a side effect of other SRIs. Over the years, it has evolved into a standard treatment for insomnia, even though there are no randomized studies that prove its efficacy for primary insomnia, and it has no FDA indication for insomnia. Since it doesn't affect GABA receptors, unlike other sedatives, it isn't addictive.

Effects on Sleep

There is a belief that trazodone improves sleep cycles, uniquely so among sedatives, the rest of which (including benzodiazepines and zolpidem and newer agents) either worsen sleep stage efficiency or are neutral at best. Specifically, the other agents add about half an hour of sleep, but at the cost of less restorative deep-stage sleep (stages 3 and 4). Trazodone instead appears to improve sleep efficiency and increases those deep sleep stages.

One blinded study found that trazodone increases total sleep time by about 50 minutes, which is about double most other sedatives. Furthermore, deep stages 3 and 4 sleep are increased from about 19% at baseline and with placebo to about 31% with trazodone. Another study found 37 minutes increased total sleep with trazodone, and an increase in deep sleep stages from 56 minutes to 87 minutes. In summary, consistently replicated randomized data indicate that trazodone improves sleep efficiency, unlike all other sedatives.

Dosing

At 50–100 mg/d, trazodone is sedating and used for sleep. Antidepressant effects occur in the 200–400 mg/d range. In bipolar illness, such doses could be destabilizing and/or cause mania.

Side Effects

The main side effects are sedation and possible priapism.

Bottom Line

- Trazodone improves sleep cycles, in contrast to all other sedatives.
- It isn't addictive.
- Higher doses may produce antidepressant effects, for better or worse (e.g., bipolar illness).

VENLAFAXINE (EFFEXOR) AND DESVENLAFAXINE (PRISTIQ)—PROBLEMATIC IN HEART DISEASE, TERRIBLE SEROTONIN WITHDRAWAL

Typical dose: 150–300 mg/d (range 75–375 mg/d) for venlafaxine; 25–50 mg/d for desvenlafaxine
Biological mechanism: Serotonin and norepinephrine reuptake inhibition
Typical side effects: Sexual dysfunction, sedation
Medically important side effects: Sudden cardiac death, hypertension
Clinically proven efficacy: FDA indications for MDD, panic disorder

Biological Mechanism

Venlafaxine has been marketed as a serotonin-norepinephrine reuptake inhibitor (SNRI), as a way to try to differentiate it from other SRIs. But in fact, venlafaxine is just another potent SRI, with some noradrenergic reuptake blockade at higher doses. It isn't the reverse: it isn't a potent noradrenergic reuptake blocker, with some serotonin reuptake blockade. In this sense, it is much more like fluoxetine (Prozac) than it is like duloxetine (Cymbalta). Fluoxetine is the classic SRI prototype, but many clinicians don't realize that it also has some norepinephrine reuptake blockade, in fact, similar in potency in animal studies to venlafaxine. In contrast, duloxetine is a much more potent norepinephrine reuptake blocker than venlafaxine, while still having some serotonin reuptake blockade (unlike the purely potent norepinephrine reuptake blocker, desipramine).

In other words, venlafaxine is much more like other SRIs than like classic noradrenergic agents such as desipramine.

Clinical Efficacy

Like other SRIs, venlafaxine has proven efficacy in MDD, mostly in moderate to severe cases, not mild MDD. There are some data showing more benefit with venlafaxine in hospitalized depression compared to other SRIs. However, specific randomized studies of venlafaxine in patients who failed SRIs found that venlafaxine is NOT more effective than other SRIs in that setting of treatment-resistant depression (unlike the adjunctive efficacy proven with aripiprazole and brexpiprazole).

It has few drug interactions and can be used without much concern about liver interactions, unlike some other SRIs.

Dosing

At low doses (37.5–75 mg/d), venlafaxine is more purely serotonergic and has anxiolytic effects. Its mean effective dose in the MDD studies was about 225 mg/d (with a range of 150–300 mg/d). Though it can be dosed higher, it hasn't been proven to be more effective for MDD above 300 mg/d than below that dose.

Cardiac Harms

Most U.S. clinicians don't realize that venlafaxine is one of the most dangerous antidepressants to use in the setting of cardiovascular disease (in contrast to other agents, like sertraline, proven relatively safe in that setting). There were some cases of sudden cardiac death with venlafaxine, which were not known until some years after its introduction to the marketplace in the 1990s. Awareness of these cases led the U.K. regulatory body to contraindicate it in 2004 in all persons with hypertension or heart disease. After some protest from clinicians and the relevant pharmaceutical company, the U.K. regulatory body revised its restriction in 2006 to restrict venlafaxine use only in persons with uncontrolled hypertension or in persons at high risk of ventricular arrhythmia.

It's well known that venlafaxine raises blood pressure. The amount of increase has been downplayed by its manufacturer, by giving a mean increase of only up to 3 mm Hg. But this average downplays the important minority of patients who have notable increases in blood pressure. In persons with hypertension, it doesn't make sense to use an antidepressant that worsens hypertension, when many other safer options are available.

Other Risks

Venlafaxine is among the worst agents for causing serotonin withdrawal syndrome, presumably due to its short half-life, which is still the case with the XR formulation. This agent also causes mania at least twice as much as is the case with other SRIs, according to randomized trials. Thus, it shouldn't be prescribed at all in bipolar depression.

Desvenlafaxine

This agent is the active metabolite of venlafaxine. Sometimes, active metabolites can have different effects than the parent drug, but this does not seem to be the case with desvenlafaxine. Except for some differences in dosing, all of the preceding benefits and harms apply to this agent as well.

Bottom Line

- Venlafaxine is more of a standard SRI than anything else.
- It has many harms, especially major cardiac risks, and is best avoided in patients with cardiac disease or hypertension.
- It has severe serotonin withdrawal syndrome and high risk of mania, and thus should not be used in bipolar illness.

ZIPRASIDONE—A COMBINED DOPAMINE BLOCKER (ANTIPSYCHOTIC) AND MONOAMINE AGONIST (ANTIDEPRESSANT)

Typical dose: 80–160 mg/d
Biological mechanism: Dopamine/serotonin blockade plus norepinephrine/serotonin reuptake blockade
Typical side effects: Akathisia
Medically important side effects: Cardiac arrhythmia

Biological Mechanism

Ziprasidone is a dopamine-2 and serotonin-2-receptor blocker, with potent norepinephrine and serotonin reuptake inhibitor effects. The latter monoamine reuptake effects are equivalent in potency to imipramine's, a classic TCA.

Clinical Efficacy

Ziprasidone is FDA-indicated for schizophrenia and mania. It has been shown to be effective in mixed depression, but it was found to be ineffective in two randomized trials of acute bipolar depression. Many clinicians have the experience that it is not effective enough for severe psychosis or mania, but it can be effective for moderate cases. It seems to have benefit for depressive states based on the mixed data just mentioned, but the negative bipolar depression studies should be noted. Its large dosing range, along with varying biochemical effects based on dose, as described later, have made it complicated to use. It has an intramuscular injectable formulation for acute agitation.

Dosing

Like most dopamine blockers, ziprasidone's dopamine blockade is dose-related in a curvilinear fashion, reaching classic antipsychotic thresholds of 80–90%, and dopamine blockade at 80–160 mg/d. In contrast, its potent norepinephrine and serotonin reuptake inhibition is present at all doses. Thus, at low doses, it has more antidepressant-like, and less anti-manic or antipsychotic, properties.

Side Effects

The most common side effect is akathisia, which is dose-related. Other Parkinsonian side effects also can occur. Ziprasidone does not have any cardiovascular or diabetes harms, nor does it cause weight gain. In the CATIE study, it was the agent with the best profile on lipid and diabetes parameters and in weight. It does increase QT length, which can increase the risk of cardiac arrhythmias. Due to is monoamine reuptake effects, it has been reported to cause manic episodes in some persons, and it may have some risk of serotonin withdrawal syndrome.

Bottom Line

- Ziprasidone has norepinephrine and serotonin reuptake blockade, like TCAs.
- It isn't effective for severe psychosis or mania, but it can help moderate states.
- It works in mixed depressive states.
- It has no metabolic harm or weight gain, but it can cause cardiac arrhythmia.

SECTION IV

Clinical Psychopharmacology of Diseases and Syndromes

16

Hippocratic Psychopharmacology

A Non-DSM Approach to Practice

A DISTINCTION CRUCIAL TO THE PRACTICE OF MEDICINE IS THE Hippocratic versus the Galenic approach. Until about 1900, the practice of medicine had been Galenic for almost two millennia. Only in the last century has medicine caught up with the profound insights of the Hippocratic method. The practice of psychopharmacology today has much in common with the practice of 19th century medicine. Table 16.1 highlights the distinction between Hippocratic and Galenic approaches to medicine.

A summary of the Galenic approach is that animal studies can reveal biological knowledge, from which one speculates on the nature of illnesses and symptoms. This biological theory—whether the "four humors" (black bile, yellow bile, blood, phlegm) or four neurotransmitters (dopamine, serotonin, norepinephrine, acetylcholine)—is used to provide a rationale for the aggressive use of many medications, which are seen as directly curative or effective in alleviating symptoms.

A summary of the Hippocratic approach is that clinical observations on humans provide the main evidence for the presence or absence of diseases. If diseases are present, the clinical observations of treatment studies will determine if effective treatments exist. If those treatments exist, and they improve on the natural course of recovery, they are given to aid natural recovery. In all other cases—where diseases are not present, or effective treatments are not clinically proven, or patients with diseases recover naturally more quickly than with treatments—treatments should not be given.

This is an essential point: the Hippocratic approach is *not* about "First, do no harm." In fact, nowhere in the Hippocratic corpus from the 5th century BC is that statement to be found. It was invented in the 19th century and later attributed incorrectly to Hippocrates.

The Hippocratic writings directly state something different: "*Practice two things with disease: Help, or at least do not harm.*"

TABLE 16.1 Hippocratic versus Galenic Approaches to Medicine

	Hippocratic approach	Galenic approach
Emphasis	Clinical observation	Biological theory
Evidence	Clinical trials/research	Animal data/biological speculation
Diagnosis	Disease-based	Symptom-based
Treatment	Conservative	Aggressive
Source of healing	Nature/God	Doctor/medication

The Hippocratic tradition is conservative, but not in an abstract sense. It is so only in relation to the concept of disease. This tradition is in fact quite aggressive about treating diseases; it emphasizes not treating conditions that are not diseases, however. The key is the presence or absence of disease. In this emphasis, the Hippocratic tradition completely contradicts the practice of contemporary psychopharmacology, which, as in the Galenic tradition, emphasizes the treatment of symptoms.

This is the key step where current psychiatry diverges from current medicine. In medicine today, it is generally considered unscientific and even inappropriate to only focus on symptoms. The primary concern is to identify diseases that may cause symptoms. Only if such diseases can be excluded can one turn to the question of whether or not to treat symptoms.

In psychiatry, in contrast, clinicians often happily treat symptoms, and ignore the whole concept of "disease." One cannot practice Hippocratically unless one takes the concept of disease seriously, and tries to match treatments to diseases, where they are proven effective. Figure 16.1 visually depicts this Hippocratic approach. Let's review the figure to clearly understand what it means to practice Hippocratic medicine, and why it is *not* "First, do no harm."

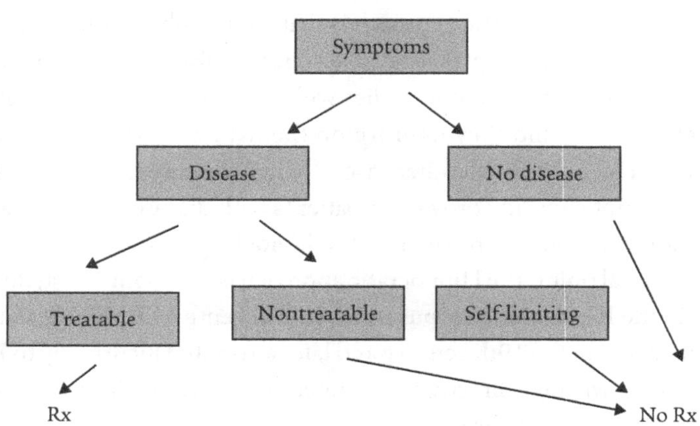

FIGURE 16.1 *Hippocratic practice.*

The patient first presents to the doctor with symptoms. The first step in the Hippocratic approach is to refuse to treat those symptoms. The doctor first investigates whether those symptoms represent a disease, or not.

Here, in this first step, one can see how current psychopharmacology immediately deviates from the Hippocratic tradition. A patient presents to a clinician today with symptoms of depression: he gets an antidepressant; with symptoms of anxiety: he gets an anxiolytic; with symptoms of poor attention or organization: he gets an amphetamine; with symptoms of mood lability: he gets a mood stabilizer; with symptoms of anger or aggression: he gets a dopamine blocker. It is routine for many patients with psychiatric diagnoses to be taking one or more of each of the drugs in each of the four classes just described. This is symptomatic, Galenic, non-Hippocratic psychopharmacology. It breaks the Hippocratic tradition from the very start.

The next step—after the all-important step of refusing to treat symptoms—is the step of seeing whether or not a disease is present. In psychiatry, this step is often ignored by practitioners who don't believe in the concept of psychiatric disease. One speaks of "mental disorders"; DSM-III and onwards has used the word "disorder" explicitly, rather than "disease," to avoid any *a priori* commitment to etiology. There are many rationales, some good, for this wish to be "atheoretical." But a harmful consequence of this DSM ideology about "mental disorder" is that it makes it impossible to practice Hippocratic medicine. The Hippocratic approach is disease-based; it requires the ability to, or at least the commitment to, identify the disease. If one rejects the whole concept of disease, then there is no hope of practicing Hippocratically.

It could be argued that there is no known psychiatric disease. This is not the case. General paralysis of the insane, a psychiatric diagnosis that was as common as dementia praecox (schizophrenia) in the early 20th century, turned out to be a disease later renamed *neurosyphilis*; psychiatrists cured that disease, and with it, cured millions of chronically psychotic individuals who were seen as hopeless. Penicillin is the most effect psychotropic medication ever discovered.

One might say that, although general paralysis of the insane might have been a disease, there are no other psychiatric diseases. This is not the case either. Schizophrenia has been well defined clinically, more or less as it is defined now, for over a century; 100 years of scientific research have identified important, replicated, definable biological mechanisms; genetic twin studies show that it is almost entirely inherited. There are good studies about its etiology based on 40-year prospective studies indicating potential second trimester infections as being important risk factors, added to baseline genetic susceptibility. As with schizophrenia, bipolar illness OCD, autism, and a few other conditions all have enough biological evidence to qualify as probable diseases by basic medical standards of disease definition. Certainly, there is much more evidence for viewing these conditions as diseases when compared to adjustment disorder with anxious mood, or brief reactive psychotic disorder, or histrionic personality disorder, or probably about 380 out of 392 DSM-IV psychiatric diagnoses.

Most DSM "disorders" are not diseases; but this does not mean that *all* of them are not diseases.

When applying Hippocratic psychopharmacology, the job of the clinician is to examine a patient's symptoms for the presence of psychiatric conditions that are well identified clinically and biologically to such an extent that they are close to medical definitions of disease.

If one can agree that at least some psychiatric conditions are diseases, then the job of the clinician is to identify these diseases first, if they are present. If present, then the next step is to assess the clinical research evidence (this would be the step called "evidence-based medicine," or EBM) to see if there are treatments that are proven effective. If so, the clinician would give those treatments. This is how a Hippocratic clinician would prescribe a medication.

Just as important—more important—is when and how a Hippocratic clinician would *not* prescribe a medication. Basically, in all of the previous steps, if the answer is "No," then a Hippocratic clinician would refuse to prescribe a medication, even despite a patient's entreaties, preferences, the culture's fads, the permission of a secular government, or the peer pressure of one's professional colleagues. If there is no identifiable disease, then the Hippocratic clinician would not prescribe. If there is an identifiable disease, but the available treatments are not proven effective or are proven ineffective, then the Hippocratic clinician would not prescribe. If there is an identifiable disease, but it is self-limiting, and naturally leads to recovery faster or to the same extent as happens with available treatments (as is the case of much "major depressive disorder"), then the Hippocratic clinician would not prescribe.

In other words, there are many, many scenarios where the Hippocratic clinician would not prescribe medications, and a few where he or she would.

This is how one causes more help than harm. Not through an abstract conservatism—the false belief in "First, do no harm"; but rather, through a disease-based commitment to treating only diseases that are treatable, and refusing to treat symptoms alone, or diseases that either will remit naturally or which are untreatable. This is how one reaches the Hippocratic goal: "Help, or at least do not harm."

There are some obvious rejoinders and clarifications that are needed. First, the Hippocratic approach is a matter of emphasis; it is not simplistic nor dogmatic. The teaching is not "Never treat symptoms." It is "Try not to treat just symptoms." The teaching is not "Never reason biologically." It is "Try to use clinical observation and research the most."

So, after the hard work of trying to identify diseases, it may be that symptoms still will need to be treated. The patient may have a terminal medical illness in which end-stage pain deserves compassionate, palliative treatment. The patient may have chronic pain syndrome of unknown etiology in which some medication-based pain treatment may be unavoidable. The patient may have anxiety as part of the personality in which some relief of symptoms may be obtained with anxiolytic medication. But in all these cases, this symptomatic treatment is provided as a last, not first, resort, and, in this Hippocratic approach, it is provided with an awareness that a very different kind of pharmacology is being practiced—not a curative one, but a palliative one. Doses will be minimized to what is possible; addictive agents will be minimized; duration of treatment will be constantly reassessed. In contrast, if a disease is present, like bipolar disorder, even toxic medications, like lithium, will be provided, and for a long duration, and at higher doses if proven effective.

NINETEENTH CENTURY DIAGNOSIS, TWENTY-FIRST CENTURY TREATMENT

The First Truth of Psychopharmacology is "Your treatment is as good as your diagnosis." Psychopharmacology is, first and foremost, *nosology*, or the art and science of diagnosis. If the diagnosis is wrong, it doesn't matter how much one knows about drugs; one can do nothing but harm the patient, without much benefit. If the diagnosis is right, then the pharmacological knowledge needed is often rather straightforward. Get the diagnosis right; then the treatment will be simple. Complex treatment often reflects poor or mistaken diagnosis.

A major problem in contemporary psychiatry is that many clinicians identify diagnosis with the DSM or *International Classification of Diseases* (ICD) symptoms of classification. This is natural. The American Psychiatric Association (APA) and its international counterparts have devised these diagnostic manuals specifically for that purpose—to tell clinicians how to diagnose. This is a major feature of late 20th century psychiatry. The third revision of the DSM (DSM-III) was published in 1980, and most of it has remained largely unchanged since that date.

But, although 1980 was a momentous year for the United States, including the election of Ronald Reagan as president, there was such a thing as psychiatry before Reagan, and even psychiatric nosology. There were other approaches to diagnosis, such as those of Emil Kraepelin and Karl Jaspers, among others, which were put aside and ignored, or completely rejected, by DSM-III in 1980. Some of those decisions were related to that time; the scientific evidence to that date may have led to some conclusions, which, with half a century of more data, may not be as defensible now. Furthermore, the entire DSM process was suffused with non-scientific, professional concerns that were unique to the American psychiatric profession when Reagan was president. They are irrelevant to world psychiatry today. A return to an analysis of some pre-1980 ideas in diagnosis may help today.

The standard approach to psychiatric diagnosis, then, is to apply DSM (now in its fifth revision, DSM-5) and ICD (now in its 11th revision, ICD-11) definitions. One then applies current biological beliefs, based on speculations from animal studies, to those DSM/ICD diagnoses. This biologically speculative approach to psychopharmacology is generally based on neurotransmitters and their effects on receptors and synapses. This might be called "synaptic psychopharmacology," and it is the core of most of the work of the middle and late periods of the 20th century, when the monoamine systems and their relationships to psychotropic drugs were delineated. The "monoamine hypothesis" of psychosis and mood conditions followed. Now, it is known that the monoamine hypothesis is false. Instead of synaptic mechanisms, research at the very end of the 20th and into the 21st century is showing that psychotropic drugs have immense postsynaptic mechanisms, at the level of the second messengers, intracellular proteins, genetic transcription, and neuroplasticity. The simplistic 20th century synaptic picture of neurotransmitters as "keys" and receptors as "locks" is less and less relevant.

In short, the mainstream practice of psychiatry today involves 20th century nosology and 20th century psychopharmacology. This textbook advocates turning the clock back on diagnosis and forward on treatment: a return closer to 19th century nosology and progress into the 21st century psychopharmacology.

The watershed period for psychiatric diagnosis was the year 1980, with the third revision of the DSM. Some history is needed to appreciate why the current DSM-5 system, little changed in its basic structure from DSM-III, may not be valid for psychopharmacology today.

Why did DSM-III happen? What led up to 1980? The standard history, which is correct in its broad outlines, is that American psychiatrists began to realize that their psychoanalytic focus of the prior half-century needed revision. From the 1920s, when Freud's ideas began to be popular, until the 1960s, there was an almost complete hegemony of Freudian ideology in American psychiatry. No other thoughts were given much credence. Kraepelin was hopelessly old-fashioned, and proven false by the id, ego, and superego. Anna Freud served as a one-person Politburo, deciding which of her father's writings would be published and how, censoring them in the process. There was an "orthodoxy," as in any religious or political sect, and "heretics." There was little to no science, in the sense of experimental research that was objective and replicable, or in the sense of clinical studies that were quantitatively analyzed by statistical methods. In the Freudian schema, diagnosis was little valued. Everyone experienced mental states on a spectrum from neurosis to psychosis, and what mattered was not the specific kinds of symptoms experienced, but rather the intrapsychic causes of those symptoms, causes that were largely uniform for all kinds of symptoms. Everything came down to unconscious emotions and their impact on mental life, including defenses to those emotions. Since all humans have unconscious emotions, all humans have some neurosis, and thus the line between health and illness was blurry if not nonexistent. The concept of "disease," accordingly, had little role.

Hence psychoanalysts thought little about diagnosis, did not study or research it, and did not emphasize the importance of classification of diagnoses. The spectrum of neurosis to psychosis was enough. With that, and the impressive edifice of psychoanalytic theory, they could practice and "diagnose" and treat everyone.

This system was accepted and practiced with little dissent for about two generations, from the 1920s to the 1960s, in the United States. Internationally, there were places where it had less influence (Germany, England) and places where it had more impact (Spain, Italy, Latin America; one could say psychoanalytic hegemony continues mostly unabated today in Argentina, for instance). There have always been skeptics; those who followed other traditions such as the socially focused eclecticism of Adolf Meyer (best exemplified by his pupil and the leader of British psychiatry, Aubrey Lewis), or the traditions of Karl Jaspers, or Kraepelin, or Carl Wernicke (best exemplified by the work of Karl Leonhard). These schools of thought persisted, as minority groups, and they began to experience a resurgence in the 1960s and 1970s that coincided with a major change in world psychiatry: the rise of psychopharmacology.

The radical third revision of the DSM was developed in 1980 to put forward an agenda; initially, there was some scientific impetus to that agenda, the laudable wish to base psychiatric diagnosis on scientific evidence that is valid—in other words, that clinicians should practice the medical specialty of psychiatry based on scientific knowledge, not ideology. The ideology of the time was psychoanalysis, thus the impetus was seen as being biological, which it was to some extent. This action met a reaction in the psychoanalytic establishment of the American Psychiatric Association (APA): the result was the compromise named DSM-III. About a dozen scientifically valid diagnoses were expanded in about two years to over 200 claimed diagnoses, including a whole category, "personality disorders," that was created overnight. Most personality disorders had little to no scientific validation at the time, and they still have very little, especially in comparison to the huge literature on dimensional nosology for personality, which continues to be rejected by DSM nosology.

The defense was that even if the DSM-III diagnoses weren't all scientifically valid, at least the new nosology was clear, and thus the diagnoses were reliable; clinicians could all agree to define them a certain way. Then those reliable diagnoses could be further studied in research to see if they were valid or not; further revisions could then replace the invalid ones with more valid ones. Reliability would lead to validity.

Over three decades later, one can say definitively that this wish has not come to pass. The fourth edition of DSM, DSM-IV (1994), was to the third edition like Stalin was to Lenin: an ideological hardening of the DSM categories, despite their poor scientific validity. The categories were expanded further to over 300, and the bar for making changes based on scientific changes was set so high that few changes were made.

Instead, a new philosophy for psychiatric diagnosis was put forward by the leadership of DSM-IV: "pragmatism." Science was barely relevant anymore. Instead, what mattered were the "pragmatic" consequences of defining psychiatric diagnoses one way versus another. Decisions were made by the DSM leadership based on what they deemed was good for patients or for the profession or for society. Such pragmatic decisions need not have anything to do with what is true. Should one define hypomania as four days versus two days, or personality disorders as having or not having sexual abuse, or allowing children to be diagnosed as having bipolar illness? On these and hundreds of other diagnostic issues, the central approach in DSM-IV was to ask the question "Is it good for us and patients or not?" The question was not "What is true?"

Reliability became an end in itself, and the profession gave up on validity. This disregard for truth partly stems from disbelief. The DSM leadership reflected much of mainstream psychiatry, which reflects much of our culture: a postmodernist cultural zeitgeist has affected Western society for the last half-century such that relativism about truth and skepticism about science have become as standard in a 55-year-old academic as in a 14-year-old teenager. Many devalue science and scientific truth; hence, it's easy to be attracted to pragmatic sophistry in psychiatric diagnosis. Yet, two decades after DSM-IV, one can say that such pragmatic nosology may well be a central reason why there has not been much progress in psychiatric knowledge and practice.

If the profession defines psychiatric diagnoses based on professional and social preferences in 1980 or 1994 or 2013, why should Nature go along? Why should the genetics or neurobiology or pharmacology of psychiatric diseases correspond with our cultural desires in a given society at a given time in human history? This is the deep conceptual problem with DSM-III and IV, and unfortunately, since it did not change in its core, DSM-5.

For these reasons, just as the National Institute of Mental Health (NIMH) has deemed DSM-5 definitions to be inadequate for scientific research, this textbook takes the approach that DSM-5 definitions are inadequate for the scientific practice of clinical psychopharmacology. Diagnostic discussions, therefore, will not be based on or limited to DSM-5 concepts.

The chapters that follow focus on the treatment of illnesses, not symptoms, following the Hippocratic tradition. While the first part of this book presented medications in their pharmacology, by their drug classes, the second part focuses on their use for illness groups. Since the same class of medications can be used for different illness groups, there will be overlap between chapters in discussion of the same classes of medications. The basic pharmacology has been described in the first part of this textbook, and that knowledge will be presumed. The focus in the following chapters is on the use of those medications for different clinical presentations.

Since treatment is only as good as the diagnosis, each section will begin with specific diagnostic considerations relevant to treatment. For the reasons given in this chapter, diagnostic discussion will not be limited to DSM definitions, but will include non-DSM definitions as well, with both approaches described and explained as needed.

SELECTED REFERENCES

Decker, H. S. (2013). *The making of DSM-III: A diagnostic manual's conquest of American psychiatry*. Oxford, UK: Oxford University Press.

Ghaemi, S. N. (2008). Toward a Hippocratic psychopharmacology. *Canadian Journal of Psychiatry, 53*(3), 189–196.

Shorter, E. (2003). *Before Prozac: The troubled history of mood disorders*. Oxford, UK: Oxford University Press.

Wootton, D. (2007). *Bad medicine: Doctors doing harm since Hippocrates*. Oxford, UK: Oxford University Press.

17

Beyond Symptoms

Diagnostic Validators

If symptoms are not the primary target for drug treatment, as the Hippocratic tradition teaches, then diagnosis becomes extremely important for the practice of clinical psychopharmacology. As discussed in the previous chapter, the importance and diagnosis entails paying careful attention to be as scientific as possible in our diagnostic system. The DSM approach has failed in this regard for the past three decades, as described there. One cannot, therefore, solely rely on DSM diagnoses in the practice of clinical psychopharmacology. A more scientific approach is needed. Yet clinical practice requires a scientific approach that is clinical, not preclinical. The NIMH solution of the Research Domain Criteria (RDoC) criteria does not address this problem, since those criteria are "preclinical," meaning that they are based on animal studies and or biological research tests, such as PET scans. These approaches are not using clinical practice, and do not help the practicing clinician at the present time or in the foreseeable future. A scientific clinical diagnostic system, not the socially constructed DSM criteria and not the clinically relevant RDoC criteria, is needed.

The solution, scientific research on clinical diagnoses, has been an approach that is based on a century of medical research, and has been well established and accepted psychiatric research for the past half-century. This approach involves the classic diagnostic validators. In this chapter, these diagnostic validators will be described, and their relevance to clinical practice of psychopharmacology will be examined.

The key insight as to the importance of diagnostic validators is the fact that clinical symptoms by themselves are inadequate, insufficient, and misleading for medical diagnosis. This is an obvious fact, and is widely accepted in medical research and practice. Pain in the chest is insufficient to diagnose coronary artery disease, since it can also be caused by musculoskeletal problems of the ribs or by gastrointestinal problems, among other possibilities. Over a century ago, in the late 19th century, clinicians like William Osler and others showed that clinical diagnosis by means of signs and symptoms at the bedside needed to be validated by an independent source of evidence. The best source, they found, was pathology at autopsy. If a patient had yellow skin and a fever, it was determined that that clinical syndrome reflected hepatitis by microscopic examination of the liver at autopsy. Some patients might have yellow skin but no fever, and an autopsy would show no abnormality of the liver. This information could then be taken back to the bedside, and used to draw clinical judgments about the relevance of yellow skin as a symptom to diagnoses of hepatitis versus other possible illnesses. Symptoms alone could not differentiate different illnesses. Pathology was the gold standard. This was called the classic clinical pathological approach to medical diagnosis.

In psychiatry, there is no gold standard. A century of research was unable to associate abnormalities in the brain at autopsy with the major psychiatric illnesses of schizophrenia and manic depressive illness. There was a need for an alternative approach, which is how the concept of multiple diagnostic validators was developed.

Let's revisit the central insight behind the need for diagnostic validators besides symptoms.

A patient has pneumonia with cough and headache. Another patient has pneumonia without a cough and headache. Are these two different "disorders"? Most clinicians would say no, because the symptoms of cough and headache do not represent a different disease.

A patient has depression with mania. Another has depression without mania. Are these two different "disorders"? These days most clinicians would say yes, because that is what the DSM has taught. Mania has a different set of symptoms than depression, one might argue. But cough and headache are symptoms, which clinicians agree do not represent a different disease.

That is the intuition behind the concept of diagnostic validators. It is not enough to say that symptoms differ and thus we have different "disorders." One has to show that those different symptoms represent some kind of different conditions or diseases.

How can we do this? Not by simply referring back to the different symptoms: that would be tautologous. There has to be some different line of evidence, separate from symptoms, that represents a different illness. In the case of pneumonia, clinicians have access to pathology: tests can show evidence of inflammation in the lung, whether or not you have a cough and fever. So those symptoms do not represent a different disease. In the case of psychiatry, there is no access to pathology (usually). So what should the independent lines of evidence be?

This is where a classic article from 1970, discussed in Chapter 46, revolutionized psychiatry. Eli Robins, who had trained in Boston, was chairman at the Washington University in St. Louis. In that era, the major U.S. cities were dominated by psychoanalytic thinking. Robins was influenced by Emil Kraepelin, the late 19th century German psychiatrist who taught that "diagnosis is prognosis"; that the course of illness tells you which symptoms represent different diseases. Robins left Boston to go to the smaller city of St. Louis, and from there, he trained a series of researchers who produced the change in U.S. psychiatry, which led to the third edition of DSM (DSM-III) in 1980. With his colleague Samuel Guze, Robins articulated four other diagnostic validators that, along with symptoms, should be used to identify whether groups of patients differ from each other enough to justify seeing them as having different diagnoses (their article focused on schizophrenia, but they later applied these principles to all diagnoses).

Those validators are as follows:

1. Symptoms
2. Course of illness
3. Genetics
4. Treatment effects
5. Laboratory tests or biological markers

The most important validator is course of illness, Kraepelin's key criterion. Some conditions are chronic, and symptoms are present all the time (like schizophrenia); others are episodic, with symptoms coming and going (like manic-depression). The next most important validator is genetics: if diagnoses are genetic, you'll find evidence in family members. Next are laboratory tests or biological markers, which are useful in research more than in clinical practice, but they can be useful clinically sometimes, as in white matter abnormalities on MRI of the brain in the diagnosis of vascular depression. Robins and Guze also referred to "delimitation from other disorders," which meant that symptoms were specific to one condition rather than another. This is not always the case, since many symptoms, like anxiety, can occur in many conditions. Since that classic study, instead of delimitation, the diagnostic validator of treatment effects has been used, although it should be used cautiously, since many drugs are nonspecific in effect, and some, like amphetamines, are even effective in normal individuals. Treatment effects can also be seen as a proxy for biological markers, but only if treatment effects are specific to an illness (like antidepressant-induced mania).

Unfortunately, these diagnostic validators have been suppressed by the evolution of DSM. Originally, these diagnostic validators were the basis for scientific justification for diagnoses in psychiatric research, leading to the original Research Diagnostic Criteria (RDC) that Robins's St. Louis group created. The RDC identified about two dozen scientifically valid diagnoses. DSM-III started with those diagnoses, and added about 270 others. In almost all cases, although the other diagnostic validators were used to justify diagnoses, only symptoms were used in the DSM criteria definitions (an exception is schizophrenia, where there is a course criterion of six months or longer for psychosis). Now we have about 400 diagnoses in DSM-5, and clinicians are used to only looking at symptoms for definitions. This leads to the perennial arguments: "Is the attentional problem ADD or bipolar disorder?" "Is the anxiety part of a major depressive disorder or generalized anxiety disorder?" "Is the sexual impulsivity a mania or a paraphilia or borderline personality?" These debates will never end as long as they are conducted on the single dimension of symptoms.

This classic paper reminds us that symptoms only go so far: as in the case of cough and fever, clinicians need to look elsewhere to know which symptoms matter diagnostically and which do not. They need to look to course of illness, genetics, and treatment effects. Clinicians should learn to use these four modified diagnostic validators in clinical practice, as will be emphasized in the chapters that follow.

APPLICATIONS TO CLINICAL PRACTICE

The application of these ideas to clinical practice would entail paying much less attention to symptoms in the context of clinical diagnosis, and instead obtaining information from family history and course of illness especially, and sometimes treatment effects, to make a diagnosis more probable than others. Symptoms are the main clinical features used for diagnostic purposes by the DSM system. Even though the other diagnostic validators—like genetics and the course of illness—are used sometimes to support the diagnostic concepts included in the DSM, those same diagnostic validators are not allowed into DSM criteria sets. For instance, sexual abuse is a clear validator of diagnosis for borderline personality, but this course criterion is not allowed in the definition of DSM criteria for borderline personality disorder. The rationale given by DSM leadership for this approach is that they want to exclude any claims to etiology, but unfortunately, this approach can lead to overdiagnosis of borderline personality in some individuals who do not have this important predictor of the diagnosis. Many other examples could be given.

The upshot of this discussion is that clinicians should look into course of illness much more carefully, as well as family history, and include that information in addition to symptoms, equally or even more importantly, for diagnostic purposes. Some examples will be given here, and will be repeated in the following chapters.

A typical scenario is a patient who presents with the clinical syndrome of a full depressive episode, and does not have any prior manic symptoms that meet full definitions for hypomanic or manic episodes. The DSM diagnosis would be "major depressive disorder." The patient would have a mother with diagnosed and confirmed bipolar illness type I. In the DSM system, this family history will be ignored completely for diagnostic purposes. In the scientific, non-DSM-based approach that incorporates all diagnostic validators, the family history would indicate that the patient's affective illness is related to bipolar illness, and not different from it. The technical diagnosis of bipolar illness using DSM definitions could not be made, but the DSM-based diagnosis of MDD, as different from bipolar illness, also would be rejected. If this patient also had an early age of onset of the first depressive episode at age 15, with multiple brief episodes lasting three months or less, the bipolar-like course of illness would be confirmed as more relevant to diagnosis and treatment, rather than the opposite approach of ignoring course and genetics entirely, as the DSM system would do in insisting on the diagnosis of MDD. In the non-DSM approach, this patient would be treated with agents that often are used for bipolar illness, like second-messenger modifiers or dopamine blockers, and would not be limited to treatment with standard monoamine agonist antidepressants, as would be the practice when focusing on the DSM diagnostic label of MDD.

Another scenario is a patient who presents with marked inattention and executive dysfunction, and is diagnosed with adult ADD. The patient denies past depressive or manic episodes or severe anxiety states. The course of illness indicates that the patient reports having had similar symptoms in childhood, although he never received clinical attention or diagnosis at that time. The patient is high-functioning as a lawyer, is successful in his life, but feels that his cognitive symptoms keep him from functioning even better. Family history identifies schizophrenia in his uncle. Since ADD is not genetically associated with schizophrenia, his family history would throw major doubt on the diagnosis of ADD. In fact, if the underlying biology of the patient's cognition is genetically related to schizophrenia, treatment with amphetamines would only worsen that underlying biology, and it could worsen some of his clinical symptoms. Further investigation of the patient's history will be warranted, and if there was evidence of paranoid features, for instance, other diagnostic possibilities will be raised, such as schizotypal personality, which is genetically associated with schizophrenia.

A third case scenario could involve a patient in her mid-30s with multiple mood swings and unstable interpersonal relationships, diagnosed with borderline personality. Assessment of the course of illness found that these symptoms were present for the past three years, but had not been present for five years before that time. Hence, the course of illness is not consistent with the long-term chronicity associated with the concept of personality disorders. Family history identifies a sister who committed suicide, and an uncle who was institutionalized with the diagnosis of manic-depressive illness in the 1950s. This family history is consistent with affective illness, not borderline personality. The course of illness also is not consistent with borderline personality. This evaluation would make the likelihood of affective illness more probable than borderline personality, once the other diagnostic validators are taken into account.

In summary, clinical diagnosis cannot be, and should not be, limited to symptoms primarily, as is common practice today. The DSM system encourages this emphasis on symptoms mainly, which leads to never-ending controversies. Many of these clinical dilemmas can be resolved by taking other diagnostic validators seriously, especially family genetics and course of illness. Clinicians are encouraged to evaluate symptoms but then also to focus on family genetics and course of illness, so as to clarify diagnoses in clinical practice. In short, the classic diagnostic validators should be used not only in research, but also in clinical practice.

SELECTED REFERENCES

Cloninger, C. R. (1989). Establishment of diagnostic validity in psychiatric illness: Robins and Guze's method reconsidered. In L. N. Robins, J. E. Barrett, eds, The validity of psychiatric diagnosis, New York: Raven Press, pp. 9–18.

Robins, E., Guze, S. B. (1970). Establishment of diagnostic validity in psychiatric illness: Its application to schizophrenia. *American Journal of Psychiatry, 126* (7): 983–7.

18

The Concept of a Diagnostic Hierarchy

A CENTRAL ASPECT OF TAKING A NON-DSM APPROACH TO CLINICAL PSYchopharmacology is the importance of tackling the "comorbidity" problem. In the DSM system, all diagnoses are created equal and clinicians are encouraged to diagnose as many disorders as possible. In practice, multiple drugs are given for multiple "disorders," thus comorbidities lead to polypharmacy. As discussed previously, since many DSM diagnoses are created for social/professional purposes, and thus overlap in content, the apparent comorbidity can lead to unnecessary treatment.

The countervailing concept to DSM's comorbidities is the idea of a diagnostic hierarchy. If a Hippocratic approach places the emphasis on diagnosis and disease, then a corollary is that diagnoses and diseases should only be identified when they are present, and not multiplied unnecessarily. The diagnostic hierarchy concept is a solution to this problem.

Two key problems for any psychiatric nosology are to set the boundary between normality/health and psychiatric illness, and to set the boundary between different psychiatric illnesses. The first is called the "false positives problem"; the second, the "comorbidity problem."

Two basic solutions have been offered in the past: diagnostic hierarchies versus diagnostic thresholds. Over time, DSM-III to DSM-5 decided against diagnostic hierarchies and for diagnostic thresholds, as solutions to these boundary problems.

This chapter examines the medical and scientific soundness of the diagnostic threshold approach, identifies the comorbidity problem, and proposed an empirically based diagnostic hierarchy approach as a solution.

THE DIAGNOSTIC THRESHOLD APPROACH

Differentiating Normality from Illness

Ever since DSM-III, psychiatric nosology has been based on the organizing principle of *diagnostic thresholds.* This view is that, as symptoms or dysfunctions increase in severity, a cutoff will differentiate those who should be diagnosed from those who should not. This is the proposed solution for dealing with the "false positives" problem of differentiating psychiatric illness form normal psychological problems in the general population. But statistical models demonstrate that this approach fails to reduce false positive rates below a floor of about 50%. Besides those statistical considerations, this approach is fraught with a conceptual problem: the fact that the association of symptomatic with functional impairment is questionable. For instance, in bipolar illness, it has been shown that despite full symptomatic recovery after an acute manic episode in almost all patients, marked functional impairment is seen in about two-thirds of those same patients. The historical example of hypertension also is important. The sphygmomanometer was discovered in the late 19th century, but for five decades, despite knowing that readings of 200–300 systolic, and above 100 diastolic, were abnormal, physicians did not treat patients with hypertension unless those measurements were associated with marked physical symptoms, such as headache. We now know that by the time such symptoms occur, hypertension usually has been present for decades, and the likelihood of stroke will be quite high. In the famous case of President Franklin Roosevelt, blood pressures of greater 200/100 were noted daily for years in the White House without any treatment being given. Even with readings near the end of his life of 300/200, Roosevelt only reported mild headache.

In short, to distinguish normality from illness, the diagnostic threshold solution has important limitations medically and scientifically.

Differentiating Illnesses from Each Other

Besides distinguishing illness and normality, nosology must distinguish illnesses from each other. In psychiatry, the principle has been the same: the standard DSM solution is to have high diagnostic thresholds to make these distinctions between psychiatric illnesses.

The symptom/function thesis is thought to handle the comorbidity problem by the following axiom: more severe symptoms with marked functional impairment should get diagnostic precedence over milder symptoms. Many clinicians intuitively practice this way. For instance, if a patient presents with severe anxiety and mild depression, clinicians tend to diagnose a primary anxiety condition, with depressive symptoms secondary to anxiety. If a patient presents with severe depression and mild anxiety, an opposite judgment is made. This is an intuitive application of the DSM approach.

A few problems arise with the assumptions of this model. If the severity of symptoms is emphasized, often patients complain of or experience a symptom as quite severe, whereas that symptom is not central to the disease: in contrast, cardinal features of a disease may not be severe at all, or may even be fully asymptomatic. For instance, a patient with autoimmune deficiency syndrome (AIDS) may complain bitterly of fever, but not of the human immunodeficiency virus (HIV) virus itself. A patient with pneumonia may complain mainly of malaise, but only have mild difficulty breathing. A patient with mania may have marked distress from poor attention, but will not see his decreased need for sleep as much of a problem. A patient with depression may have much worse insomnia than anhedonia.

In short, to distinguish illnesses from each, the diagnostic threshold solution continues to have important limitations medically and scientifically.

The Comorbidity Problem

By focusing on diagnostic thresholds alone, and rejecting the concept of diagnostic hierarchies, the DSM system produces the well-known problem of comorbidities. For instance, most persons who meet those affective illness diagnostic definitions also meet anxiety disorder diagnostic definitions.

The DSM approach to comorbidity is a misuse of the term. As originally invented in 1970 by Feinstein, "co-morbidity" meant the co-occurrence by chance of two independent and separate diseases, such as gout and dementia. It did not mean giving two names to a set of overlapping symptoms, such as diabetes being comorbid with hyperglycemia. In medicine, the "morbidity" reflects presence of disease, and "comorbidity" means presence of multiple, different diseases. In psychiatry, the concept of "disease" has been downplayed, and instead, the vaguer term "disorder" is used, and the concept of comorbidity thus loses its moorings. It becomes instead a reflection of overlapping symptom presentations in different DSM defined "disorders," which may reflect the same disease, or no disease at all.

Proponents of the DSM approach argue that we cannot know if and when diseases are present, thus all symptom presentations should be diagnosed, even if they routinely overlap with each other. This produces many comorbidities, which, according to the DSM philosophy, is not a problem. Instead it is to be encouraged, such that in the future, research may clarify which comorbidities are real, and which reflect common underlying conditions. This approach can be questioned on multiple grounds, including the failure to achieve much change in basic DSM categories, such as mood and anxiety conditions, over decades, despite extensive clinical research.

More practical immediate consequences follow from the DSM approach to encouraging comorbidities. One potentially harmful direct consequence is polypharmacy. Patients who get multiple diagnoses frequently get multiple medications, one or more for each diagnosis. This phenomenon has been widely remarked upon, and quantified. One reason for its occurrence is that the United States Food and Drug Administration (FDA) only gives marketing approvals for drugs that are tied to DSM "disorders." Hence, pharmaceutical companies are encouraged by our current nosology to produce a different drug for each different "comorbidity," despite the fact that the latter conditions may be different labels for many of the same symptoms. A recent review found that use of almost all psychotropic drug classes has increased notably in the past decade. Some experts emphasize the need to treat each comorbidity separately with different medications, such as the recommendation to give specific anxiolytic treatments for the anxiety symptoms that occur in bipolar illness.

This DSM-based comorbidity/polypharmacy syndrome can be seen as another consequence of the basic DSM organizing principle of diagnostic thresholds, and rejection of diagnostic hierarchies. In the remainder of this paper, the concept of diagnostic hierarchies will be described and explained and its application to current psychiatric nosology explored.

THE DIAGNOSTIC HIERARCHY APPROACH

Conceptual Basis for Diagnostic Hierarchies: Not Limited to Etiology

A "diagnostic hierarchy" means that some diagnoses should be subsumed under other diagnoses. The reason for such privileging of one diagnosis over another is presumed to be etiological. Thus, if we know that one disease is caused by etiology X, then the symptoms of that disease should not be separately diagnosed as representing other putative diseases. The common example in psychiatry is neurosyphilis, where symptoms of mania and depression and dementia occur. Such persons are not diagnosed with neurosyphilis plus bipolar illness plus major depressive illness plus dementia. Rather, one diagnosis excludes the others.

The most common criticism made of diagnostic hierarchies in psychiatry is that they are "arbitrary." This is so because etiologies are unknown or debatable (except neurosyphilis).

This criticism assumes that only etiology can be a basis for a diagnostic hierarchy. There are many medical illnesses in which etiologies are unknown, but in which diagnostic hierarchies make clinical and scientific sense. For instance, the etiology of diabetes is unknown, as is the etiology of hypertension, as are the etiologies of most epilepsies. But diabetes would be ruled out before diagnosing psychogenic polydipsia. Hypertension would be ruled out before diagnosing tension headache. Epilepsy would be ruled out before diagnosing syncope. The general principle, in all these conditions for which etiologies are not known, is that these illnesses have many symptoms, and they should be ruled out before other conditions with fewer symptoms are diagnosed. In short, polysymptomatic illnesses should be ruled out before conditions with one or just a few symptoms are diagnosed.

In the examples just given, although etiologies are not known, pathophysiologies often are known (e.g., for diabetes, hypertension, and epilepsies). Similarly, despite our not knowing their etiologies, much neurobiological knowledge exists regarding the pathophysiologies of major psychiatric illnesses, like schizophrenia and manic-depressive illness, that could be placed at the top of a diagnostic hierarchy.

This conceptual basis for diagnostic hierarchies also addresses a second critique sometimes made, to the effect that diagnostic hierarchies are said to imply "pure" or "ideal" types, the notion being that we have conditions that are clearly identifiable and unambiguous, and then other conditions are viewed as less important in some way. This is not the case in medicine, and need not be so in psychiatry, as explained. Diagnostic hierarchies can be based on differentiating polysymptomatic conditions from those with fewer symptoms, not implying that one is "purer" than the other, but that more symptoms are present in one case than the other, with a pathophysiological basis that is sound, with or without a known ultimate etiology.

In sum, a diagnostic hierarchy concept is not solely dependent on knowledge of etiology, nor does it imply knowledge of some pure or ideal state. Rather, differential diagnosis based on ruling out broader polysymptomatic conditions before diagnosing narrower conditions can be the basis for legitimate diagnostic hierarchies.

Can Diagnostic Hierarchies Be Validated?

If it is admitted that diagnostic hierarchies can be applied legitimately in the absence of knowledge of etiology, the next question is whether or not they can be or have been validated empirically.

There is some scientific research on this matter in psychiatry. For instance, the classic U.S.–U.K. Diagnostic Project used the Present State Examination (PSE), a 1970s diagnostic program that had an influence on Research Diagnostic Criteria (RDC), which in turn influenced DSM-III categories. A total of 397 patients were organized into four basic syndromes, with the following hierarchy: first, "delusions of disintegration" (meaning "delusions of control . . . and hallucinations"); second, "integrated delusions" (meaning "delusions of persecution, grandeur, or contrition"); third, "neurotic symptoms" (meaning "obsessional, phobic, and hysterical symptoms"); and lastly, "dysthymic states" (meaning "states of anxiety, depression, and elation"). The hypothesis, based on earlier studies, was that if any patient had a symptom, or met the definitional criteria, for classes higher on the hierarchy, that patient would also have symptoms or meet definitions for all classes below that level on the hierarchy. Thus if someone had delusions of control, she would also have integrated delusions, neurotic symptoms, and dysthymic states. Similarly, if someone had no delusions at all but had neurotic symptoms, that person would also have dysthymic states.

Two kinds of hierarchies were used: (a) broad hierarchies—in which any symptom in any of the four classes would identify a person as having that class of symptoms; (b) narrow hierarchies—in which a certain number of symptoms was required for each class to meet a diagnostic threshold. The result was that 76% of subjects in the broad approach, and 81% in the narrow approach, were able to be classified in a hierarchy model. In other words, the hierarchy model was validated most subjects.

Another analysis of this dataset provides further evidence for how to validate diagnostic hierarchies empirically. The patients in this dataset were reanalyzed using eight definitions divided into four broad groups: Depression, Mania, Schizophrenia, and Other Diagnoses (mainly "neuroses other than depressive," which represented anxiety conditions, "personality syndromes, alcoholism, and combinations of these"). In the two categories defined as "Depression" and "Other Diagnoses," over 90% of patients fit the hierarchy model described here well. Only about half of patients with mania or schizophrenia fit the proposed hierarchy model, though (48% for schizophrenia,

55% for mania). Of these "non-conforming" patients, many (72% with the broad hierarchy, 47% with the narrow hierarchy) had delusions but no "neurotic symptoms" (i.e., depression, anxiety, or mania). Translated into current terms, these patients were psychotic without severe mood states, which is the basic definition of schizophrenia. These results suggest, therefore, that the proposed hierarchy was not empirically correct: mood states should not be placed below psychotic states on a diagnostic hierarchy.

Other studies from that era and later confirmed this conclusion. The notion that "first-rank symptoms" were positive and specific for schizophrenia was disproven; about 25% of manic patients also had those psychotic symptoms. The opposite hierarchy was thus empirically established; in psychotic patients, one had to rule out mania, even in the presence of first-rank symptoms, before diagnosing schizophrenia.

These studies demonstrate that diagnostic hierarchies can be, and have been, empirically validated.

An Empirically Based Diagnostic Hierarchy

Given these empirical studies, Box 18.1 proposes an empirically based diagnostic hierarchy for psychiatric nosology, based on the organizing principle that polysymptomatic conditions with well-established pathophysiologies should be higher on the diagnostic hierarchy than conditions with fewer symptoms.

BOX 18.1
A HIERARCHY OF DIAGNOSIS

- Affective illnesses:
  - Bipolar illness
  - Unipolar depression
- Psychotic conditions:
  - Schizoaffective illness
  - Schizophrenia
- Anxiety conditions:
  - OCD
  - PTSD
- Other:
  - Personality
  - ADD

Psychotic symptoms often happen in affective illness, but mood episodes frequently happen in psychotic illness. The latter scenario is currently captured with a separate diagnosis, "schizoaffective illness." Thus, the empirical data support a diagnostic hierarchy where affective illnesses sit above psychotic illness, and where schizoaffective illness sits above schizophrenia. Panic attacks, obsessive-compulsive symptoms, and generalized anxiety frequently happen during manic and depressive episodes, as well as during psychotic episodes. Thus, the empirical data support a diagnostic hierarchy where anxiety conditions are placed below affective and psychotic illness.

Some aspects of an empirical diagnostic hierarchy may be controversial, but this should be able to be adjudicated with appropriate research studies. For instance, the placement of ADD below mood and anxiety illnesses is based on the general principle that polysymptomatic conditions should be higher on a diagnostic hierarchy than narrower conditions. Affective illnesses have been well established to cause attentional impairment in particular, and cognitive impairment in general. Psychotic illnesses are also well associated with attentional and cognitive impairment. Anxiety conditions have been shown to impair attention and cognition. Attentional/cognitive impairment in ADD, on the other hand, has not been shown to cause psychotic states. Thus, psychotic illnesses are empirically proven to be higher than ADD in a diagnostic hierarchy. If some wish to argue otherwise, they would need to provide empirical evidence of a causal relationship of ADD producing mood, anxiety, or psychotic conditions.

Regarding personality disorders, some studies are interpreted as showing that personality illnesses, especially borderline personality, truly exist independent of other psychiatric diagnoses, such as MDD. Other studies disagree. For instance, in one study of patients who met criteria for both MDD and borderline personality disorder, when they were treated with antidepressants and followed up one year later, 67% had improved such that they were not experiencing major depressive episodes at the time. In most of those patients, borderline personality disorder diagnostic criteria were no longer met. Since personality illnesses are defined as being pervasive and traitlike, rather than episodic, these high cure rates would seem to support a diagnostic hierarchy where affective illness sit above personality illnesses.

The Concept of a Diagnosis of Exclusion

A final nosological approach to appreciating the concept of diagnostic hierarchies involves the often loosely used concept of "diagnoses of exclusion." In the history of medicine, having diagnoses of exclusion originally meant ruling out all known diseases before making a given diagnosis. In psychiatry, hysteria was the classic diagnosis of exclusion. For instance, Richard Cabot, in his *Differential Diagnosis* (2nd edition, 1912), advised readers to exclude many physical causes before concluding that a convulsive attack was "due to hysteria." Essentially, a diagnosis of exclusion was a diagnosis made *negatively*, by ruling out other conditions, rather than *positively*, by identifying its own diagnostically specific features.

With that definition, for instance, bipolar illness cannot be said to be a diagnosis of exclusion relative to personality disorders, as some claim. Mania has its own diagnostically specific criteria, most of which are not part of DSM criteria for personality disorders. Since mania can be positively diagnosed independently of personality disorders, bipolar illness is not a diagnosis of exclusion for personality disorders. On the other hand, DSM major depressive episodes are defined in the same way for both bipolar illness and MDD. The difference is that in bipolar depression, past mania is present (a *positive* finding), and in MDD, past mania is *not* present (a *negative* finding). Hence, using the classic medical definition, MDD is a diagnosis of exclusion relative to bipolar illness, because it is negatively diagnosed after positive symptoms of mania are ruled out. This general logic would place MDD below bipolar illness on a diagnostic hierarchy, and it would exclude any claim to placing personality disorders above bipolar illness or MDD on a diagnostic hierarchy. In other words, the logic of medical diagnosis, which has been established for centuries and is widely accepted in the medical profession, provides a basis for non-arbitrary judgments about a diagnostic hierarchy for psychiatric conditions such as bipolar illness, MDD, and personality disorders.

A diagnostic hierarchy approach could help clinicians to be achieve more effectiveness with fewer medications and less misdiagnosis. For instance, if mistaken comorbidity definitions are put aside, clinicians could find that some medications have more benefits by improving the underlying primary illness that causes apparently "comorbid" symptoms. For instance, lithium, which has negligible direct anxiolytic effects, has been shown to improve anxiety symptoms in persons with bipolar illness by improving the mood episodes that cause those anxiety symptoms.

Clinicians would also be influenced to give more attention to the primary psychiatric illness underlying apparent comorbid symptoms. For example, in the current anti-hierarchical DSM approach, patients with bipolar illness receive mood stabilizers for much shorter durations, and in fewer trials, than antidepressants, anxiolytics, and amphetamines given for comorbid anxiety and cognitive symptoms. This dilemma is worsened when treatments for comorbidities worsen the underlying primary illness, which, in a negative feedback loop, can inadvertently worsen the comorbidities. Again, using bipolar illness as a common example, many patients are treated with antidepressants for comorbid anxiety symptoms, which can produce worsened anxiety if the antidepressant causes or worsens underlying manic episodes with associated anxiety. Adults and children diagnosed with bipolar illness often receive the comorbid diagnosis of ADD, are treated with amphetamines, and in about one-half of cases, according to one study, develop manic episodes, which produces more inattention.

If they used an empirically validated diagnostic hierarchy, clinicians also would be less likely to make misdiagnoses. In the current DSM anti-hierarchical system, depression as a syndrome is commonly diagnosed as MDD, without ruling out bipolar illness first. This leads to marked under-diagnosis, with 40% of bipolar patients initially misdiagnosed as having MDD, analogous to the 1970s problem of under-diagnosis of affective illness relative to schizophrenia for psychotic symptoms. This misdiagnosis is not just a matter of poor clinical judgment; it is encouraged by the non-hierarchical organizing principle of DSM.

Researchers also are influenced by the DSM approach in a potentially unscientific manner. For instance, family genetic studies do not apply a hierarchical approach, and thus do not bother to rule out diagnoses, which may explain the genetic findings, rather than the specific condition that is claimed to be genetic. In studies of adult ADD, for example, very high heritabilities are reported, around 80%, similar to bipolar illness and schizophrenia, which are the only other major psychiatric illnesses with such a high heritability. (MDD, in contrast, has a heritability of only 40%.) However, adults who participated in those studies can also be diagnosed with bipolar illness, and still be included in the genetic studies of ADD. In other words, the "comorbidity" of bipolar illness is not an exclusion criterion for diagnosing ADD and including such "ADD" subjects in family history genetic studies. If the empirically based diagnostic hierarchy proposed in this chapter is correct, then the apparently high genetic heritability of adult ADD could simply reflect the underlying primary disease of bipolar illness. Hence, it would not be surprising to find identical heritabilities in studies of apparent adult ADD and other studies of bipolar illness.

SUMMARY

The diagnostic hierarchical approach argues that certain diagnoses should not be made (those lower on the hierarchy) if other diagnoses are present (those higher on the hierarchy). The DSM system is based on the organizing principle of diagnostic thresholds and rejects the alternative principle of diagnostic hierarchies. The medical and scientific soundness of diagnostic threshold was examined and found to be wanting. In contrast, medical and scientific evidence in favor of diagnostic thresholds was identified. It was suggested that application of the concept of a diagnostic hierarchy as an organizing principle for psychiatric nosology, in place of diagnostic thresholds alone, can compensate for many of the harmful clinical and scientific consequences of the DSM approach, especially polypharmacy and misdiagnosis.

SELECTED REFERENCE

Surtees, P. G., & Kendell, R. E. (1979). The hierarchy model of psychiatric symptomatology: An investigation based on present state examination ratings. *British Journal of Psychiatry, 135*, 438–443.

19

Treatment of Affective Illnesses

DIAGNOSTIC CONSIDERATIONS

Classically, depression was characterized by the slowing down of one's thoughts, feelings, and movements. In other words, depression involved psychomotor retardation. Classically, mania was characterized by the speeding up of one's thoughts, feelings, and movements. In other words, mania involved psychomotor activation. Thus, psychomotor aspects can be seen as central to these conditions. The term "mood disorders" is a misnomer if interpreted, as is commonly the case, to mean that mood is central to diagnosis. In fact, mood is variable in the phenomenology of these conditions, and the most consistent clinical features for diagnosis are psychomotor changes. One can have depression without any sad mood at all; instead, anhedonia is present. One can have mania without any euphoric mood at all; instead, irritability is present.

Manic-Depressive Illness

The pre-DSM-III concept of manic-depressive illness (MDI) was defined by Emil Kraepelin in 1898 and later editions of his textbooks, and used as thus defined for about century, until DSM-III in 1980. The Kraepelinian definition of MDI was that any recurrent mood episodes of any kind, depressive *or* manic, constituted the diagnosis of MDI. This is *not* the same thing as bipolar disorder, which became official with DSM-III, which meant the presence of depressive AND manic episodes, not depressive *or* manic episodes. In other words, MDI meant bipolar illness *plus* unipolar depressive illness. That is, it represented what is defined by DSM terms as bipolar disorder *and* most of MDD (Figure 19.1).

MDI was defined by *recurrence* of mood episodes as its diagnostic standard, not *polarity* of mood episode. As long as recurrent episodes occurred—i.e., they came and went and were repeated—the diagnosis was MDI. It did not matter if the diagnosis reflected 100 depressive episodes and zero manic episodes, or 100 manic episodes and zero depressive episodes. The diagnosis of MDI was the same in both cases. In other words,

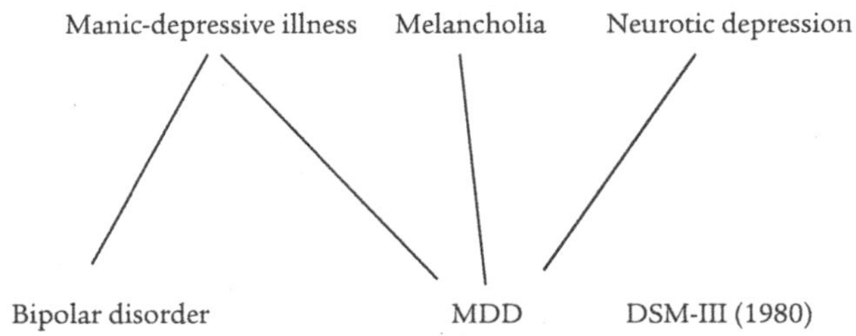

FIGURE 19.1 *Manic-depressive illness equals "bipolar disorder" plus "MDD."*

bipolar and unipolar courses were subtypes of the same illness, MDI, rather than two separate purported illnesses, as in the DSM system.

One reason that Kraepelin deemphasized polarity and focused on recurrent course of illness was his observation, along with others', that most mood states were neither purely depressive nor manic, but rather mixed. Kraepelin defined six different types of mixed states, building on Weygandt, as opposed to the two purely depressive or manic states. Mixed states were the most common presentation of MDI, thus it was not possible to define the illness by polarity, since most mood states were not at one pole or the other. DSM-III tried to ignore this problem by refusing to define mixed episodes, and by defining manic episodes very narrowly as being severe and lasting one week or longer. This definition, which conflicted with a large literature on mixed states and hypomanic episodes, was partially rectified by DSM-IV, which accepted a definition of milder hypomanic episodes and introduced a definition of mixed episodes. However, hypomanic episodes were cut off at four days, without any scientific evidence for that cut-off duration, and mixed episodes were defined narrowly (requiring the presence of full syndromal mania and depression at the same time). DSM-5 has broadened the mixed definition somewhat, as noted, but it did not change the hypomania duration definition, despite absence of evidence for the four-day cut-off and the presence of some data supporting a shorter cut-off of two days. Furthermore, the definition of mixed states proposed by DSM-5 has been criticized as being primarily conceptual (focused on the concept of "non-overlapping" symptoms), as opposed to extensive empirical evidence that most mixed states are broader and characterized primarily by psychomotor excitation—like rapid thoughts, marked rage/irritability, agitation, and impulsivity—added to depressive features. These empirically based mixed features are not part of the DSM-5 definition, but are central to the non-DSM concept of mixed depressive and dysphoric manic states.

Mixed States

The most common approach to the description of the phenomenology of mood conditions contrasts depression and mania. While this clinical distinction can and should be made, it is not easy to make. It also is important to acknowledge that the phenomenology of mood conditions involves the frequent, if not usual, admixture of manic and depressive symptoms at the same time—called "mixed states." In this scenario, a full-blown clinical depression may be present, but some manic symptoms may also be

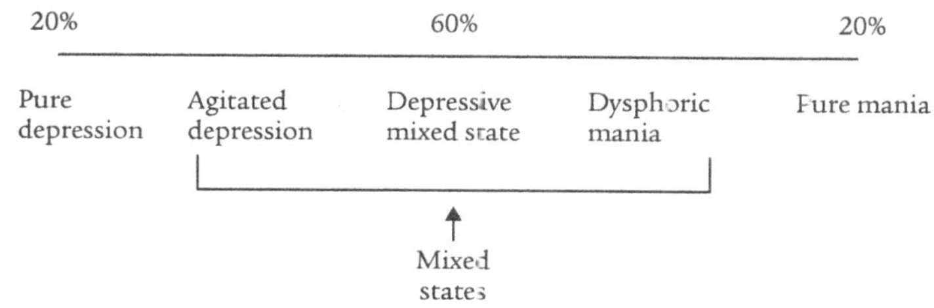

FIGURE 19.2 *Mood episode spectrum.*

present, such as rapid thoughts, increased sexual drive, and marked anger and mood lability. Another variety involves classic psychomotor retarded depression, lasting weeks to months, interspersed with very brief bursts of manic symptoms lasting hours to days. The manic variety involves a full-blown manic episode, but with the presence of sad mood or suicidal thoughts or other potential depressive symptoms such as guilt or low self-esteem.

When defined in this manner broadly, mixed states have been reported to be the most common presentation of mood states. This broad definition includes concepts such as agitated depression and dysphoric mania. If defined this way, mania and depression would be seen as uncommon pure variants of mood states, while the most common mixed states are a mixture of two (Figure 19.2).

If this phenomenology is correct, then it has important implications for classification of diagnoses. The current diagnostic system is based completely on the distinction of depression and mania. If manic versus depressive states cannot be distinguished in most cases, then the current diagnostic system would be very difficult to implement validly. Put otherwise, the frequent presence of mixed states would invalidate the diagnostic system built on a mania versus depression dichotomy. The concept of mixed states is discussed in more detail in Appendix I of this book.

Temperament

The concept of affective temperaments dates back at least 200 years, and was systematized about a century ago by Emil Kraepelin and Ernst Kretschmer. In Kraepelin's texts, we read about "manic temperaments" and "depressive temperaments." Kretschmer developed these concepts, which eventually led to the concepts of hyperthymia and dysthymia, respectively. The main idea is that manic and depressive states present not only in episodes of attacks of severe symptoms, but also as mild symptoms that are present all the time, as part of the baseline personality of an individual. Thus, the temperaments can be defined as mild versions of mood states, but they go beyond that initial concept to include basic differences in personality traits and in energy levels, as expressed in sleep patterns and behaviors, such as sexual and social or work-related activities. Hence, the following brief descriptions apply.

Hyperthymia involves a mild manic state as part of one's basic temperament. Such persons are high in energy, need less sleep than most people (often only four–6 hours nightly), have high sex drives, are highly social and extroverted, often workaholics, and often humorous. They are described as the life of the party, as fun-loving, and can engage in risk-taking behaviors that others avoid, such as skydiving, bungee-jumping, motorcycle riding, or airplane flying. They dislike routine, and are spontaneous. They can be quite anxious and inattentive.

Dysthymia is the reverse, a mild depressive state as part of one's basic temperament. Such persons are low in energy, need more sleep than most people (often 10–12 hours nightly), have low sex drives, are socially anxious, introverted, low in work productivity, and not humorous. They avoid risk-taking behaviors, are devoted to routine, and can be obsessive. They can be quite anxious but not usually inattentive.

Cyclothymia involves constant alternation between mild manic and depressive states on a day-to-day, or a few days at time, basis. Such persons go up and down in mood and energy and activity levels, though they can be generally mostly extroverted and productive and social. They tend to be risk-takers at times, and are unpredictable and spontaneous. They can be quite anxious and inattentive.

In the original view of Kraepelin and Kretschmer, these temperaments are mild variations of manic-depressive illness. They are not separate or independent diseases or disorders, as the DSM system sets them up. They are part of the same condition, just mild versions, *formes frustes*, as in the French term. This is no different than saying that mild adrenal insufficiency is related to but not the same as Addison's disease; or that mild hypothyroidism is related to but not the same as Grave's disease. Affective temperaments are different in severity but not in kind from severe depressive or manic illness.

This perspective differs from the DSM-III–based view of dysthymia and cyclothymia as "Axis I" conditions, rather than aspects of personality. Further successive DSM revisions have ignored hyperthymia completely. A useful resource is the TEMPS (Temperament Evaluation scale from Memphis, Pisa, and San Diego) scale, which is the most validated research scale to assess affective temperaments. As an aid to clinical diagnosis, a short self-report TEMPS scale can be invaluable.

By the Numbers

How frequent are mood temperaments? It depends partly on how they are defined. In one study, they were defined as 75% or more items being endorsed on the TEMPS scale. Using that definition, about 40% of patients in a mood disorder clinic met the definition of cyclothymia. About 15% met the definition of hyperthymia, and 10% were definable with dysthymia.

About 50% of patients did not have any full mood temperament. If they endorsed mood temperament criteria, they did so only in fewer than 50% of items. Thus, they might have some mood temperament features, but not enough to meet the full definition of any one. If the cut-off is put at a lower threshold of 50% of items, then the majority of persons with mood conditions—about 80%—meet the definition of a mood temperament.

Population prevalence studies are limited, but genetic studies that have looked at mood temperaments have noted that they are the most frequent diagnoses in family members of persons with mood illnesses. These family members don't have full-blown depressive or manic episodes. Thus, since mood conditions occur in about 5–10% of the general population in the United States (about 5–10% for MDD and 1–2% for bipolar illness), one could infer that mood temperaments occur in about 10–20% of the general population, at least in the United States. In many cases, they occur by themselves, meaning that no other diagnoses are present. In other cases, they occur as the baseline temperament in between full depressive or manic episodes in persons with mood illnesses.

Neurotic Depression

Besides MDI, the other major non-DSM classification in mood conditions is neurotic depression. This diagnosis was made commonly before DSM-III in 1980, and it was targeted specifically for exclusion from DSM-III. It was defined, as with MDI and unlike DSM definitions, primarily by its course, rather than cross-sectional symptoms. Neurotic depression reflected a mood condition that was not severe, episodic, or recurrent—like MDI—but rather chronic and constant, but mild to moderate in severity. The mood symptoms were never manic, but rather depressed and anxious. Brief exacerbations could occur to higher severity, usually in the setting of psychosocial stress, but these periods of worsening were brief, usually days to weeks, followed by a return to a chronic baseline. In the United States, the terms "neurotic and psychotic" were used in the mid-20th century loosely, based on psychoanalytic assumptions about the severity of repressed unconscious emotions. In Europe, the terms were used phenomenologically, with *neurosis* simply reflecting anxiety with some admixture of mild depressive symptoms, and *psychosis* reflecting the presence of delusions or hallucinations.

There was a robust debate about the validity of neurotic depression as a diagnosis in the 1970s, especially in the United Kingdom but also in the United States. Since the term was used differently in the two nations, the debate was not the same exactly. In the United Kingdom, neurotic depression became identified with "exogenous" or "reactive" depression, while psychotic depression was defined as "endogenous." Since MDI was always seen as a biological, and thus "endogenous," disease, neurotic depression was seen in Europe as an entirely different kind of depressive condition than MDI. However, not all depressive episodes in MDI were psychotic, which led to the problem of how to differentiate non-psychotic depression in MDI (both bipolar and unipolar subtypes) from neurotic depression. In the U.K. debate, the focus was on the exogenous versus endogenous distinction—i.e., on whether psychosocial stressors could be shown to differ in non-psychotic depressive states. As this factor was thrown into doubt based on research, the concept of neurotic depression was weakened accordingly. The definition of endogenous depression based primarily on the course of illness did not receive adequate attention, though.

In the United States, the concept of neurotic depression fell into disfavor as being Freudian, even though it did not have psychoanalytic roots in Europe. In the course of DSM-III debates and decisions, as now documented in new historical research, the evolution of neurotic depression was as follows: it was replaced initially by the term "minor" depression, as opposed to "major" depression, which was to be reserved for the more severe mood states of MDI (renamed "bipolar disorder" and "unipolar major depressive disorder"). Psychoanalytic groups in the United States objected to the term "unipolar" as

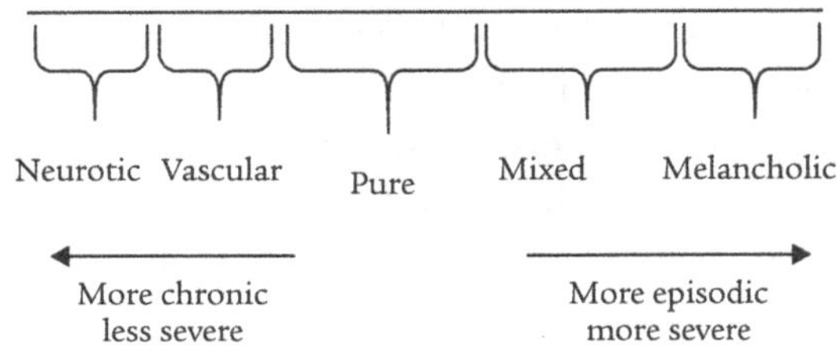

FIGURE 19.3 *The MDD spectrum.* SOURCE: *Adapted from Ghaemi SN, Vohringer PA, Vergne D. Psych Clinics North Am. 2012;35(1):73–86.*

being seen as "endogenous," and thus leading to likely drug as opposed to psychotherapy treatments. Those same groups objected to the term "minor" as likely to result in minor insurance reimbursement. Thus, all the proposed terms were lumped eventually into the diagnosis of "major depressive disorder." There was still reluctance in the American clinical community to give up the term "neurotic depression," so additional diagnoses were created or redefined—namely, generalized anxiety disorder and dysthymia—to compensate clinicians for giving up the concept of neurotic depression.

In sum, it can be seen that the MDD concept itself is an amalgam of a number of different kinds of depressive states, which, before 1980, were viewed as different conditions. If these depressive conditions are not the same, as DSM assumes, then their differentiation becomes important for treatment. Figure 19.3 depicts the major subtypes of MDD that lie on the spectrum that is lumped together in DSM-5 as one diagnosis.

A POST-DSM CLASSIFICATION

After almost half a century of more research and clinical experience, one might ask how well DSM-based definitions of mood disorders have held up. The main question relates to the radical distinction between MDI, as a single broad disease, versus two different and separate bipolar and unipolar conditions. The bipolar/unipolar dichotomy was justified in the 1970s, leading up to DSM-III, based on differences in the classic diagnostic validators of course, genetics, biological markers, and treatment response. In other words, the claim that the presence or absence of manic episodes marked different diseases was supported by observations of differences in course, genetics, biology, and treatment between bipolar and unipolar groups. In particular, bipolar illness had an early age of onset (mean age about 19 years, versus about the late 20s for unipolar depression), brief depressive episodes (three months or less on average in bipolar illness, versus 6–12 months on average in unipolar depression), highly recurrent course (more frequent episodes in bipolar than unipolar illness, with rapid cycling, defined as four or more episodes yearly happening in about 25% of bipolar illness cases, but in less than 1% of unipolar depression cases), genetic specificity (manic episodes were found in families of persons with manic episodes, but not in families of persons with unipolar depression), and differential treatment (antidepressants for unipolar depression versus neuroleptics and lithium for mania).

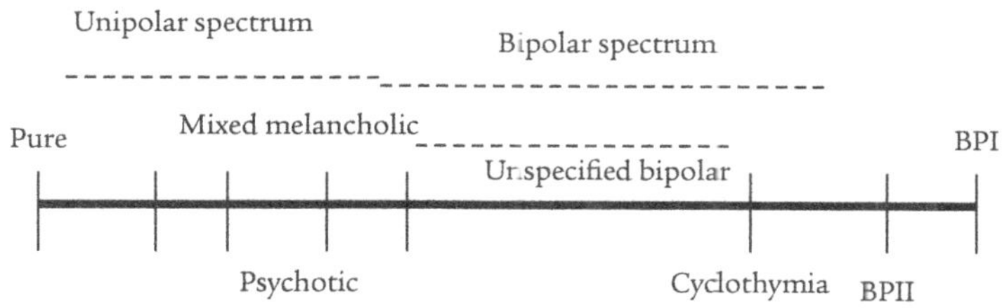

FIGURE 19.4 *The manic-depressive spectrum.*

In the intervening half-century, all of these distinctions have been weakened and/or refuted. Regarding the course of illness, the common diagnosis of MDD in children, far below the mean onset of the late 20s, conflicts completely with the rationale that bipolar illness and MDD differ on that course criterion. Brief depressive episodes that occur multiple times yearly are commonly diagnosed in patients with MDD, whereas such a course of illness should be rare if MDD were a different illness than bipolar disorder. Genetic studies have found high rates of depressive episodes, without mania, in persons with bipolar illness, and also frequent occurrence of bipolar illness in relatives of those with unipolar depression. Treatment now overlaps considerably, with neuroleptic agents proven effective not only for mania but also for depression, in both bipolar and unipolar types. Lithium has been well known to be effective not only for mania but for depression, in both bipolar and unipolar types.

In short, the bipolar/unipolar distinction, now calcified in DSM-III through DSM-5, has not been supported by further research in mood disorders, and in fact, that research could be used to support the original MDI perspective of one broad mood illness.

Another perspective taken on this research would be to maintain the bipolar/unipolar dichotomy but to recognize that it is not a strict distinction, but rather that there is one mood spectrum, with extremes of classic bipolar and unipolar cases, but with many cases in the middle of that spectrum. Some have called this concept a "bipolar spectrum" or a "manic-depressive spectrum." Such views would incorporate both the original MDI concept and the later observations of bipolar and unipolar variations (Figure 19.4).

The DSM approach to diagnosis generally is opposed to spectrum concepts, on *a priori* "pragmatic" grounds of wanting to have a high threshold for psychiatric diagnosis to avoid "overdiagnosis." Separate from the fact that this belief reflects stigma of psychiatric illness, it is not based on empirical evidence, but rather reflects a conceptual assumption. For that reason, the scientific evidence supporting spectrum concepts in mood disorders was rejected in the DSM-5 process.

Differential Diagnosis

The differential diagnosis of mood conditions involves distinctions within the mood dichotomy (bipolar versus unipolar), and distinctions with other conditions based on overlapping symptoms, such as personality changes (borderline, antisocial, narcissistic personality disorders), delusions or hallucinations (schizophrenia and/or schizoaffective illness), and cognition (ADD). An important aspect to approaching differential diagnosis is the concept of a diagnostic hierarchy, which has been rejected by DSM nosology. In the hierarchy approach, diagnoses with multiple symptoms should be diagnosed preferentially to diagnoses with fewer symptoms. Thus pneumonia would be the only diagnosis in a case of fever with lung infection, as opposed to "fever disorder" comorbidity. Since mood disorders cause personality changes, delusions, and cognitive effects, they should be diagnosed instead of assuming the presence of personality disorders, schizophrenia, and/or ADD. Furthermore, the assumption of "comorbidity," which is encouraged by the DSM approach, would be challenged by a hierarchical concept. Multiple diagnoses would not be made unless other symptoms could be shown to exist independently of the mood condition.

Unipolar versus Bipolar

In the DSM polarity-based nosology of mood disorder, the differential diagnosis of unipolar versus bipolar illness rests completely on the identification of manic or hypomanic episodes. Most patients present for treatment in the depressive phase; thus differential diagnosis rests entirely on past manic/hypomanic episodes. Unfortunately, patients deny having manic episodes about half the time, due to lack of insight. Such impaired insight is even worse in hypomania. Thus, in most cases, patients will deny manic/hypomanic episodes, leading to underdiagnosis of bipolar illness and overdiagnosis of MDD, which has been shown empirically. Interviewing should include family and friends, who report manic symptoms more accurately than patients, to correct for this diagnostic bias. Patient self-report is not sufficient to rule out past manic/hypomanic episodes.

A non-DSM-based approach would emphasize all diagnostic validators, including course of illness and genetics and not just symptoms, to differentiate bipolar from unipolar depression. The depressive states themselves are somewhat different, with more melancholia, mixed states, and delusions/hallucinations in bipolar than in unipolar depression. Family genetics of bipolar illness would argue against the legitimacy of diagnosing MDD in a depressed person. A course of illness with early age of onset (i.e., 20 years or earlier), brief depressive episodes (three–6 months or less), and high recurrence (multiple depressive episodes yearly) all would argue for the diagnosis of bipolar illness and against unipolar depression.

The therapeutic relevance of this distinction, as discussed in more detail later in this Chapter, is that antidepressants appear to be mostly ineffective in acute bipolar depression, and in prophylaxis. They also can cause acute manic/hypomanic episodes, and, more importantly, have been shown to worsen the long-term course of bipolar illness in some subjects, especially those with a rapid-cycling course. In rapid-cycling cases, randomized data show that more mood episodes, including depressive states, occur over time with antidepressants than if those agents are discontinued or foregone altogether.

Borderline, Narcissistic, and Antisocial Personality Disorders

Bipolar illness and borderline personality share some features, and differ in others. This topic is discussed in more detail in Appendix II; a brief summary is provided here.

Shared features include rapid mood swings, unstable interpersonal relationships, impulsive sexual behavior, and suicidality. DSM-III through DSM-5 criteria for borderline personality are met with the preceding four criteria, along with one more out of nine total criteria. Thus, using DSM definitions, most persons with bipolar illness would meet borderline criteria automatically. This apparent "comorbidity" is questionable, due to overlapping diagnostic definitions. True comorbidity would be definable with the other five borderline criteria, which are less common in bipolar illness, especially dissociative states and self-mutilations. If sexual trauma is added, which is not even one of the DSM criteria for borderline personality, then it has been shown that specific differentiation of bipolar illness from borderline personality is feasible. Furthermore, the presence of bipolar family genetics would strongly argue for bipolar illness and against borderline personality, with the former being about twice as heritable genetically as the latter.

When manic, or as part of hyperthymic or cyclothymic temperament, persons with bipolar illness have high self-esteem, which can get reflected in lack of empathy towards others and a range of selfish behaviors. If seen through a Freudian and DSM-based lens, many clinicians misdiagnose such persons as having narcissistic personality disorder (NPD), characterized by pervasive pattern of grandiosity, need for admiration, and low empathy. This approach would ignore the diagnostic validators that would support mood illness, such as family bipolar genetics, and other manic symptoms that are irrelevant to NPD, such as high energy levels and a decreased need for sleep. It is relevant that NPD has been invalidated by research with diagnostic validators, because it cannot be distinguished from several other personality disorders (i.e., borderline, histrionic, dependent, antisocial). The DSM-5 Personality Disorders Task Force recommended removal of NPD, but this recommendation was opposed vociferously by professional leaders who had been involved with the introduction of personality disorders in DSM-III, and was eventually rejected by the APA Board of Trustees. Thus, the scientific legitimacy of NPD as a diagnosis is questionable.

In contrast, antisocial personality has been diagnosed and validated for a century or more in psychiatry. Again, there is overlap with manic behaviors, which can be aggressive and impulsive, leading to legal troubles. If those behaviors are viewed solely from a social perspective, the antisocial diagnosis may seem relevant. Such an approach would be corrected if other diagnostic validators were taken into account, again emphasizing family bipolar genetics, but also course of illness with different behaviors in and out of mood episodes, as well as the presence of other manic symptoms that are irrelevant to antisocial personality, such as high energy levels and decreased need for sleep.

Schizophrenia/Schizoaffective Illness

When delusions or hallucinations are present, the differential diagnosis of mood conditions includes schizophrenia and schizoaffective illness. Delusions or hallucinations occur in about one-half of manic states, and about 10% of depressive states, somewhat more in bipolar than unipolar illness. When present, such symptoms are qualitatively similar to the delusions or hallucinations of schizophrenia, and thus can be mistaken for the latter. Furthermore, negative symptoms of schizophrenia like apathy, lack of affect, low energy, and social isolation can look like symptoms of depression episode. In both conditions, cognitive impairment is present. This misdiagnosis was common throughout the 20th century, when schizophrenia was diagnosed cross-sectionally by the presence of delusions/hallucinations (as Eugen Bleuler popularized) as opposed to longitudinally by a chronic declining course (as Emil Kraepelin taught). This course was key, in the Kraepelinian view: dementia praecox was chronic, and manic-depressive illness was episodic. The Bleulerian view was disproved by the seminal U.S.–U.K diagnostic project and other research, which led to the return to the Kraepelinian course criterion with DSM-III in 1980.

Some recent genetics studies indicate common genetic etiologies for schizophrenia and affective illness, which some interpret as challenging the nosological dichotomy. Other genetic studies differentiate the two basic diagnostic groupings, as do other diagnostic validators such as course and neuroimaging.

Some patients share features of both conditions, defined in the DSM system as schizoaffective disorder. Various studies of the classic diagnostic validators suggest that schizoaffective illness does not breed true, and does not appear to represent a valid third psychotic disease. Instead, it likely is sometimes a more severe variant of affective illness and sometimes a less severe variant of schizophrenia. In some cases, it could represent the chance comorbidity of schizophrenia and affective illness in the same person.

The topic of schizoaffective illness is discussed in more detail in Appendix III.

Attention Deficit Disorder (ADD)

Depressive and manic states are characterized by impaired concentration, as well as executive function impairment, and abnormal working and short-term memory. These cognitive states are also present in ADD, leading to the diagnosis of ADD in persons who have manic and depressive symptoms. This misdiagnosis would be common especially in hyperthymia and cyclothymia, where chronic problems with attention are present due to constant manic and depressive symptoms. Using the hierarchy concept, such persons would be diagnosed preferentially as having mood conditions; using DSM definitions, the comorbidity of both diagnoses would be asserted. In contrast to bipolar illness definitions, which have remained restrictive, DSM-5 broadened the diagnosis of childhood ADD, requiring fewer criteria to be met and extending the age of onset range from a maximum of six years to 12 years. DSM-5 also formalized a definition of ADD in adulthood as well.

Again, differential diagnosis would be assisted by attention to all diagnostic validators, not just symptoms; thus family genetics of bipolar illness would argue against the ADD diagnosis, as would recurrent depressive episodes. Since amphetamines are used to treat ADD, and they have been associated with worsening of manic states as well neurotoxicity in animal studies, the differential diagnosis has important practical implications.

This topic is discussed in more detail in Appendix IV.

TREATMENT

Given the diagnostic considerations, the treatment of affective illnesses using the most current scientifically valid diagnostic concepts is much more complex than the simple application of the DSM pragmatism of MDD versus bipolar disorder. In the DSM approach, the matter is simple but doomed. Either the patient is "only" depressed, and thus has MDD, and receives "antidepressants" (sometimes "adjunct" with dopamine blockers), or the patient also has manic or hypomanic episodes, and thus has bipolar illness, in which cases mood stabilizers also are given (usually along with "antidepressants" and dopamine blockers). This approach is simple, but ineffective. It produces the pseudo-problem of "treatment-resistant" depression or bipolar illness, where the patient fails to respond to most of the various "antidepressants" and other agents alone and in combination with each other.

This is a classic case of breaking the Hippocratic insight that the treatment is only as good as the diagnosis. Where the diagnosis is false, no treatment will work. The problem is not "treatment resistance" but diagnostic invalidity.

The alternative approach would give up the DSM-based MDD versus bipolar ideology, and take seriously the scientific evidence for MDI as a unifying overall spectrum diagnosis, with the most common presentation of mixed states, and the important presence of affective temperaments. All these diagnostic aspects of MDI would be distinguished from neurotic depression. Monoamine agonists would be found to have a limited utility, mostly short-term, for only some kinds of non-mixed depressive episodes. Second-messenger modifiers would be found to the most effective agents for long-term prevention of mood episodes of any kind. Dopamine blockers would be the most effective agents for acute mixed states, and sometimes in long-term use. Affective temperaments improve mainly with low-dose second-messenger modifiers if manic symptoms are present, and modestly with low-dose monoamine agonists if dysthymia alone is present. None of those agents would be needed in neurotic depression, where psychotherapies would be as effective.

In the rest of this Chapter, detail will be provided to explain the preceding approach treatment to affective illnesses.

Antidepressant Efficacy in MDD

There are two major sources of evidence for antidepressant efficacy in MDD. One source is a huge number of pharmaceutical industry research studies that are most accessible through the FDA database. A number of researchers have analyzed that FDA database, in meta-analyses that have received notable public attention. The second major source is the largest recent NIMH-funded comparative study of multiple antidepressants in MDD, the Sequenced Treatment Alternatives for Resistant Depression (STAR*D) study. Each source will be examined here in turn.

The FDA Database of Pharmaceutical Industry Studies of Antidepressants in MDD

By far the largest source of evidence regarding the efficacy of monoamine agonists involves the research done by pharmaceutical companies. Those companies do this research to be able to sell their drugs on the market. Such sales occur only after FDA approval. If medications are effective in at least two trials, such approval is usually granted. However, if medications are ineffective in multiple other trials, such negative studies do not count against approval of those medications by the FDA, as long as at least two studies are positive. If fewer than two studies are positive, then negative trials would count against indication. If a medication reaches the marketplace, a pharmaceutical company is obligated to provide all of its studies, positive or negative, to the FDA. However, no functional company is obligated to publish any studies in scientific journals. From an economic perspective, it can be seen that there are reasons to publish positive trials in scientific journals, but there are equal reasons not to publish negative trials. If the medication does not come to the marketplace, then a pharmaceutical company is not obligated to provide all of its studies, including all of its negative trials, to the FDA, nor is it obligated to publish those trials. Hence, if the medication does not reach the marketplace, there could be ample evidence of inefficacy that would not be accessible to clinicians in any way.

For the previous reasons, evidence of lack of efficacy in negative trials also would not be accessible to clinicians through scientific journals. The only means of access to such data would be through Freedom of Information Act (FOIA) requests to the FDA. Such requests have been made by researchers, and important analyses of the FDA database have been published.

The first such analysis identified 74 randomized clinical trials of antidepressants and MDD. These studies involved 12 different agents in 12,564 patients. The researchers initially examined the frequency of positive to negative trials among the studies in the published scientific literature. They found that 94% of the published trials were positive. Hence, by relying on the scientific literature, researchers and clinicians would conclude that the vast majority of studies of antidepressants demonstrated efficacy for treatment of acute depressive episodes in MDD. When examining the FDA database, though, researchers found many negative unpublished studies. When the scientific published literature was combined with the negative unpublished studies in the FDA database, the overall result was that 51% of all the studies that had been conducted were positive, and 49% were negative. In other words, when access was obtained to negative unpublished studies, the appearance of an overwhelmingly effective class of medications disappeared. Instead, medications were equally likely to be ineffective as effective in the 74 RCTs (Figure 19.5).

Part of the same database, consisting of 47 RCTs of SRIs, was reanalyzed by another group examining, not whether the studies were positive or negative, but rather the mean change in the depression rating scale with antidepressant versus placebo in each study. In this influential meta-analysis, the authors reported an overall mean difference between antidepressant and placebo of 1.8 points on the Hamilton Rating Scale for Depression (HRSD). There was substantial improvement with both groups, but the difference between groups was not large. Converted to a standardized effect size, the overall difference was 0.32 using Cohen's d, which is considered a small effect. The authors then compared the overall result with a definition of clinically meaningful improvement for depression, given by the United Kingdom National Institute for Clinical Excellence (NICE), which was set at a three-point difference between drug and placebo using the HRSD.

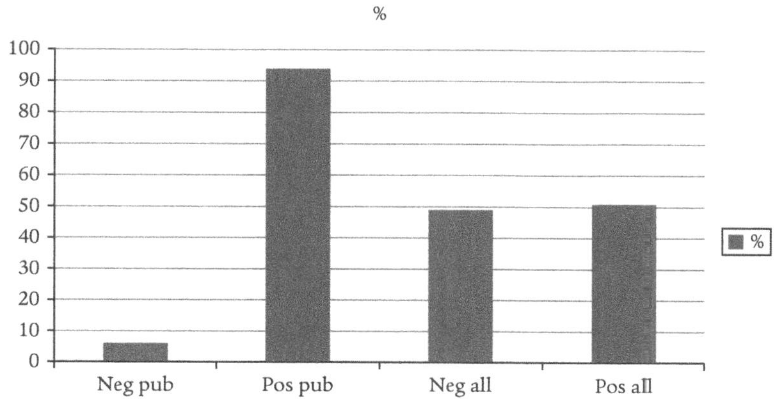

FIGURE 19.5 *Negative publications: Antidepressants.* SOURCE: *Turner EH, et al. N Engl J Med. 2008;358(3):252–260.*

Given that the overall observed difference was smaller than three points on that scale, the authors concluded that there was not clinically meaningful improvement overall with SRI antidepressants in the treatment of acute MDD.

This finding was interpreted in the public media as meaning that a full analysis of all the studies of antidepressants in MDD, including the unpublished negative studies in the FDA database, shows that these agents were not clinically effective overall. The authors concluded that most of the benefits seen with these agents were a placebo effect, which could be obtained with psychotherapy treatment, instead of SRI medications, more safely and equally effectively.

This conclusion is not supported by a central analysis in the same paper, though. This analysis involves a comparison of initial severity of depression with antidepressant versus placebo response. As seen in Figure 19.6, both treatments were very effective, with standardized effect sizes around 1, which is considered large. But it is important to note that the benefits seen with antidepressants were consistent for mild, moderate, and severe depression. In contrast, the benefits seen with placebo was strong for mild depression, but decreased linearly with moderate and severe depression. The decrease in placebo effect led to a larger difference with antidepressants, such that in the severely depressed category, the difference between drug and placebo exceeded the NICE standard, and thus could be considered clinically meaningful. In a reanalysis of this study, conducted by the author of this textbook, it could be shown that the difference between antidepressants and placebo also exceeded the NICE standard in the moderate depression category, when HRSD scores were adjusted for baseline severity, and thus relative improvement was assessed as opposed to absolute improvement.

Hence, an objective reading of this meta-analysis does not demonstrate that antidepressants are ineffective in general, in most cases of depression. It shows, in fact, that antidepressants are clinically meaningfully effective for both moderate and severe depression. However, the lack of benefit in mild depression is clear, and consistent no matter how the data are analyzed. Furthermore, the majority of studies in the analysis belonged in the mild depression category.

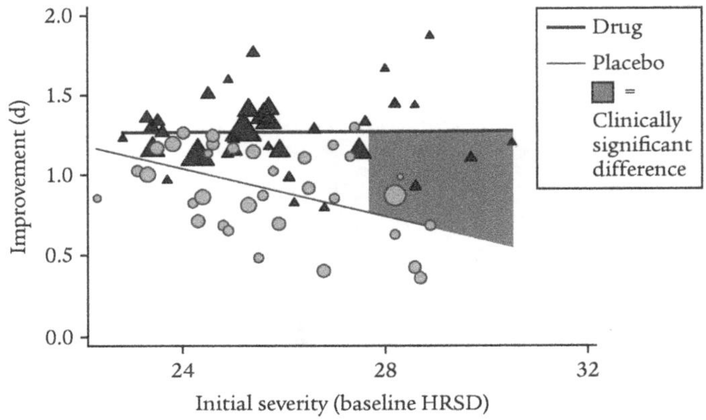

FIGURE 19.6 *Antidepressant meta-analysis: Do they work?* SOURCE: *Kirsch, et al. PLoS Med. 2008;5(2):e45.*

It is relevant to point out that this apparent lack of benefit in mild depression involved relative benefit, not absolute efficacy. In other words, it was not the case that patients with mild depression did not improve with antidepressants; rather, they improved a great deal with antidepressants, and equally so with placebo. Thus there was no difference between the two groups, but all patients improved. This observation is important, because these studies do not show that antidepressants failed to improve patients, but rather the meta-analysis shows that antidepressants improve most patient outcomes, but that the improvement for mild depression was not due to the pharmacological effects of serotonin reuptake in addition, since it occurred equally well with inert placebo.

A final point is important in this meta-analysis. Figure 19.6 helps clarify the clinical experience of many clinicians. Clinical experience involves the straight-line of antidepressant benefit. If the placebo sloping line was removed from Figure 19.6, it would appear that antidepressants are very effective for all severity levels of depression. This is clinical experience, since placebo is not given in clinical practice. The importance of these RCTs is that the presence of the placebo arm allows clinicians to examine whether the benefits seen in practice are due to the pharmacological effect of the medications given, or follow from other causes. The answer is that the benefits seen with antidepressants can be attributed to serotonin reuptake in moderate to severe depression, but not in mild depression. The clinical conclusion would follow that such agents could be defended for short-term treatment of acute depression and moderate to severe cases, but that they should not be given for mild depression, since such patients will improve no matter what.

The Placebo Effect

Can one then conclude that such cases of mild depression should be treated with psychotherapy, as a reflection of the placebo effect? To answer this question, it is important to examine what we mean by the placebo effect, discussed in more detail in Chapter 40. As discussed there, placebo effects have multiple aspects. One aspect, certainly, can involve psychological expectation and the therapeutic relationship with the clinician. But this feature is not the sole aspect of the placebo effect, nor is it the most powerful aspect, depending on what condition is being examined. For objective outcomes, such as mortality and cancer, the psychological aspects of the placebo effect have little influence, as has been shown in many studies. In contrast, for subjective outcomes, such as the experience of depression or pain, the psychological aspects of the placebo effect have been shown to be important. Nonetheless, even in depressive illness, a second important feature of the placebo effect is the natural history of the illness. If a condition is recurrent and episodic, then it will come and go naturally. Hence, the placebo effects will be elevated because they will reflect the natural waxing and waning of episodes of that illness. Unipolar depressive illness is recurrent and episodic, thus the natural history of recovery in that illness will be an important aspect of placebo effects observed. Similarly, neurotic depression is not episodic, but it is mild, with brief exacerbations, and the natural history of that illness would be expected to produce a high placebo effect given the brevity of exacerbations. In other words, the marked improvement of symptoms in the mild depression category with placebo could be due to the natural history of neurotic depression or mild unipolar depressive illness, and cannot be solely attributed to the psychological aspects of clinical treatment. This conclusion would argue against a simple recommendation of psychotherapy in those cases.

Another line of evidence that would argue against simply equalizing psychotherapy and the placebo effect has to do with waitlist studies, in which a no-treatment arm can be compared to placebo. In those studies, as shown in Figure 19.7, it is found that nontreatment, in which even in an inert placebo pill is not given, is more effective than placebo. In fact, the benefits seen involved a mean improvement on the HRSD of about four points, and a standardized effect size of 0.49. These benefits are larger than the improvement seen with antidepressants versus placebo. The improvement seen with non-treatment exceeds the NICE criterion and is more clinically meaningful than the

Study name	Std diff in means	Standard error	Variance	Lower limit	Upper limit	Z-value	p-value
	Statistics for each study						
Arean et al 1993	0.079	0.265	0.070	−0.440	0.598	0.295	0.766
Boton et al 2003	0.341	0.091	0.008	0.183	0.519	3.747	0.000
Clarke et al 1999	1.047	0.283	0.080	0.492	1.602	3.700	0.000
Cohen et al 2010	0.247	0.321	0.103	−0.382	0.876	0.769	0.442
Diamond et al 2002	0.263	0.301	0.091	−0.327	0.853	0.874	0.382
Mufson et al 1999	0.788	0.277	0.077	0.245	1.331	2.845	0.004
Nezu et al 1986	−0.058	0.483	0.233	−1.003	0.891	−0.116	0.908
Nezu et al 1989	1.009	0.438	0.192	0.151	1.867	2.304	0.021
OLeary et al 1990	1.388	0.479	0.229	0.449	2.327	2.898	0.004
Wright et al 2005	0.271	0.311	0.097	−0.339	0.881	0.871	0.384
	0.486	0.122	0.015	0.246	0.725	3.977	0.000

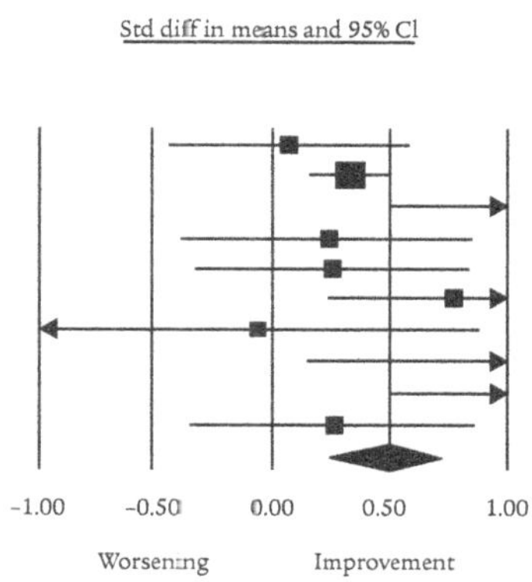

FIGURE 19.7 *Forest plot for effect sizes of wait-list control conditions. 10 trials (n = 340) with mean sample size of 32.2 ± 51.6 patients, duration 10.0 ± 3.7 weeks, and dropout rate of 18.6%. Baseline HAMD score was 21.0 ± 5.0. Mean improvement in HAMD scores was 4 points, with standardized effect size = 0.49, which meets the NICE criterion for clinically meaningful benefit.* SOURCE: *BR Rutherford et al. J Psychiatr Res. 2012;46:697–702. Permission to reprint from Elsevier.*

benefits seen with antidepressants themselves. One might conclude, therefore, that instead of being given antidepressants or psychotherapies, patients with mild depression can be reassured that their brief exacerbations would resolve, and no further immediate treatment would need to be provided, except for follow-up if symptoms should persist or worsen.

*The STAR*D Study*

The second major source of scientific evidence regarding the potential efficacy of antidepressants in MDD, after the pharmaceutical industry–based studies located in the FDA database, involves the NIMH-sponsored STAR*D study. The importance of this study is that it was conducted by academic clinicians, not by pharmaceutical companies. Furthermore, it was designed to be able to compare antidepressants in common use, which was not usually the case in the single-drug versus placebo designs used by the pharmaceutical industry for marketing purposes. And lastly, the STAR*D study was specifically designed to obtain the data regarding the relative efficacy of antidepressants in treatment-refractory depression (TRD). An analysis of the STAR*D study is provided here, followed by a more general discussion of TRD.

This study was one of three classic NIMH-sponsored studies at the end of the 21st century, one each in MDD, bipolar illness, and schizophrenia. In the MDD study, called STAR*D, a sequential large, randomized clinical trial (RCT) was conducted. Before STAR*D, there were few RCTs comparing antidepressants to each other, and hardly any looking at outcomes after multiple failed trials.

The STAR*D protocol was as follows: First, patients were treated openly with citalopram. If they failed to respond, they were then randomized double-blind to a different monoamine agonist or combination with two monoamine agonists (or other adjunctive agents like buspirone). If they failed this second trial, they were randomized to switching to tricyclic antidepressants (TCAs) or augmentation with lithium or thyroid hormone. If they failed this third trial, they were randomized to a MAOI or the combination of venlafaxine plus mirtazapine (Figure 19.8).

Response rates are shown in Figure 19.9, and further described later in this Chapter in "By the Numbers." As can be seen, treatment response was good in the first two episodes,

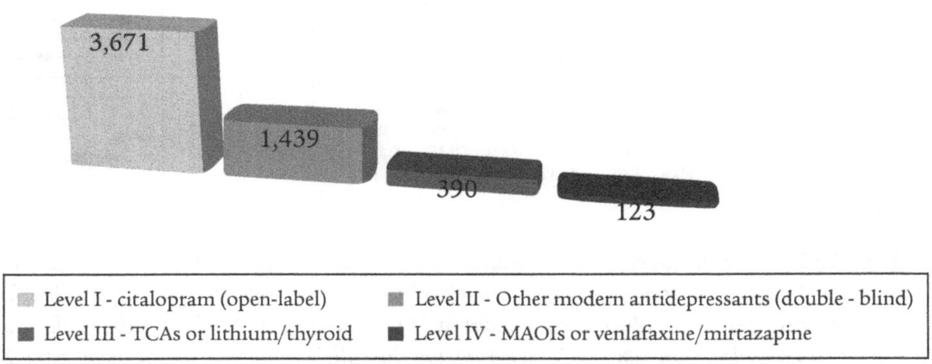

FIGURE 19.8 *Four levels of STAR*D, with sample sizes.*

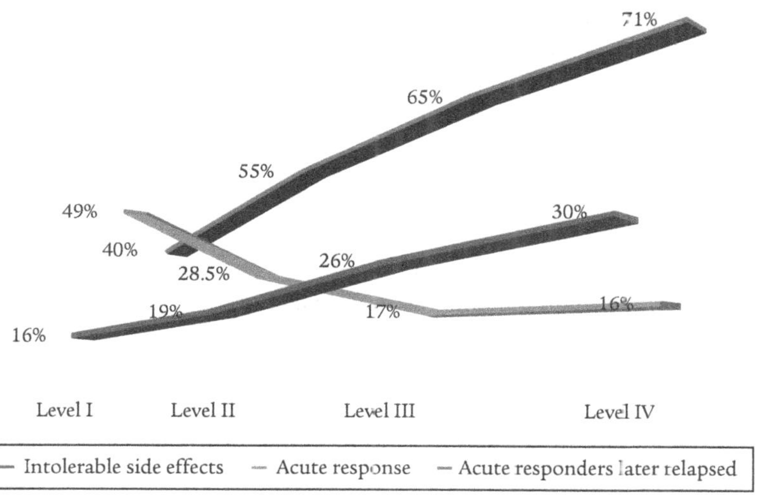

FIGURE 19.9 *Treatment response, long-term relapse, and side effect rates in STAR*D.*

but fell by half thereafter. By the fourth monoamine agonist trial, only 15% of subjects responded to any new treatments, even the most potent agents known, the MAOIs. Furthermore, even if patients responded, about 40–70% relapsed within one year, even if they stayed on the same agents that led to acute response. If intolerable side effects are included, about 20–30% of patients could not remain on their monoamine agonist treatments due to severe side effects (more with the older agents than with newer ones).

In sum: The good news was that about 60–70% of patients responded eventually for the acute depressive episode, if multiple different agents were used. The bad news was that this response fell off markedly after the first few trials, and, furthermore, only about one-third stayed well for the long term, defined as just a year of staying well.

Some researchers and clinicians have interpreted the STAR*D results in a manner similar to what is presented here. The STAR*D researchers themselves adamantly try to interpret their results in as positive a manner as possible.

The case remains, however, that before STAR*D, much higher response rates were cited. After STAR*D, such optimism cannot be supported by this scientific evidence.

Bottom Line

- STAR*D demonstrated good acute response rates in the 60–70% range but low long-term prevention rates in the one-third range.
- After multiple failed antidepressant trials, further agents had a very low likelihood of acute treatment response (about 15%).

By the Numbers

Given these data, what should clinicians tell their patients regarding the probabilities of responding to "antidepressants" for MDD?

Here are some statistics to remember and to cite with patients based on the STAR*D study. These numbers apply to standard monoamine agonists (antidepressants) used to treat MDD:

- Combining two monoamine agonists, or augmenting them (with lithium or thyroid hormone) is similar in efficacy to switching from one monoamine agonist to another.
- With the first monoamine agonist used to treat the first acute depressive episode, the likelihood of clinical response is about 50%.
- With the second monoamine agonist used to treat the first acute depressive episode, the likelihood of clinical response again is about 30%.
- After two failed trials of monoamine agonists for an acute depressive episode, the likelihood of response with a third or fourth agent (even adding lithium or an MAOI) is cut in half to about 15%.
- Of those who respond acutely to a monoamine against for an acute depressive episode, the likelihood that they will stay well for a year staying on the same medication is 50% or less.
- Apart from efficacy, about 20–30% of patients will not be able to tolerate side effects in each antidepressant trial.
- In short, using multiple monoamine agonists, about two-thirds of patients will eventually respond for the acute depressive episode.
- However, half of those patients will relapse within a year. Thus using multiple monoamine agonists, only about one-third will respond and stay well in the long term.

"Treatment-Resistant" Depression

> *All who drink of this remedy recover in a short time, except those whom it does not help, who all die. Therefore it is obvious that it fails only in incurable cases. —Galen*

It's well-known that TRD is a major problem in clinical psychiatry. It's also widely accepted that there is no illness in which 100% of patients respond to appropriate treatments. In other words, even when a disease is correctly diagnosed, and effective treatments are proven to exist, it is never the case that every single person who has that disease will always respond to effective treatments. In this sense, there always can be treatment-resistance in any illness.

But, in most illnesses, if the disease is correctly diagnosed, and the treatments are proven effective, a minority of cases should be treatment-resistant. By definition, if an effective treatment exists, it will be effective for the majority of cases.

TRD is a different story: one could argue, based on our best studies, that the majority of patients who are diagnosed these days with MDD, and treated with the class of agents that are proven effective for that treatment ("antidepressants," or monoamine agonists), are treatment-resistant.

How can that be? If the diagnosis is right, and treatments are proven effective, why are a majority treatment-resistant? These considerations raise an alternative hypothesis—it might not be that the illness is resistant to otherwise correct treatments; it could be that the wrong illness is being treated with the wrong class of drugs.

The quote from Galen states the conceptual assumption underlying TRD. The unstated belief, usually completely unconscious to clinicians, is that the MDD diagnosis is correct, and the drugs are just weak. In fact, it could be that the MDD diagnosis is weak, and the drugs are just fine, seeming ineffective because they are being used for the wrong disease.

The possibility of misdiagnosis always is cited in TRD, but this possibility is not taken seriously in most cases. It is listed as one among a dozen reasons for TRD, and given the same emphasis as medication non-compliance, substance abuse, poor therapeutic alliance, and so forth. Misdiagnosis—or perhaps more correctly, the invalid concept of "major depressive disorder"—should be seen as the most important cause of TRD, based on Galen's assumption, unconsciously held by many clinicians. Galen's fallacy is obvious: "this illness should respond to this kind of treatment; if it doesn't, then the patients were incurable," or, to use modern terms, "treatment-resistant." The clear assumptions are (a) the illness is correctly diagnosed, and (b) the treatments work for that illness.

In TRD, both assumptions are often false. Frequently, TRD is present because the "MDD" diagnosis is mistaken. Also, even when MDD is correct using DSM definitions, TRD is present simply because "antidepressants" are less effective than often presumed for MDD. These two points require a discussion of the misdiagnosis literature and a critical analysis of the classic STAR*D study.

In the long list of causes of TRD, a misdiagnosis usually is one of many. But some research suggests that one-third to one-half of all cases of TRD reflect misdiagnosis, a frequency that is much greater than the many other individual causes that are raised. Thus, when TRD is observed, misdiagnosis should be examined carefully and seen as the most likely factor, far above other possible causes. In other words, other possibilities should not receive the same priority as misdiagnosis, which needs to be ruled out carefully before other possibilities are considered.

Among the other conditions that are misdiagnosed as MDD, the most common is bipolar illness, especially the type II subtype. Hypomanic, and sometimes manic, episodes are missed in clinical histories, often because patients lack insight into those symptoms and do not report them to clinicians, and sometimes because clinicians do not ask about or recognize those manic/hypomanic episodes.

When bipolar illness is misdiagnosed as MDD, TRD can result because monoamine agonists have been shown to be ineffective in bipolar depression, in meta-analyses and multiple RCTs, as opposed to MDD, where monoamine agonists have been shown to be effective over placebo (at least acutely).

Hence TRD is not TRD when it represents misdiagnosis. It is not that the depression is "refractory" to treatments, it is refractory to the wrong treatments. Such patients respond well to a number of dopamine blockers and mood stabilizers, which are proven effective in bipolar depression.

The STAR*D study was an NIMH-sponsored study published in the last decade, reviewed in detail before. As described there, a key finding of that study (although not one accepted by many of the researchers involved with it) was that monoamine agonists are not as effective as often presumed. Specifically, as noted above, only about one-third of patients responded to the whole panoply of monoamine agonists with long-term response. This is much less than the 60–80% efficacy range that many of us often cited before STAR*D. One special observation of concern was that about one-half of patients who responded acutely for a current depressive episode would still relapse within a year, despite staying on the same medication that had improved their acute depression. In other words, monoamine agonists seemed much more effective short-term than long-term; acutely, than in maintenance prevention.

Therefore, the fact that many patients with MDD get better temporarily, but then relapse despite staying on monoamine agonists, is not an unusual observation. This happens in about one-half of patients. Another quarter of patients never seem to respond to any monoamine agonist at all, even short-term.

It seems that about one-third of cases of TRD conservatively can be stated to reflect misdiagnosed bipolar illness. Another one-half of cases reflect the inherently low long-term efficacy rate of monoamine agonists in MDD. The remainder of patients, a small group of 20% or so of subjects, may be truly refractory for other reasons, most commonly medication non-compliance, concurrent substance abuse, concurrent borderline personality, or concurrent psychotic symptoms.

The two biggest factors, though, which explain the vast majority of cases, are misdiagnosed bipolar illness and the limited long-term efficacy of so-called antidepressants. In the case of misdiagnosis, patients can improve with a change in treatment strategy toward mood stabilizers and/or dopamine blockers. In the case of low long-term antidepressant efficacy, a larger clinical question is raised about whether and for how long such agents should be used. This question has not been asked and answered sufficiently in the scientific literature on depressive illnesses. It suggests that TRD is the rule rather than the exception in antidepressant treatment of MDD.

Bottom Line

- "TRD" blames the illness instead of the drugs.
- The largest class of causes for TRD is misdiagnosis, especially for bipolar depression.
- The second-largest class of causes for TRD is the inherently low efficacy of "antidepressants" for long-term maintenance prevention of MDD.
- In the case of misdiagnosis, treatment should shift to mood stabilizers and/or dopamine blockers.
- In the case of low maintenance efficacy in MDD, given STAR*D results, TRD is the rule rather than the exception in antidepressant treatment of MDD.

Treatment of Acute Mood States: Bipolar Depression and Manic Episodes

Antidepressants for Bipolar Depression

The use of antidepressants in bipolar depression is extremely common, yet it has little scientific evidence to support it. In fact, antidepressants are the most commonly used class of medications in bipolar illness, given to about 50% of patients treated for that diagnosis in the United States. In contrast, the most proven effective treatment in bipolar illness, lithium, is given to only about 10% of patients treated for that diagnosis in the United States.

This common practice occurs despite the fact that there are very few RCTs that support benefit with antidepressants in bipolar depression. And there are many RCTs that show that antidepressants are ineffective in bipolar depression. Why is there this disconnection between evidence and practice? The reluctance to stop using antidepressants in bipolar illness needs to be understood, not only in the context of their probable inefficacy, but also in the context of the evidence for some harms, such as causing mania, and causing more mood episodes over time. We will review the scientific evidence first, followed by an examination of the clinical reluctance to implement that evidence.

Beginning with RCTs of acute bipolar depression, there have been numerous meta-analyses of antidepressants in acute bipolar depression over the last decade. In the most recent such review, about half a dozen trials met inclusion criteria, and overall, antidepressants weren't statistically better than placebo. It's a standard approach in evidence-based medicine not to prescribe treatments that are proven ineffective. So why do clinicians and many experts still use and recommend antidepressants in acute bipolar depression? Whatever their reasons, they can't base their judgments on these RCTs.

Turning to RCTs of maintenance prevention of mood episodes in bipolar illness, a meta-analysis found that antidepressants weren't better than placebo, when used with mood stabilizers, in prevention of mood episodes in bipolar illness. Most of these studies involved older classes of antidepressants, such as the TCAs. There are very few studies of the newer antidepressants, like the SRIs, in long-term treatment of bipolar illness. There is in fact only one placebo-controlled maintenance trial of any SRI in bipolar illness. In that study, citalopram was equivalent to placebo. In other words, there are no studies—zero—that show that any modern antidepressant is more effective than placebo in prevention of mood episodes in the maintenance phase of treatment of bipolar illness.

Clinicians often refer to "manic induction with antidepressants." Usually the term "manic induction" isn't well defined. Acute mania related to antidepressants can be defined as occurring within a few months after starting treatment. It's important to distinguish between immediate and long-term harms with antidepressants. Acute mania isn't the major problem with antidepressants. Long-term worsening of mood episodes, usually depressive rather than manic, is a bigger problem, as discussed further later.

Do antidepressants cause acute mania? If limited to looking at randomized trials, some experts would answer in the negative, because many report equivalent rates of mania in subjects treated with antidepressants versus placebo, therefore a causal connection can't be established for antidepressants. Yet those RCTs aren't set up to identify and test the hypothesis that antidepressants cause mania. Rather, they're designed to test the hypothesis of efficacy with antidepressants over placebo, not worsening with mania. The frequency of antidepressant-induced mania is about 10–30% with SRIs and 25–50% with TCAs, thus only part of the overall sample would experience this outcome. Since these studies are powered for efficacy in the whole sample, not side effects in part of the sample, these RCTs don't have statistical "power"; this means there aren't enough patients in the studies to observe enough manic episodes to make a statistical distinction between antidepressants and placebo. This is the classic statistical fallacy—called the "false negative bias"—of saying that "nothing happens" when your study is too small to see if something happens. Furthermore, in many of those RCTs, patients received antimanic medications, such as neuroleptics or mood stabilizers, which would reduce the frequency of antidepressant-induced mania even more.

Nonetheless, even with these design issues, there are numerous randomized trials—involving TCAs—that show higher rates of mania with antidepressants over placebo. The reason those studies are statistically significant has to do with the larger effect size of frequency of antidepressant-induced mania with TCAs (in 25–50% range, as opposed to about half that rate with SRIs). Also, randomized data show twice as much mania with venlafaxine compared to other new antidepressants, like sertraline or bupropion.

Some experts argue that antidepressants only cause mania in monotherapy, not when combined with mood stabilizers. This is not true, as the preceding TCA data included concomitant mood stabilizer treatment with lithium, and mania still was caused by TCAs more than with placebo. Then experts will say that SRIs and other new agents do not cause mania in monotherapy; again, this claim is questionable, given the numerical increase in mania in some studies with SRIs, and the lack of statistical power to assert that statistical non-significance means that nothing happened.

With this context, the following conclusions are reasonable: Antidepressants (like TCAs) have been proven to cause mania in RCTs (in about 25–50% of subjects). SRIs have about half that rate (10–30%). Rates are even lower with concomitant use of mood stabilizers or neuroleptic agents, and also lower in type II (5–10%) than in type I bipolar illness (10–50%). But there is a causal association in all cases; the claim of no effect is weak scientifically. The specific modern antidepressants that have been shown to have the lowest risk of causing acute mania in randomized trials are paroxetine and bupropion.

Rather than acute mania, the most important harm associated with antidepressants in bipolar illness is long-term worsening, meaning they cause more and more mood episodes over time. These mood episodes tend to be depressive rather than manic, which leads to the paradoxical fact that antidepressants worsen depression long-term in bipolar illness. In some patients, this long-term worsening leads to a rapid-cycling course, meaning four or more mood episodes yearly. Typically, these patients are labeled as having "treatment-refractory" bipolar illness, while in fact they often aren't treatment-refractory. Rather, their bipolar illness has been worsened by the mood-destabilizing effects of antidepressants, counteracting the benefits of mood stabilizers. It's not that these patients have failed to respond to multiple mood stabilizers, as is often assumed, but rather that the constant use of long-term antidepressants impedes the mood stabilizers from working. A full and fair trial of a mood stabilizer in this setting must happen in the absence of any antidepressants. Therefore, the recommendation would be to stop antidepressants, and then resume mood stabilizers, including those that had been used the past, and frequently a much better response occurs.

The RCT evidence for these observations begins with studies from the 1970s, which used the on–off design to show that when patients with rapid-cycling bipolar illness received TCAs, their cycling worsened, whereas when they were switched to placebo, their cycling improved. Three decades later, two maintenance RCTs of modern antidepressants in bipolar depression examined outcomes in rapid-cycling versus non–rapid-cycling subgroups. In both studies, patients with rapid-cycling bipolar illness had more depressive episodes if they continued antidepressant use "long-term," defined as up to one year, as opposed to either not being treated with antidepressants at all, or stopping antidepressants after the acute phase. Thus all three RCTs on this topic have found that antidepressants are associated with rapid cycling bipolar illness. Some experts refer to observational data suggesting otherwise, but a basic principle of evidence-based medicine is that randomized data are more valid than observational data, as we'll discuss more later, therefore the latter can't be used to refute the former.

Since rapid cycling occurs in about one-quarter of patients with bipolar illness, it's reasonable to conclude that antidepressants worsen bipolar illness overall in at least 25% of subjects. In short, the most valid available scientific evidence indicates that antidepressants cause or worsen rapid-cycling bipolar illness.

Given this scientific evidence, it is reasonable to consider why clinicians, and also many bipolar experts, use or recommend these agents. A common view among bipolar experts is that if clinicians continue to use these medications, despite the scientific evidence to the contrary, they must know something. Perhaps clinicians see some real benefit that isn't captured in the RCTs. This is a possibility. But one would think that after 30 years of research in many RCTs conducted by researchers who generally have been very positively disposed towards antidepressants, some benefit would have shown up. Another hypothesis could be made that is much more consistent with the basic principles of scientific research and clinical medicine. This hypothesis, as discussed in Chapter 4, has to do with the concept of "confounding bias." Confounding bias reflects the idea that there are many factors in clinical practice that influence the results seen. Clinicians as well as patients don't necessarily know which factors are in play. For instance, it may seem that coffee causes cancer, as repeatedly shown in many huge observational studies. But this association between coffee and cancer is not causal, because of the confounding factor of cigarette smoking. People who drink more coffee also tend to smoke cigarettes, and the latter factor is causal for cancer. Similarly, the fact that clinicians think that antidepressants are associated with improvement in bipolar depression doesn't mean that there is a causal association. The whole point of randomization is to get rid of all the other confounding factors in clinical practice so that a causal scientifically valid judgment can be made. Placebo is a stand-in for natural history, not merely a reflection of psychological wishes, as is commonly assumed. If one has an illness that improves in many people over time, then one has to show that medication does better than the natural course of recovery. Over a century of natural history research, long before any treatments were available, shows that the natural history of bipolar illness is such that episodes last two to four months for mania and three to six months for depression. The reason these mood states are called "episodes" is because they have a natural end, as well as a beginning. They will end, even without any treatment, in three to six months for bipolar depression. Thus, when a clinician gives an antidepressant to a patient with bipolar illness who has been depressed for two months, the natural history of that depressive episode would be such that it would end within two more months, even if no antidepressant had been given. The clinician's interpretation of antidepressant benefit is disproven by the randomized trials that show the same benefit with placebo.

Unfortunately, many bipolar experts tend to ignore the reality of confounding bias in their interpretation of the disconnection between the research studies and clinical practice on this topic. Clinicians haven't been aware enough of the reality of confounding bias in the assumptions they make based on their clinical experience. Both groups would do well to be more cautious in assuming clinical effectiveness when scientific evidence demonstrates the contrary.

Regarding the issue of harm with antidepressants, clinicians tend to be more open to the notion that these drugs cause mania, as opposed to experts who mistakenly ignore the false negative bias of RCTs that are not statistically powered to assess manic induction with antidepressants. Clinicians can't ignore the reality of patients' getting markedly manic soon after starting antidepressants. In contrast, the long-term worsening of mood episodes caused by antidepressants can be hard for clinicians to identify, since those episodes occur a year or longer after antidepressant treatment began. A direct association can be hard to confirm in the real world of clinical practice, where medications are changed frequently, and where many stressors and life events occur over years of follow-up. The RCTs of maintenance treatment in bipolar illness come to the rescue by clearing out confounding factors and demonstrating a causal association between antidepressant use and long-term worsening of bipolar illness with a rapid-cycling course.

Another factor that may be relevant here is that clinicians and patients may be misled by the English language. As discussed in the first Chapter of this textbook, the word "antidepressant" is misleading, because it implies, to clinicians and patients alike, that these medications should be useful for any kind of depression, despite the fact that the research literature indicates that they aren't effective for bipolar depression, and as discussed in this Chapter, they may not be very effective for many types of MDD. This text recommends the phrase "monoamine agonists" as a more neutral term, leaving open the clinical question of which conditions this class of medications can help. For instance, monoamine agonists appear to be more consistently helpful for anxiety than for depressive symptoms; thus the phrase "antidepressant" rather than "anxiolytic" sends clinicians and patients in the wrong direction.

Once, upon hearing a lecture on this topic, including all the preceding studies, an older clinician left the room and commented to a colleague, "The studies may be this way, but I'm still going to use antidepressants." Although clinical practice has its strengths, it also has its limitations. The main limitation of clinical practice involves confounding bias: the many competing, conflicting, and often unknown factors that influence outcomes in the real world. If clinical practice is the art of medicine, and randomized trials are the science of medicine, then these two aspects should be seen as complementary. The art of medicine is strengthened by the science, and science needs to be applied with the most effective art possible. William Osler put it this way: *Medicine is the lifelong attempt to correlate art with science.* Notice that it isn't the other way around. Science isn't there to correlate with art. It's not the job of research to confirm what clinicians already believe, but rather, more often, to refute clinical beliefs. Science is about falsifying our hypotheses, not simply confirming them.

What about type II bipolar depression? It's commonly believed by many clinicians that type II bipolar depression is more responsive to antidepressants than type I bipolar depression. This impression is based partly on a number of RCTs that report benefit with antidepressants. A key concern about those studies is that they are "enriched," which means that patients are preselected to respond to the antidepressant being studied, before the study even begins. This preselection of treatment response in a study of treatment response prejudges the matter. This research design problem hasn't been appreciated by the FDA, which accepts enriched studies for indications for treatment. The same critique holds for maintenance trials of antipsychotics in bipolar illness, some anticonvulsants in bipolar illness, and antidepressants in MDD. This critique has been described in the scientific literature, and in Chapter 6. Here the main point to make is that the apparent efficacy of antidepressants in some bipolar type II studies may be overstated because of the bias of the enriched research design. Furthermore, when antidepressant efficacy has been examined in RCTs of bipolar depression comparing type I and type II subgroups in the same trial, no differences exist. In other words, antidepressant efficacy in type II bipolar depression was the same as in type I bipolar depression, which means it was equally low in both groups.

In summary, the scientific literature of randomized trials most simply supports the conclusion that antidepressants are ineffective at best and harmful at worst in bipolar illness. Many clinicians will disagree with these judgments and many experts will seek to interpret the data as positively as possible. When randomized trials repeatedly show that a class of medications aren't effective, it's important to draw the simple clinical conclusion that they shouldn't be prescribed routinely. In the case of bipolar depression, it may be that the profession has been giving a pass to antidepressants because they have been so popular for so long with both clinicians and patients.

Bottom Line

- Antidepressants are proven ineffective in treating the acute depressive episodes of bipolar illness.
- Antidepressants are proven ineffective in treating and preventing future depressive episodes of bipolar illness.
- Antidepressants are proven to cause acute mania in bipolar illness.
- Antidepressants are proven to cause more and more mood episodes, mostly depressive, over time in about one quarter of patients with bipolar illness.
- Antidepressants are ineffective at best and harmful at worst in bipolar illness.

By the Numbers

Given these data, what should clinicians know and tell their patients regarding the probabilities of harms with "antidepressants" for bipolar illness?

Here are some statistics based on a range of research studies. These numbers apply to standard monoamine agonists (antidepressants) used to treat bipolar illness.

- The risk of acute mania with the TCAs is about 50%.

- The risk of acute mania with SRIs in type I bipolar illness is about 10–30%.
- The risk of acute mania with SRIs in type II bipolar illness is about 5–10%.
- The risk of long-term worsening of bipolar illness, with rapid-cycling course, is about 30% with any antidepressants in type I or type II bipolar illness.
- These risks are reduced by a factor of about one-half for acute mania if concomitant mood stabilizers or neuroleptics are given.
- The risks for long-term rapid cycling are not reduced if concomitant mood stabilizers or neuroleptics are given.
- About 50% of unipolar depressive episodes are mixed states, which is similar to the rate in bipolar depression.

Treatment of Bipolar Illness with Dopamine Blockers (Antipsychotics)

Traditional dopamine blockers have been and are still widely used in the treatment of mood conditions, mainly bipolar illness. However, two double-blind studies have demonstrated that traditional dopamine blockers added to lithium are ineffective in the prevention of mania in bipolar disorder compared to lithium alone. In fact, the use of dopamine blockers simply tended to worsen long-term depression. Thus, outside of treating acute mania, these agents are simply not proven effective in the long-term prevention of mania, and may actually cause or worsen depressive symptoms in patients with mood disorders. In addition to limited evidence regarding their efficacy in bipolar disorder, the safety of traditional dopamine blocker use remains controversial. Numerous studies have suggested that patients with bipolar disorder may be at increased risk for the development of EPS and TD, compared to patients with schizophrenia, when treated with traditional dopamine blocker agents. It is generally agreed that traditional dopamine blockers should be avoided or used only temporarily in patients with bipolar disorder. However, until recently, manic inpatients treated with traditional dopamine blockers ostensibly for acute mania generally were not tapered off their traditional dopamine blockers after the acute manic episode resolved.

Given the disadvantages of traditional dopamine blockers, newer dopamine blockers have emerged as a much preferable alternative in mood disorders. There is a biochemical rationale why this may be the case. Mechanistically, dopamine blockade probably confers an antimanic effect. Since traditional dopamine blockers only possess dopamine blockade effects, they tend to bring mood down from mania, but they continue to exert a downward effect on mood, leading to depression in many persons. Serotonin-2 receptor blockade may produce some antidepressant effects, by means of increasing neurotransmission along 5HT-1 receptors, which is the serotonin receptor system thought to mediate antidepressant effects. Yet 5HT-2 blockade by itself is likely to be weak in its antidepressant effects; standard antidepressants that share this mechanism also have other effects (such as serotonin reuptake blockade for nefazodone, or alpha-2 adrenergic blockade for mirtazapine).

Newer dopamine blockers differ in their other effects, which may be relevant to antidepressant properties. In addition to 5HT-2 blockade, risperidone is a strong alpha-2 blocker (which blocks a negative feedback loop, resulting in increased serotonergic and noradrenergic transmitter availability). Olanzapine increases frontal lobe serotonin neurotransmission preferentially, which may assist with antidepressant efficacy. Ziprasidone is a rather potent blocker of serotonin reuptake, at a level in vitro similar to that of tertiary TCAs. Some combination of these kinds of effects with antidopamine effect may allow atypical dopamine blockers to exert antimanic effects without leading to depression (which is the clearest clinical effect observed in bipolar disorder). Furthermore, this biochemical profile could explain mood-stabilizing properties with this class.

Acute Mania

Consequently, numerous double-blind studies have been conducted with olanzapine and risperidone in acute mania, and one double-blind study each has been conducted with clozapine, quetiapine, and ziprasidone. All of these studies have found these agents effective in treating acute mania. The entire class clearly seems effective as antimanic agents.

Initial randomized clinical trials found that risperidone and olanzapine produced fewer EPS in acute mania than haloperidol. This finding was not surprising, but it was important, since all previous comparisons had occurred in schizophrenia, and we know that patients with bipolar disorder are likely to be more sensitive to EPS.

However, in the CATIE study, there were no or minimal differences in EPS between second generation dopamine blockers and perphenazine (Trilafon). Yet low doses of perphenazine were used, and somewhat lower akathisia rates were seen with quetiapine than with perphenazine.

One of the key findings with most of these studies is that modern dopamine blockers treat acute mania without any worsening of depression. In other words, resolution of acute mania is not followed frequently by switch into acute depression. This finding differs from the research with traditional dopamine blockers in bipolar disorder, many of which were associated with a depressogenic effect.

Prophylaxis of Bipolar Illness: Are Antipsychotics "Mood Stabilizers"?

The view taken here is that dopamine blockers are not "mood stabilizers" if by that it is meant that their maintenance studies demonstrate efficacy in the prophylactic phase of treatment. These maintenance studies, which are "enriched" randomized discontinuation trials (RDTs), are questionable in validity, as discussed in detail in Chapter 6.

In that critique, the RDT design was seen as invalid because it measures the same acute treatment response twice: before and after randomization. It preselects treatment responders for a drug, then tests that same response again, always finding a positive result. It is as if chocolate cake lovers were tested for whether they love chocolate cake.

In natural history terms, these RDTs do now show prevention of new episodes six months or longer after the acute phase. Almost all the relapses are in the first six months, which still reflect the acute episode that existed before the maintenance trial began. In bipolar illness, another way of examining this matter is to see if new episodes of the opposite pole to the index episode (the acute phase just before the maintenance trial began) are being prevented, since after six months, almost all episodes are of the opposite pole. Thus, if a study begins with a dopamine blocker given for acute mania, and then treatment responders are included in a maintenance trial, one test of true prevention of a new episode would be prevention of the opposite pole, a depressive episode, which would be the next phase of illness. Among dopamine blockers, this design critique applies to all claims of maintenance efficacy in bipolar illness.

An example is the aripiprazole maintenance study, which received an FDA indication. Acutely manic patients were preselected for aripiprazole response, then randomized for up to six months to stay on or come off that agent. Aripiprazole only prevented manic, not depressive, episodes. Why? Is it simply because it works well for mania, not depression? This is highly unlikely, given that aripiprazole has been proven effective for acute depressive episodes in MDD. In fact, it was ineffective in one placebo-controlled trial of acute mania. In contrast, the results would make sense if they simply reflected the fact that the study was not long enough to assess new mood episodes, and that its lack of efficacy in the opposite phase of illness simply indicated that it wasn't preventing new mood episodes.

This controversy can be addressed also as a matter of the English language. In a prior issue, as discussed in Chapter 1, the term "antipsychotic" is not a scientifically and clinically accurate term. The author of this text prefers the term "dopamine blockers." These agents often are effective in non-psychotic conditions, like depression and mania. The term "dopamine blocker" was suggested it because it is true, although it is not reflective of all of the biological effects of these agents, and it is neutral as to clinical effect. The term "mood stabilizer" also is meaningless scientifically. These medications do not "stabilize" mood; rather, they treat both acute depressive and manic episodes, and they prevent those mood episodes. What distinguishes these agents clinically to the greatest degree from other classes of medications is their long-term prevention of mood episodes. So the term "mood stabilizer" really does not capture what these medications do. A more neutral term that reflects their biological mechanism is "second-messenger modifier."

So the question "Are antipsychotics mood stabilizers?" can be translated more neutrally and scientifically to the question "Are dopamine blockers second-messenger modifiers?" When restated this way, the answer is obvious. Dopamine blockade is not the same thing as second-messenger modification. Just to clarify: dopamine blockade happens at the synapse and is associated with improvement primarily in psychotic or manic symptoms. It's an acute effect. Second-messenger modification happens postsynaptically and it relates mainly to long-term changes in neurons and their connections with other neurons. Those biological effects would correlate more with long-term clinical effects of prophylaxis of mood episodes. In other words, the basic biological effects of these two different classes of medications differ and correlate with differences in clinical strengths, with acute symptom benefit for dopamine blockers and long-term prophylaxis for second-messenger modifiers. Therefore, at one level we can assert that antipsychotics aren't mood stabilizers simply because dopamine blockers aren't second-messenger modifiers.

In sum, the view is that antipsychotics are not mood stabilizers because "enriched" maintenance randomized discontinuation trials are inherently invalid based on their preselection of acute treatment efficacy, followed by reassessing acute treatment efficacy.

They don't assess new mood episodes in the maintenance treatment of bipolar illness. Because they involve a tautology, they never fail. The FDA approves this design, but it doesn't appreciate the invalidity of how this design is used in psychiatric maintenance studies. This error benefits the pharmaceutical industry, but misleads clinicians and patients into major errors in long-term treatment of bipolar illness.

Given these considerations, this text strongly recommends that clinicians shouldn't consider dopamine blockers as equal to or better than standard second-messenger modifiers, like lithium. These maintenance studies don't justify replacing lithium with quetiapine, or replacing valproate with olanzapine. Rather, the latter agents could be used short-term, preferably, and if used long-term, they should be seen *as adjuncts only* to second-messenger modifiers, not as "mood stabilizers" by themselves, that could be effective for bipolar illness *in place of* standard second-messenger modifiers like lithium, valproate, lamotrigine, or carbamazepine.

Bottom Line

- "Antipsychotics" are not mood stabilizers because they have not been proven to prevent new mood episodes in believable maintenance studies.
- "Enriched" maintenance studies are not valid, preselecting acute treatment response and then assessing the same thing.
- Dopamine blockers are not second-messenger modifiers; their different biological mechanisms reflect different clinical effects.
- Dopamine blockers should be used mainly short-term; if used long-term in bipolar illness, they should be used *as adjuncts to* second-messenger modifiers, *not as replacing* the latter.
- If you like chocolate cake, you're going to like chocolate cake. This doesn't mean that chocolate cake is inherently better than vanilla cake.

By the Numbers—Natural History of Mood Episodes

For over 100 years, manic-depressive illness has been defined, but for most of that time, no effective treatments existed. Thus, there is an extensive research literature on the natural course of this condition, especially based on the late 19th and early 20th century work in Germany inspired by Emil Kraepelin and his coworkers. Here are some statistics based on those research studies. These time-frames all apply to *the untreated duration of mood episodes, with their spontaneous recovery naturally, without any treatment at all.* (For a review of these sources, see the "Natural History" chapter in *Manic-Depressive Illness*, 2nd edition, 2007, by Frederick K. Goodwin and Kay R. Jamison.)

- The natural duration of an acute depressive episode in unipolar depression is six to 12 months.
- The natural duration of an acute depressive episode in bipolar depression is three to six months.
- The natural duration of an acute manic episode in unipolar depression is two to four months.

- The typical patient with bipolar illness has one episode per year.
- The typical patient with unipolar depression has an episode every three to five years.
- After an acute manic episode, over 90% of patients will have a second mood episode within five years.

Dopamine Blockers for Acute Bipolar Depression

FDA-indicated medications for acute bipolar depression are quetiapine (Seroquel), olanzapine-fluoxetine combination (Symbyax, also called OFC), and most recently, lurasidone (Latuda). Two medications that do not have FDA indications, ziprasidone (Geodon) and aripiprazole (Abilify), also have a scientific rationale for efficacy in bipolar depression. Of these agents, quetiapine and OFC have, by far, the worst risks, especially if used long-term (given that they worsen metabolic syndrome and cardiovascular risks). Hence, lurasidone, aripiprazole, and ziprasidone—not quetiapine or OFC—are recommended as the primary dopamine blocker treatments for bipolar depression.

Studies using dopamine blockers exist mainly for *acute* bipolar depression, meaning a current severe clinical depressive episode that usually lasts one to six months untreated. The usual duration of treatment, in standard FDA studies, is six to eight weeks.

Thus, to the extent there is scientific evidence of efficacy of dopamine blockers in bipolar depression, that evidence exists for about two months of treatment, not two or 20 years. In other words, this research evidence, if valid, would instruct clinicians to treat bipolar depression with dopamine blockers for two months, then stop those agents. To say that dopamine blockers should be continued, evidence of maintenance efficacy would be needed, which was critiqued before. It is worth pointing out that there are no data on OFC for maintenance treatment (olanzapine is not the same), and that the aripiprazole maintenance study found that it was *not* effective in prevention of bipolar depressive episodes (efficacy was present only in prevention of manic episodes). The Second Fallacy of Psychopharmacology should not be forgotten: *Long-term preventive efficacy cannot be assumed from acute efficacy data.*

Olanzapine-Fluoxetine Combination (OFC)

The main study that led to FDA indication for OFC proved that olanzapine did *not* work for treating bipolar depression, and the amount of data supportive of OFC is rather small in size and less definitive than many might suppose. In fact, the "OFC" (olanzapine/ fluoxetine combination) study was designed originally to prove the efficacy of olanzapine alone, not OFC. The study was powered statistically for that purpose: 370 subjects were randomized to olanzapine, and 377 to placebo. Luckily for the manufacturer, a small sample of 86 subjects also was randomized to OFC. Olanzapine alone showed benefit over placebo using p-values, but the "effect size" was tiny: a very small improvement in the Montgomery Asberg Depression Rating Scale (MADRS) of about two points: one for sleeping more and another for eating more. Sedation and increased appetite are side effects of olanzapine, not proof of its efficacy for bipolar depression. The FDA reached the same conclusion.

Olanzapine was shown *not* to be effective in acute bipolar depression, despite its "statistically significant" benefit over placebo. In contrast, OFC showed efficacy, including for standard mood symptoms of sad mood and low interest and low energy, albeit in a small sample of 86 subjects. Should a drug get an FDA indication when its only data involve fewer than 100 subjects treated in the effective arm in one randomized clinical trial? Usually, the general FDA rule is that companies need to show efficacy in two randomized clinical trials before an indication will be given. Exceptions are made, though, especially for clinical conditions in which few or no treatments already are approved. This was the case for acute bipolar depression in 2003. No FDA indications existed at that time for any drug. (Keep in mind that "antidepressants" are not FDA-indicated as having efficacy for bipolar depression). So the FDA gave approval for OFC based on one RCT, with a small sample, even though the study was never designed for that purpose. Now that two other agents are approved for bipolar depression, if the same OFC data were presented to the FDA today, the FDA probably would reject it as insufficient to be given an indication for bipolar depression. But OFC is now grandfathered into its FDA indication. And, going by the mere fact of FDA indication, many clinicians will draw the mistaken conclusion that the scientific evidence for efficacy of OFC in bipolar depression is as good as that for quetiapine or lurasidone.

Quetiapine

Acute bipolar depression studies with quetiapine are, superficially, more straightforward than with OFC. Astra Zeneca planned two large eight-week trials of quetiapine alone versus placebo, and the drug worked in both cases, with large effect sizes of benefit that included core mood symptoms (like anhedonia, low energy, and sad mood). The FDA provided the bipolar depression indication. As clinicians and patients know, quetiapine is an extremely sedating drug. It has potent antihistaminic, antiadrenergic, and anticholinergic effects. One would tend to notice taking it. Some academic leaders involved in the quetiapine studies acknowledge that it's likely that those RCTs weren't truly blinded: patients could tell when they took quetiapine, and when they didn't (received placebo). Unblinded studies tend to increase treatment effect sizes, hence the quetiapine studies probably overestimate its benefits. This doesn't mean quetiapine isn't effective in bipolar depression at all. It means that the claim that it is *especially* effective, more so than other agents, may be inflated based on sedating non-mood effects. In sum, quetiapine showed benefit; but is it as big of a clinical benefit as it seems, or an inflated effect of a highly sedating drug?

Lurasidone

This newest FDA-indicated agent was shown effective in two- to six-week RCTs of bipolar depression. It isn't sedating, and other aspects of study design seem valid.

Aripiprazole

The manufacturer conducted two eight-week trials of this agent for bipolar depression. In both cases, repeatedly, the drug was better than placebo from weeks 1 through 6, but at week 8, placebo showed a benefit that reduced the overall effect size and led to a *p*-value above 0.05 (see Figure 19.10).

FDA indication wasn't given since the study was designed with the *a priori* outcome of improvement at eight weeks. It could be held that aripiprazole was effective in bipolar depression, because the benefits seen at four and six weeks are more meaningful scientifically than the final eight-week endpoint. This is because the duration of a study should be adjusted to the duration of an illness. There is no general rule that a study should be long, or that the longer the study, the better it is. Mania RCTs are only three weeks in duration, because manic episodes are short, lasting two to four months untreated according to

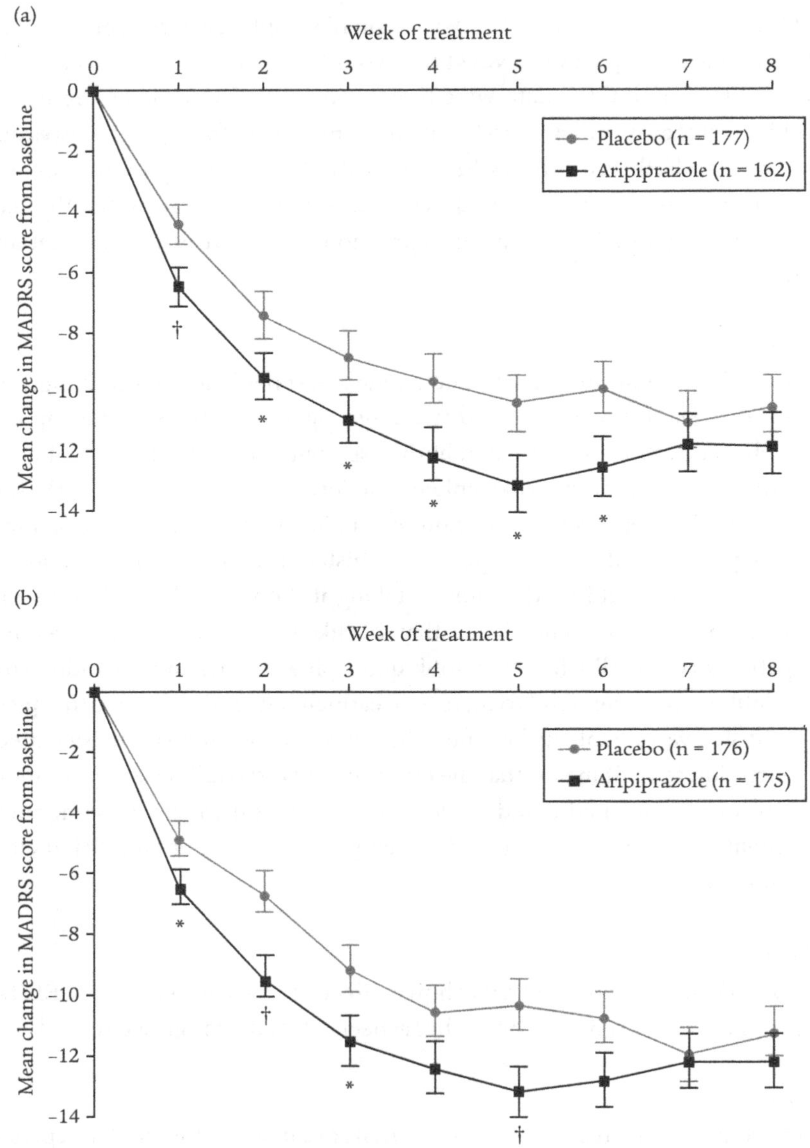

FIGURE 19.10 *Aripiprazole efficacy in two RCTs of acute bipolar depression.*

some studies. Unipolar depression studies are eight weeks long because unipolar depressive episodes are long, lasting six to 12 months untreated. But bipolar depressive episodes, though longer than mania, are shorter than unipolar depressive episodes. According to a century of natural history data dating back to Kraepelin, bipolar depressive episodes tend to last two to six months, and fewer in those with rapid-cycling course (about one-quarter of bipolar subjects). So, if one conducts a trial that is eight weeks long, in a condition where a substantial minority of patients is improved by one to three months, there will be a "placebo" rate of improvement, due to natural remission, that is high. This makes it difficult to show drug benefit. Thus six weeks is more scientifically valid than eight weeks for the duration of a bipolar depression trial. That mistake has confused some clinicians into thinking the drug has no benefit for a condition in which it showed benefit. This is why the lurasidone studies were six weeks long. And this is why the aripiprazole study's effect at four and six weeks shouldn't be ignored. If aripiprazole improves depressive symptoms, it isn't surprising that other studies found it to be effective in unipolar depression, leading to FDA indication as augmentation of antidepressants.

Lastly, although this text takes the approach that biological rationale should not be the primary factor in treatment decisions, biological mechanisms are relevant for interpreting clinical trial data. Aripiprazole is a moderate dopamine agonist. Dopamine agonists (like amphetamines and bupropion) improve depressive symptoms. In contrast, olanzapine and quetiapine have little monoamine agonist effects (minor effects were shown retrospectively in some animal studies later conducted by their companies), and certainly not as much as aripiprazole (or ziprasidone).

Ziprasidone

Based on its biological mechanism, if any dopamine blocker is going to be effective for depressive symptoms, it should be ziprasidone. It's the only modern dopamine blocker that also is an SRI and an NRI. Its effects are about as potent as standard SRIs' and TCAs'. The trouble is that Pfizer conducted two RCTs of ziprasidone versus placebo in acute bipolar depression, and it didn't work. Unlike aripiprazole, there wasn't benefit at some weeks but not others. There just wasn't benefit. This should seem odd: drugs without strong monoamine agonism, like quetiapine, are supposedly "antidepressant" in their effects, while drugs with strong classic antidepressant mechanisms, like ziprasidone, are not. How can this be?

The concept of "mixed states" is explained further later. It could be that the apparent "antidepressant" effect of dopamine blockers has to do partly with dopamine blockade itself, which is effective for mixed manic/depressive states, rather than with mood-elevating monoamine agonism effects of classic SRIs/NRIs. In other words, dopamine blockade provides benefit for mixed states—this is well known. *Most "bipolar depression" is, in fact, a mixed state,* as described later. Hence, almost any dopamine blocker should help, not just quetiapine or OFC. This hypothesis could be tested directly by studying ziprasidone (or any antipsychotic) in patients selected for "mixed depression." Indeed, in such a randomized trial, ziprasidone was effective, better than placebo, in an overall sample of 73 subjects. This result is similar in size to the OFC study arm ($n = 86$). In other words, the widespread use of OFC is based on an amount of scientific evidence that is similar to what exists for ziprasidone for mixed depression, even though the latter never obtained FDA indication because it was going to be a generic agent by the time these data were obtained. This is another example of why FDA registration should not be the primary guide to assessing scientific evidence when comparing medications.

The axiom of Paracelsus was that all drugs are toxic; it's only the dose and indication that make them therapeutic. In the aripiprazole studies of bipolar depression, secondary analyses found that in those treated with *lower* doses (5–10 mg/d), aripiprazole was *more* effective than placebo; it was in the higher dose group (>10 mg/d) that placebo seemed similar to aripiprazole. In the lurasidone monotherapy studies, the low-dose arm (20–60 mg/d; mean dose 32 mg/d) was equivalent in efficacy to the high-dose arm (80–120 mg/d; mean dose 82 mg/d). A similar principle may apply with ziprasidone. At low doses (<80 mg /d), patients can show good improvement for bipolar depression; it could be that *higher* doses are *less* effective. This observation seems to contradict the common clinical intuition that *more is better.* This idea is may seem sound logically, but it is unsound biologically. A biological explanation may be as follows: At lower doses of all dopamine blockers, there is less dopamine blockade. It's commonly believed that about 80–90% dopamine blockade is needed for full antipsychotic effect.

What is relevant to treating psychosis may not be relevant to non-psychotic bipolar depression. It could be that only about 50% or so of dopamine blockade is sufficient to get benefit for the mixed depressive state in bipolar depression. Thus, higher doses of dopamine blockers may confer no further mood benefit. Turning to the dopamine agonism of aripiprazole and the serotonin/norepinephrine reuptake blockade of ziprasidone, these effects are present to the same extent at any dose, including low doses.

So it could be that low doses provide a good amount of "antidepressant"-like monoamine agonism, with sufficient dopamine blockade for manic symptoms; while higher doses might just produce more and more dopamine blockade, which might just produce more antimanic effect, moving the mood down, rather than elevating it. These biological explanations may or may not be correct, but the approach of this text is to emphasize the clinical research evidence, which indicates *more* benefit in bipolar depression with *lower* doses of dopamine blockers. Thus clinicians should avoid using the high doses shown effective for schizophrenia and mania as their standard for treating bipolar depression.

In weighing risks and benefits, Osler's dictum that the art of medicine is the art of balancing probabilities also comes into play. Clinicians shouldn't use only the drugs that are FDA-indicated, and hence marketed to them. They should compare the scientific evidence of all drugs, take into account comparisons of side effects among drugs with scientific evidence of efficacy, then weigh the probabilities of benefits versus harms. Quetiapine has notable and long-term metabolic syndrome and harmful cardiovascular effects. So does olanzapine. When these known common harms are taken into account, the benefit/harm calculation tilts in the direction of lurasidone, aripiprazole, and ziprasidone. These three agents are left mainly with the risk of akathisia, which can present as worsened agitation and/or suicidality. Akathisia is dangerous, and immediate intervention is needed, either by stopping the dopamine blocker, or by lowering its dose and/or adding a counteracting agent, like propranolol, as discussed in Chapter 10.

Bottom Line

- Recommended agents for bipolar depression are lurasidone, aripiprazole, and ziprasidone.
- Low doses should be used. Akathisia is the main problem with these agents.
- The benefit of quetiapine is probably overestimated in its studies.
- Olanzapine alone is proven ineffective.
- Dopamine blockers may mostly help "bipolar" depression when it represents "mixed depression," the combination of severe depression with some manic symptoms.

Treatment of Mixed States

The preceding discussion of dopamine blocker efficacy in bipolar depression, along with limited antidepressant efficacy in MDD, raises the question of the diagnostic limitations. In other words, it could that the diagnosis of MDD or bipolar depression does not lend itself to adequate treatment with a single drug class, such as the monoamine agonists. The diagnostic subtype of "mixed states" was mentioned earlier and can be seen as a specific kind of depressive state that responds poorly to monoamine agonists, and more effectively to dopamine blockers. In Appendix I, the concept of mixed states is discussed in more detail diagnostically. Here, treatment aspects of mixed states will be examined.

As a reminder, the DSM system defines mania as diagnosable only if it lasts seven days or longer, and hypomania as occurring when manic symptoms occur for a shorter amount of time: four days or longer. But what if manic symptoms occur for three days and 23 hours? Or two days, or one day or 12 hours, or three hours? The current mainstream DSM approach, preached now for four decades, tells clinicians to ignore all manic symptoms, as if they didn't matter at all, or didn't happen at all, if they last three days and 23 hours or less.

In Appendix I, a number of scientific studies are examined that show that this claim appears to be false: that manic symptoms of any duration, occurring in a clinical depressive episode, are similar to manic symptoms of longer duration, occurring in hypomanic or manic episodes. This similarity is based on the scientific standards of diagnostic validation: genetics, course, and treatment effects.

In other words, it doesn't matter whether manic symptoms are brief or long-lived; they have the same genetics, course, and treatment effects. This means they are not different diagnoses, but the same diagnoses. Put otherwise, DSM-based bipolar diagnoses cannot be shown to change into different diagnoses when manic symptoms are less than four days to one week in duration. Or to restate, there is zero evidence to support the DSM cutoff of four days or longer for manic symptoms, as representing a bipolar diagnosis as opposed to non-bipolar diagnoses.

If one takes manic symptoms seriously, then, at all times, and refuses to ignore them as DSM wishes when they are less than four days in duration, then one would pay attention to diagnosing those depressive states with manic symptoms as "mixed states," the term that Kraepelin and others used for these common mood states. If these mixed-state concepts could be valid, then their treatment implications may be relevant: Which treatments worsen and which treatments improve mixed states?

Perhaps the most important relevance of the mixed state concept is that antidepressants worsen these states. Since most mixed states are diagnosed in current practice as "major depressive episodes," and antidepressants are given for such purported major depression, it would be quite important if it were true that these clinical presentations instead are mixed states that worsen with antidepressants.

Antidepressants are known to cause mania, but many clinicians don't realize that the main kind of manic state produced is a mixed state; in other words, manic symptoms and depressive symptoms mixed together. These mixed states are the highest-risk states for suicide, which is one reason why antidepressants can cause suicidality.

Antidepressant-induced mania is about four times more likely in persons with mixed states, as defined by having multiple manic symptoms for any duration, along with depression (Angst's "bipolarity specifier"; see Appendix I). In a study using Koukopoulos's definition of mixed states (depression with psychomotor excitation, usually marked anger; see Appendix 1), antidepressant-induced mixed depression was associated with over twice as many suicide attempts, when compared with spontaneous mixed states (occurring without antidepressant use).

So the first and most important step of understanding mixed states is to conclude that antidepressants shouldn't be used, and if they are present, they should be stopped. If antidepressants add "fire" to mixed states, dopamine blockers are the "water brigade." There are only two medications proven in randomized studies to improve mixed depressive states, specifically in so-called MDD (i.e., unipolar mixed states): ziprasidone and lurasidone. Probably all dopamine blockers are beneficial, but these two are the best-proven.

In contrast to monoamine agonists ("antidepressants"), which have been proven ineffective in mixed depressive states, and in fact worsen them, dopamine blockers are effective and improve mixed depressive states. There may be some special utility to the dopamine blockers that have some monoamine agonist properties also (meaning they are either partial dopamine agonists, like aripiprazole and brexpiprazole, or they are SNRIs, like ziprasidone).

Lurasidone has been shown to be effective in a large randomized trial of DSM-5–defined MDD with mixed features, which is a narrowly defined mixed state concept (see prior issue). Despite this efficacy greater than placebo, the FDA did not grant an indication to allow the manufacturer to market this agent for unipolar mixed states.

In mixed manic episodes, it has been shown that divalproex and carbamazepine are more effective than lithium. Whether this enhanced efficacy translates into mixed depressive episodes is unknown, but it may. Since the mixed depressive concept has been ignored for decades, no randomized research has been conducted on it with these agents. However, it may be reasonable to extrapolate from studies of mixed manic episodes, and from manic episodes in general. We know that valproate and carbamazepine are more effective in treating acute mania than placebo, and they work reasonably rapidly. Lithium is proven effective also, but works somewhat more slowly. Lamotrigine has repeatedly been proven ineffective for acute mania, as well as repeatedly proven ineffective for acute depressive episodes (whether bipolar or unipolar). Thus it may be rational to conclude that lamotrigine is not effective for acute mixed depressive states, since it is ineffective for all acute mood episodes. In contrast, valproate and lithium probably are effective, as is lithium. Given some uncertainty about the extent of benefit with these agents, though, it may be wise to use dopamine blockers along with them, or even in place of them, for more severe acute mixed depressive states.

Nonetheless, these agents are likely to have a role in long-term prophylaxis of mixed states, even if they are not sufficiently effective for improving acute mixed symptoms. With the exception of lamotrigine, which is proven less effective in preventing manic than depressive episodes, there is no evidence that the other three second-messenger modifiers ("mood stabilizers") are more or less effective than each other in prevention of manic episodes. Thus it would seem reasonable to conclude that any of them could be used for prevention of mixed states.

Bottom Line

- The treatment of mixed states begins with the avoidance and discontinuation of monoamine agonists (antidepressants).
- Monoamine agonists are ineffective, and double the suicide attempt rate in mixed states.
- Dopamine blockers, specifically ziprasidone and lurasidone, are the most proven treatments for acute mixed depressive states.
- Second-messenger modifiers also are effective, especially for prophylaxis, with the likely exception of lamotrigine, which probably is ineffective acutely in mixed depressive state.

Efficacy of Lithium and Anticonvulsants

In Chapter 25, there is extensive discussion of lithium's potential benefits for suicide prevention, and in Chapter 11, its potential dementia prevention benefits were discussed. In this chapter, the discussion will focus on the effects of lithium and other anticonvulsants on mood states.

One of the most obvious aspects of understanding lithium has to do with the awareness that there are dozens of randomized clinical trials that show benefit with lithium in prevention of mood episodes in manic-depressive illness. This is a simple statement, but it cannot be said of the vast majority of psychotropic drugs. Most medications are proven effective in a few randomized clinical trials, often the minimum of two RCTs required for FDA indication. Usually those studies are conducted by the manufacturer of the drug. In the case of lithium, dozens and dozens of studies have been conducted over literally half a century with replication by many different research groups. In fact, lithium is the only psychotropic medication that came to the U.S. market without being promoted by any pharmaceutical company. The extent of proof of lithium's efficacy is unrivaled.

The prophylactic benefit of lithium in manic-depressive illness proven in multiple studies in the 1960s and 1970s involved patients who would today be diagnosed with unipolar depression as well as bipolar illness. Thus, lithium has been proven to prevent mood episodes not only in bipolar illness, but also in unipolar depression.

Besides this long-term benefit, there have been many studies of lithium in acute mood episodes of both mania and depression. It has proven effective in both cases, with the proviso that it is somewhat slower in effect for acute manic episodes than dopamine blockers. For acute depressive episodes, it was studied mainly as an adjunctive agent to monoamine agonists in unipolar depression, but often in monotherapy in bipolar depression. It has been proven effective overall in both cases, although it may be slower in effect than some monoamine agonists in unipolar depression.

The one setting in which lithium has been proven to be less effective than other agents is for acute mixed episodes. For mixed manic states, valproate has been shown to be more effective than lithium in RCTs. It is likely that carbamazepine also is more effective than lithium for mixed episodes.

It often is held that lithium is less effective in rapid-cycling bipolar illness than anticonvulsants. However, unlike mixed episodes, there is no difference among these agents in rapid-cycling bipolar illness.

Rapid-Cycling Bipolar Illness

Rapid-cycling does not mean that moods cycle rapidly. That is English, not science. "Rapid-cycling," in the scientific use of the term, means having four or more mood episodes in a year, which means that the episodes can last three months. This is not about moods "cycling" over hours. That is "mood lability," which is part of mixed states, not rapid-cycling. The difference is important. Rapid cycling is often missed because clinicians may not pay attention to the fact that patients have episodes lasting a few weeks, a few times in a year. That is rapid cycling.

The importance of the diagnosis is that it means that there is an *absolute* contraindication to the use of antidepressants, under any circumstances at all. This is because antidepressants cause rapid cycling; they worsen it, as discussed previously in this chapter. Put another way, the only intervention shown to improve rapid cycling is antidepressant discontinuation.

If antidepressants are stopped or aren't being used, clinicians still are faced with the reality that rapid cycling is a major poor prognostic factor. It was originally defined in people who did not respond to lithium. So lithium is ineffective by itself. This inefficacy has been interpreted to mean that other agents are more effective than lithium in rapid cycling. This misconception is disproven. Lamotrigine was studied and proven ineffective, equal to placebo, in two randomized trials of rapid-cycling. Valproate was shown to be equal to lithium in the largest randomized trial of rapid cycling. Carbamazepine also is equal to lithium in rapid cycling in head-to-head.

In short, nothing works in rapid cycling—except stopping antidepressants. After that, since no single mood stabilizer is effective, it is logical to combine mood stabilizers. Valproate plus lithium have been proven more effective together than when used alone. Often, patients tend to need one dopamine blocker added to two standard mood stabilizers.

Even so, improvement in rapid-cycling is slow and should not be judged on the basis of what happens over a month or two with a current mood episode. One can assess efficacy only by seeing if four or more mood episodes in a year decrease in frequency. This means one has to look at multiple episodes, over six to 12 months, before a drug's efficacy in rapid cycling can be evaluated. This requires patience on the part of patients and clinicians.

The Bipolar Affective disorder: Lithium/anticonvulsant Evaluation (BALANCE) study, discussed in Chapter 46, is a project that is relevant to the concept of using combination mood stabilizing agents in rapid-cycling bipolar illness. That large RCT showed that the combination of lithium plus valproate was more effective than either agent alone, in general. The study was not specifically limited to rapid-cycling bipolar illness, but it included about one-quarter of patients with that course of illness. In general, combined lithium plus valproate seemed effective in those patients versus either agent alone. Furthermore, the BALANCE study showed more efficacy with lithium in depression and mania prophylaxis. This finding contradicts common beliefs that lithium may be more effective for manic and depressive symptoms.

Lamotrigine

Among anticonvulsants, lamotrigine has become widely used, at least in the United States, and a separate discussion of its strengths and weaknesses is warranted. In a discussion of lamotrigine, it is important to address some marketing phrases that have filtered deeply into clinical practice. Specifically, the notion of "stabilizing from below" versus "from above," as introduced in Chapter 11, will be examined again.

Consider the following case vignettes:

Case 1. A man in his mid-40s has a two-decade history of manic and depressive episodes. He is treated for his bipolar illness with lamotrigine 200 mg/d, and lithium 600 mg/d (level 0.6). He experienced breakthrough depression, and his new psychiatrist recommended olanzapine/fluoxetine combination (OFC). The consultant recommeded to increase lithium instead of adding OFC. The treating psychiatrist responded that lithium is more for "top-down" control, while lamotrigine is for "bottom-up" control. He was skeptical that increasing lithium would help with further depression prophylaxis.

Case 2. A man in his mid-30s has rapid-cycling bipolar illness type I. He has six mood episodes yearly, alternating between brief hypomanic states and longer depressive episodes, lasting one month or so each. His life is very disrupted. He is treated with lamotrigine 200 mg/d plus lithium 900 mg/d (level 0.6; higher doses could not be tolerated) for eight months, without benefit. Lithium was switched to divalproex (1000 mg/d, level 65) added to lamotrigine, without benefit. Pregabalin was added, without benefit. His psychiatrist was avoiding antidepressants and dopamine blockers. Theonsultant recommended switching from lamotrigine to lithium, combined with divalproex, and adding a dopamine blocker. The psychiatrist refused, insisting that the patient needed more mood stabilization "from below" as opposed to more "anti-manic" medication.

These two cases demonstrate how false pharmaceutical marketing continues to influence clinical decision-making years after a drug, now generic, is marketed no longer.

The author of this textbook was present at the creation: one of the investigators in the first maintenance studies of lamotrigine, and a member of its national advisory board over a decade ago. At the time, lamotrigine had a problem: it was proven ineffective for acute mood states of all varieties—depressive or manic. It was further proven ineffective in acute depression in both unipolar or bipolar illness. All these negative randomized studies had been conducted by the manufacturer, but they didn't plan to publish them anytime soon. They didn't even tell the academic members of the national advisory board. A few years later, in the setting of a lawsuit against another agent owned by the same manufacturer, a judge ordered the manufacturer to put all its material online for the public to see. That is when these negative studies came to light, though most still remain unpublished, except for a summary of them published by author of this text based on the court-ordered website data.

These negative studies provide the context for the marketing decisions made by the manufacturer regarding their two positive prophylaxis studies with lamotrigine. In those two maintenance studies of bipolar I illness, lamotrigine was more effective than lithium and placebo, and it received an FDA indication. The marketing question was "How do you persuade clinicians to prescribe a drug for prevention when it isn't effective for the acute episode?"

The solution was a marketing slogan: "Stabilizing from below." As many clinicians know, this slogan was based on the observation in the lamotrigine maintenance trials that this agent was more effective than lithium and placebo in the prevention of depressive episodes, but less effective than lithium and placebo in the prevention of manic episodes. The origin of the marketing slogan came from an academic consultant: lamotrigine stabilizes "from below" and lithium stabilizes "from above."

The slogan could translate into persuading clinicians to give lamotrigine in their patients with mostly depressive episodes, which, not by coincidence, is the case in the vast majority of persons with bipolar illness. Clinicians were convinced, by a phrase, that lamotrigine should be preferred to lithium in the vast majority of persons with bipolar illness. And this effect was achieved despite the fact that lamotrigine was completely ineffective (repeatedly shown to be the same as placebo in randomized trials) for treating acute bipolar depression (a fact kept hidden from clinicians by not publishing those negative studies).

The claim that lamotrigine is more effective than lithium for depressive episode prophylaxis can be challenged based on the validity of the research method used in those maintenance studies: the "enriched" design. As described in Chapter 6, this method involves preselecting treatment responders to the medication being studied (i.e., lamotrigine) for the maintenance study. Those who had failed to respond to lamotrigine before the maintenance study began would be excluded from the maintenance study. Yet lithium was not similarly preselected so as to include only lithium responders in the maintenance study.

In the two prophylaxis trials, patients were initially treated with lamotrigine for an acute mood episode, in one trial, depression, and in the other trial, mania. This treatment occurred openly and was not part of the randomized maintenance trial itself. All this initial treatment was just for preparation to enter the actual research study: the randomized maintenance trial. If patients improved and tolerated lamotrigine, they were then entered into the research study; i.e., the randomized maintenance trial, where they were randomly assigned to stay on lamotrigine or to switch to lithium or to switch to placebo.

Notice that these were all patients who at least tolerated lamotrigine and improved, and then they stayed on it. If they didn't stay on it, they were switched to lithium (or placebo), but they had not been recently treated with lithium and preselected to improve on lithium and to tolerate it. In other words, it should be clear to readers that this is not a fair comparison. About half the patients tolerated and responded to lamotrigine in the prior two to three months, and this "enriched" group of responders was then compared to people given lithium *de novo*, as opposed to also being preselected to having just improved with lithium over the prior two to three months.

An unfair comparison produces biased results. Thus, one cannot fairly say that lamotrigine was more effective than lithium in depression prophylaxis, when the sample was biased to include only prior lamotrigine responders but it was not biased to include only prior lithium responders.

It is notable that, even with this heavy bias in favor of lamotrigine, lithium still was more effective than lamotrigine in mania prophylaxis. Clinicians can believe that result because it means that, even with a strong handicap, lithium still beats lamotrigine for mania prophylaxis. But the opposite is not the case. Since lithium was being studied with a strong handicap, one cannot accept the findings at face value that lithium was less effective than lamotrigine for depression prophylaxis. Hence the lithium versus lamotrigine comparison cannot be accepted at face value given these concerns.

Furthermore, one should not ignore the rest of the scientific literature:

First, in unipolar depression, dating back to the 1950s, there are many randomized trials that show that lithium is very effective in prevention of depressive episodes, greater than placebo. There also are many randomized trials supporting acute efficacy of lithium in a current major depressive episode, in both unipolar depression and bipolar depression. These positive results in many studies contrast with the consistently negative results of lamotrigine for the acute depressive episode, in both unipolar and bipolar depression. In other words, outside of the two Glaxo studies, the rest of the scientific literature is much more supportive of greater depression treatment and prevention benefit with lithium, rather than lamotrigine.

Second, the best recent study to compare to the lamotrigine manufacturer's trials is the large U.K.-based BALANCE study, discussed previously, which compared lithium with divalproex in maintenance treatment of bipolar illness. That study was not enriched, and not biased to either agent. In BALANCE, lithium was *more* effective in prevention of depressive episodes than in prevention of manic episodes. Given that the BALANCE trial is more valid (less biased) than the lamotrigine manufacturer's enriched trials, it argues for the reverse: lithium is not an agent that mainly stabilizes "from above," if one wishes to use the marketing slogan: lithium also "stabilizes from below."

In sum, lithium robustly prevents depressive and manic episodes, whereas lamotrigine is better at the former than the latter. There are no head-to-head valid data that lamotrigine is better than lithium, or vice versa, in depression prophylaxis in bipolar illness.

Bottom Line

- "Mood stabilizing from below" is a false marketing slogan.
- Lithium is highly effective in depression prophylaxis in bipolar and unipolar illness.
- Lamotrigine is not proven to be more effective than lithium in depression prophylaxis in bipolar illness, using unbiased research designs.

SELECTED REFERENCES

Ghaemi, S. N. (2007). *Mood disorders: A practical guide*. 2nd edition. Philadelphia, PA: Wolters Kluwer.

Ghaemi, S. N. (2008). Why antidepressants are not antidepressants: STEP-BD, STAR*D, and the return of neurotic depression. *Bipolar Disorder, 10*(8), 957–968.

Rush, J., et al. (2006). Acute and longer-term outcomes in depressed outpatients requiring one or several treatment steps: A STAR*D report. *American Journal of Psychiatry, 163*(11), 1905–1917.

20

Anxiety Conditions

DIAGNOSTIC CONSIDERATIONS

Anxiety is the "fever" of psychiatry. It is common, bothersome, and nonspecific. It happens with depression, psychosis, and mania, and is a personality trait. In short, anxiety is all over the place. In fact, the philosopher Søren Kierkegaard saw anxiety as *the* central human emotion, part of mere existence. If you exist, you're anxious. If it is normal to be anxious, then how are we to make sense of anxiety in psychiatry?

If anxiety is present, does it immediately mean that a person has an anxiety "disorder"? If so, then if Kierkegaard was right, all of humanity has an anxiety disorder. Half a century of extensive personality research has proven Kierkegaard right. Perhaps the most replicated normal human personality trait is a trait for anxiety. If anxiety is a personality trait, then we all have it; or, more properly put, we all have some of it. So it isn't valid to identify anxiety as anxiety "disorder" automatically. The questions should be "How much anxiety?" "And in what context?"

Five different categories are suggested here:

1. A personality trait
2. Part of affective illness (unipolar or bipolar)
3. Part of psychotic illness (schizophrenia)
4. Part of anxiety illnesses (OCD and PTSD) or specific phobias (especially in children)
5. Existential anxiety (part of life)

Anxiety as Personality Trait

In the mid-1950s, a transplanted German psychologist in postwar London had a strange idea. Hans Eysenck was coming of age at the peak of Freudian influence. The Freudian view was that personality was all about childhood experiences, conscious or unconscious, related to one's parents and in one's social world. In other words, personality was all about environment. There might be other conditions—like schizophrenia—that could be seen as biological. But personality was quintessentially environmental.

Eysenck had an odd idea: What if personality also was biological, at least in part? Eysenck began to use new statistical methods to answer this question. "Factor analysis" was a quantitative method that allowed researchers to look for basic qualities that could be pulled together from a mass of data. Using that approach to personality questionnaires, Eysenck identified three basic personality traits that could be seen repeatedly in many studies of the normal population. People didn't seem so unique as Freudian ideas suggested: coming from different family backgrounds and different cultural settings, they still had the same basic traits in factor analysis of personality questionnaires. No Oedipus complex showed up in those factor analyses, no unconscious sexual traumatic experiences. This is not to say that such possibilities didn't exist; they obviously can't be captured in personality questionnaires. But whether or not we all suffer from Oedipus complexes and unconscious sexual conflicts related to our parents, we *also*, at least, have identifiable personality traits that are replicated across large populations.

There were three traits: a trait for anxiety—which Eysenck called "neuroticism"; a trait for sociability, which he called "extraversion"; and a trait for abnormal thinking, which he called "psychoticism." Later researchers reinterpreted psychoticism as a trait that is not so much about thinking patterns, but rather about openness to experience, or willingness to be curious about new experiences, or to take risks. Stated positively, this third trait is about "openness to experience"; stated negatively, it's about risk-taking behavior. In the past half century, Eysenck's basic work has been confirmed in literally hundreds of studies in dozens of cultures in many thousands of persons in the normal population. These three personality traits, defined one way or the other, have stood up. The most common terminology is "NEO," standing for Neuroticism, Extraversion, and Openness to Experience.

This background is useful to understand how the idea of anxiety as a personality trait, or neuroticism, is among the most well-established scientific concepts in psychology. We all have anxiety, these studies show, in a normal curve, just like height or weight and other biological traits of the normal population. Most of us have anxiety to a middling degree, near the mean of the normal curve, at or around the 50th percentile. Figure 20.1 demonstrates the features of a normal curve.

By definition, a small percentage of about 2% have a lot of anxiety (two standard deviations above the mean) and about 2% have very little anxiety. A much larger group of another 14% is one standard deviation to each side; this group, on the high side, is still quite anxious compared to most people. These persons are high in neuroticism; we call them "neurotic" colloquially, or "worry-warts." An equal percentage are low in neuroticism; they're Buddha-like, super-calm persons.

The first step to understanding anxiety is comprehending the fact that by far the largest portion of the population, about 16%, has high anxiety as part of a "normal" personality trait. This is not an illness, nor a "mental disorder": it is a normal variation in a normal personality trait in the normal population.

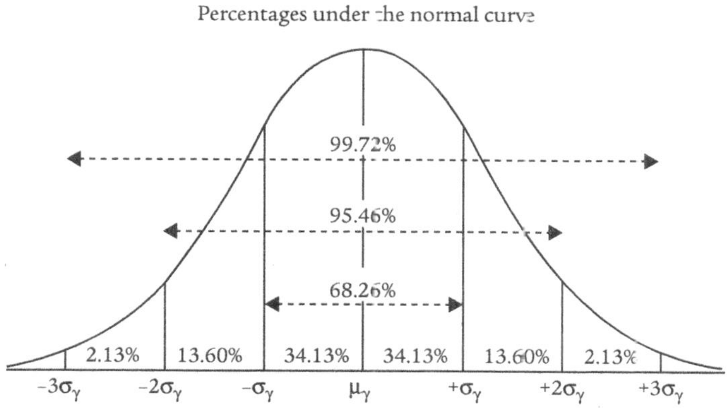

FIGURE 20.1 *Percentages under the Normal Curve.*

Part of a Mood Illness

After this large group of almost one-fifth of the general population, which has high anxiety as a normal personality trait, the next-largest group would be persons with mood illnesses—namely, unipolar and bipolar illness—which is thought to represent about 10% of the general population in the United States and in most Western nations. Anxiety is a frequent symptom of both depressive and manic/hypomanic episodes. When people have those episodes, they have marked anxiety. It's commonly said that if anxiety persists at one's baseline personality, in between mood episodes, then it's independent of the mood illness. This can be the case; people with mood illnesses may also have, independently, high neuroticism as a personality trait. But there is another possibility: they could have mood temperaments. About one-half of persons with mood illnesses also have mood temperaments: namely, dysthymia (constant mild depressive symptoms), cyclothymia (constant mild manic and depressive symptoms), and hyperthymia (constant mild manic symptoms). So, even in between mood episodes, many people have mood symptoms as part of their usual temperaments, as part of their personalities. In these cases, anxiety can be present, still secondary to the mood symptoms. Many persons with cyclothymic temperament, for instance, often have anxiety symptoms as well. When cyclothymia improves with low-dose mood stabilizing agents, anxiety also improves. In other words, the anxiety isn't independent of mood temperament.

Part of a Psychotic Illness

Perhaps the least common kind of anxiety occurs in schizophrenia and schizoaffective conditions. In the Freudian era, the term "psychotic anxiety" was used, and it is observed that many persons with schizophrenia, especially early in the course of the illness, will be notably anxious and agitated. A subgroup develop frank obsessive-compulsive disease later in the course of the schizophrenia disease process. This illness occurs, as is well known, in only about 1% of the population. It is relevant to realize that, despite these people's flat affect, anxiety can be part of the illness of schizophrenia.

An Independent Anxiety Illness or Disease

If a person has a lot of anxiety, but doesn't have a mood illness or mood temperaments or schizophrenia—after assessing all these other causes of anxiety—it is possible that this person has a specific anxiety condition. Dividing anxiety conditions into three categories that are well validated scientifically, there are:

- Specific phobias: These are the most common kinds of specific anxiety conditions, typically about public speaking, height, airplanes, animals or snakes, and so on. Specific phobias are common in childhood, but some types—especially public speaking—persist in adults also. Behavioral therapy methods are effective.
- Post-traumatic stress: After the experience of a major trauma, anxiety symptoms follow, both acutely and long-term, related to flashbacks and nightmares. This is not a disease, in the biological sense where a genetic or biological cause has a natural course that might interact with, but does not require, life events. Instead, PTSD is a psychological response to extremely stressful experiences. It occurs in about 10–20% of persons who experience major traumatic events, like childhood sexual abuse or war. Overall, PTSD in the United States is diagnosable in about 5% of men and 10% of women.
- Obsessive-compulsive disease: This condition is a genetic disease, or the result of streptococcal infection, occurring mainly in childhood, and persisting in some persons into adulthood. One might say it is the only pure anxiety disease. A common error is to diagnose the disease of OCD when anxiety symptoms of OCD occur as part of mood or psychotic illnesses. In those cases, once again, when the underlying illness is treated, and mood or psychotic symptoms completely resolve, OCD symptoms also resolve. One review suggests that about one-half of cases of apparent comorbidity of OCD with bipolar illness in fact represents OCD symptoms as part of mood episodes of bipolar illness, which resolve, *without specific anti-OCD treatments*, when the mood episodes resolve. Like schizophrenia, the independent disease of OCD is uncommon, happening in about 1% of the population.

Existential Anxiety

Not all anxiety is normal; certainly there are four major kinds of abnormal anxiety, as described. But some anxiety is normal, which could be seen in the concept of the normal curve. Another way of thinking about how anxiety can be normal is in terms of psychological development: the Freudian notion that we go through life stages has a rationale. There is childhood, then adulthood, then late life. And in each phase, there are transitions that can be difficult: adolescence, midlife, late-life illness.

Losses occur, and death is present in the end. This is what Kierkegaard and others, like the psychiatrist Karl Jaspers, meant by the normal anxiety of existence. The existential psychiatrist Viktor Frankl, who was imprisoned in Auschwitz, noted that the healthiest prisoners were the anxious ones; they survived. It was the calm, apathetic ones who perished. The pale DSM term is "adjustment disorder," which is both weak and false. Anxiety in the face of unavoidable life crises—in someone who isn't high on neuroticism as a personality trait and who doesn't have manic-depression, schizophrenia, OCD, or PTSD—is no disorder: it's human existence. And it's healthy.

A LITTLE HISTORY ON GENERALIZED ANXIETY DISORDER

Readers will note, after all this discussion on anxiety, that this text has not mentioned "generalized anxiety disorder" (GAD) or "panic disorder" or "social anxiety disorder." There is a reason for this, which a little history can explain. These three terms, which are the most common DSM diagnoses made in persons with anxiety symptoms, were created with DSM revisions, beginning in 1980 with DSM-III. As described in the previous chapter, none of these terms was used for a century in favor of another concept: "neurotic depression." As reviewed well in new historical writings using the minutes of the DSM-III task force, and interviews with participants in that process, we now know that the creation of GAD in particular involved finding a political compromise to allow for the removal of the term "neurotic depression." As described in Chapter 16, the DSM-III leadership wanted to remove neurotic depression, but many of the psychoanalysts who were rank-and-file members of the American Psychiatric Association (APA) resisted this radical change. Neurotic depression had a Freudian basis in unconscious conflicts, and it was their main insurance reimbursement code. The term "major depressive disorder" was created broadly to include those with neurotic depression, but some psychoanalytic psychiatrists still felt that the importance of anxiety was not captured by the MDD category. The DSM-III leadership then invented the term "generalized anxiety disorder" for those same patients; the criteria were created to capture the neurotic depressive presentation, hence they overlap in most symptoms with MDD. But a little more emphasis is placed on anxiety. Clinicians could replace neurotic depression with not one, but two, codes: MDD comorbid with GAD.

There was still opposition. Literally about a week before the final vote by the APA assembly on passing DSM-III, Spitzer went to a psychiatric dictionary and found the term "dysthymia," which had meant a mood temperament of mild chronic depression occurring in persons with manic-depressive illness. The term was hardly known in American psychiatry in 1980. Spitzer resuscitated it and redefined it to reflect chronic mild depression in general, unrelated to bipolar disorder. He argued to the APA assembly that now *three* codes could be given in the old neurotic depression patients: MDD and comorbid dysthymia ("double depression" some now call it) and comorbid GAD: three diagnoses in place of one.

Still the APA general assembly hesitated. In the final hours of the vote on DSM-III, another final compromise was brokered. The new category of dysthymia would be included with a parenthesis next to it as follows: "Dysthymia (neurotic depression)." The term "neurotic depression" was, after all these controversies, included in DSM-III in the end, but only as if it were a synonym for dysthymia (which it isn't). Someone joked, "DSM-III passed the APA assembly vote because of a parenthesis." Seven years later,

DSM-III quietly removed the parenthesis of neurotic depression from the dysthymia category.

"GAD" or Personality?

This brief history can highlight for readers that the origin of GAD is based on professional and social considerations, not on scientific studies. As reviewed earlier, the scientific evidence base is extremely strong for mild constant anxiety as part of an extreme of a personality trait. The scientific evidence base for GAD in the past 30 years is weak. When thinking of diagnostic validators that demonstrate that a condition is a different valid diagnosis compared to other conditions, the scientific consensus is to examine symptoms, genetics, course, and biological markers. GAD does not differ from MDD on most of its symptoms; genetic data indicate that GAD has low genetic heritability (about 30%) and cannot be differentiated genetically in twin studies from MDD; its course is constant, which is similar to that of personality traits; and its biological markers are nonspecific markers of stress, such as elevated adrenal activity; there are no specific definable biological markers that differentiate it from mood illnesses or other conditions. In short, the evidence for the validity of GAD as an independent, valid clinical construct is weak both historically and scientifically.

Anxiety be seen in the five constructs presented at the start of this chapter, with the chronic mild anxiety that DSM-5 continues to label as GAD seen as usually part of the personality trait of high neuroticism.

A Comment on Panic Disorder and Social Anxiety Disorder

These terms were also created for DSM-III in 1980 or in later revisions. Panic attacks and social anxiety usually happen in persons also diagnosed with GAD, or often as part of mood or psychotic illnesses. It is the same with these anxiety states as with any anxiety symptom: they often represent other conditions, like mood illnesses, or they are simply part of the high anxiety state of persons who have a high score on the baseline personality trait of neuroticism. As with GAD, if the scientific literature is examined in the four diagnostic validators, there is very weak scientific ground to claim that panic "disorder" or social anxiety "disorder" are valid independent clinical constructs. (In other words, these conditions do not differentiate well from other diagnoses or from personality traits on symptoms, course, genetics, and biological markers.) Thus, panic attacks and anxiety in social settings can be interpreted being anxiety symptoms that occur as part of other anxiety states (like OCD or PTSD), as part of other illnesses (like mood conditions), or as simply expressions of the heightened tendency to anxiety of some persons with the personality trait of high neuroticism.

TREATMENT

Given the diagnostic considerations, it may not be surprising that treatment recommendations will be limited. The simplest summary of the treatment of anxiety states is that symptomatic benefit can be obtained with some medications, especially the class of benzodiazepines, but this symptomatic benefit is limited, and does not involve any deeper disease modifying effect. An important exception to this statement involves the treatment of the disease of OCD with high-dose SRIs, which appear to have a more profound and disease-modifying effect in this condition.

This review of treatment studies will separately discuss GAD, social anxiety, panic attacks, and OCD.

In GAD, there have been 23 RCTs with 2,336 subjects comparing the benzodiazepines diazepam, lorazepam, and alprazolam, versus placebo. The overall benefit seen was a RR 0.78 (95% confidence intervals [CI], 0.62–1.00). In other words, there was a 22% decrease in GAD symptoms, but the confidence intervals touch the null value of one, which means that there might have been no benefit at all. No study exceeded six months in duration.

There are many studies of SRIs in GAD. A recent review identified 22 studies overall, with venlafaxine having the most studies. As with studies of monoamine agonists in MDD, it should be kept in mind that this published literature is biased in favor of positive studies, and the number of unpublished negative studies of SRIs in GAD is unknown. With that important limitation, benefit was seen in the published literature with almost always agents in almost all trials. Exceptions include two negative trials of paroxetine versus placebo, and one negative trial of venlafaxine.

Other agents that have been studied are pregabalin, gabapentin, and quetiapine, mostly by their manufacturers. Seven such RCTs were conducted with pregabalin, with all published as positive except for one. One published positive trial has been reported with gabapentin. Four RCTs were conducted with quetiapine, all reporting benefit. Despite these positive trials, the FDA did not grant quetiapine an indication for the treatment of GAD.

Almost all the studies tend to be 8 to 12 weeks in duration, with only three studies lasting up to 28 weeks. Thus long-term efficacy any medications, including SRIs, in GAD beyond six months has absolutely no basis in any scientific evidence involving randomized clinical research data.

A recent review of randomized trials of medications for social anxiety disorder identified 32 trials with SRIs, 11 trials with MAOIs (six with moclobemide, five with phenelzine), and five each with benzodiazepines (four with clonazepam) and anticonvulsants (three studies with pregabalin, one with gabapentin, and one with levetiracetam). In these published randomized trials, the most studied agent was paroxetine (12 trials). All agents show benefit. Again, as with all literature use of RCTs where many of the studies are conducted by the pharmaceutical industry, it is likely that many negative studies are unpublished and not available in the scientific literature., The true effect size of benefit with these agents is unknown, given the likelihood of many unpublished negative studies.

In panic disorder, many studies conducted of both SRIs and benzodiazepines, as well as with other monoamine agonists such as tricyclic antidepressants and monoamine oxidase inhibitors. A Cochrane Collaboration systematic review identified 35 randomized clinical trials for panic disorder in 5,365 subjects. Overall, monoamine agonists and benzodiazepines were the same in treatment response. SRIs were better tolerated than tricyclic antidepressants, and benzodiazepines appeared to be somewhat better tolerated than SRIs. Again, readers should keep in mind that this systematic review is limited to the published literature, with many studies being supported by pharmaceutical manufacturers, who had no obligation to publish negative trials. Thus the likely effect sizes are smaller, given probable unknown, negative unpublished studies.

In OCD, the Cochrane collaboration database analysis identified 17 RCTs of SRIs versus placebo in 3,097 subjects. Notable benefit was seen, although all studies were short-term, usually 6 to 12 weeks in duration, with no proof of long-term benefit. Among the SRIs, the highest number of studies conducted was with fluvoxamine and sertraline (five studies each). Paroxetine and fluoxetine each had three studies. Benefit was reported in all cases; negative unpublished studies are unknown.

In sum, the scientific evidence for efficacy of psychotropic medications for anxiety conditions is mostly limited to positive published studies, mostly conducted by the manufacturers of those agents. The likelihood of unpublished negative studies must be taken into account. Nonetheless, symptomatic benefit is reported with most medications studied, although it must be emphasized that almost all trials are short-term. Proof of long-term efficacy and safety is lacking for most medications given for anxiety conditions or symptoms.

SELECTED REFERENCES

Amerio, A., Odone A., Liapis C. C., Ghaemi S. N. (2014). Diagnostic validity of comorbid bipolar disorder and obsessive-compulsive disorder: a systematic review. *Acta Psychiatrica Scandinavica, 129*, 343–358.

Baldwin, D. S. et al. (2011). Evidence-based pharmacological treatment of generalized anxiety disorder. *International Journal of Psychopharmacology, 14*, 697–710.

Bighelli, I., et al. (2016). Antidepressants and benzodiazepines for panic disorder in adults. *Cochrane Database of Systematic Reviews*, Issue 9, Art. No.: CD011567.

Martin, J. L. R., et al. (2007). Benzodiazepines in generalized anxiety disorder: heterogeneity of outcomes based on a systematic review and meta-analysis of clinical trials. *Journal of Psychopharmacology, 21*, 774–778.

Mayo-Wilson, E., et al. (2014). Psychological and pharmacological interventions for social anxiety disorder in adults, *Lancet Psychiatry, 1*, 368–376.

Somroo, G. M., et al. (2008). Selective serotonin reuptake competitors versus placebo for obsessive-compulsive disorder. *Cochrane Database of Systematic Reviews*, Issue 1, Art. No.: CD001765.

21

Treatment of Personality

DIAGNOSTIC CONSIDERATIONS

Personality always has been an important aspect of psychiatric diagnosis and practice. In the DSM era, personality has been conceptualized, like everything else, through the prism of "disorders," a deliberately vague term. One feature of personality "disorders" is its commitment to a categorical concept. Your personality is either "normal" or "disordered." Besides this approach, there is another approach, long established in the experimental psychology (not psychiatry) literature: the concept of personality traits, or dimensions. In this view, personality traits are present in everyone, occurring on a normal curve, with all of us having more or less of a trait. At the extremes, personality traits can be seen as "abnormal," but not in a categorical sense, not as being *qualitatively* different than normality.

PERSONALITY TRAITS

Over the past century, many experimental psychology studies have established that human personality can be identified in the general population as having a few basic traits. These studies name these traits somewhat differently, but they cover similar features. As discussed in the prior chapter, there is a general personality trait of anxiety, labeled as "neuroticism" by the psychologist Hans Eysenck. There is another general personality trait of interpersonal skills, which Eysenck called "extraversion," contrasting with introversion. A third general trait has to do with curiosity or risk-taking, as opposed to being routinized; it has been called "openness to experience." These three basic traits—Neuroticism, Extraversion, and Openness to Experience—have been called the NEO scale. Twin studies demonstrate that these three traits are about half genetic and half environmental. This is similar to other partly genetic traits or conditions like physical weight or hyperlipidemia. Since these conditions have a genetic aspect, they can be seen as the biological aspect of personality. The term "temperament" often is used for the biological part of personality.

There is a completely different way to look at personality, the one that is more familiar in psychiatry, since it's enshrined in DSM. Personality "disorders" were first introduced in 1980 with the third revision of DSM, and were based mostly on psychoanalytic theory. It's important to note that of the ten DSM personality disorders, seven do not have good scientific evidence of empirical validation, as defined by nosological validators demonstrating that they can be distinctly identified from each other and from other diagnoses. These include *paranoid, schizoid, avoidant, narcissistic, histrionic, obsessive-compulsive,* and *dependent*. Three personality disorders had, and have, some empirical basis outside of pure psychoanalytic theory: *antisocial, borderline,* and *schizotypal*.

Antisocial personality has the longest history: it has been described in psychiatry since at least the 19th century, and often termed "psychopathy" or "sociopathy." The basic idea was that there might be some psychiatric condition that relates to being a criminal, or having criminal tendencies. These persons tend to lack "conscience," are unethical towards others, and use others purely for their own wishes. This general attitude frequently can lead to violence and crime. Whether or not there is a biological cause to this type of personality has been a topic of long debate. The general consensus tends to be that early childhood neglect is a major factor.

Borderline personality as a concept was more complex. The term "borderline" stems from the notion that these patients are at the "border" between neurosis and psychosis. The psychoanalytic tradition didn't care much for diagnosis. It only conceived of two major diagnostic groupings, depending on reality testing: psychosis and neurosis. The neurotic patient mostly was in touch with reality but had some unconscious emotional conflicts that aroused anxiety and depressive symptoms. The psychotic patient was less in touch with reality and had unconscious emotional conflicts that aroused delusional or hallucinatory symptoms. The difference was in degree, not kind. There was a single continuum for neurosis to psychosis, and at the borderline from one to the other, there were patients who were usually neurotic, but who could become, under the right circumstances, somewhat psychotic. The psychoanalysts had a practical test for this type of patient: she (usually she was female) would enter psychoanalysis as a somewhat normal neurotic person; but after some time on the couch, she would become psychotic. In other words, psychoanalysis would diagnose the borderline patient by making her worse.

Psychoanalysts used the phrase "psychotic" loosely: it simply meant being out of touch with reality to a greater degree than whatever would be termed "neurotic." And the term "psychosis" was more or less identified with the older concept of the diagnosis of schizophrenia. So, an early term from the 1950s for what would later be called borderline personality was "pseudoneurotic schizophrenia": these patients seem neurotic in daily life, but they're really schizophrenic (psychotic) underneath it all. In the 1960s, the psychoanalyst Otto Kernberg coined the term "borderline personality organization," which was taken up in the 1970s by John Gunderson, who, with others, persuaded the DSM-III leadership to introduce the new diagnosis of "borderline personality disorder."

It requires a great deal of allegiance to the DSM insistence on the word "disorder" to categorize schizotypal personality as a "personality disorder," but the concept has empirical validation as a mild version of schizophrenia, which occurs in families with the genetics of that disease. It has no origin in psychoanalytic theory.

DSM-5: NO CHANGE

An odd thing happened in 2013; over three decades after these 10 personality disorders were introduced based mostly on psychoanalytic theory in 1980, DSM-5 changed nothing. It's odd, because DSM leaders tended to pay homage to science, and the scientific evidence for personality traits is huge, but for most personality disorders is slight. Indeed the DSM-5 personality disorders task force recognized this fact, and over about five years of preparation, it recommended that the 10 original personality disorders be reduced to six, and that personality traits be added to DSM-5. There was some question about which traits and how to define them, but the DSM-5 personality disorders experts admitted that it was time to introduce personality traits into psychiatry. Half a century of replicated research should be sufficient to make this change in psychiatric diagnosis.

In the final weeks of the DSM-5 approval process, this recommendation was rejected by the DSM-5 Scientific Advisory Board and the American Psychiatric Association Board of Trustees (leading academics and APA activists, most of whom were not personality research experts). The reasons have been made public: there was strong opposition by leaders from the era of DSM-III, and APA leaders determined that personality traits would be too complicated for psychiatric clinicians to understand. This failure to accept well-proven science occurred despite the fact that the DSM-5 field trials showed that even after three decades of usage, psychiatrists mostly disagreed about how to use personality disorder criteria. In other words, they have poor reliability (consistency of agreement among clinicians when applied to the same patient). The only exception was borderline personality.

So DSM-5 didn't change the basic structure of DSM-IV, which was basically the same as DSM-III. The ten personality disorders live on. Personality traits remain unknown in DSM-based psychiatry.

A POTENTIAL SOLUTION

Clinicians are left with a dilemma: Should they follow the science of personality traits, or should they continue to repeat three decades of psychoanalytic theory–based definitions of personality disorders?

The perspective of this text is that the concept of personality traits is more clinically helpful because it is more scientific than the concept of personality "disorders." Of the latter, the three empirically proven ones may be clinically worthwhile: antisocial, borderline, and schizotypal. But schizotypal personality is not really a personality disorder, and antisocial personality is a complex phenomenon that ties into crime and legal aspects of psychiatric practice. Only borderline personality would seem to stand as a personality condition on its own.

If clinicians are willing to think about personality in terms of traits, and not just DSM-based disorders, then each patient can be examined for some of the basic personality traits. The three-item NEO could be used as a basic screen. For each patient, after some period of clinical evaluation, you can determine whether they are high or low or in the middle on each trait for neuroticism (anxiety), extraversion/

introversion, and openness to experience. This approach will open clinicians up to the many combinations of traits that patients can have, as opposed to the unreliable attempt to push them into one DSM personality disorder category or another. Furthermore, the concept of personality traits is less pejorative and stigmatizing than the DSM personality disorders concepts, and it allows for linking traits to variants of normality. This can enable freer dialogue and discussion about a patient's personality, how it influences one's life, and what might be done.

TREATMENT

The practical consequence of the DSM-based personality disorder concept was, from the beginning, that it would lead to psychotherapy treatments. In the last two decades, symptom-based medication treatment also has become the norm. The personality trait approach would be more realistic and more conservative.

Some psychotherapies, like cognitive behavioral therapy (CBT), are not very effective for changing personality, but are more helpful for acute symptoms, such as panic attacks or a current depressive episode. High neuroticism as a personality trait (often labeled "generalized anxiety disorder" using DSM terms) is not responsive to CBT. Even long-term psychotherapies, such as psychoanalytically oriented therapy, don't have much impact on making someone more or less extroverted, or more or less open to experience. Psychoanalytic psychotherapies can have many benefits, and produce insights or awareness about oneself, but one's basic personality doesn't change much, whether with psychotherapies or with medications.

One could conceive the use of medications for personality traits in this manner: they move patients from the extremes of the normal distribution curve toward the middle. But the effects are modest; they don't remove symptoms completely; rather, at best, they make symptoms somewhat less severe. This kind of thinking about medications would lead to more caution since the modest benefits might not outweigh even modest risks.

In all, personality traits can be a useful way to capture many of the problems presented by patients, without mistakenly labeling them as personality disorders that may not be valid, and without leading to excessive or probably ineffective psychotherapies and/or medication treatments.

REVIEW OF TREATMENT STUDIES

Given these diagnostic considerations, this text recommends avoiding aggressive, intensive, or frequent use of psychotropic medications for DSM-defined personality disorders. A review of the limited benefit of those agents would support this recommendation.

As will be discussed also with post-traumatic stress disorder (PTSD) in chapter 24, the treatment literature on medications in personality disorders is quite weak and does not support the widespread usage of psychotropic medications for this indication. There are very few randomized trials of medications in any personality disorder except for borderline personality. This discussion will be limited to that indication.

A classic early placebo-controlled randomized trial conducted at the NIMH in 1988 compared the anticonvulsant carbamazepine, alprazolam, the MAOI tranylcypromine, and the traditional dopamine blocker trifluoperazine. Overall, it found improvement in the dopamine blocker and anticonvulsant arms, especially in impulsive behavior and self-harm, whereas the alprazolam-treated patients had an increase in impulsive behavior. Patient and physician report of improvement was documented, and differences were observed in that physicians felt that patients improved better on dopamine blocker and anticonvulsants whereas patients felt they improved more with the antidepressant tranylcypromine. Although mood improved with the antidepressant, decrease in self-harm and impulsive behavior was not seen. In the intervening decades since this classic study, randomized trials of borderline personality have tended to be conducted by academic researchers, not the pharmaceutical industry, and thus have tended to be small, usually with inconclusive results.

A recent systematic review provides more specific detail on the medication study in RCTs of borderline personality disorder. Fluoxetine has been studied in four RCTs, with sample sizes ranging from 17–40 subjects per trial. Three out of four studies found some benefit with anger or impulsivity. There has been one RCT of fluvoxamine, with similar benefits, and no further RCTs of any other SRI in borderline personality. There has been one RCT with lithium and two with carbamazepine, with sample sizes in the 10 to 20 subject range, with reported benefit for anger/irritability, and self-mutilation. Three RCTs have been conducted with valproate, with the largest sample involving 52 subjects, all showing benefit for irritability and impulsivity. Two RCTs exist with lamotrigine with sample sizes of up to 28 subjects, which showed benefit for anger and impulsivity. This was also the case with three RCTs of topiramate with up to 56 subjects.

The randomized clinical trial literature in borderline personality is most extensive with dopamine blockers, especially with olanzapine, in which seven trials have been conducted. Again trials tend to be small, and most find some benefit in anger and impulsivity. Similar benefit has been reported in single RCTs with aripiprazole and risperidone, and two RCTs with haloperidol. One small RCT with ziprasidone failed to find benefit versus placebo in 16 subjects.

There has been some interest in the use of the opiate antagonist naloxone for self-cutting, but the only randomized trial of this topic involved nine subjects and did not find any benefit for dissociative symptoms or self-cutting. There have been two randomized trials of omega-3 fatty acids in borderline personality, with 49 subjects in the largest trial, reporting some benefit in aggressive and depressive symptoms.

A summary of the preceding studies in the Cochrane collaboration database of systematic reviews identified 28 randomized trials and 1,742 total subjects with borderline personality. Where benefits were reported over placebo, they occurred mostly with second-generation dopamine serotonin blockers, mood stabilizers, and omega-3 fatty acids. However, these benefits were not replicated in most cases, with the exception of olanzapine. Regarding harm, there was some evidence, after meta-analytic summation of results, of increased self-harming behavior with olanzapine. There are very few head-to-head studies comparing medications directly, and when they were conducted, no differences were observed, often because of very small sample sizes. Overall, this evidence is very weak to support any substantial scientific basis for clinical effectiveness of psychotropic medications in borderline personality disorder.

SELECTED REFERENCES

Bellino, S., et al. (2011). Pharmacotherapy of borderline personality disorder: A systematic review. *Current Medicinal Chemistry, 18,* 3322–3329.

Cowdry, R. W., & Gardner, D. L. (1988). Pharmacotherapy of borderline personality disorder: Alprazolam, carbamazepine, trifluoperazine, and tranylcypromine. *Archives of General Psychiatry, 45,* 111–119.

Stoffers, J., et al. (2010). Pharmacological interventions for borderline personality disorder. *Cochrane Collaboration Database of Systematic Reviews,* Issue 6, Art. No.: CD005653.

22

Schizophrenia and Schizoaffective Conditions

THE DIAGNOSIS AND TREATMENT OF SCHIZOPHRENIA HAS A LONG HISTORY, with interesting diagnostic aspects, and slow but consistent work on treatment. In this chapter, diagnostic aspects of schizophrenia and schizoaffective illness are examined first, followed by further discussion of treatment with modern dopamine blockers.

SCHIZOPHRENIA

Diagnostic Considerations

The original name for schizophrenia was "dementia praecox," by which Emil Kraepelin meant a range of psychotic symptoms that began in adolescence ("praecox"), and remained present chronically throughout life, with gradual worsening of function ("dementia"). Before Kraepelin, different psychotic states were identified (hebephrenia, catatonia, paranoia), which he pulled together in the single dementia praecox diagnosis. Kraepelin's view was that the specific symptoms' variations didn't matter; they all started in adolescence, were chronic, and worsened in function; they were the same illness.

Kraepelin put these views forward in the 1890s. Within two decades, though widely accepted, they were transformed by the Swiss psychiatrist Eugen Bleuler, a prominent leader in academic psychiatry. Bleuler (the mentor of Carl Jung) was influenced by Freud and applied Freudian ideas to psychosis. Bleuler felt that symptom differences in Kraepelin's dementia praecox mattered, specifically that the flatness of affect of these patients was central to the illness. They had a splitting ("schizo-") of their affect from the thoughts in their head ("-phrenia"), hence the new diagnostic term. These psychotic symptoms were auditory, and tended to be in the third person, with a running commentary on the patient's behavior. Bleuler's schizophrenia was much broader than Kraepelin's dementia praecox. No longer did patients need to begin with the illness in adolescence; it could be diagnosed in a middle-aged person for the first time. Nor need it be chronic; the symptoms could go away and come back later. Nor was there a decline in function; some patients recovered completely and permanently.

For most of the 20th century, Bleuler's concept held sway, until the 1970s, when researchers showed that Bleuler's definition, then the status quo in American psychiatry, led to the diagnosis of schizophrenia in manic states that might only last a few days, preceded and followed by complete normality. Similarly, psychotic symptoms that occurred only during depressive episodes were mislabeled "schizophrenia." Since new treatments then were available—the neuroleptics—but they had serious long-term risks, like TD, it was important to know who had a long-term need for treatment for psychosis, and who did not. The classic U.S.–U.K. diagnostic project identified the overly broad sweep of Bleulerian schizophrenia and led to the return to a "neo-Kraepelinian" definition in the West, codified in 1980 in DSM-III. Again, there was a requirement for chronic decline in function, which ruled out brief psychotic symptoms during affective episodes. This return to a Kraepelinian view did not lead to a change in the diagnostic label, though. Bleuler's "schizophrenia" label continues to be used, even though it is meant these days to reflect something closer to Kraepelin's "dementia praecox."

DSM-III and DSM-IV maintained some of the non-Kraepelinian aspects of diagnosis by listing the symptom variations as subtypes: paranoid, catatonic, undifferentiated, simple, and residual. DSM-5 has dispensed with these subtypes, to the consternation of some experts, especially in Europe. A particular concern that has been raised is that the diagnosis of catatonia is now absent from the DSM system, since it is no longer an aspect of schizophrenia. Furthermore, many experts hold that catatonia is not, and never was, simply a kind of schizophrenia.

A final important diagnostic consideration is the concept of "schizoaffective illness." In clinical practice in many settings in the United States, this diagnosis is made more commonly than that of schizophrenia proper.

SCHIZOAFFECTIVE ILLNESS

Soon after Kraepelin put forward his diagnostic concepts of dementia praecox (DP) and manic-depressive illness (MDI), he was opposed by those who felt the distinction was wrong. Some held that the two major diagnoses were too broad: many different diseases existed within each of the larger diagnoses (e.g., bipolar and unipolar illness instead of MDI; catatonia and paranoia instead of schizophrenia). Others held that the two major diagnoses were too narrow: only one unitary psychosis existed, subsuming both DP and MDI.

This latter unitary-psychosis view was supported by family history and course-of-illness studies, but the strongest support was symptomatic: by the 1930s, clinicians identified patients who had symptoms of both schizophrenia and affective illness, hence the "schizoaffective" label. The term was codified in DSM-III in 1980, and has changed little since then.

Yet research on the schizoaffective picture suggests that one thing is clear: it is not a valid separate diagnosis. Hence, if the label is used, it should be understood as a clinical picture, not a disease. Patients present with these symptoms, but this presentation is not its own separate disease. (In Appendix III, the clinical and research rationale for this judgment is provided.) This conclusion would have important implications for treatment and for interpretations on prognosis.

TREATMENT

Schizophrenia has been the most studied psychiatric illness. For over a century, a great deal of attention has been given to research on the biology and treatment of this condition. Despite this extensive research database, it is unfortunately true that most treatments for schizophrenia are symptomatic and modest in effect. They are important nonetheless, especially during acute exacerbations of psychosis, but they have not had extensive benefit in modifying the disease or altering the course of the illness, unlike the larger benefits seen with lithium and mood stabilizers in bipolar illness. The extent to which the dopamine blockers are helpful in schizophrenia, and not, requires careful discussion.

It is important to begin by noting that the inherent chronicity of schizophrenia confers treatment resistance to all treatments. It should not come as a surprise that the dopamine blockers are not very effective in the treatment of schizophrenia, since no treatments are very effective in this chronic condition. As with Alzheimer's dementia, the failure of treatments is not a reflection of the weakness of those treatments, but rather of the chronicity of the disease. This reality is reflected in the standards used by researchers and the FDA in the determining that treatment benefit is seen with medications for schizophrenia. Treatment response in antipsychotic trials of schizophrenia and schizoaffective illness is defined by a 20% reduction in psychosis symptom scales, such as the Positive And Negative Symptom Scale (PANSS). This 20% reduction is a much lower threshold than the 50% reduction required in mood rating scales for studies of medications in mood conditions. This lower standard is a reflection of the inherent chronicity and treatment refractoriness of schizophrenia. Hence, it should be kept in mind that when studies report treatment response in schizophrenia, they are referring to a mild improvement in symptoms.

With this qualification, there are many studies with dozens of dopamine blockers, conducted over decades, that demonstrate that these agents are more effective than placebo in treating acute psychotic symptoms in schizophrenia. These benefits are more robust for "positive" symptoms of delusions and hallucinations than for "negative" symptoms of flatness of affect or apathy, or for cognitive impairment symptoms. Yet the improvement seen in delusions and hallucinations, especially during acute hospitalizations, has been dramatic and clear in the past few decades.

The most important question in relation to efficacy is whether dopamine blockers are effective outside of cute reduction of positive psychotic exacerbations. In other words, do they alter the course of the illness or confer any other longer-term benefit?

A central resource to answer this question is a large meta-analysis conducted by James Hegarty and colleagues about two decades ago. This classic study was titled "100 Years of Schizophrenia," because when it was published, it sought to examine a century of research on the outcome of this condition ever since its initial description by Kraepelin in the 1890s. In an effort that required digging up studies in old journals in multiple languages, 320 studies from 1895–1992, with 51,800 subjects, were included in the project, which was one of the first meta-analyses in psychiatry. The main question was whether schizophrenia improved or not. This question involves the effect both of natural history and of treatments. Before the 1960s, dopamine blockers were not available to be used in the treatment of schizophrenia. Hence, the meta-analysis was able to compare outcomes in the pre-treatment era versus the treatment era. For much of the 20th century, there was great debate about whether schizophrenia was incurable or not. Kraepelin's view was that schizophrenia was chronic and deteriorating, and thus did not improve with treatment. It was analogous to the dementia that his research group discovered in older persons, named after his colleague Alois Alzheimer.

In contrast, other researchers reported in the mid-20th century that many patients with schizophrenia appeared to improve, especially after receiving either psychoanalytic psychotherapy or other kinds of social interventions. After the introduction of the dopamine blockers in the 1950s and 1960s, some researchers also reported massive benefit with those agents. This meta-analysis was complex because it involved hundreds of studies in many countries using different criteria both for the definition of the diagnosis of schizophrenia and for the definition of improvement in outcome. For the purposes of the study, "good" outcomes were defined variably as examined in different ways in different studies. For instance, some studies considered a good outcome to be "discharged from hospitalization," while other studies in another setting defined a good outcome as "improved function" or being "able to live independently." These varying definitions of outcome should be kept in mind, since in no case was a good outcome defined as "complete remission of all symptoms and recovery of completely normal function." Nonetheless, with the relatively low standards of good outcomes defined, the meta-analysis found that overall, about 40% of patients with schizophrenia appeared to improve when followed for about five years. In other words, even with a low standard for the definition of "improvement," the majority of patients with schizophrenia did not improve. The authors then examined whether improvement rates differed during the pre-treatment and treatment eras. Surprisingly, they found slightly lower rates of improvement during the treatment era from 1960–1990, with only 36% improvement in studies during that period. This outcome rate compared unfavorably with higher improvements in the 1920–1960 period of 48%. Somewhat more surprisingly, when these rates were compared to outcomes from 1890–1920, the overall recovery rate of 35% observed was almost exactly the same as the rates seen in the treatment era. The researchers noted that diagnostic definitions changed during the three treatment periods they described. In the 1890–1920 era, the Kraepelinian definition of schizophrenia, which was narrow and required chronicity of psychosis and deterioration as part of the diagnosis, was used. In the 1920–1960 era, a Bleulerian definition of schizophrenia, which was broad and did not require chronicity, was used. In the

1960–1990 era, there was a return to the Kraepelinian definition. Therefore, the authors observed that the differing outcome rates seen correlated best with diagnostic definitions. If the narrow chronic Kraepelinian definition was used, only about one-third of patients improved. If the broad Bleulerian definition was used, probably including many patients with schizoaffective illness or even bipolar illness, about one-half of patients improved. The use or non-use of dopamine blocker treatments did not appear to influence outcomes as defined in these studies. In other words, the dopamine blockers did not appreciably alter the course of schizophrenic illness, even though they provided clear benefit for acute symptom exacerbations. Besides this lesson, the larger lesson of this classic meta-analysis of outcomes in schizophrenia is that diagnostic definitions powerfully predict outcomes. This lesson is important in terms of the impact of DSM definitions on the outcomes seen in clinical practice, as described in Chapter 16. These diagnostic definitions appear to be even more important than treatment effects of specific drug classes.

This observation is consistent with the teaching of Dr. Edwin Cassem of Massachusetts General Hospital, codified in this text as the First Truth of Psychopharmacology. "How good is your treatment?" Dr. Cassem asked residents on rounds one day. He answered the question himself: "It's as good as your diagnosis."

A second key source of evidence regarding the treatment efficacy of dopamine blockers in schizophrenia is the classic NIMH-sponsored Clinical Antipsychotic Trials of Intervention Effectiveness (CATIE) study. In that study, 1,432 patients with schizophrenia were double-blind randomized to 18 months of treatment with a range of different dopamine blockers. "Treatment response" was defined at a low bar as treatment discontinuation. Rather than using standard psychosis symptom-rating scales, partly for practical reasons since the study was so large, the judgment was made that a pragmatic outcome could be defined as treatment discontinuation, assuming that patients would continue with their treatments if they had benefit, and would stop those treatments if they did not have benefit. All patients were supervised in clinical settings, and thus continuation or discontinuation of treatment in this study was not dependent on the patient's opinion alone, and thus did not reflect treatment noncompliance. The primary outcome was time to discontinuation, with more benefits seen with olanzapine as opposed to other agents. In the study, 64% of subjects discontinued olanzapine, as opposed to 74% with risperidone, 75% with the traditional neuroleptic perphenazine, 79% with ziprasidone, and 82% with quetiapine. Overall, 74% of all subjects discontinued dopamine blocker treatment over 18 months or less.

As can be seen with these results, about three-quarters of patients with schizophrenia these days do not respond to any dopamine blocker given, even with the very low threshold definition of simple medication continuation over one year. These results are consistent with the meta-analysis of outcome just described, even in the pre-treatment era, where it was observed that with Kraepelinian definitions, only about one-third of patients improved by natural history or with dopamine blocker treatment. In the CATIE study, with similar Kraepelinian definitions, only about one-quarter of patients improved with dopamine blocker treatment, which is lower than natural history rates of improvement in the early 20th century.

After CATIE, the next most influential recent RCT in schizophrenia probably is the Cost Utility of the Latest Antipsychotic Drugs in Schizophrenia Study (CUtLASS) from the United Kingdom. In CUtLASS, 227 patients with schizophrenia were randomized to treatment with first- and second-generation dopamine blockers for one year. Similar outcomes were seen in the PANSS and quality-of-life scales in both groups of treated subjects. Side effects were also reported to be similar, thus the researchers concluded that the older dopamine blockers are just as effective and safe as the newer ones. In a second phase of the study, 136 subjects were randomized to treatment with clozapine versus other second-generation dopamine blockers, and clozapine was found to be more effective in reducing symptoms, but less effective in improving quality of life. The judgment that new dopamine blockers, which are more expensive, need not be used unless older agents fail can be questioned, since the study did not assess long-term risks such as TD. TD has been shown to be much higher in prevalence with the first-generation dopamine blockers than with the second-generation agents, and thus long-term treatment over five years or more would seem to be more harmful in effect with older than with newer agents. This study does not disprove the literature that demonstrates more harm, at least with TD, with the older than newer dopamine blockers. The result regarding clozapine is important, since that agent has been proven to be the most effective dopamine blocker. It is, however, also associated with the highest rates of metabolic syndrome and cardiovascular disease. Along with marked weight gain and risk of agranulocytosis, these medical risks and harms negatively influence quality-of-life with clozapine. Although it is an important agent in the most severe cases of schizophrenia and schizoaffective illness, this study highlights the fact that symptom benefit may not be associated with improved quality of life.

Besides long-term outcome, a final line of evidence regarding the efficacy of dopamine blockers for schizophrenia as a disease has to do their effects on the brain. This literature is growing and suggests that, not only is there no benefit for brain structures with dopamine blocker treatment, there appears to be some harm.

In a study of 211 patients with schizophrenia, who were followed after their first episode with MRI scans over a mean of seven years (up to 14 years), researchers observed that longer follow-up was associated with smaller brain volumes and more cortical atrophy. In other words, over time, schizophrenia had a chronic and deteriorating neurological effect on the brain, as Kraepelin had predicted. The researchers also found that treatment with dopamine blockers had an independent effect of causing more cortical atrophy. This effect was present with both first- and second-generation agents. Illness severity, controlling for treatment, also had an independent effect, with more severe symptoms being associated with more cortical atrophy over time.

A meta-analysis of 30 longitudinal MRI studies with a mean of over one year of follow-up compared cortical atrophy in 1,046 patients with schizophrenia versus 780 controls. Progressive cortical atrophy was observed during follow-up, and was most associated with dopamine blocker treatment. Such atrophy was not strongly associated with either severity of illness or duration of illness.

In sum, although a larger literature demonstrates that neurodegeneration probably is part of the illness of schizophrenia, it appears that dopamine blocker treatment hastens or worsens the process of progressive cortical atrophy over years of long-term treatment of this illness. Such neurodegenerative worsening does not necessarily appear to be better with second-generation dopamine blockers compared to earlier agents.

A conclusion that could be given to this discussion of treatment of schizophrenia with dopamine blockers is that this chronic and deteriorating condition is difficult to treat, and apparently, most of the benefit of dopamine blockers is for immediate symptom relief of positive psychotic symptoms. In long-term treatment, there is not good evidence that they alter or improve the overall course of illness, and there is evidence that they may worsen the underlying neurological abnormalities that are present in this condition. In brief, they have important symptomatic benefits, but no disease-modifying effect in this illness.

SELECTED REFERENCES

Fusar-Poli, P., et al. (2013). Progressive brain changes in schizophrenia related to antipsychotic treatment? A meta-analysis of longitudinal MRI studies. *Neuroscience and Biobehavioral Reviews, 37,* 1680–1691.

Hegarty, J. D., et al. (1994). One hundred years of schizophrenia: A meta-analysis of the outcome literature. *American Journal of Psychiatry, 151,* 1409–1416.

Ho, B.-C., et al. (2011). Long-term antipsychotic treatment and brain volumes. *Archives of General Psychiatry, 68,* 128–137.

Jones, P. B., et al. (2006). Randomized controlled trial of the effects on quality of life of second versus first generation antipsychotic drugs and schizophrenia. *Archives of General Psychiatry, 63,* 1079–1087.

Lieberman, J. A., et al. (2005). Effectiveness of antipsychotic drugs in patients with chronic schizophrenia. *New England Journal of Medicine,* 353(1), 209–1223.

23

Addictions

Addictions come in two basic types: those that exist independently of other psychiatric conditions, and the addictions that are caused by other psychiatric conditions. The first kind can improve with addictive behavior treatment, such as Alcoholics Anonymous 12-Step–style approaches. The second kind can also improve that way, but they are more likely to improve if the underlying psychiatric illnesses that cause or promote addictive behaviors are treated. In other words, the concept of a diagnostic hierarchy is again relevant, as explained in Chapter 17. If the addictive behavior happen as part of other illnesses, then it is not necessarily a separate illness in itself. (Just as fever occurring with pneumonia is not a separate fever "disorder.")

SECONDARY ADDICTIONS: SELF-MEDICATION

Khantzian coined the phrase "self-medication" in the 1980s to describe how many persons who abuse substances do so to manage painful subjective affects. This insight is important, but it extends beyond psychological experience to psychiatric diagnosis. It appears to be the case that many persons abuse substances as a consequence of another underlying psychiatric disease. In other words, as with anxiety and depression and agitation, the presenting clinical experience may be an effect of another cause, rather than a cause by itself.

Extensive research now exists to flesh out the frequency of substance abuse as self-medication for another underlying psychiatric illness. The most common psychiatric disease that causes addictive behaviors is bipolar illness (60% also have addictions), followed by severe unipolar depression (40% substance abuse prevalence), then anxiety conditions and schizophrenia. Since many addictive drugs can cause depressive symptoms, anxiety, or even psychosis, the key treatment question is whether patients should be treated by 12-Step approaches and/or rehabilitation counseling alone, or whether such psychosocial interventions should be combined with medications for their psychological symptoms.

If mania or psychosis is present, it is reasonable to treat patients with mood-stabilizing agents, as in the treatment of bipolar illness. This is because few addictive agents cause mania (while many cause depression or anxiety). Of the agents that cause mania (like cocaine or amphetamines), it is difficult to defend the view that manic episodes are solely secondary to the addictive behavior, unless every single manic episode is immediately preceded by cocaine or amphetamine use, and no drug use happens at any other time when manic episodes are not present. This course is rarely the case. So mania always should be treated with mood stabilizing agents, whether addictive behaviors are present or not. Usually, those patients have addictive behavior secondary to bipolar disease, rather than the reverse.

If depression or anxiety is present, it may make sense to take the opposite approach: one would avoid routinely using antidepressants and benzodiazepines for depressive and anxiety symptoms in the presence of addiction. Sometimes a separate depressive or anxiety disease may be present, in which case those agents may be needed, but this should not be assumed routinely in most patients. How can a clinician figure this out? One approach would be to give addiction treatments initially for some amount of time, without antidepressants or anxiolytic treatments; if there is no progress after sufficient time (which depends also on patient compliance; in the best-case scenario, six months or more of addictive behavior treatment would seem rational), then antidepressant or anxiolytic treatment can begin.

PRIMARY ADDICTIONS

It certainly is the case that, whatever the cause, addictive behaviors can take on a life of their own; the person becomes addicted, meaning that the brain changes, with dopamine system involvement, such that even if the underlying cause is removed (e.g., their bipolar disease is treated to remission), the person may still remain addicted, especially to drugs like heroin or cocaine. In those cases, specific addictive behavior treatment should be given along with medications for bipolar disease. Many people who have bipolar disease and alcoholism or other drug abuse experience remission of their compulsion when their bipolar disease is effectively treated, without necessarily needing formal addictive behavior treatments (such as 12-Step groups).

The most effective direct treatments for addictive behavior are 12-Step programs and individual substance abuse–specific counseling. Specific medication treatments for narcotic dependence exist, such as naltrexone and gabapentin, but they are modestly helpful at best.

Other "addictions" besides street drugs or alcohol, like sexual compulsions (paraphilias), internet use, cellphone, and food compulsions can be seen as primary addictions, and directly treated with variations on 12-Step programs. But the clinical judgment that they are primary should only be made after treatable secondary causes, most importantly bipolar disease or psychotic illnesses, are ruled out, and sufficiently treated first if present.

PSYCHOPHARMACOLOGICAL TREATMENT

Given these considerations, specific medications shown to have some benefit for addictions will now be examined.

For alcohol abuse and dependence, there is some evidence that gabapentin can be helpful for alcohol abuse and withdrawal. In one randomized trial, high-dose gabapentin at 1800 mg a day produced improvement in heavy drinking in 44% of a sample, compared to 22% with placebo.

Divalproex has been shown to help alcohol abuse in the setting of concomitant bipolar illness, without significant elevation of liver enzyme tests. This benefit with divalproex may be higher when combined with lithium. Substance abuse in general is a poor prognostic factor in bipolar illness, an outcome observed in many studies of lithium effectiveness. There is a widespread misconception, though, that lithium specifically is ineffective in the setting of comorbid bipolar illness and substance abuse. This has never been proven. Carbamazepine and divalproex are also less effective for bipolar illness in the setting of substance abuse than otherwise, reflecting the generally negative impact of substance abuse on outcome in bipolar illness, whatever the treatment. Nonetheless, combining divalproex with lithium has been shown to be more effective for substance abuse itself than lithium alone, in the setting of concomitant bipolar illness.

There is no evidence that SRIs or other monoamine agonists are helpful for substance abuse, dependence, or withdrawal. Benzodiazepines are used for alcohol withdrawal and can be very important and lifesaving in severe cases. Of course, benzodiazepines are discouraged in the setting of active alcohol abuse.

In cocaine abuse, it has been shown that GABAergic agents like gabapentin and anti-glutamatergic agents like topiramate may have some benefit in reduced cocaine use among addicts. The available randomized data on these findings are small and mostly unreplicated.

Regarding abuse of other substances, like amphetamines and hallucinogens, there is no appreciable research literature on possible effective psychotropic treatment.

Regarding marijuana, there is a great deal of controversy about its addictiveness. There is good biological and clinical evidence that marijuana is an addictive substance, although not as potent as some other agents. Even though it is increasingly legalized in some parts of the world, legalization should not be mistaken for safety. Similarly, tobacco and alcohol are legal but not safe substances. Used in small amounts in moderation, their harm may be limited. But when used frequently and in higher amounts, they are harmful. The same logic holds for marijuana. Current marijuana available in the United States appears to be highly potent, much more so than in prior decades. Thus even small amounts can produce major effects. An increase in car accidents, often fatal, has been noted in some states that have legalized marijuana. Regarding long-term effects, it has been shown that early exposure to marijuana in adolescence and young adulthood is associated with longer-term cognitive effects, including some decline in neuropsychological testing. Marijuana is known to directly increase paranoia and depression, and thus may worsen acute symptoms in individuals with underlying affective or psychotic illness. Marijuana does have direct anxiolytic effects, which leads to its frequent use for self-medication of anxiety symptoms, themselves typically caused by underlying affective or psychotic illness.

12-STEP PROGRAMS AND MEDICATIONS

In the addiction community, there often is a strong resistance to the "medical model." If by the "medical model" is meant a complete and constant presumption that all addiction is a physical disease, then this rejection could be defended based on available research. However, any such medical model is a mere straw man. The approach suggested here is that some, not all, addictions are due to other underlying diseases of the mind. These conditions commonly involve bipolar illness, unipolar depression, or schizophrenia. Other psychiatric conditions, like PTSD, may not be medical diseases per se, but they may be life experiences that lead to self-medication of subjective pain, as Khantzian so well described.

This disease-oriented approach applies to perhaps one-half or so of cases of substance abuse. The other half are not caused by underlying psychiatric disease, but probably reflect the more standard scenario for which 12-Step programs are best applied. The most common scenario here may involve recreational use, either due to the pure enjoyment of the subjective high of addictive drugs, peer pressure during adolescence and young adulthood, other social factors such as drinking with work colleagues, or other cultural factors, such as general socialization in the setting of alcohol and drugs. In these scenarios, recreational alcohol and drug use turns into addiction in some people because of the inherent biological effects of these agents on the pleasure centers of the brain, as is increasingly well-established in neuroimaging studies. There is no medication that can cure this kind of substance abuse, and any benefits seen are modest and symptomatic. The various studies described previously are of this character. In this setting, the skepticism of 12-Step advocates regarding medications is well-placed.

One might insist, though, that in the secondary addictions, such skepticism is ill-placed. If substance abuse occurs because the patient has manic or depressive states, such abuse will not go away until that manic-depressive disease is treated with lithium or other second-messenger modifiers. Even the best 12-Step program and the most devoted attempts by the patient are likely to fail in the long run.

Even though for almost a century many clinicians have advocated 12-Step programs, it has been noted that the long-term recovery rates are low. Many have been resigned to this outcome. But one explanation might be that the rejection of any medical approach would produce low overall results if indeed a substantial portion of individuals with substance abuse are self-medicating for underlying psychiatric disease. If clinicians can differentiate between primary and secondary addictions, and appropriately treat those who have underlying psychiatric disease and secondary addictions, while providing effective 12-Step treatment for those with primary addictions, better overall results might be achievable.

A final comment may be relevant for those who are exposed to the current prevalent opinion in the United States that "substance abuse is a disease." The discussion here may appear to contrast with that viewpoint since two types of substance abuse are being described, one that is caused by other psychiatric diseases, and another that is not a disease in itself, but a long-term result of recreational use followed by biological dependence. In the first case, substance abuse itself is not the disease, but rather the effect of another disease. In the second case, substance abuse cannot be called a "disease" in the traditional sense of the term, meaning an abnormality of an organ or part of the body that is either genetic or environmentally caused in such a way that it produces a consistent clinical syndrome. There are many problems of the body that involve external injuries, which are not diseases. For instance, a brain tumor is a disease; but a traumatic injury to the brain is not a disease. Both conditions may produce similar neurological symptoms. In the case of primary substance abuse, an external event (repeated recreational use) produces a biological result (effects on the brain circuitry leading to addiction). This pathogenesis is more similar to an external injury than to an internal disease process. In any case, once the addiction takes on a life of its own, it functions as if it could have been a disease, and it requires treatment. It is important to note, though, that this primary addictive condition had an original environmental origin, not a purely biological one, which is why 12-Step programs can be effective by attending to the environmental contexts in which addiction began, continued, and grew out of control.

SELECTED REFERENCES

Khantzian, E. J. (1997). The self-medication hypothesis of substance use disorders: A reconsideration and recent applications. *Harvard Review of Psychiatry*, *4*(5), 231–244.

Mason, B. J., et al. (2014). Gabapentin treatment for alcohol dependence: A randomized clinical trial. *JAMA Internal Medicine*, *174*(1), 70–77.

24

Post-traumatic Stress

DIAGNOSTIC CONSIDERATIONS

The concept of trauma has been a central feature of psychiatry and psychology ever since a century ago, when a Viennese neurologist concluded that many of his young female patients with hysteria had experienced childhood sexual abuse. Freud's analysis, which he later modified to mean fantasies of childhood sexual experience, opened the gates to a century of attention to experiences of childhood, especially traumatic ones. The concept of trauma soon was extended to adults, mainly soldiers. In fact, a major impetus to the rise and acceptance of Freudian thinking had to do with "shell shock" in World War I. German and Austrian government officials realized that traditional psychiatric methods didn't explain or help the soldiers who had developed intense fear and depression, whereas psychoanalytic ideas seemed tailor-made for them. During the war period, the German authorities even sponsored one of the first and largest psychoanalytic congresses. "Hysteria," "shell shock," "war neurosis"—it all became mutated in DSM-III's radical revision of 1980 into "post-traumatic stress disorder" (PTSD).

When DSM-III radically changed diagnoses in American psychiatry, one of its main goals was to remove directly Freudian or psychoanalytic causes from diagnostic definitions. The term "neurosis" was removed in general for that reason. In contrast, psychoanalytic ideas were reintroduced in psychiatric diagnoses more descriptively with new diagnostic terms that had never existed before, such as borderline personality disorder and PTSD.

The original definition of PTSD included the important description that the traumatic experience must be something that was outside the bounds of usual human experience. This definition was used for two reasons: one was that military trauma, as in Vietnam, was an important influence on the drafters of DSM-III's definition of PTSD, and military trauma, by definition, is not a routine experience that happens to the general population; it is a unique experience that happens to some soldiers during periods of war.

Another factor was the (mistaken) belief that childhood sexual trauma was uncommon. We now know that childhood sexual trauma happens in about 10–20% of the general population (less in males, more in females). As a result, by DSM-IV in 1994, a strong movement existed to remove the descriptor limiting trauma to unusual human experiences. The matter has not changed with DSM-5. Now trauma is defined as any terrible event that causes PTSD symptoms. This tautological definition has led to a common conflation of life events with trauma, defined by DSM-IV and DSM-5 in a much broader interpretation by adding the phrase "serious injury," so that the definition reads "exposure to threatened death, serious injury, or sexual violence. . . ." Studies on PTSD using current definitions report that the most common traumata are car accidents.

Another way of seeing the matter is that what has been termed "life events" are now seen as traumata. "Life event" is a more neutral descriptor for the experiences described here. It has been shown in extensive research that clinical depressive episodes are preceded by life events in the prior 6–12 months in the vast majority of cases. As noted, such life events are not unusual experiences, but rather the typical stresses of life.

Those who prefer to take a social or psychological orientation to psychiatry see those life events as "causes" of the depression that follows. A similar perspective is seen with proponents of PTSD: the traumata are "causes" of PTSD. The problem is that everyone experiences those life events; but 90% of the population never develops clinical depression. Similarly with PTSD: about 80–90% of persons exposed to severe trauma do not develop PTSD. This means that the underlying biological susceptibility of the individual to depressive episodes or to PTSD is the deciding factor, not the occurrence of life events or trauma.

This evolution has led to a shift in the PTSD literature from a sole focus on risk factors to protective factors. What are the protective factors that keep persons mentally healthy? The basic term used to explain such protection from PTSD is "resilience," a phrase that has become part of popular culture now. A scientific approach to the concept of resilience would focus on personality, or temperament, as the baseline susceptibility of a person to PTSD, which would then interact with traumata, or life events. Some people are more susceptible, and some less so, to PTSD, given the same traumatic experience. This baseline susceptibility is often seen as being related to personality traits, with depressive-type personality traits predisposing one to PTSD: if one is nervous or anxious or sad (e.g., has the mood temperament of dysthymia or the illness of recurrent unipolar depression), one is more likely to develop PTSD. In contrast, manic-like personality traits appear to protect against PTSD: if one is high-energy, sociable, has lots of friends, is future-oriented, is humorous, and is other-oriented—then one is less likely to develop PTSD. The psychological literature tends to examine these "positive" traits one by one, and it has been seen as part of a general approach to emphasizing strengths and positive aspects of one's personality (hence the "positive psychology" movement). These traits can also be seen in the clinical tradition as part of the manic side of mood symptoms, which can be positive and beneficial. Therefore, these protective personality traits can be seen in the mood temperaments of hyperthymia (constant mild manic symptoms) or cyclothymia, or even in frank bipolar illness.

The clinical relevance of the preceding discussion is as follows: If a person has an apparently harsh life event, this by itself is not sufficient to presume that person has PTSD. Instead, one should look at the other three diagnostic validators (besides symptoms): course of illness, genetics, and biological markers/treatment response. Does the person have family genetics of manic-depressive illness or severe depressive disease? If so, current depressive symptoms probably stem from the same biological cause, not from PTSD. Does the person have past repeated depressive episodes with many different life stressors? Then the current depression is probably another manifestation of the underlying depressive disease, with the life events being "triggers," not traumatic causes, of the underlying depressive disease. If someone has no prior depressive episode and no family genetics of severe mood disease and then has a sudden extreme traumatic experience, such as military combat or sexual trauma, then new depressive and anxiety symptoms probably do represent PTSD. Similarly, if someone has childhood sexual or extreme physical abuse, and no family genetics for mood disease, then lifelong anxiety and depressive symptoms are likely to be related to PTSD.

Classic PTSD symptoms are dissociative—flashbacks and nightmares—and these do not happen by themselves in non-PTSD conditions like manic-depressive illness. The presence of severe dissociative symptoms by themselves would increase the likelihood of PTSD. However, it should be noted that dissociative experiences of a milder nature, like depersonalization, can happen with panic attacks and marked anxiety; and such anxiety can be caused by depressive or even manic episodes; thus, even in the presence of dissociative symptoms, one should rule out severe mood episodes and pay attention to other clues for a non-PTSD diagnosis, such as psychiatric genetics and the course of illness.

TREATMENT

If PTSD is correctly diagnosed, what should clinicians do? There is extensive research now with many medications in randomized trials, and the general results are that most medications in PTSD are modestly effective at best. Their effects are symptomatic only, which means they do not get at the cause, and they only superficially help the painful symptoms. Such effects may be better than nothing, but one should not have an inflated expectation of the effects of medications in PTSD: they are symptomatic, temporary, and modest.

The real treatment, as Freud discovered, is psychotherapy. There may be different ways to conceive how to conduct this psychotherapy; the Freudian approach is insight-oriented, but other approaches may also help. The supportive and empathic aspects of psychotherapy are also important. Benefits are not rapid, and require long-term treatment, as Freud emphasized. In some persons, improvement is only modest, but in others, major benefits can occur. The U.S. Veterans Administration now recommends psychotherapy, not medications, as first-line treatment for PTSD.

Thus, clinicians should be careful not to overuse medications in PTSD, since benefits are minimal and side effects correspondingly will outweigh the modest benefits. Drug effects, if present, are only short-term in any case. Long-term improvement, and more than minimal benefit, will be obtained mainly by psychotherapy. Clinicians should put the emphasis there, rather than on medications. In doing so, clinicians should be careful to avoid overdiagnosis of PTSD by mistaking all life events for traumata, and they should pay close attention to genetics and course of illness to make sure that they are not missing manic-depressive illness or other psychiatric conditions. In the case of manic-depressive illness, in particular, the distinction is especially important because the treatments are opposite: medications are central, and psychotherapies are less effective in manic-depressive illness, whereas medications are peripheral and psychotherapies are central to the treatment of PTSD.

The limited nature of the PTSD drug-treatment literature is highlighted in a recent consensus statement of the PTSD Psychopharmacology Working Group, titled: "It is time to address the crisis in pharmacotherapy of posttraumatic stress disorder." The consensus statement highlights the fact that there is an obvious immediate need to pay more attention to PTSD treatment in the United States, given the rise of combat-related trauma in the last decade in military veterans. It noted that the first RCT of PTSD occurred in 1988, which gives an indication of how little research has been conducted of high quality in this field in the past. Furthermore, it was noted that SRIs, like sertraline, have been found to be ineffective, equivalent to placebo, in male military veterans with PTSD. In other words, although it is known that SRIs have limited benefit symptomatically in general PTSD overall, they may be entirely ineffective in the subset of military veterans who are of male gender. Yet military patients and the Veterans Administration hospitals in the United States who are diagnosed with PTSD are prescribed antidepressants about 70% of the time. SRIs are the most commonly prescribed class of medication for such veterans with PTSD, despite the fact that they appear to be entirely ineffective. Among other classes of medications, in the last decade, anticonvulsants are prescribed to about 25% of veterans with PTSD, antipsychotics to about 22%, benzodiazepines to 30%, opioids to 37%, stimulants to 2%, and lithium to 1%. The consensus experts noted that no class of medication used for PTSD in veterans meets the standard definition of well-proven efficacy based on large RCTs.

Recent randomized trials conducted by the pharmaceutical industry with potentially new treatments for PTSD include an analog of the steroid precursor dihydroxyepiandrostenidione (DHEA), cyclobenzaprine, and other novel agents. All those studies were terminated for poor enrollment, or found no benefit compared to placebo.

While it is important to emphasize the very weak nature of efficacy with any drug treatment in PTSD, it is nonetheless relevant to point out a few symptomatic uses of two other medications with impact on the sympathetic nervous system. The alpha-adrenergic blocker prazosin is often found to be helpful for treatment of nightmares and insomnia. It can reduce blood pressure and cause cognitive impairment, however. Beta-blockers, like propanolol, have been found to be helpful in general, and more specifically for acute stress reactions in the traumatic event.

BOTTOM LINE

- Today, many stressful life events are seen as trauma.
- If most life events are viewed as causal traumata, PTSD will be overdiagnosed.

- Almost 90% of people who experience trauma do not develop PTSD.
- The underlying biological susceptibility of a person is the deciding factor, not trauma.
- Resilience, often related to manic symptoms, reflects low underlying susceptibility
- Medications should be used conservatively if at all; they are effective modestly at best.
- Psychotherapies should be the main emphasis in treatment of PTSD.

SELECTED REFERENCE

Breuer, J., Freud, S. (1895, 2000). *Studies on hysteria*. New York: Basic Books.

Krystal, J. H., et al. (2017). It is time to address the crisis in the pharmacotherapy of posttraumatic stress disorder: A consensus statement of the PTSD Psychopharmacology Working Group. *Biological Psychiatry, 82*(7), e51–e59.

McHugh, P. R., Treisman, G. (2007). *PTSD: A problematic diagnostic category. 21*(2): 211–222.

SECTION V

Special Topics in Psychopharmacology

25

Carcinogenicity of Psychotropic Drugs

THE USE OF PSYCHOTROPIC MEDICATIONS HAS DRAMATICALLY INCREASED over the past two decades. In the United States, in 2005, approximately 27 million people were treated with antidepressants, compared to 13.3 million in 1996, corresponding to an overall increase of 74%. The majority of U.S. prescriptions for psychotropic drugs happen at the primary care level, usually for anxiety and depressive symptoms and their physical correlates. Given the extensive use of these agents, carcinogenic risk should be carefully weighed when prescribing long-term drug therapies. From a public health perspective, even a small increased risk factor, when applied to a large population, will produce many preventable cases of disease.

During the FDA approval process for psychotropic drugs, a series of safety studies are required. All drugs are examined with similar preclinical paradigms in these safety studies. Carcinogenicity is one of the outcomes assessed. In the published scientific literature, some concerns have been raised about the potential carcinogenicity of some psychotropic drugs. However, clinical studies are variable, and they rarely control for a myriad of potential confounding factors. Preclinical studies are extensive and use different methodologies, making comparisons between studies difficult. Furthermore, the non-publication of negative studies creates a potential bias in assessing the published scientific literature. Thus, the FDA-based studies can provide a database that can be examined in which all agents are studied similarly, thereby allowing comparisons within and between drug classes. This chapter summarizes the FDA preclinical evidence to assess and compare carcinogenic risk among and between drug classes, especially with the most commonly used current psychotropic drugs.

Data on carcinogenicity outcomes, including tumor-promoting activity and frequency of tumor incidence, were retrieved from animal studies conducted in vivo. Descriptive analysis was carried out, and findings pooled by drug class. The following drug categories were considered: antidepressants, antipsychotics, benzodiazepines and sedatives-hypnotics, amphetamines and stimulants, lithium and anticonvulsants. For each drug, the number of studies reporting positive or negative risk of carcinogenicity

TABLE 25.1 Preclinical Studies: Carcinogenicity of Antidepressants

Antidepressants	Carcinogenesis	Risk
Citalopram	(++)	High
Fluoxetine	(++)	High
Fluvoxamine	(–)	Low
Paroxetine	(+)	Intermediate
Sertraline	(++)	High
Viloxazine	?	Unknown
Duloxetine	(–)	Low
Mirtazapine	(++)	High
Venlafaxine	(–)	Low
Nefazodone	(–)	Low
Trazodone	?	Unknown
Bupropion	(+)	Intermediate

?: Not tested

+ = one positive study

– = one or more negative studies

++ = replicaed positive studies

were compiled. No data were available for some agents, mostly older drugs that entered the U.S. market before current FDA efficacy and safety procedures were implemented in the 1960s and 1970s.

Among antidepressants (Table 25.1), 63.6% (7 out of 11) of examined agents were associated with carcinogenicity, with 45% (9/20) of all studies being positive for carcinogenicity. Specific agents associated with carcinogenicity were mirtazapine, sertraline, paroxetine, citalopram and escitalopram, duloxetine, and bupropion. Agents not associated with carcinogenicity were fluoxetine, venlafaxine, trazodone, and imipramine.

Among antipsychotics (Table 25.2), 90% (9/10) of examined agents were associated with carcinogenicity, with 69.6% (16/23) of all studies being positive for carcinogenicity. All these agents were associated with carcinogenicity except clozapine.

Among benzodiazepines and sedative-hypnotics, 70% (7/10) of examined agents were associated with carcinogenicity, with 55% (11/20) of all studies being positive for carcinogenicity. Specific agents associated with carcinogenicity were clonazepam, zolpidem, zaleplon, diazepam, eszopiclone, oxazepam, and midazolam. Agents not associated with carcinogenicity were lorazepam, alprazolam, and triazolam.

Among amphetamines and stimulants, 25% (1/4) of examined agents were associated with carcinogenicity, with 10% (1/10) of all studies being positive for carcinogenicity. Only methylphenidate was associated with carcinogenicity, in one out of three studies of that agent. Amphetamine salts, modafinil, and atomoxetine were unassociated with carcinogenicity.

TABLE 25.2 Preclinical Studies with Typical and Atypical Antipsychotics

Antipsychotics	Carcinogenesis	Genotoxicity	Risk
Haloperidol	(+)	(-)	Intermediate
**Perphenazine	?	*(-)	Low
Chlorpromazine	?	(++)	Intermediate
Trifluoperazine	(+)	?	Intermediate
Pimozide	(+)	(-)	Intermediate
Fluphenazine	*(-)	(++)	Intermediate
Mesoridazine	(-)	?	Low
Clozapine	(-)	(-)	Low
Risperidone	(++)	(-)	High
Olanzapine	(++)	(-)	High
Quetiapine	(++)	(-)	High
Ziprasidone	(+)	(++)	High
Aripiprazole	(++)	(++)	High

? Unknown

** Few studies available*

***: Only antipsychotic evaluating genotoxicity in psychiatric patients*

+ = one positive study

– = one or more negative studies

++ = replicaed positive studies

Among anticonvulsants, 85.7% (6/7) of examined agents were associated with carcinogenicity, with 64.3% (9/14) of all studies being positive for carcinogenicity. The only agent not associated with carcinogenicity was lamotrigine. Specific agents associated with carcinogenicity were valproate, carbamazepine, gabapentin, pregabalin, oxcarbazepine, and topiramate.

No data were available for lithium in the FDA-based safety information.

If all examined psychotropic agents are combined, 71.4% (30/42) of agents had some preclinical evidence of carcinogenicity. If all specific experimental studies of those agents are combined, evidence of carcinogenicity is found in 43.7% (38/87) of studies.

Overall, new-generation dopamine blockers and anticonvulsants showed the highest evidence of carcinogenicity among psychotropic drug classes, with most drugs being carcinogenic in FDA-based preclinical studies. Antidepressants and benzodiazepines were next (half carcinogenic), and amphetamines (with the exception of methylphenidate) were least. If all examined psychotropic agents are combined, about 71% of agents had some preclinical evidence of carcinogenicity.

By agent, almost all atypical antipsychotics (with the exception of clozapine) and anticonvulsants (with the exception of lamotrigine) were carcinogenic in at least some preclinical studies. A majority of antidepressants (63.6%) and anticonvulsants (70%)

were also carcinogenic. Among the amphetamines/stimulant drug class, only methylphenidate had some evidence of carcinogenicity.

The relationship of these results to the published scientific literature is complex. Published preclinical animal studies vary, with some studies showing reduced cancer risk with some drug classes, such as antidepressants, based on proven beneficial immunological effects (e.g., enhanced natural killer cell activity). Other studies, as in the FDA-based studies, show direct carcinogenic activity in animals exposed to some antidepressants.

Clinical studies also are very variable. The only meta-analysis of the topic examined breast and ovarian cancer with antidepressants, and found a relative risk of 1.10. This small increased risk may be important for public health, and the authors interpreted the results in that manner, along with analyses of possible non-publication of harmful data based on associations with the pharmaceutical industry. But a 10% increased relative risk can easily be accounted for by the myriad potential confounding factors that exist in observational practice, such as smoking, diet, and other environmental risk factors, none of which was controlled in the meta-analysis. Specific clinical studies, some of which are positive and others negative, suffer from the same problem of major confounding bias.

The FDA-based analysis presented here has the advantage of being systematically the same for all agents, and unaffected by publication bias. Furthermore, by being limited to preclinical animal settings, where other environmental risk factors can be controlled or minimized, it is less susceptible to confounding bias. While the relevance of these animal findings for human studies remains to be established, these basic science findings should not be ignored. An example of a potentially notable cause of carcinogenicity with a widely used drug class, despite absence of clear evidence of risk in observational clinical practice, is the case of hormone replacement therapy (HRT). In the United States, for decades, HRT was prescribed to nearly 40% of women in postmenopausal age until evidence from a large clinical trial demonstrated a small but real increased risk of breast and uterine cancer associated with HRT. Taking into consideration the rate of prescription of HRT at the time, about 5,000 breast cancer deaths per year were attributable to HRT. After the findings of the trial were disseminated, HRT prescription rates decreased, as did breast cancer incidence.

In conclusion, although this FDA-based analysis is limited to animal studies, it is relevant for planning clinical studies, and should be part of the basic science information used by clinicians and patients for an appropriate informed consent process of potential harms and benefits in clinical decision-making.

SELECTED REFERENCES

Amerio, A., et al. 2015 Carcinogenicity of psychotropic drugs: A systematic review of US Food and Drug Administration-required preclinical in vivo studies. *Australia & New Zealand Journal of Psychiatry*, *49*(8), 686–696.

Cosgrove, L., et al. (2011). Antidepressants and breast and ovarian cancer risk: A review of the literature and researchers' financial associations with industry. *PLoS ONE*, *6*(4), e18210.

26

Seasonal Affective Illness

SEASONAL AFFECTIVE ILLNESS IS BEST UNDERSTOOD NOT AS A SEPARATE disease from other affective conditions, but rather as seasonality in affective illness. All human beings are sensitive to light; the impact of light is hardwired in neuroanatomy, with transmission from the retina through optic nerves to the lateral geniculate nucleus, and the suprachiasmatic nucleus, which controls the sleep–wake cycle. The body has intricate circadian rhythms that are regulated by the interaction of light with this neuroanatomy. Thus, everyone is affected by light, or its absence.

Persons with mood illnesses, though, are more sensitive to light than others: too much light, shortening the sleep–wake cycle, causes manic symptoms; too little light, lengthening the sleep–wake cycle, causes depressive symptoms. In the spring and summer, there is too much—in the fall and winter, not enough—light. One thus needs to modulate light exposure to avoid causing manic symptoms in spring/summer and depressive symptoms in fall/winter. *Mood episodes go together, so if you want to prevent winter depression, you should also try to prevent summer mania.* In this chapter, the concept of seasonal affective illness is examined, and its interaction with medication treatment is discussed.

The best metaphor for seasonal affective illness (SAI) is hibernation, which can be thought of a biological correlate of wintertime depression. Unlike people with classical depression, who typically eat less and sleep less, people with SAI eat and sleep more, much like animals hibernating in winter. Many persons with SAI don't realize they have depression, because their mood isn't depressed (i.e., they don't feel sad). Yet they feel tired and uninterested in usual activities (anhedonic) and have greater appetite and sleep, thereby meeting clinical depression criteria.

Initial studies of SAI, which defined the condition, were conducted at the NIMH in the late 1970s; the first report involved 29 patients, 93% of whom were diagnosed with bipolar illness. They had depressive episodes in the fall and winter and hypomanic/manic episodes in the spring and summer. In other words, SAI occurred almost entirely in persons with bipolar illness. Thus, from the beginning, SAI was not a newly discovered disease distinct from other affective illnesses, but rather a course pattern in persons with already known affective illness. This rediscovery of seasonality in affective illness at the NIMH occurred almost a century after its clear description in the classic German psychopathology literature, by Emil Kraepelin and others. Kraepelin classically showed, as described in Chapter 26, that there is a peak of suicidality that correlates with the seasons too: there is a peak in the spring in particular, along with manic episodes, which he though was related to mixed states.

DSM revisions since the 3rd edition in 1980 have taken a different view; they have assigned a different label to seasonality, "seasonal affective disorder" (SAD), as if it were separate from other affective conditions. In DSM-5, SAD is now a specifier for depressive and bipolar illness "with seasonal pattern." This usage is more consistent with the scientific literature.

Still, many people have seasonal mood changes but don't have full clinical depressive or manic/hypomanic episodes. If defined as never having any full mood episodes of any kind in their lifetime, such persons can be said to have "winter blues," which correlates with latitude. In areas with little light during winter, near the poles of the earth, the population with winter blues can be large.

TREATMENT

The treatment of seasonal mood episodes is not, in the first instance, lightbox therapy. Rather, since seasonal mood episodes occur as part of affective illness, bipolar or unipolar, the main treatment involves treating the underlying affective illness. Light and the seasons are *triggers* for timing of mood episodes, like stressful life events. They are not the sole cause. The underlying susceptibility to mood episodes, which is the affective illness itself, needs treatment with second-messenger modifiers or monoamine agonists.

Lithium, for instance, has many circadian effects biologically. The *CLOCK* gene, which regulates circadian rhythms, is used in an animal model of mania. Animals with this gene removed are hyperactive, with decreased need for sleep. Lithium normalizes this behavior in the animal model. Manic-depressive illness is a disease of cyclicity, characterized by recurrent mood episodes that come and go. This cyclicity is probably related to underlying abnormalities in circadian rhythms. Lithium and other second-messenger modifiers can normalize these rhythms, and thereby exert beneficial effects in mood episode prevention.

Some of the medical benefits of lithium, in possible dementia prevention and decreased medical mortality, also may relate to its circadian benefits. Circadian rhythms are tied closely to many bodily functions. Steroid hormones, for example, vary in amount in the body over 24 hours based on circadian cycles. When a person is depressed or manic, these cycles are disturbed, and instead of the usual ups and downs of release, steroid hormones are produced at a more constant and higher rate, which is likely to cause damage leading to heart disease and dementia. Many studies show that poor sleep patterns, whether insomnia or just sleeping too little (less than eight hours nightly), are associated with poor medical outcomes and increased mortality.

When giving medications for unipolar depression or bipolar illness, it is important for clinicians to be aware of any seasonal patterns of episodes. If these are not taken into account, it could be that patients routinely improve from depression in the spring or summer. Clinicians may use multiple agents without benefit throughout the fall and winter, and then the patient improves in the spring, after getting a new medication. That medication will be seen as "causing" improvement, whereas in fact, spring did. The patient relapses again in a few months in the fall, despite continuing the "effective" medication, and clinicians might think there is "poop-out." In fact, the medication might not have been effective at all, and any ascribed benefit to it was misplaced. Clinicians should pay attention to natural history of seasonality so as to attribute possible medication benefit appropriately.

Also, when patients are known to be at high risk of relapse into depression in the fall/winter, clinicians and patients can have more appointments around that time, or possibly change medications to prepare for that period of relapse. For instance, mood-stabilizing doses might be increased in the summer in preparation for fall depression. Or, if antidepressants are given short-term, they might be given in late summer in preparation for fall depression, rather than in the spring, when they are more likely to precipitate manic episodes instead. Among antidepressants, bupropion XL is FDA-indicated for prevention of seasonal affective disorder.

LIGHT PRECAUTIONS

In addition to the preceding adjustments with medications, there are some behavioral interventions that are important in managing seasonality of affective episodes. In fall and winter, there is much less light than in spring and summer, and those who are sensitive to this reduction in light may become depressed. Accordingly, during these seasons, it is essential to maximize their exposure to what light there is. The light that is most needed is the light that causes awakening in the morning, which serves to entrain the daily circadian cycle. Therefore, the first—and single most important—action to take is simply to lift the bedroom shades so as to obtain as much of the early morning light as possible. This step, in itself, is a major help to many people experiencing fall/winter depression. If it does not provide enough relief, another step that can be taken is to minimize sunglass wearing during the day so as to maximize exposure to the available daytime light. Because the most light is available around noon, it is helpful to take a walk at this time on sunny days. It is important to take reasonable care of one's eyes and skin to avoid long-term damage. Once one feels better, one can start wearing sunglasses again as much as feasible.

In spring and summer, there is a relative excess of light. Those who are sensitive to it may experience manic symptoms, which can be mild (hypomania) or severe (mania). The first and most important precaution to be taken here is the opposite of that for fall/winter depression—namely, to reduce early morning light exposure, either by using room-darkening shades or by sleeping with an eye mask. This simple step is very important and can stop spring/summer manic symptoms by itself. Efforts should be made to decrease exposure to the sun through the rest of the daytime as well, and sunglasses should be worn outdoors at all times. In those with bipolar illness, it is important to remember that prevention of spring/summer mania will help prevent fall/winter depression. By not going up in the summer, patients are less likely to go down in the winter. Another major reason to take spring/summer light precautions is that springtime mixed episodes are a major cause of suicide.

If these behavioral interventions are insufficient for fall/winter depression in particular, then light therapy can be instituted. There are two forms: light boxes and dawn simulators. Light therapy can be thought of a replacement for sunlight. Because the sun is missing for part of the morning in fall/winter, the light box should be used during the morning to replace that absent sunlight; use during the afternoon or evening is ineffective. The sun does not come out at 3:00 PM or 8:00 PM, so the use of more light box therapy at those times is unsound biologically, and unhelpful clinically. Only morning light is needed and is helpful for normalizing circadian rhythms.

In most cases, 30 minutes daily is sufficient; the dose (time) can be decreased or increased as needed. Unlike medications, light therapy exerts a rapid effect, usually within one to two weeks. If no benefit is achieved in that time frame, the treatment can be stopped. A light box should be treated like the sun. Do not look directly into it, just as you should not look at the sun; otherwise corneal damage ensues. Rather, the light box should be put on a table while eating or reading and the light should be received indirectly. Dawn simulators differ from traditional light boxes in that they come on gradually, like an alarm clock, at times when the sun would normally have risen in the spring and summer. This gradual increase in light exerts a waking effect, mimicking a natural sunrise. It can be seen as a more natural approximation of the effect of light on circadian cycles. Even if the eyes are closed, light will enter through the eyelids. Some studies suggest that dawn simulators have efficacy similar to that of traditional light boxes.

Until recently, it was thought that light therapy was effective only in persons with seasonal affective illness. However, a recent study in non-seasonal unipolar depression found that the addition of light box treatment to fluoxetine was mildly more effective than fluoxetine alone (with placebo). This was the first randomized trial to assess benefits of light therapy outside of SAI and it suggests benefits even outside the fall/winter time frame. Further study will be needed to confirm or refute this initial finding.

Light boxes have a purely antidepressant effect, which means they can cause mania. Thus, though they can and should be used in bipolar illness, combined with second-messenger modifiers, they should be stopped if manic symptoms occur. Also, their use should stop, if there is benefit for winter depression, sometime in February. The use of light boxes should not continue into April, since they could exacerbate mixed states and possibly increase the risk of suicide.

A common therapeutic misconception, stemming from the view that SAI is a distinct "disorder" separate from other affective illnesses, is the belief that light boxes are an alternative to medications. Once it is understood that SAI is a course pattern within affective illness, it becomes obvious that many patients also need medications, with light boxes as adjuncts to medications. In fact, given that SAI is part of a mood cycle that includes spring/summer manic symptoms, not just fall/winter depression, most patients would probably benefit from year-round use of second-messenger modifiers or mood stabilizers (like lithium or lamotrigine), with light boxes being used, if needed, only if behavioral light precautions fail to further ameliorate the seasonal pattern of mood episodes when employed in addition to standard mood stabilizers.

In summary, SAI is not a separate disease process; rather, it represents seasonality in affective illness. It is not solely about depression, but is often part of a mood cycle that moves from spring/summer manic symptoms into fall/winter depressive symptoms. When symptoms are mild, they tend to represent winter blues, a condition related more to latitude than to any underlying disease. When full clinical episodes occur, SAI is often part of a larger manic-depressive illness. Behavioral light precautions are the best initial intervention and often are sufficient by themselves, alone or combine with medications. If needed, light boxes also can be effective for fall/winter depression.

BEHAVIORAL INTERVENTIONS FOR SEASONAL AFFECTIVE ILLNESS

For the Fall–Winter (September–January)

In winter, there is not enough light. Therefore, people sleep in the morning longer than they should, and that will throw off their circadian rhythms. They need to increase their light exposure.

Specific approaches include:

- *Keep shades and curtains open at night*, to maximize morning light exposure. This is the simplest thing to do to reduce risk of winter depression.
- Don't wear sunglasses in routine activity, or use them less than one normally would (or limit only to driving). Go for walks around noontime, without sunglasses, for up to an hour.
- Go to bed at a regular time at night. Wake up at a regular time in the morning; use an alarm.
- For light therapy: The usual dose is 10,000 lux (most light boxes are at that dose). There are many companies that make them. *Use indirect light*; do not look into the light box directly (treat it like the sun). One should have a light box on the table while reading or eating in the morning. The dose is 30 minutes, on average, as long as depression persists. Use the light box daily initially, and then reduce use to every other day for prevention. *Use the light box in the morning (before 10:00 AM)*: remember that you are trying to replace the morning sunlight, which declines in winter.

For the Spring/Summer (March–August)

In summer, there's too much light; so people tend to sleep in the morning less than they should, throwing off their circadian rhythms.

To decrease light exposure:

- Wear sunglasses at all times.
- *Wear an eye mask to sleep,* or get room-darkening shades.
- *Close curtains at night, to minimize morning light.*
- Go to bed at a regular time at night. Wake up at a regular time in the morning, but not early.

SELECTED REFERENCE

Magnusson, A., & Boivin, D. (2003). Seasonal affective disorder: An overview. *Chronobiology International, 20,* 189–207.

27

Suicide

ABOUT 41,000 PERSONS KILL THEMSELVES EVERY YEAR IN THE UNITED States. That comes out to over 100 persons daily, about 5 persons per hour. The World Health Organization (WHO) estimates that about 1 million people in the world commit suicide yearly. Suicide is to psychiatry what mortality is to medicine: preventing it is the ultimate goal and responsibility in treating psychiatric illnesses. Clinicians may or may not succeed in making people happier, or more functional, or more satisfied with their lives. But clinicians ought to at least help keep patients alive.

Besides psychiatric explanations, there was a prominent social explanation for suicide, dating to the French sociologist Emile Durkheim. His impression was that suicide had increased in frequency in the 19th century compared to what was presumed to be the case in earlier centuries. He drew a simple conclusion: that suicide is the result of modern life. The big difference between modernity and the Middle Ages is industrialization; we work in factories and offices in cities where we avoid each other and where we are separated from families of origin. "*Anomie*" was the word Durkheim coined: meaning our modern sense of isolation and alienation from each other and from the verities of the past.

Many have debated Durkheim's claim, but it's clear that some related claims are wrong: they confuse correlation with cause. Some thought that living in cities caused suicide, since suicide rates are much higher in cities than in the countryside. Of course, there are more people in cities, too, and those with psychiatric illnesses are often brought to cities, or decide to go there, to seek treatment at medical centers. This latter point is important—a common mistake some clinicians make about suicide. Antidepressants were introduced decades ago; suicide rates went down. But you can't draw a causal relationship. The connection isn't necessarily causal. These are called "secular" factors in suicide: social and cultural changes that can affect the entire population, and possibly affect those more prone to suicide negatively. Two relevant secular factors are poverty and sunlight.

One way of addressing these complex social factors is to examine national rates of suicide: Greenland has by far the highest rate of suicide in the world, followed by Lithuania, South Korea, Guyana, Kazakhstan, Slovenia, Japan, and then a number of other East European countries. The lowest rates in the world are in Nepal, preceded by Haiti, Grenada, other Caribbean islands, and then Egypt and multiple Middle Eastern states. Examining this list, poverty doesn't stand out as a risk factor: Japan is wealthy but has a high suicide rate; Haiti is quite poor but has low suicide rates.

Another secular risk factor, sunlight, turns out to have a much stronger effect than poverty on risk of suicide. There is a direct correlation, though small, between more sunlight and more suicide. There is a much larger correlation between the season of the year and suicide, with springtime being the highest risk, followed by fall. In the spring, there is rapid increase in sunlight as winter transitions to summer; in the fall, there is a steep decline in light, as summer transitions into winter. In both cases, it seems that the *slope* matters: when there is a change in light, people become more suicidal. People with mood illnesses especially appear to be more sensitive to these seasonal changes in light. The slope upwards, from less to more light in April and May, seems to be the most harmful change: one can infer that winter depression is shifting to summer mania, with many people developing mixed mood states, which are the most likely mood states to produce suicide.

"Psychological autopsies" involve taking cases of suicide and trying to identify common correlates. In this research, the following correlations have been found at the time of suicide: clinical depression, the use of antidepressants, anxiety, past suicide attempts, financial or marital/romantic problems, alcohol and substance abuse, male gender, access to firearms, social isolation, older age, white race; and in the United States, German or northern European ethnicity. In studies where many suicidal risk factors are identified in at-risk persons, though, most such persons still don't commit suicide. So these risk factors are about relative risk, not any predication that all or even most such persons would commit suicide.

It's easy to overestimate or underestimate these risk factors. Take past suicide attempts: it's rational to view them as a risk factor for suicide. But about one-half of persons who kill themselves do so with the first attempt. For half of all suicides, the first time is the only time. One can't predict their cases by past attempts.

Take anxiety: as discussed in the text, anxiety is a basic personality trait, with a normal distribution. About one-fifth of the general population has "high" anxiety based on being in the top two standard deviations of the normal curve. But much less than 1% of the general population commits suicide. Anxiety by itself is a poor suicide predictor.

PSYCHIATRIC DISEASES

Of all the risk factors from the psychological autopsies, the most common and predictive appears to be clinical depression. Not only is it present in the vast majority of completed suicides, it works the other way around: a good number of persons with severe clinical depression eventually commit suicide (in contrast to those with the traits of anxiety and being white or being northern European in ethnicity). It turns out that up to 20% of persons with severe clinical depression eventually commit suicide. This is a very large number, in contrast to anxiety. It is more if people have bipolar illness, as opposed to unipolar depression, and more if they've ever been psychiatrically hospitalized as opposed to solely needing outpatient treatment. If they were only outpatients with less severe depressive episodes, and no manic periods, the suicide rate can go down to a 2% lifetime prevalence. So a major risk factor for suicide is the presence of the bipolar or severe unipolar depressive diagnosis. Then one can start adding other important risk factors.

It was mentioned that suicide attempts aren't present in half of patients, but when present, suicide attempts are important predictors: almost 10% of persons who make a suicide attempt will kill themselves within the following decade.

It is suggested that clinicians should focus on the necessary (but insufficient) conditions for suicide: they should pay attention to past suicide attempts, be on high alert with all clients with severe depression or bipolar illness. Treat those conditions appropriately for suicide prevention, which, as we'll see, doesn't involve most of the medications we use, like antidepressants, but rather a drug most clinicians avoid: lithium, as discussed further later.

Another at-risk clinical group involves those who engage in self-cutting or other self-harm (burning themselves with cigarettes, head-banging). Called "parasuicide," this kind of self-harm doesn't have the intent to end one's life. It's most common in borderline personality, happening in about 60% of persons with that condition. It tends to be associated with a history of past sexual abuse, but not invariably so. It's unclear whether these persons are at high risk of completed suicide, if they don't make more typical suicide attempts like overdose. As noted previously, if they do also make standard suicide attempts, like overdose, they do have a notable risk of future suicide.

ANTIDEPRESSANTS: CAUSES OR CURES?

There has been a great debate about whether antidepressants cause or prevent suicide. As discussed later, the evidence from the FDA database shows that SRIs increase the risk of suicide in young adults and children (although not in middle age or older persons). Critics have claimed that suicide rates went down when antidepressants were introduced widely in the 1970s through the 1990s. It's claimed that suicide rates went up after the FDA black box warning when antidepressant use declined in adolescents and children. It's claimed in some analyses of insurance records that suicide rates don't go up after antidepressants are given, but rather decline. These reports use non-randomized, observational data to contradict the FDA-based randomized data. This way of thinking ignores the concept of the "confounding bias," which is the central reason why clinicians need to pay more attention to randomized studies than to anything else, including their own clinical experience, as described in Chapter 4. As noted, social factors can affect suicide, thus population-based rises or declines cannot be directly linked to antidepressant use.

In fact, randomized data with antidepressants repeatedly demonstrate they contribute little to no appreciable suicide prevention, although the harm of causing actual suicide also seems to be very low in frequency. In sum, SRIs do not provide major benefits in prevention of suicide, and they appear to have a risk of some harm in younger persons.

If clinicians wish for drugs with a robust benefit shown to prevent completed suicide, there are only two agents shown to do so, lithium and clozapine. If focusing on randomized trials, clozapine has only one study, and it showed reduction in suicide attempts but not in completed suicide. Lithium has four placebo-controlled randomized trials, which, taken together (as described later), demonstrate almost 90% reduction in completed suicide.

In short, there is something like a cure for suicide, if clinicians are willing to use it, as will be explained later in this chapter.

Bottom Line

- There is a social component to suicide, but the most important cause appears to be psychiatric disease, especially manic-depressive illness.
- The most important predictors are severe depression and suicide attempts.
- Parasuicidal self-harm may not predict suicide without other risk factors.
- Antidepressants don't prevent suicide, and they hasten it in some persons.
- Lithium and clozapine have anti-suicide effects, with lithium being the only drug to prevent suicide definitively in randomized clinical trials.

DO ANTIDEPRESSANTS CAUSE OR PREVENT SUICIDE?

In the preceding discussion, it was held that antidepressants are at best neutral, and at worst harmful, in the prevention of suicide. Furthermore, lithium is said to be a very effective agent in suicide prevention. In the rest of this chapter, the scientific evidence concerning these two claims will be examined.

There are two major sources of evidence to answer this question: (1) the FDA meta-analysis of all randomized clinical trials (RCTs) conducted by the pharmaceutical industry in major depressive disorder (MDD); and (2) the largest NIMH-sponsored RCT of suicidality with SRIs in adolescents, the Treatment of Adolescent Depression Study (TADS).

FDA Analysis of Suicide and Antidepressants

In the 1990s, pharmaceutical companies were encouraged by the FDA to conduct randomized clinical trials (RCTs) on antidepressants in children and adolescents. The wish was to make these agents, believed to be so effective for MDD in adults, available to children, too. The agents were only somewhat effective. As the FDA examined side effects in these trials, it identified some evidence of suicidality, defined as worsened suicidal ideation or suicide attempts. This is when the FDA decided to meta-analyze the data from all the studies that the companies had done (which they were legally obligated to provide to the FDA, although they have no legal obligation to make those data available to the public or the scientific community). When the FDA statisticians conducted those analyses, they found the results that they later published (Figure 27.1).

The FDA and its advisors then voted to institute a black box warning in the SRI package inserts saying these agents may cause or worsen suicidality. All this occurred in 2004, and it led to a major backlash from the psychiatric community, especially from child psychiatry clinicians. Nonetheless, the FDA had an impact, and antidepressant use has declined in the last decade in children.

In this meta-analysis, a few points are important:

1. All the studies were conducted quite similarly for FDA approval, being of similar duration, with the same rating scales, and similar inclusion and exclusion criteria. Hence, they are comparable, and the meta-analysis has limited "heterogeneity." In other words, this review is about as valid as a meta-analysis can get.
2. There were no suicides, as many of the opponents of the FDA black box always point out. But these RCTs were conducted for FDA approval of drugs for kids. The last things drug companies could afford would be a suicide in an RCT. The media backlash that would ensue would cost a lot of money. Suicidal ideation is a major exclusion criterion for these studies. In short, the patients were selected carefully to be highly *non-suicidal*. And yet some of them became suicidal, as shown in these data. This argues for these data being even more, not less, concerning.
3. The absolute rates matter. The meta-analysis shows about a 67% increase in suicidality with SRIs over placebo. But the absolute rates were about 2% with SRIs versus 1% with placebo. In other words, about 1% of children will get more suicidal with SRIs, as opposed to placebo (mainly a stand-in for natural history).

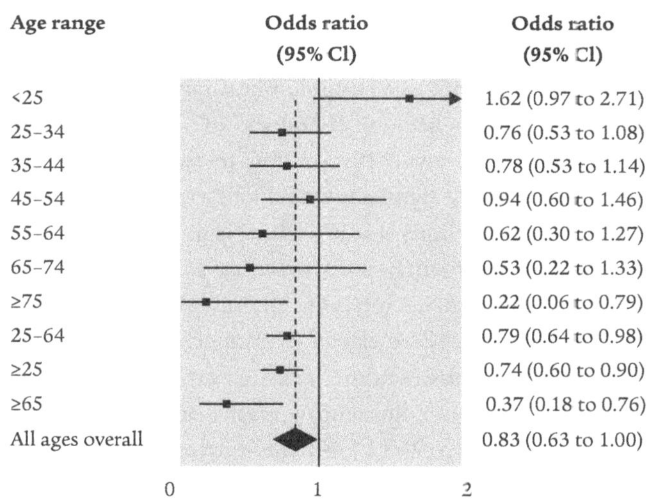

FIGURE 27.1 *Suicidality risk with SRIs by age.* SOURCE: *M Stone et al. Risk of suicidality in clinical trials of antidepressants in adults: Analysis of proprietary data submitted to US Food and Drug Administration. BMJ 2009;339:b2880. Reprinted with permission of The BMJ.*

Put otherwise: 99% of children will not get more suicidal. This absolute rate provides a clinical context for decision-making. This doesn't mean one should completely ignore these data. There is an increased risk of suicidality here, but it doesn't apply to most patients. Nonetheless, the 1% matter, especially when death is the result.

4. But will any child die? Many assume not, since no one died in these eight-week trials. That assumption ignores the research literature that about 10% of persons who make suicide attempts will eventually kill themselves. One can calculate the "number need to harm" using these figures, which is done later.
5. In another FDA analysis of all their antidepressant studies in adults, increased suicidal risk is only present for young adults under the age of 25 and for children. There is a notable increased risk there, but a decreased risk in all older adult groups, such that there is an overall decreased risk of suicidality with antidepressants of 17% (odds ratio of 0.83, which is 17% decreased risk compared to the null value of 1). What does this mean? Early onset of depression (under 25 years) was said to reflect a higher probability of bipolar illness, as opposed to unipolar depression. This raises the question that perhaps antidepressants are causing suicidality in young adults and children because "depression" in those ages is not "MDD" but rather bipolar illness.

The Treatment of Adolescent Depression (TADS) Study

Another approach to the problem would be to conduct a larger RCT to try to answer the question, with a specific plan to look at suicidality as a secondary outcome (unlike all the studies in the FDA database). This led to the NIMH-sponsored Treatment of Adolescent Depression Study (TADS). Even there, though, where no pharmaceutical influence existed based on funding, the investigators appear to under-report the suicidal risks of fluoxetine by over-reliance on hypothesis testing methods.

In that study, 479 adolescents were double-blind randomized in a factorial design to fluoxetine versus cognitive behavioral therapy (CBT), versus both, versus neither. Response rates were 61% vs. 43% vs. 71% vs. 35%, respectively, with differences being statistically significant. Clinically significant suicidality was present in 29% of children at baseline (more than most previous studies, which is good because it provides a larger number of outcomes for assessment); and worsening suicidal ideation or a suicide attempt was defined as the secondary outcome of "suicide related adverse events" (no completed suicides occurred in 12 weeks of treatment). Seven suicide attempts were made, six on fluoxetine. In the abstract, the investigators reported improvement in suicidality in all four groups, without commenting on the differential worsening in the fluoxetine group. The text reported 5.5% (24) suicide-related adverse events, but it did not report the results with RR (relative risks) and CIs (confidence intervals).

When the author of this text analyzed those data that way, I saw the following risk of worsened suicidality: with fluoxetine, RR 1.77 [0.76, 4.15]; with CBT, RR 0.85 [0.37, 1.94]. The paper speculates about possible protective benefits with CBT for suicidality, even though the CIs are too wide to infer much probability of such benefit. In contrast, the apparent increase in suicidal risk with fluoxetine, which appears more probable based on the CIs than in the CBT effect, is not discussed in as much detail. The low suicide attempt rate (1.6%, $n = 7$) is reported, but the overwhelming prevalence with fluoxetine use is not. Using effect estimate methods, the risk of suicide attempts with fluoxetine is RR 6.19 [0.75, 51.0]. Due to the low frequency, this risk is not statistically significant. But hypothesis testing methods (*p*-values) are inappropriate here; use of effect estimation shows a large, six-fold risk, which is probably present, and could be as high as 51-fold. In short, fluoxetine had about a six-fold increased risk of suicide attempts, a huge effect size.

Hypothesis-testing methods, using *p*-values, are biased toward the null hypothesis, meaning they tend to say that nothing is happening unless there is overwhelming evidence otherwise. Effect estimation methods, less biased and more neutral, tell another story. For side effects in general, especially for infrequent ones like suicidality, effect estimation stories are closer to reality.

An Oslerian Approach to Antidepressants and Suicide

Recalling Osler's dictum once again that the art of medicine is the art of balancing probabilities, we can conclude that the antidepressant/suicide controversy is not a question of yes or no, but rather of whether there is a risk, quantifying that risk, and then weighing that risk against benefits.

This effort has not been made systematically, but one researcher made a start in a letter to the editor commenting on the TADS study. Carroll noted that the number needed to harm (NNH) for suicide-related averse events in the TADS study was 34 (6.9% with fluoxetine versus 4.0% without it). The NNH for suicide attempts was 43 (2.8% with fluoxetine versus 0.45% without it). In contrast, the benefit seen with improvement of depression was more notable; the number needed to treat (NNT) for fluoxetine was 3.7. So about four patients need to be treated to improve depression in one of them, while a suicide attempt due to fluoxetine will only occur after 43 patients are treated. This would seem to favor the drug, but we are really comparing apples and oranges: improving depression is fine, but how many deaths due to suicide from the drug are acceptable?

One has to now bring in other probabilities besides the actual data from the study (an approach related to Bayesian statistics): epidemiological studies indicate that about 8% of suicide attempts end in death. Thus, with an NNH of suicide attempts of 43, the NNH for completed suicide would be 535 (43 divided by 0.08). This would seem to be a very small risk; but it is a serious outcome. Can we balance it by an estimate of prevention of suicide?

The most conservative estimate of lifetime suicide in unipolar MDD is 2.2%. If we presume that a part of this lifetime rate will occur in adolescence (perhaps 30%), then an adolescent suicide rate of 0.66% might be viable. This produces an NNT for prevention of suicide with fluoxetine, based on the TADS data, of 560 (3.7 divided by 0.0066).

One could do the same kind of analysis using the FDA database cited previously, which found an NNH for suicide attempts of 100 (higher than the TADS study). If 8% of those patients complete suicide, then the NNH for completed suicide is 800 (100 divided by 0.08).

So one life is saved out of every 560 treated, but one is taken out of every 535, or possibly every 800 patients. Applying Osler's dictum about the art of medicine meaning balancing probabilities, there seems to be about neutral overall effect. It is also possible that the actual suicide rates used here are too conservative, and that antidepressants might have somewhat more preventive benefit than suggested, but even with more benefit, their relative benefit would still be in the NNT range of over 100, which is generally consider minimal. Overall, then, antidepressants have minimal benefits, at least, in relation to suicide. They can increase suicidal risk, but again infrequently.

At some level, the controversy about antidepressants and suicide has to do with mistaken abuse of hypothesis testing statistics. The proponents of the association argue that anecdotes are real, and not refuted by the RCTs. They are correct. Their opponents claim that the amount of risk shown in RCTs is small. They also are correct. Both sides err when they claim their view is absolutely correct.

When effect estimation methods are applied, one observes see that there is no scientific basis for any general controversy. There is a real risk of suicide with antidepressants, but that risk is small, and equal to or less than the probable benefit of prevention of suicide with such agents.

Overall, antidepressants do not have a major suicide benefit. Their use should be on other grounds (e.g., quality of life, side effects, medical risks).

Bottom Line

- Antidepressants cause and prevent about one suicide in every 500 adolescents or young adults.
- They thus both cause and prevent suicide, but their net effect is neutral.

LITHIUM: META-ANALYSIS FOR PREVENTION OF SUICIDE

Lithium is the only medication ever proven to prevent suicide in double-blind placebo-controlled randomized clinical trials. This is an exceedingly important statement that needs to be explained. It means that, among all psychotropic agents, only lithium is proven to prevent suicide. The main evidence for this claim is found in a meta-analysis of this topic.

In that meta-analysis, 48 RCTs were included, with 6,674 participants. Let's focus on the placebo comparisons, which are four RCTs. Overall there was a 87% decreased risk of suicide (odds ratio 0.13), which means that only about one in ten persons committed suicide who would have committed suicide without lithium. (There were zero suicides in the lithium arm versus six suicides in the placebo arm.) (Figure 27.2). Contrast this large effect size with the modest 17% decrease in suicidality (not completed suicide) with antidepressants in the second figure of the prior article. Since only about 5–10% of persons who make suicide attempts eventually commit suicide, the antidepressant benefit for completed suicide is not more than about 1% at best. This contrasts with 87% with lithium. In other words, lithium is about 90 times more powerful in prevention of suicide than antidepressants.

Study	No of events/total: Lithium	No of events/total: Control	Peto odds ratio fixed (95% CI)	Weight (%)	Peto odds ratio fixed (95% CI)
Versus placebo					
Bauer 2000	0/14	1/15		16.8	0.14 (0.00 to 7.31)
Lauterbach 2008	0/84	3/83		49.8	0.13 (0.01 to 1.27)
Prien 1973a	0/45	1/39		16.7	0.12 (0.00 to 5.91)
Prien 1973b	0/101	1/104		16.8	0.14 (0.00 to 7.02)
Subtotal	0/244	6/241		100.0	0.13 (0.03 to 0.66)

Test for heterogeneity: $\chi^2 = 0.01$, df = 3, p = 1.00, $I^2 = 0\%$

Test for overall effect: Z = 2.47, P = 0.01

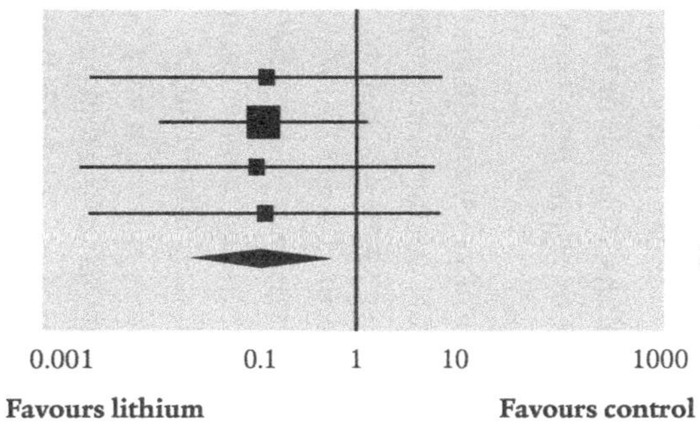

FIGURE 27.2 *Lithium in the prevention of suicide in mood disorders.* SOURCE: *Cipriani et al. Lithium in the prevention of suicide in mood disorders: Updated systematic review and meta-analysis. BMJ 2013;346:f3646. Reprinted with permission of The BMJ.*

Other aspects of this meta-analysis are interesting: Parasuicidal self-harm was not affected by lithium (odds ratio [OR] 0.60, CI 0.27–1.32). The benefit seen with lithium was present also in unipolar depression (OR 0.36), with a 64% decreased suicide rate. Lithium also generally had lower suicide rates than most active comparators, including other agents known to be effective in bipolar illness, like carbamazepine. Other studies have compared lithium and valproate, and again, lithium seems to have a preferential anti-suicide effect in bipolar illness, while suicide rates are not decreased by valproate.

The importance of this meta-analysis is that it combines different RCTs to demonstrate statistical efficacy for prevention of completed suicide. In all RCTs, researchers tend to design inclusion and exclusion criteria so as to avoid suicide or other major harms. Since there is careful scrutiny of research by many groups, at least in the West, a suicide in a double-blind trial would receive negative attention from institutional review boards (IRBs; ethics committees), university administrators, and possibly the media. Studies also tend to be short, usually a few months, or a year or two at the longest. Suicide is uncommon enough, and especially so in the short time frames in most studies. Thus it is very difficult to study in a RC paradigm.

There has never been a RCT specifically designed to prevent suicide. (One study with clozapine was designed to assess suicide attempts, not completed suicide). It probably would be seen as unethical to design such a study. So, if we ever obtain RCT data about suicide prevention, it would have to occur in studies in which suicide just happened, unfortunately. These suicides are needed as outcomes, otherwise one could never know whether a drug could prevent them, compared to other comparators (such as other drugs or placebo). This is why this meta-analysis is important.

Lithium has been around for decades, and there have been 48 RCTs of it, and there have been some suicides. So it is only in this setting that one could possibly even try to answer the question of whether lithium prevents suicide. All this description is meant to explain how hard it is to answer this kind of research question with randomized data. When we have them, we should appreciate how important and rare they are. It's also relevant that there are hundreds of studies with antidepressants, also over decades, like lithium. Yet the meta-analysis of antidepressant data shows the reverse of the lithium data: there was not 90% reduction in completed suicide, but about 70% increase in suicidal thinking or behavior in those below age 25. Yet antidepressants are used widely, while lithium is avoided widely.

For suicide prevention, these randomized studies of lithium and of antidepressants demonstrate that the reverse—using lithium more widely and using antidepressants less—would be more consistent with our best scientific evidence.

A final point is that these studies tended to use standard doses of lithium. There is an extensive literature on examining the effects of lithium in areas of the world where there is a "high" amount of lithium in the drinking water. "High" means about 1–2 mg/d of lithium (compared to standard doses of around 900 mg/d). Even at these very low doses (1–2 mg/d), the lithium in the water studies showed notable evidence of decreased suicide rates associated with "high" lithium in the water, compared to other regions with low or no lithium. Those studies were observational, and thus could be affected by confounding factors, but some did control for some predictors, like urban versus rural location and socioeconomic status.

If randomized studies didn't exist, one couldn't be certain that this lithium effect was causal, as discussed previously. But since we have randomized data that lithium prevents suicide, it's likely these epidemiological data are also valid.

In short, lithium may prevent suicide even at very low doses, down to a few milligrams per day. Concerns about side effects and toxicity, discussed later, relate to much higher doses (usually about 900 mg/d).

Bottom Line

- Lithium is the only drug proven to prevent suicide in RCTs versus placebo
- It has a large effect size of almost 90% reduction in suicide risk.
- Lithium may prevent suicide in many persons even at very low doses.

LITHIUM IN THE DRINKING WATER AND SUICIDE

This discussion is now extended to research on very low doses of lithium in drinking water, and its apparent anti-suicide benefits. We think about certain minerals as being essential for life, like calcium and magnesium, needed for normal heart rhythm. There's sodium and potassium, needed for cell membrane function. These are all basic ions, part of the periodic table of chemical elements. They are essential for life; but we don't think of them as toxic or dangerous. Yet too much magnesium or potassium causes cardiac arrhythmia, leading to immediate death. Too much calcium can cause delirium, and too much sodium causes swelling of the brain.

Lithium is also an essential mineral, needed for viability of life. If you have none, zero, then the organism's ability to live is harmed. We all know too much is toxic, so it is often seen as dangerous. Yet we don't seem to fear potassium or calcium in the same way.

All drugs are toxic; only the dosing and indication makes them therapeutic. That's the old maxim, dating back to Paracelsus. But the maxim applies not just to drugs; it applies to the chemical elements themselves, the basic building blocks of biological life. One could say instead, "All elements of chemistry are toxic; it's only their amount and combinations that make them therapeutic."

First, let's appreciate that lithium is essential for life. Chemists and geologists study such matters by exposing animals to a diet deficient in or wholly lacking a certain element. They then compare those animals to others who are fed a diet rich in the element. If one group dies more quickly than the other, then the element is deemed to be essential for the viability of the animal.

With lithium, this research has been conducted with sheep. It turns out that sheep deprived of any lithium have much shorter lifespans than sheep who eat the usual amount of lithium in the diet. These animal studies provide a context for studies of the effects of lithium in drinking water.

Lithium seeps from rocks into the ground, where it is taken up into water, or into vegetables. It is consumed by animals and humans through eating vegetables or meats of other animals who have eaten vegetables. Eggs, for instance, have a notable amount of lithium. All this depends, of course, on the source of such food. Since food is shipped to different parts of the world, a better measure of local lithium supply is the drinking water, which tends to come from local sources.

In the last 50 years, about ten different studies have been conducted on the biological, medical, and social effects of lithium in drinking water. To give a sense of these studies, let's take the first, from 1970, which looked at lithium levels in the 100 largest American cities. It found lower overall mortality in areas with higher lithium levels; much of this benefit was related to less death from cardiovascular disease. Another study, in 1972, compared different counties in Texas. More recently, a 2009 study in Japan looked at over 1 million people; four reports in 2011–2012 came from Japan, England, and Austria; and a new Texas study was published in 2013. These studies mainly focused on suicide, and, rather consistently, they found lower suicide rates in the regions where lithium levels were higher in water compared to the regions with lower lithium levels.

The most obvious question in such population studies is the issue of confounding bias. What other factors in these populations could affect suicide rates? Could it be that the lithium association is spurious because of those other factors? As described in Chapter 27, there are many known risk factors for suicide, such as depression and social isolation, which cannot be assessed in such large national studies. Some proxy measures can be assessed, though, such as living in cities versus rural areas, or measures of poverty and unemployment rates in areas being studied. Some of the recent studies controlled for those social factors. Still, since randomized analysis is impossible in studies of entire countries, we will be left with some uncertainty in such large-scale analyses. With that caveat, controlling for some social confounding factors, there still is an association between more lithium and less suicide.

The fact that lithium has been proven to prevent suicide in randomized clinical trials, as reviewed in the meta-analysis just described, is the main scientific rationale for accepting the likely validity of that same association in the multiple studies of lithium in drinking water. In other words, the water studies don't "prove" that lithium prevents suicide. We already know that is the case with the meta-analysis of RCTs of bipolar illness. What the water studies strongly suggest is that very low doses of lithium could be sufficient for such suicide-prevention purposes. We now turn to the meaning of the concept of "very low dose" lithium.

If this association is real, then we can turn to characterizing what it might mean in clinical settings. Clinicians who prescribe lithium are used to thinking of standard doses as around 900 mg/d, which produces blood levels of about 0.6–1.0, which is proven therapeutic for acute mania or prophylaxis of bipolar illness. Lower doses are seen as "low"; thus, for clinicians a dose of 300 mg/d of lithium carbonate would be seen as "low" or "subtherapeutic." Most would consider that dose clinically ineffective.

However, when you start to think about lithium doses from the perspective of the normal diet, rather than prescribing pills for bipolar disease, then the concepts of "low" and "high" begin to change. In the normal diet, we consume about 1 mg/d of elemental lithium. In the water studies, "high" amounts of lithium meant more than that amount. Thus, about 5 mg/d of elemental lithium would be considered high by dietary standards. This kind of dose produced apparent suicide-prevention benefit.

It is important to translate elemental lithium into lithium compounds. For lithium carbonate, 100 mg/d of that compound is equivalent to 18.8 mg/d of elemental lithium. Thus, the "high" dietary amount of 5 mg/d of elemental lithium translates into about 25 mg/d of lithium carbonate. This dose would be considered vanishingly low by clinicians, who would think of 300 mg/d as "low." In fact, 300 mg/d of lithium, which is about 56 mg/d of elemental lithium, is quite high. It is 56 times the normal amount consumed in the diet. The "standard" lithium dose of 900 mg/d of lithium carbonate translates to 169 mg/d of elemental lithium, which is extremely high, using the standards of naturally consumed lithium.

In other words, if the suicide-prevention studies of lithium are correct, clinicians may be justified in rethinking their conception of lithium dosing, and coming to the conclusion that there is almost no minimum to lithium dosing. Any amount of lithium is better than none, at least for suicide prevention. This perspective would be justification for giving very low doses of lithium.

Another aspect of the water studies is that they showed suicide prevention in the general population, not just people with bipolar illness. Thus, they can provide justification for considering lithium in all suicidal persons, irrespective of diagnosis. Given the risks of toxicity and side effects, if lithium is effective in very low doses for suicide, such dosing could allow for more feasible use in a wide range of populations at risk for suicide, such as military veterans and athletes with chronic traumatic encephalopathy (CTE). In other words, don't think of lithium for suicide prevention as only being limited to bipolar illness.

A word of caution regarding "parasuicide," such as self-mutilation and self-cutting. The meta-analysis of RCTs showed that lithium did NOT reduce parasuicidal behavior. Thus, these considerations apply to serious suicide risk, such as overdoses or hanging or other such behavior, and do not apply to persons who only engage in self-mutilation, such as in many cases of borderline personality.

Bottom Line

- Studies of lithium in drinking water show that its anti-suicide effects are present in the general population.
- Lithium should be considered for suicide prevention broadly, not limited to mood conditions.
- It can be given at very low doses, equivalent to about 25 mg/d of lithium carbonate.

Low to Very Low Doses of Lithium

The lithium in water studies suggest that more than 1 mg/d of elemental lithium can be effective for suicide prevention. If we take 5 mg/d of elemental lithium as a clearly "high" amount from a dietary perspective, that translates to about 25 mg/d of lithium carbonate. The smallest pill size of lithium carbonate in the United States is 150 mg/d. Thus a half pill taken every other day should be equivalent to 37.5 mg/d, which would approximate the lithium in water dose of somewhat more than 5 mg/d of elemental lithium.

At least two other approaches exist:

- *Lithium citrate* is available as 300 mg/d in 5 ml liquid form. Thus 1 ml in a dropper would be equivalent to 60 mg/d. Taken every other day, the dose would approximate 30 mg/d of lithium citrate, which is equivalent to about 5 mg/d of elemental lithium.
- *Lithium orotate* is available as an OTC preparation, with the standard 120 mg/d pill size being equivalent to 5 mg/d of elemental lithium. Its safety is little studied, unlike lithium carbonate's, but it is widely used by many in the general population, and it has the advantage of not requiring a prescription or pill-cutting (as with lithium carbonate) or taking a liquid formulation (as with lithium citrate).

SELECTED REFERENCES

Cipriani, A., et al. (2013). Lithium in the prevention of suicide in mood disorders: Updated systematic review and meta-analysis. *British Medical Journal, 346,* f3646.

Mauer, S., et al. (2014). Standard and trace dose lithium: The systematic review of dementia prevention and other behavioral benefits. *Australia and New Zealand Journal of Psychiatry, 48,* 809–818.

28

Children

DIAGNOSTIC ASPECTS OF THE TOPIC OF ADD ARE EXAMINED IN DETAIL IN Appendix III. In this chapter, other aspects of psychopharmacological treatment of children are considered, specifically for diagnoses or symptoms of depression, manic states, anxiety, and behavioral problems, as well as autism and OCD. In the last part of this chapter, the use of amphetamines for ADD symptoms is examined through a detailed evaluation of the most definitive RCT on that topic, the Multimodal Treatment of ADHD (MTA) study.

AGITATION

Perhaps the most common presentation of any psychiatric issue in children involves agitation. Like anxiety, the second most common presentation, agitation is not itself an illness. It is the effect of some other cause. DSM terms like "oppositional defiant disorder" and "conduct disorder" are simply adjectives masquerading as nouns. They are bureaucratic ways of stating that the patient is agitated. This agitation can reflect an underlying disease that could be schizophrenia, bipolar illness, unipolar depression, OCD, autism, epilepsy, or a range of other possibilities.

A central problem with the practice of child psychiatry is that the patient is a runner in motion, and the clinician is a photographer who gets nothing but blurred pictures. The picture does not become clear until the patient is no longer a child, when the course of the illness expresses itself explicitly in young adulthood, as schizophrenia, bipolar illness, unipolar depression, or other conditions. Until that time, the child psychiatrist is only guessing, and knowing so, it behooves the clinician to look for clues wherever possible. Symptoms, like agitation, are too non-specific to be very meaningful clues of the ultimate underlying diagnosis. Better sources are genetics, course of illness, and possibly treatment effects.

If agitation occurs in the setting of a child with a family history of bipolar illness, then it probably reflects manic-like symptoms, and a rational judgment could be made for treatment with low-dose second-messenger modifiers like lithium or divalproex. If agitation occurs in the setting of a child with a family history of schizophrenia, then the likelihood of the latter diagnosis is markedly increased, and the beginning of low-dose antipsychotic treatment to affect the prodrome of schizophrenia could be justified. If agitation occurs in a child with no family history of any psychiatric illness, or with unclear family history, then the clinician and the family need to have a careful risk–benefit discussion about symptomatic treatment of agitation. Such treatment usually involves low-dose dopamine blockers and or anticonvulsants, and the clinical judgment about treatment will have to pay attention to side effects. Low doses and shorter durations of treatment would be advisable. Common medications used for such symptomatic treatment are low-dose risperidone 0.5–2.0 mg a day, divalproex 500–1000 mg per day, or aripiprazole 2–5 mg per day. Clinicians would be advised to avoid other medications in these classes with many more side effects, especially of the medical kind, such as cardiac arrhythmias or cardiovascular disease. These would include amphetamines, olanzapine, clozapine, and quetiapine.

ANXIETY

Besides agitation, anxiety is a very common presentation in children. It is perhaps the most non-specific symptom of all. Anxiety and agitation often go together, but not always. One can be agitated and highly anxious, or not very anxious at all. One can be anxious but not agitated at all. Anxiety itself, representing a sense of worry and physiological activation, is too non-specific to be diagnostically meaningful. The diagnostician of the developing child cannot get a clear picture of the runner in motion. The clinician is advised to turn to the genetics of the family and the course of illness, as much as is available, to make the best clinical judgment regarding diagnosis. If anxiety occurs in a child with a family history of bipolar illness, then it probably reflects manic or depressive symptoms, and a rational judgment could be made for treatment with low-dose second-messenger modifiers like lithium or divalproex. If anxiety occurs in the setting of a child with a family history of schizophrenia, then the likelihood of the latter diagnosis is markedly increased, and the beginning of low-dose antipsychotic treatment to affect the prodrome of schizophrenia could be justified. If anxiety occurs in a child with no family history of any psychiatric illness, or with unclear family history, then the clinician and the family need to have a careful risk–benefit discussion about symptomatic treatment of anxiety. Most clinicians would prescribe low doses of SRIs in preference to benzodiazepines and children. It is thought that the latter agents cause a kind of paradoxical disinhibition. This may be the case, based on clinical experience, but the research evidence for this belief is limited. Some children may be able tolerate low doses of benzodiazepines, and may indeed do better with those agents than with SRIs. The use of low-dose SRIs in children with family genetics for bipolar illness is something that should be avoided. The fact that SRIs are associated with increased risk of suicidality in children, as discussed in the previous chapter, should give pause to the routine use of these agents for anxiety. If given, low doses and shorter durations of treatment would be advisable. Other alternatives besides benzodiazepines could be gabapentin or antihistamines. When used symptomatically, the types of agents that could be given include citalopram, 10 mg per day; fluoxetine, 10 mg per day; sertraline, 25–50 mg per day; lorazepam, 0.5–1 mg per day; clonazepam, 0.5–1 mg per day; gabapentin, 300–900 mg per day; and hydroxyzine, 25–50 mg per day.

OBSESSIVE-COMPULSIVE DISORDER

Frequently, the anxiety presentation in children evolves into a full-blown obsessive-compulsive illness. This OCD is quite common, and in many children, it eventually goes away. Sometimes it occurs as part of depressive or manic episodes in children with bipolar illness or unipolar depression, and sometimes it can be part of a psychotic illness. It can also occur as a long-term consequence of severe streptococcal infection. OCD also can be part of a neurological process that could include Tourette's syndrome, and other neurobehavioral abnormalities. Again, the key job of the clinician is to try to identify the most probable underlying illness. Family genetics is the number-one source of evidence, followed by course of illness. As in the case of anxiety and agitation, treatment should be guided by that family history. Where there is no such family history of another psychiatric illness, or where the family history is unclear, then direct treatment for the OCD can be given with SRIs in standard doses. These would include fluoxetine, 20–80 mg per day; sertraline, 50–200 mg per day; paroxetine, 20–60 mg per day; and other SRIs. It should be noted that dopamine blockers, like risperidone or olanzapine, have been shown to have anti-OCD effects as well, at least as adjuncts, and possibly by themselves. Where OCD is present and the patient is highly agitated, and other risk factors exist such as bipolar family history, high-dose SRIs are not likely to be helpful. In these cases, OCD symptoms could be addressed directly with low- to medium-dose dopamine blockers by themselves or in addition to other agents that might be used for bipolar illness.

DEPRESSION

Despite the many controversies in child psychiatry related to ADD and mania, it has been overlooked that the most straightforward and common issue psychiatrically in children is depression. Most clinicians do not realize, as described in Chapter 18, that the whole concept of MDD was based on differences in the course of illness with bipolar subjects (in addition to genetic differences). Bipolar illness was supposed to begin earlier in life than unipolar depression, about age 20 in the former versus around age 30 in the latter. Furthermore, depressive episodes were brief and frequent in bipolar illness, and long and less frequent in unipolar depression. They lasted for a few weeks to a few months in bipolar illness, as opposed to six months or longer in unipolar depression.

It has become commonplace to diagnose children with MDD, in direct contradiction to the whole concept of MDD, which is not supposed to begin until the latter part of the second decade of life. Furthermore, these children are diagnosed with MDD even though they have brief depressive episodes lasting weeks to months at the longest, and they are often defined to have rapid-cycling illness, meaning multiple depressive episodes per year. This is the case despite the fact that, in the original research differentiating bipolar illness from MDD, rapid cycling was found to occur in about 25% of persons with bipolar illness, but was not reported to occur with MDD.

These studies were done mostly in the 1960s and 1970s, leading to the diagnostic definitions of MDD in DSM-III in 1980, which have not changed in any important fashion in the intervening four decades. The common diagnosis of MDD in children with brief and rapid episodes of depression leaves contemporary clinicians with two options: either this diagnosis of childhood depression is mistaken, or the DSM distinction between bipolar illness and MDD is mistaken. In either case, the diagnosis of childhood MDD is not a straightforward matter.

The idea that childhood-onset depression is not MDD, but reflects either bipolar illness or something related to bipolar illness, has been supported by studies in recent decades, which are consistent with the earlier studies in the 1960s and 1970s. These recent studies indicate, for instance, that 12-year-old children with depressive episodes but no manic or hypomanic episodes will eventually develop manic or hypomanic episodes with about 10 years of follow-up in about 40% of cases. This is a very high transition rate from apparent unipolar depression to bipolar illness. Other research on young adults finds that individuals with severe depression but no manic or hypomanic episodes diagnosed in their early 20s will develop manic or hypomanic episodes with about 15 years of follow-up in about one third of cases. In short, depressive episodes that occur in childhood, and into adolescence and young adulthood, really represent bipolar illness (meaning these patients will eventually develop manic or hypomanic episodes) in up to about one-half of cases.

This matter is important regarding the debate about childhood bipolar illness, because the controversy here is not whether or not the child is experiencing mania, but rather whether or not the child's depressive condition is occurring in the setting of bipolar illness. It might be said that even if one grants that about one-half of these children have bipolar illness, the other half would be said to have unipolar depression. Again, it is important to remember that the whole distinction between bipolar and unipolar depression involves differential courses of illness, as well as differential genetics. If the course of illness overlap so much that about one-half of patients possess a certain variety of illness and the other half has the other variety, then it seems to be difficult to claim that two illnesses are present as opposed to one; that is, manic depressive illness (MDI).

In addition to these considerations about age of onset, genetics are also an important diagnostic validator to bring into clinical valuation. A family history of bipolar illness is an important predictor of eventual bipolarity. In children with depression and a family history of bipolar disorder, serious consideration again should be given to the use of lithium or anticonvulsants, with or without dopamine blockers, as opposed to the routine prescription of monoamine agonist antidepressants.

MANIA

Most psychiatrists agree that bipolar disorder can be adequately diagnosed using standard adult criteria in adolescents. There is disagreement about whether it can be diagnosed in preadolescents. Available studies suggest that standard adult criteria are recognizable in adolescents. However, these adolescents demonstrate mainly mixed manic symptoms (about 80% of adolescents), rather than pure manic symptoms (about 40% of adults). Like adults, adolescents can demonstrate periods of wellness in between periods of mood episodes. Since the manic phase is of the mixed varieties, bipolar adolescents are predominantly depressed. They are depressed during their major depressive episodes, which can be lengthy, and they are depressed during their mixed episodes. To detect the difference, the clinician needs to rely on assessments of energy and other behaviors. In mixed episodes, bipolar adolescents are "wired," agitated, demonstrate decreased need for sleep, and are "hyperactive." In pure major depressive states, they have low energy and are tired. The primary behavioral manifestations of mania in adolescence are sexual excesses or impulsivity with drugs or alcohol.

Preadolescents, in contrast, often do not demonstrate the adult criteria for a manic episode. They do express symptoms of depression, but manic symptoms mainly reflect the classic psychopathological concept of psychomotor excitation: anger, mood lability, agitation, hyperactivity, and violent or destructive behavior. Rapid-cycling course, meaning multiple episodes in a year, is common. Since preadolescent children do not generally engage in sexual behavior, they are not able to express the sexual behavioral symptoms of mania, and, like adolescents, they are of course unable to express the adult-related work, spending, and travel symptoms. Thus the only behavioral symptoms of note might be non-specific hyperactivity and aggression, which are often misdiagnosed as the claimed "hyperactivity" of ADHD.

In recent years, there has been great controversy about this diagnosis in children, and the majority of child psychiatrists appear to refuse to make this diagnosis in the preadolescent age group. This anti-bipolar approach is especially prevalent in Australia and the United Kingdom, and many parts of the United States.

It could be argued that this overly intense controversy is based on excessive reliance on symptoms for diagnosis. As noted in Chapter 16, symptoms are only one of four criteria for diagnostic validity, the others being genetics, course, and treatment response. It is reasonable to assess a preadolescent child for excitatory symptoms, and then to proceed to the other three criteria to attempt to differentiate incipient bipolar illness from other conditions. The first, and perhaps most important, criterion to address, after identifying the excited clinical picture, is the family history. If a family history of bipolar illness is present, especially in parents or siblings, then the likelihood of bipolar illness in the depressive or excited preadolescent child is high.

Academics can engage in these controversies for entire careers. But clinicians and patients need to make decisions. Even if one is not convinced fully of a diagnosis of bipolar illness, it seems unreasonable to refuse to try a mood stabilizer under any circumstances. Frequently, such patients receive SRIs and amphetamines repeatedly and over years. Yet a single second-messenger modifier is not tried. Furthermore, if tried, lithium or anticonvulsants are almost always added to amphetamines or antidepressants, which would counteract the benefits of the mood stabilizing agents, as discussed in Chapter 18. Therefore, it is important to try second-messenger modifiers without antidepressants or amphetamines. In other words, the latter agents need to be stopped. Many clinicians are unwilling to take this approach. Patients and clinicians could consider at least taking a pragmatic approach, such that if multiple SRIs and amphetamines have failed to help a child, then perhaps at least one trial of a mood-stabilizing agent, without amphetamines and SRIs, would be warranted. If it succeeded, all the better. If it failed, then clinicians could return to the attitude of not using mood-stabilizing agents.

If used, low-dose second-messenger modifiers could be given as follows: lithium 300–600 mg per day, divalproex 500–750 mg per day, carbamazepine at standard doses of about 600 mg per day. Lamotrigine could also be given at standard doses, but should preferably be given only in settings where manic symptoms are not predominant. Furthermore, there is increased risk of Stevens-Johnson syndrome in children compared to adults, and thus lamotrigine would not be the preferred first-line mood-stabilizing agent of choice. This textbook recommends lithium first, followed by divalproex, followed by lamotrigine and carbamazepine in the treatment of manic symptoms or states in children and adolescents. Of course, dopamine blockers could also be used, but mainly as adjuncts to the second-messenger modifiers. Among these, low-dose risperidone and aripiprazole probably have the most benefit with the least side effects. Again, agents that cause marked weight gain and metabolic syndrome, like olanzapine and quetiapine, would be avoided in most cases.

The use of low doses should be emphasized, because many clinicians are very reluctant to use lithium or other mood-stabilizing agents because of their fears of toxicity. These fears are relatively unfounded, because the main medical risks of lithium, such as chronic renal insufficiency, occur in the long term, meaning over two decades or so. In the case of children with marked psychomotor excitation, treatment may not last longer than weeks to months, thus long-term concerns are irrelevant until one reaches the long term. Besides this logic, the concerns of clinicians regarding toxicity should be lessened if it were understood that low doses of lithium or divalproex could be effective enough in many children with manic or mixed states. The insistence on "therapeutic" standard levels of lithium and divalproex in children is misplaced. Those levels are based on studies of adults in severe acute mania. They may not be relevant for depressive or prophylaxis indications, and they may be less relevant in children and older persons. As stated in Chapter 11, clinicians should treat to clinical effect, not blood levels. Therefore, they should begin with low doses of lithium and divalproex in children and adolescents, and they will find that many of those patients will improve. In those who do not, clinicians can increase the dose to standard levels that are believed to be therapeutic in adults with acute mania.

PRODROMAL SCHIZOPHRENIA

Recent years have seen increasing interest in identifying prodromal schizophrenia and potentially preventing full-blown, severe onset of that chronic illness. That research identified adolescents in particular who appeared to have early-onset brief or attenuated psychotic symptoms, and often had a family history of schizophrenia. There have been three randomized trials of low-dose dopamine blockers for prodromal psychosis with the outcome of eventual full psychotic illness. Two studies were with risperidone, and one with olanzapine, with benefits seen more in the olanzapine study. Several studies have looked at cognitive behavioral therapy for prodromal psychosis, with reported benefit compared to non-treatment. Another study found that treatment with omega-3 fatty acids in those adolescents identified with prodromal schizophrenia led to improved longer-term outcomes versus untreated patients. A follow-up study on omega-3 fatty acids compared to intensive cognitive-behavioral case management failed to find a difference between the groups, which may be due to the benefit of the psychosocial intervention, making it difficult to see a difference. Given these studies, though, interventions that are rather benign such as long-term treatment with omega-3 fatty acids, or interventions that are limited in risk, such as low-dose dopamine blockers (such as risperidone 0.5–2.0 mg per day), could be reasonably considered in high-risk adolescents with prodromal schizophrenia-like symptoms. The growing interest in prodromal psychosis led to a movement to consider adding the diagnosis of prodromal schizophrenia to DSM-5, but this addition was rejected by many who oppose new diagnoses, and eventually did not enter the main body of DSM-5.

AUTISM

Autism is another important presentation in children. Sometimes it can reflect prodromal negative symptoms of later schizophrenia. Usually it is thought to reflect neurological abnormalities of unclear etiology leading to a lack of social connection as a primary pathology, often associated with later behavioral problems. Treatment remains symptomatic, with the limited benefits seen with all agents in purely symptomatic treatment. Given some harms with all psychotropic medications, the risk–benefit ratio of such symptomatic treatment needs to be assessed carefully by clinicians and patients. Psychosocial interventions at present are likely to be the most important approaches to ameliorating the effects of this condition during development in childhood.

THE USE OF AMPHETAMINES IN ADD: AN EXAMINATION OF THE MTA STUDY

In discussing amphetamine treatment of ADD, it is worthwhile to examine in detail a classic NIMH-funded study that is the longest and largest randomized trial of the efficacy of amphetamines in childhood ADD: the Multimodal Treatment of ADHD (MTA) Study. It is cited widely as showing more benefit with those medications than with psychosocial interventions. In fact, this is not the case for functional outcomes. Moreover, the study provides important safety data that contradict other widely held beliefs; namely, it shows that substance abuse rates do not decline with amphetamine treatment of ADD; furthermore, it provides evidence for a harmful effect of shortened height as a side effect of this medication class in growing children.

Children aged 7–10 with ADD were recruited (mean age 8.5 years, total sample = 579). They were double-blind randomized to one of four arms of treatment: medication (73% methylphenidate, 27% other amphetamines), intensive behavioral management, both, or neither ("standard community care"). Average dose of methylphenidate was 30.5 mg/d. It was well tolerated, with 86% of children having no or mild side effects.

At the end of 14 months of double-blind treatment, the children who received methylphenidate were almost one inch shorter than those who did not receive it (4.25 vs 6.19 cm difference, equal to 0.76 inch difference). In a range of 19 outcomes, benefits were seen in 10 outcomes. ADD symptoms improved more with medications than with behavioral management. Both treatment groups did better in most cases than standard community care.

However, *functional improvement was not statistically significantly different between medications and behavioral management.* These functions included: academic achievement, oppositional/aggressive behaviors, social skills, and parent/child relations.

This is a key finding: in the longest randomized trial of amphetamines versus behavioral management, it is NOT true that amphetamines were more effective for functional outcomes. It is true that amphetamines were more effective for symptoms of ADD: namely, children were felt or were observed to be more attentive and less agitated.

But when it comes to whether they did better in school, or had better social relationships at school or home, behavioral interventions were just as good as medications, and better than standard community care.

The importance of this matter is that one often hears statements by ADD experts to the effect that the MTA study showed that amphetamines were superior to psychosocial interventions in general. This is not true as stated. For functional outcomes, which is a key rationale for prescribing, amphetamines were *not* more effective than behavioral interventions.

After the one-year randomized study, patients were allowed to receive whatever treatment they or their clinicians wanted, in an open, unblended, non-randomized manner, for two more years. Now keep in mind that at the two- and three-year outcomes, the results are no longer randomized, thus there is possibility of "confounding bias," which means that others factors may influence results besides the treatment given (this is the whole point of randomization: to control for other confounding factors such that the randomized arms can be seen as causal in their effects on outcomes; see Chapter 5). Nonetheless, despite needing to think about confounding factors, two- and three-year outcomes provide important information on the long-term efficacy and safety of amphetamines versus behavioral interventions for ADD.

At three years' follow-up, with subjects now at a mean of about 12 years old (mean, 11.9 years), all groups showed similar improvement. In other words, the amphetamine group no longer was better than other groups for symptoms, nor were medication and behavioral intervention arms more effective than community care for functional outcomes. All groups had similar outcomes. Now the authors went to great lengths to keep you from drawing the wrong inference that medications are ineffective. They wrote: "It would be incorrect to conclude from these results that treatment makes no difference or is not worth pursuing." They are right, because of confounding bias; the results are no longer randomized, anyone can get any treatment they wish, which means that some of the non-medication arm subjects would now be receiving medications, and some of the medication arm subjects would now be receiving behavioral interventions. It is worthwhile noting exactly how this played out.

In the behavioral arm, where patients initially were randomized only to behavioral interventions, and zero amphetamine use, three-year outcome found that 45% of patients had begun to receive amphetamines, added to their behavioral interventions.

In the combination arm, where 100% of subjects were randomized to receive amphetamines plus behavioral management, three-year outcome found that medication use had decreased to 71% of patients. In the standard community care arm, where doctors could do whatever they wanted, medication use stayed stable at three years (going from 60% to 62%).

What do these results mean? One way of looking at it is that in all treatment arms, medication use stabilized out at about 1/2–2/3 of subjects. In other words, patients and doctors judged that medications were needed and helpful in many, but not all, patients.

Another way of looking at these results involves focusing on the behavioral intervention arm. Three-year outcomes suggest that if one tries to provide good behavioral intervention to patients, without any amphetamines at all, only about one-half of ADD children will eventually need medications. To put it another way, one can avoid the need to use amphetamines at all, even for the long-term, in one-half of children, if adequate behavioral interventions are provided.

What about side effects at three years? The MTA results are usually interpreted as good news, because the 0.75-inch growth impairment plateaued at three years; there was no further difference in height between medication and non-medication groups. The authors and many experts often cite these data to assert that we need not worry about shortened height as a long-term risk with amphetamines.

But this conclusion is inconsistent. If the results cannot be interpreted as showing lack of efficacy with medications (since all groups had similar outcomes at three years), they also cannot be interpreted as showing lack of harm with medications (since all groups had similar height changes at three years). Put differently, the results do *not* show that there is no height risk; they simply are uninformative since the three-year results are non-randomized and there is similar medication use in all four groups, thus one can no longer draw causal inferences about medication effects between groups.

All one can say is that when assessed during randomized treatment, amphetamines shorten height by almost one inch per year. One cannot know if this effect persists or goes away after multiple years.

There is another two- to three-year analysis that deserves more attention than it receives: the effect of amphetamine prescription on substance abuse. It is commonly stated, based on observational data, that amphetamine prescription leads to *less* substance abuse in persons with ADD. But observational data are non-randomized data, and non-randomized data are prone to confounding bias, as discussed. Therefore, one cannot draw causal inferences. If, in adolescents with ADD, those who received amphetamines had less substance abuse than those who didn't receive amphetamines, it may have been because clinicians gave amphetamines mainly to those who didn't have evidence of substance abuse. The causal link can go in any direction. Only randomization can allow causal assertions in a simple manner.

The MTA study is useful in this regard again, because it is the longest randomized trial of amphetamines. Its non-randomized outcomes at two and three years are more dependable than most studies', since they follow up on an initial randomized period of treatment of one year, which is much better than studies that are purely observational from the get-go.

With that context, let's ask what happened in MTA with substance abuse. At one year, in the pure randomized follow-up period, there was no difference in substance abuse rates between amphetamine-treated children and those treated with behavioral interventions. In other words, the most definitive interpretation is that amphetamines were neutral. They did not worsen substance abuse rates, but they also *did not improve* substance abuse rates, contrary to common claims. At three years of follow-up, again there were no differences between the groups, but this doesn't mean that there was no risk, for the same reasons given previously regarding similarities in efficacy and height at three years. At two years of follow-up, there was *more* substance abuse in amphetamine-treated children than in non–amphetamine-treated children. This finding in the MTA study contradicts the common claim that amphetamines reduce substance abuse. In fact, using the best data on the topic, which is the MTA study, the most objective interpretation of these data is that amphetamines do not reduce the risk of substance abuse. They may have no effect, or they may *increase* risk, but there is no evidence in this study that they decrease risk of substance abuse.

BOTTOM LINE

- The MTA study is the longest randomized trial of amphetamines in childhood ADD, with a one-year randomized period, and two more years of non-randomized outcomes.
- The main finding, contrary to the emphasis of its authors and experts, is that amphetamines are NOT more effective than behavioral interventions for functional outcomes in ADD, such as academic achievement and social relationships.
- Amphetamines were shown to shorten height by about 3/4 inch in one year.
- Substance abuse was not decreased with amphetamine treatment, and was increased at two-year outcomes.
- If behavioral management is given, medications can be avoided entirely in almost one-half of children for the long term.

SELECTED REFERENCES

Ghaemi, S. N., Martin, A. (2007). Defining the boundaries of childhood bipolar disorder. *American Journal of Psychiatry*, 164: 185–188.

Jensen, P. S., et al. (1999). Multimodal treatment of children with ADHD. *Archives of General Psychiatry, 56*, 1073–1086.

McGorry, P. D., et al. (2017). Effect of ω-3 polyunsaturated fatty acids in young people at ultrahigh risk for psychotic disorders. The NEURAPRO Randomized Clinical Trial. *JAMA Psychiatry, 74*(1), 19–27.

Woodberry, K. A., et al. (2016). Progress and future directions in research on the psychosis prodrome: A review for clinicians. *Harvard Review of Psychiatry, 24*(2), 87–103

29

Older Persons

In the older patient population, some special considerations are entailed for clinical psychopharmacology. This age group can be defined as persons at age 70 and above, although some of these principles may apply to individuals in their 60s or even their 50s, if they are medically compromised or otherwise fragile physiologically. In treating older persons, these principles are relevant to the use of psychotropic medications, based on some basic facts about aging:

1. Physiological changes lead to pharmacokinetics effects, such that doses of medications should generally be halved;
2. These pharmacokinetic changes also lead to the need to dose medications about half as frequently;
3. Normal aging related changes in bodily organs are such that potentially dangerous medical harms from medications notably increase in older persons.

In sum, the use of psychotropic medications in older persons should be at much lower dose, shorter duration, and decreased frequency than in young or middle-aged adults (Table 29.1). In this chapter, the background to these recommendations, and specific details related to drug classes, will be discussed.

PHARMACOKINETICS

As discussed in Chapter 2, the pharmacokinetics of medications are influenced primarily by the kidney and liver. Kidney function declines with age. One rule of thumb is that renal excretion is decreased by about 1% per year after age 40. It is estimated that about two-thirds of older persons have 50% or more decreased renal excretion than younger age groups. In other words, when a medication is dosed in such older persons, twice as much of it stays in the body as is the case with younger persons. This is one rationale why in general, dosing of medications in older persons should be about one-half of the dosing used

TABLE 29.1 Psychotropic Medications in Older Persons

	Advantages	Disadvantages	Comments
Second-messenger modifiers	Useful for prevention of mood episodes.	Lithium toxicity more common. Drug interactions with carbamazepine problematic. Divalproex causes cortical atrophy.	Lamotrigine probably most tolerable.
Dopamine blockers	Useful for management of acute mania and agitation.	Probably not effective long-term in monotherapy. Clozapine and olanzapine have metabolic risks. Quetiapine associated with notable sedation and risk of falls. Risperidone associated with possible stroke. More EPS in the elderly. QTC prolongation with ziprasidone and iloperidone.	Aripiprazole and other newer agents most tolerable.
Monoamine agonists	May be helpful for acute depressive and anxiety symptoms.	Numerous cardiac risks with most agents in this population. Many agents have drug interactions.	None are benign.

in younger persons. Furthermore, hepatic metabolic function decreases somewhat with age, such that it has been estimated that hepatic metabolism of drugs via the cytochrome P450 enzyme system is decreased by about 30–40% in older persons. Keep in mind that all of these changes are part of normal aging. Therefore, there will be no abnormalities in kidney or liver function tests. The serum creatinine will be normal, as will hepatic function tests. These tests are normal because there is a great redundancy in kidney and liver anatomy and physiology. In other words, the body is supplied with many more kidney and liver cells that it needs to function with normal health. Even though kidney cells are dying gradually over time, such that by the eighth or ninth decade of life, over half of one's kidney cells may be nonfunctioning, the other half of those cells are sufficient to provide adequate function such that overall bodily health remains normal. More sensitive testing of kidney and liver function will show the decline described here, but again, this is part of normal aging and does not lead to toxic or harmful consequences in the body under normal circumstances. These changes are relevant to clinicians who are prescribing medications, though, in terms of adjusting dose and duration of treatment downwards, so as to maintain medication use in the established safe range.

THE BLOOD–BRAIN BARRIER

The blood–brain barrier becomes more porous with normal aging. This means that substances can diffuse from the bloodstream into the central nervous system (CNS) more easily as one ages. Normally, the blood–brain barrier consists of membranes and protein pumps which protect cerebrospinal fluid (CSF) from the range of substances that may enter the bloodstream. For instance, there is a sodium potassium pump that functions to pump lithium out of the CSF and back into the bloodstream. Thus, the reason why it is said that the therapeutic level of lithium is 0.8 is because this is the therapeutic serum level in the bloodstream. It takes a level of 0.8 in the serum in young and middle-aged persons for a level of 0.4 to be achieved in the CSF and thus inside the brain. The blood–brain barrier combats the ability of lithium to diffuse from the bloodstream into the CSF, and pumps about half of the lithium back into the bloodstream, allowing one-half into the CSF. In older persons, the ratio of lithium in the serum to the CSF is about 1:1. So a serum level of 0.8 in older persons will produce a CSF level of same amount. In contrast, in younger persons, a serum level of 1.6, which would be considered toxic, would be required to obtain a CSF level of 0.8. Thus a serum lithium level of 0.8 in older persons is toxic.

These age-related changes are not taken into account in laboratory value ranges given in test results. Hence, clinicians cannot rely on laboratory ranges sent to them in test results marked as normal or abnormal, based on the usual ranges supplied, since those ranges are based on persons in the middle range of age in the lifespan. In other words, those laboratory results apply to individuals generally speaking between the ages of 20 and 60. They do not apply to children or older persons. Clinicians need to adjust in their own minds for the correct serum levels for lithium in older persons. It is known that these normal age-related changes in the blood–brain barrier are increased in persons with neurological diseases, such as dementia. Some research suggests that changes in the blood–brain barrier in normal aging begin in the hippocampal area, and are worse with mild cognitive impairment.

SENSITIVITY TO MEDICAL HARM

The major organs of the body gradually decline in function in normal aging. Again as noted above, this decline in function is such that it does not typically lead to clinical symptoms or problems in the healthy aging individual. When medications are prescribed, however, these changes of normal aging need to be taken into account. Besides the liver and kidney changes mentioned before, other organs such as the heart and lungs can be increasingly sensitive to medications during the aging process. Some psychotropic medications can be associated with occasional liver effects, for example, such as carbamazepine or divalproex, yet those hepatic effects are infrequent and reversible in younger and middle-aged persons. By the decade of the 50s or later, however, the same persons who may have tolerated those medications without hepatic problems could then develop more notable hepatic side effects, including not only elevated liver enzymes, but also frank clinical hepatitis, sometimes severe enough to require hospitalization. For this reason, this textbook recommends using carbamazepine, for instance, in younger persons mainly, and not routinely above the age of 55.

Similarly, the heart may be more sensitive to side effects associated with certain medications that may be less frequent in younger persons. For example, methylphenidate and other amphetamines are associated with some risk of cardiac arrhythmias. This concern has been discussed and studied mostly in children, because these agents have tended to be used for attention deficit disorder (ADD) in the past primarily in children. Now that these agents are used increasingly in adult ADD, researchers have begun to assess cardiac side effects in the adult and older population as well. One recent study found less risk of cardiac side effects with methylphenidate in children as opposed to adults. In the adult population in the study, which was a middle-aged population, the risk of sudden cardiac death associated with methylphenidate was almost double. A systematic review of about a dozen studies on this topic confirmed more risks in adults than in children.

These basic principles can be applied now to specific drug classes and the use of psychotropic medications for various clinical conditions.

DEPRESSIVE STATES

First-episode depression can occur in persons older than age 60, representing a second peak of incidence (the first occurring around age 30). It used to be thought that any mood episodes occurring for the first time after age 40 are primarily secondary to underlying medical illness. It is true that such a course should engender careful examination of potential medical etiologies. In the past, some centers used to test all new mood disorder patients of any age with an MRI of the head, a sleep-deprived electroencephalogram (EEG), and neuropsychological testing. While economic factors have led to less testing in younger patients who develop primary mood disorders in their 20s and 30s, it is still reasonable to conduct such testing where feasible, especially in new-onset mood disorders after age 40.

When depression begins in middle-aged or older persons, the clinical investigation should assess whether the cause of such depression has to do with brain based abnormalities in relation to vascular depression, or whether that depression is secondary to psychosocial influences. It is often thought that such depressive episodes may accompany the losses of aging associated with grief for the deaths of family and friends, physical impairment in daily activities, loss of work-related satisfaction, and isolation. In this setting, psychotherapies, especially of the supportive kind, would make sense.

Concurrent medical illnesses, especially cardiac and oncological diseases, are also highly associated with depression. It can be unclear whether depressive symptoms are causes or effects in relation to these medical illnesses, but even if depression is the effect of medical illness, it appears the depressive symptoms worsen outcomes of many medical illnesses. For example, it has been shown that patients have more cardiovascular morbidity and mortality if they have depressive symptoms than if they do not, corrected for other cardiac risk factors such as lipid levels and hypertension and diabetes. In other words, it is clear that depressive symptoms themselves are harmful medically. Unfortunately, as discussed later, attempts to improve those depressive symptoms with antidepressant medications have not led to clear evidence of improvement in medical outcomes.

Another important scenario is late-onset depression in the setting of long-standing affective temperaments; i.e., cyclothymia, hyperthymia, or dysthymia. In these persons, 40, 50, 60, or more years can pass with constant mild depressive symptoms as part of the baseline personality of the individual. Then in middle age or later years, a first severe depressive episode occurs. In this setting, the apparent late-life new-onset of depression is in fact the evolution of a mild depressive or manic temperament into a later full-blown depressive episode. In other words, the actual age of onset of the affective illness is not the first depressive episode, but the beginning of the affective temperament, which usually dates back to childhood. It is important to note that late-onset depression often happens after lifelong mild manic temperaments like hyperthymia or cyclothymia, not just after lifelong mild depressive symptoms of dysthymia.

Cases have been observed of first-episode mania at age 85 years, with normal brain MRI and no medical cause, in a person with lifelong hyperthymia who had been a very wealthy, successful business man for decades.

More commonly, the presentation involves first-episode depression at or around retirement, in a highly successful person, with normal brain MRI and medical workup. Depression is attributed to psychosocial causation due to retirement, but preexisting cyclothymia or hyperthymia could be an important factor in the predisposition to depression after retirement in one person, while another retires happily. Further discussion of affective temperaments and their treatment is provided in Chapter 19.

VASCULAR DEPRESSION

Perhaps the most important cause of new-onset depression in middle-aged and older persons is vascular depression. This concept is relatively new and only beginning to be explored and understood, but it is increasingly important. "Vascular depression" is defined as depressive symptoms or episodes beginning in the fourth or fifth decade of life or later, without prior history of depression. These depressive symptoms or episodes are associated with white matter abnormalities in the brain, which consist of small microvascular strokes, reflecting cerebral hypertension. Typical risk factors are preexisting hypertension and/or diabetes and/or vascular disease. It is important to note that cerebral vascular hypertension may be present in the absence of generalized hypertension. In other words, it could be that the small blood vessels of the brain may suffer from elevated blood pressure, leading to closing of the blood vessels and consequent neuronal death in the regions around those small blood vessels. This process could occur only in small blood vessels deep in the brain, leading to white matter abnormalities, and not occur in the large blood vessels in the brain typically associated with more severe stroke symptoms such as the carotid artery. Furthermore, the small vascular changes may occur in the brain without elevated blood pressure in the vasculature in the rest of the body, such as in the brachial artery, where the diagnosis of hypertension is assessed. Hence, it could be the case that a patient could have vascular depression with white matter abnormalities in the brain due to cerebrovascular hypertension and yet not be diagnosable with hypertension in the brachial artery; most clinicians would not diagnose that patient or treat that patient with antihypertensive agents. Diabetes is an important risk factor because it is specifically associated with small vessel disease, which would increase the risk of white matter abnormalities in the brain. Occasionally, white matter abnormalities in the brain will be noted in individuals with depression who do not have any of these risk factors. In fact, white matter abnormalities can be found in the brain and some persons who do not have depression at all. This is why radiologists and neurologists tend to see white matter abnormalities as variants of normal unless there is clinical evidence of any other illness. When patients have depression, though, white matter abnormalities should be seen as associated with the observed clinical syndrome of depression. It's also relevant that white matter abnormalities in the brain are associated with increased risk of dementia; i.e., vascular dementia. The mechanisms for this risk could include both the direct effect of depression as well as the effect of cerebrovascular small vessel disease.

There are very few studies assessing the treatment of vascular depression, but the general clinical consensus is that vascular depression is associated with a poor prognosis. Monoamine agonists appear to be less effective in vascular depression than in non-vascular depression. Given the pathophysiology of underlying cerebrovascular hypertension, it would appear to make sense that aggressive antihypertensive treatment could slow the progress of vascular depression, and/or prevent future worsening of it, and/or augment any potential benefit with monoamine agonists. If patients are diagnosed with hypertension and are taking antihypertensives already, it makes sense for clinicians to increase the antihypertensive dose as tolerated to achieve blood pressure readings that are as low as acceptable in the body, in the hope that levels will decrease in the brain sufficiently. This aggressive antihypertensive treatment may help vascular depression, although there are no studies of this topic yet. In patients who do not have a prior diagnosis of hypertension, and do not have generalized hypertension as measured by the brachial artery, the treatment of vascular depression with antihypertensive agents might still make sense physiologically, although again, there are no studies, and many clinicians probably would tend to avoid using antihypertensive agents outside of the standard clinical indication for generalized hypertension. Until studies are conducted on this very important topic, this textbook raises this idea as an option for clinicians and patients to consider.

MONOAMINE AGONISTS AND ANTIDEPRESSANTS

When using monoamine agonists in older persons, clinicians should pay attention to the pharmacokinetic principles described previously. These medications should be given in general at about half the dose and half the frequency given in younger persons. Medications with very long half-lives, like fluoxetine, should be avoided. Due to the need to take medications for other medical illnesses, psychotropic medications that have many drug interactions should be avoided also. These agents would include fluoxetine, paroxetine, and fluvoxamine. Given the sensitivity of the brain as part of the aging process, older persons are more sensitive to cognitive side effects of medications, like sedation. Thus medications that are sedating and have anticholinergic effects, which can cause impaired cognition, should be avoided; these include mirtazapine, venlafaxine, paroxetine, and TCAs. The medications that affect specific organs in potentially harmful ways are concerning, such as TCAs, which can cause cardiac arrhythmias; venlafaxine, which also can cause sudden cardiac death; or citalopram, which has been found to be associated with cardiac arrhythmias as well. It is important to note that bupropion, which has been considered safe in older persons, is an amphetamine in its pharmacological structure. Since amphetamines are associated with cardiac arrhythmias, with increasing risk as one ages, it is probably wise to avoid bupropion in older persons as well. This caution also applies to amphetamines in general, which many clinicians view as safe in older persons. Given the cardiac risks with these agents, it would seem rational to view these agents as relatively unsafe in older persons.

It also is notable that all SRIs increase the risk of osteoporosis (and thus fractures) and cause some thinning of the blood (and hence bleeding risk). Furthermore, some of these agents increase carcinogenicity risks in animals, as discussed in Chapter 25, with some human epidemiological studies also raising the possibility of increased cancer rates.

When going through each agent and its specific risks, a consensus has evolved that sertraline may be a first-line SRI in older persons, especially in the setting of cardiovascular disease. However, as discussed in Chapter 32, the Sertraline Against Depression and Heart Disease in Congestive Heart Failure (SADHART) study of that agent in cardiovascular disease is not as benign as it has been interpreted, with evidence of doubled stroke risk and slightly more cardiovascular mortality with sertraline than with placebo. Given all of these concerns, SRIs and other monoamine agonists cannot be seen as benign in older persons.

MANIC STATES

Usually, mania in older persons occurs in those with long-standing bipolar illness (though sometimes not previously diagnosed, or misdiagnosed in the past as unipolar depression). Sometimes, new late-onset manic episodes occur secondary to underlying etiologies such as thalamic stroke or white matter infarcts.

As described previously, life-long affective temperaments, usually cyclothymia or hyperthymia, predispose to later mood episodes, not only depression but also mania. After decades of mild manic symptoms as their baseline personality, a person can develop a first full manic episode in middle age or in late decades of life. Medical workup will be negative, and hospitalization even can occur.

Whatever the etiology, as with younger persons, the treatment of bipolar illness should include a standard proven second-messenger modifier, such as lithium, divalproex, carbamazepine, or lamotrigine. Choosing among these agents is somewhat more complex, though, in older persons, as described in the following section.

SECOND-MESSENGER MODIFIERS

As described before in relation to the blood–brain barrier, special care should be taken in the use of lithium in older persons. Declining renal function also is important. Both of these factors make older persons especially sensitive to lithium and prone to lithium toxicity. For these reasons, it is best to avoid lithium in older persons, or to use it in low doses and levels.

It bears repeating that the older patient requires much lower serum lithium levels in the blood to achieve the same CNS lithium levels that are obtained only with higher serum lithium levels in younger persons. So a serum lithium level of 0.4 in an older person is basically therapeutic and similar in effect to a serum lithium level of 0.8 in a younger adult. As a corollary, a serum lithium level of 0.8 in an older adult can be toxic, equivalent to almost twice that level in a younger adult. Unfortunately, many clinicians are fooled by standardized laboratory ranges that report "therapeutic" levels often in the 0.6–1.2 range, which is incorrect for older persons. If lithium is used in older persons, it should usually be used at "low" levels, which are in fact therapeutic levels.

In contrast, divalproex levels appears to be largely the same in older as younger persons. Divalproex is therefore in some ways safer, with its wider therapeutic dose range leading to fewer medical complications in older persons than often occurs with lithium. Unfortunately, divalproex is associated with cortical atrophy in older persons, based on a study of mild cognitive impairment. Animal data also indicate that divalproex has some neurotoxic effects. Hence, while it may be safer for many organs in the body, and less risky regarding toxicity than lithium, divalproex is more harmful to the brain than lithium and other options. Carbamazepine is usually not helpful due to its many drug interactions, given the need for polypharmacy for multiple medical conditions in most older persons. Many clinicians use oxcarbazepine as an alternative to carbamazepine, given its lack of drug interactions, but as discussed in Chapter 19, it is not an effective agent for bipolar illness. Risks of hyponatremia still need to be monitored with that agent as well.

Given these considerations, lamotrigine can be seen as, in general, the safest mood stabilizing agent for older persons. As with younger people, the risk of rash and Stevens-Johnson syndrome exists and should be taken into account. Assuming an older patient does not have drug allergies or other special risk factors, though, lamotrigine would have few risks overall. The main problem is that lamotrigine is not very effective for patients who have many manic episodes, or severe manic symptoms. In these patients, in older age, lamotrigine's safety may be irrelevant, since it may not be effective. For these patients with manic morbidity, divalproex probably would be the agent in which benefits exceed harms most appreciably.

ANXIETY STATES

As with younger persons, anxiety occurs in older individuals usually as an effect of some other cause, rather than as a cause itself. Bipolar illness and unipolar depression can both lead to marked anxiety as part of those mood states, and affective temperaments like hyperthymia or cyclothymia can be associated with concomitant anxiety as a constant or baseline state. Besides these scenarios, some individuals who may have high neuroticism as a personality trait will continue to have notable anxiety into older age. In some persons, anxiety seems to begin or worsen in the older decades of life. It is possible that brain aging can make such persons more vulnerable to anxiety. As with younger persons, the best intervention is to treat the underlying cause, which typically involves treating the underlying mood illness. Where there is no mood illness or affective temperament, then the decision clinically again becomes one of weighing risks and benefits of purely symptomatic treatment with benzodiazepines or low-dose SRIs. In younger persons, there may be more benefit to benzodiazepines in the sense that the long-term withdrawal syndrome risks may be worse with SRIs, and in the setting of bipolar illness, benzodiazepines would not worsen that illness, unlike SRIs. These considerations apply to younger persons without substance abuse histories. In older persons, the use of benzodiazepines can be much more complicated, due to an increased potential for delirium, as described later, as well as an increased risk of falls. It also is not straightforward to use low-dose SRIs in older persons, given the many medical and cardiovascular risks associated with the majority of these agents, as discussed.

DEMENTIA AND DELIRIUM

Perhaps the most common presentation of psychiatric symptoms in older persons has nothing to do with primary psychiatric illnesses, like mood or anxiety states, but rather relates to delirium and/or dementia. Delirium occurs in individuals who have some susceptibility to disorientation. In the aging brain, due to loss of neurons, insults to the brain can lead to disorientation. These can be medical insults, such as hypoxia, or they can be external insults such as the effects of prescribed medications. Among psychotropic medications, the types of effects that produce delirium are anticholinergic, antihistaminic, and antiadrenergic effects. Therefore, medications that have these effects, like olanzapine or mirtazapine, can cause delirium. Benzodiazepines also can cause delirium, due to their GABAergic effects. It is common to have milder cases of delirium in the outpatient setting, or in assisted living or nursing home contexts. In such cases, delirium may come and go at different times of the day, such as "sundowning" at night, and intermittent dopamine blocker treatment often is given. Other non-psychotropic medications that commonly cause delirium include opiate medications and steroids.

Dementia frequently is associated with behavioral agitation. Sometimes this agitation involves the occurrence of delirium on top of dementia. Sometimes the behavioral changes appear to be part of the dementing process. It is common for dopamine blockers to be used for these behavioral symptoms, as discussed in the following section.

DOPAMINE BLOCKERS

The usual treatment for delirium involves high-potency dopamine blockers, such as haloperidol or risperidone. Some clinicians use high doses of such agents, especially intravenously with haloperidol, in the hospital setting for very severe delirium. It is best to avoid agents with anticholinergic and antihistaminic effects, such as olanzapine and quetiapine. A dilemma can arise since older persons are also more sensitive to EPS, such as Parkinsonism and akathisia, which may be especially prevalent with high-potency dopamine blockers.

Certain specific cautions are in order. Risperidone has been associated with a possible increased risk of stroke in older persons, with an FDA black box warning to that effect; it is unclear to what extent this association is causal. Otherwise, low-dose risperidone is often well-tolerated for agitation. Quetiapine has notable antiadrenergic effects, which can lead to notable sedation and orthostatic hypotension. Given the major mortality risks associated with falls in older persons, this risk of orthostasis needs to be carefully considered and monitored. Low doses of aripiprazole or ziprasidone may be well tolerated. The lack of metabolic harms (increasing diabetes and cardiovascular risks) with ziprasidone and aripiprazole in particular, and newer dopamine blockers, may make them most useful.

Clinicians should also pay attention to the cardiovascular and diabetes risks of some dopamine blockers, especially so in this age group, given that cardiovascular morbidity and mortality as well as diabetes risks increase notably in older persons. Since the most common cause of death is cardiovascular disease, wherever feasible, clinicians should not add to that risk by prescribing dopamine blockers that cause cardiovascular harm, like clozapine, olanzapine, and quetiapine.

SELECTED REFERENCES

Downing, L. J., Caprio, T. V., & Lyness, J. M. (2013). Geriatric psychiatry review: Differential diagnosis and treatment of the 3 D's—delirium, dementia, and depression. *Current Psychiatry Reports, 15*, 365.

Klotz, U. (2009). Pharmacokinetics and drug metabolism in the elderly. *Drug Metabolism Reviews, 41*(2), 67–76.

Montagne, A., et al. (2015). Blood–brain barrier breakdown in the aging human hippocampus. *Neuron, 85*(2), 296–302.

Schelleman, H., et al. (2012). Methylphenidate and risk of serious cardiovascular events in adults. *American Journal of Psychiatry, 169*(2), 178–185.

Westover, A. N., & Halm, E. A. (2012). Do prescription stimulants increase the risk of adverse cardiovascular events? A systematic review. *BMC Cardiovascular Disorders, 12*, 41.

30

Women

USE OF PSYCHOTROPIC AGENTS IN WOMEN INVOLVES CERTAIN ASPECTS that are unique to the pathophysiology of women. This chapter will examine special issues for women, such as pregnancy, postpartum depression, menopause, menstrual cycles, and potential differential treatment effects.

PREGNANCY

Many experts recommend that most psychotropic medications can be continued during pregnancy. For instance, many SRIs and dopamine blockers are viewed as safe in pregnancy. However, this judgment of safety is based on immediate effects that can be observed during or soon after pregnancy is over; i.e., presence or absence of birth defects. This assessment does not tend to entail effects that can happen a few years after delivery. For instance, it has been found that some medications, like divalproex, can have long-term effects three to five years after birth, involving some evidence of low IQ or neurodevelopmental delay. Thus, the judgment of safety should be understood to be short-term only. Long-term safety is unknown for most psychotropic medications.

It is difficult also to draw causal conclusions about the safety or lack thereof of psychotropic medications during pregnancy since there are very few, if any, randomized trials of medications during pregnancy. Due to the special nature of pregnancy, most of the research on this topic is observational, and not randomized. Thus the potential problem of confounding bias exists with almost all research studies on pregnancy.

One of the questions raised during pregnancy has been the clinical lore that women during pregnancy have fewer psychiatric symptoms than before afterward. Some women report a sense of subjective well-being during pregnancy that is higher than their baseline. Some clinicians have judged that depression is less likely during pregnancy, due to this subjective improvement in mood. The theorized biological basis for this pregnancy effect has been that estrogen, which is thought to exert an antidepressant effect, is markedly increased during pregnancy. The clear clinical problem of postpartum depression is hypothesized to be related to the sharp decline in estrogen that happens at and after delivery.

This clinical opinion has been studied in some observational studies in which it has been found that relapse rates into depression during pregnancy do not appear to be notably different than relapse rates before or after pregnancy. These observational studies suggested that the clinical lore of enhanced well-being during pregnancy may not be the case, or at least may not protect against depressive relapse. This is one reason why some perinatal psychiatry experts recommend continuation of antidepressants during pregnancy on a routine basis.

It is important to divide pregnancy risks into the three major trimesters. During the first trimester, major organ formation occurs, and any harmful drug effects will lead to major organ malformations. These tend to be rather serious results such as anencephaly, or somewhat less serious but clear abnormalities such as Ebstein's anomaly, associated with lithium. Unless pregnancy is planned, it is usually the case that a woman will not realize she is pregnant until she is well into her first trimester. Thus, any medications can potentially have first-trimester effects, so it is difficult to fully prevent harm.

Most medications of concern in psychiatry have second-trimester effects. These include anticonvulsants and benzodiazepines, which can cause neural tube defects. During the second trimester, one of the major processes that occurs is brain development. During this trimester, there is migration of cortical neurons, for example, and general maturation of the brain. Other organs in the body have been fully formed, but final maturation of those organs tends to occur in second trimester. The only organs that are not fully developed until the third trimester are the lungs, and the third trimester is mostly devoted to lung maturation.

When considering the effects of psychotropic medications on fetal development, it is relevant to think about which trimester is being discussed and which effects could occur. Usually, the first trimester is already underway by the time pregnancy is discovered, and in the third trimester, there is no major organ effect that is important. Hence the main trimester of concern tends to be the second trimester. Since benzodiazepines and anticonvulsants are the main medications that have effects in the second trimester, these tend to be the medications that are stopped during pregnancy. It should be noted that the main anticonvulsants that have been associated with neural tube defects are divalproex and carbamazepine. It appears that lamotrigine does not have notable neural tube defects based on its pregnancy registry.

Looking at the major drug classes, the preceding considerations explain the usual recommendations that are given during pregnancy. Antidepressants tend to be continued, while anticonvulsants, except for lamotrigine, tend to be stopped, as are benzodiazepines. Lithium tends to be continued past the first trimester.

Regarding dopamine blockers, there is a great deal of experience with haloperidol and with some other older dopamine blockers such that many clinicians continue those agents during pregnancy. Many of the second-generation dopamine blockers have been studied in pregnancy registries, and generally are reported to be safe by their manufacturers. Again, however, this judgment of safety is observational and based on short-term effects only.

Many clinicians focus on FDA Category assignment given to different medications. It should be kept in mind that these Category assignments are based on poor outcomes reported to the FDA, which are purely observational and can be affected by many confounding factors, including non-reported cases. These category assignments are not the most valid measures of safety during pregnancy from a scientific perspective. Nonetheless, there may be at least medicolegal reasons to pay attention to some category assignments from the FDA regarding pregnancy.

The FDA categories are as follows: Category A refers to drugs thought to be safe with no known adverse effects. Category B refers to drugs that are not known to have any risks in humans. Category C refers to drugs for which there is insufficient research to be able to make a judgment regarding safety. Category D refers to adverse effects having been found in humans. In the American College of Obstetricians and Gynecologists (ACOG) guidelines on psychotropic drugs, benzodiazepines are listed as Category D. Other agents used for sleep, such as eszopiclone (Lunesta) and Zaleplon (Sonata), are listed as Category B, and zolpidem (Ambien) as Category C.

Divalproex and carbamazepine and lithium are all listed as Category D, while lamotrigine is listed as Category C. This categorization is not clinically accurate since lithium has many fewer risks than divalproex or carbamazepine.

All antidepressants are listed as Category C except for bupropion (Category B). All amphetamines, including methylphenidate and its variants, are listed as Category C. It is interesting that bupropion is an amphetamine but is listed as Category B. All dopamine blockers are listed as Category C except for clozapine (Category B).

What guidelines can be given to clinicians regarding decision-making about continuing or discontinuing psychotropic medications before, during, and after pregnancy, given these considerations? One approach would be to make decisions regarding continuation of psychotropic medications during pregnancy in reference to the natural history of the illness being treated. The most difficult decision-making scenarios would involve chronic severe illnesses, such as schizophrenia or epilepsy, in which complete discontinuation of medications would not seem to be a viable option. For other illnesses that are mild, but chronic, such as generalized anxiety or affective temperaments, it may be reasonable to come off medications during pregnancy, since symptoms are not naturally severe otherwise. For other illnesses that are severe, but episodic, like bipolar illness and recurrent unipolar depression, it may be reasonable to come off medications if the natural history of the illness would suggest that remission could persist for nine months or longer. This last scenario may be feasible if the affective illness is well treated, and the patient has been in remission for some time before a planned pregnancy. For example, suppose a woman with bipolar illness has been treated with divalproex for 10 years and has not had any mood episodes for the prior five years. If she has been completely stable for five years, it is unlikely that she will relapse into a mood episode immediately upon discontinuation of her divalproex. It is likely that she will have at least a few months or longer of natural remission. The natural history of the patient can inform the decision-making. Suppose in this case the patient had had three episodes of her lifetime, one at age 17, another at age 20, and a third at age 25. Now she is 30 years old, and considering pregnancy. Her natural history is such that she tends to go three years in remission before having an episode. Since she has been five years in remission, it is likely that discontinuation of divalproex will not lead to mood episode relapse in the following nine months of pregnancy. Therefore, she and her clinician could potentially make the judgment that it would be reasonable to come off divalproex a few months before planning a pregnancy, and continue to stay off of it throughout pregnancy as long as she does not have a relapse into a mood episode. A backup plan should be put into place such that other medications could be instituted should a mood episode occur. For instance, a dopamine blocker could be given if a manic episode were to occur, and an antidepressant could be given if a depressive episode should occur. In contrast, if a patient had rapid-cycling bipolar illness, and had mood episodes every two to three months, then discontinuation of divalproex or any other psychotropic medication would be likely to lead to a mood episode relapse during pregnancy. This fact would not necessarily mean that divalproex should be continued during pregnancy, given its clear risks, but the decision-making would at least be informed with a high probability of relapse should divalproex be stopped, and other effective medications not given.

In other words, the decision whether to continue or discontinue medication during pregnancy is a contextual one. There is no general rule that would absolutely prohibit or absolutely ordain the use of psychotropic medications during pregnancy. Some perinatal psychiatry experts contend that medications should be continued in the vast majority of cases during pregnancy, albeit using ones that have lower fetal risks, but the preceding considerations would suggest that this general rule need not apply, and that such decisions should be made contextually in relation to the natural history of the illness and the patient's specific response to medications prior to pregnancy.

If this approach were taken, the general perspective would be that, all other things being equal, it would be best to take as few medications as possible during pregnancy, and preferably none. This approach could be feasible in patients with milder and/or episodic psychiatric illnesses that are well controlled for a long period of time before pregnancy. It would not be recommended in patients with severe chronic psychiatric illnesses or with those with highly episodic or relatively uncontrolled symptomatology prior to pregnancy.

Another aspect that is relevant to possible psychotropic medication discontinuation before during pregnancy is the viewpoint that, if psychotropic medications are discontinued, then increase in anxiety or depressive symptoms or relapse into mood episodes or psychosis are harmful experiences not only for the mother, but also for the fetus. It is held that these psychopathological states lead to overactivation of the hypothalamic pituitary adrenal axis (HPA-axis) that results in increased steroid hormone production. Steroid hormones cross the blood–brain and placental barriers easily. They could then cause direct damage to the fetus, in various ways. The perspective here is that continuation of medication, even with a small amount of possible harm, outweighs the potential harm of psychopathological worsening of the underlying psychiatric illness, including its physiological effects via the HPA-axis. This perspective may be correct, but it does not obviate the approach of making decisions regarding possible medication discontinuation based on the natural history of the illness of the patient. Where there is a reasonable likelihood of natural remission lasting six months or longer, then the continuation of medications just may not be necessary. However, if there is a serious risk of relapse that is probable based on the natural history during the six-month to nine-month period of pregnancy, then the considerations given here would argue for continuation of medication treatment in some way to minimize the pathological harm of psychiatric illness relapse, not only for the mother, but also for the fetus.

If medications were discontinued just before pregnancy, it should be appreciated that a full nine months without medication use is not necessary. The most important trimesters are the first and second trimesters, as described. In women who might be in remission but in whom there is some risk of relapse that increases after six months, it may be reasonable to come off medication only during the first and second trimester and then to resume medications in the third trimester. Also, since the highest risk is postpartum, at least for the mother, then it is important to resume medications in the third trimester, or just before or at delivery, or just after delivery. This resumption of medication will be very important in terms of reduction of risk of postpartum depression, discussed further later.

The resumption of medications at delivery raises the question of breast-feeding. On this topic, there have been numerous studies assessing the extent to which psychotropic medications of various kinds cross the placental barrier or cross into milk and are transmitted to the baby. In general, researchers have suggested that an infant serum level 10% or higher than the mother's level could be a potential clinical concern. Another rule of thumb is that the smaller the molecule, the more likely it will be transmitted into milk. Lithium, which is an ion, crosses the milk barrier easily and is transmitted in notable amounts from the bloodstream of the mother into the milk supply of the baby. It is estimated that about one-half of the serum levels of lithium in the mother is transmitted into the breast milk and exposed to the baby. Medications that are highly plasma protein–bound do not tend to diffuse into the breast milk. For example, sertraline is 98% plasma protein–bound and does not transfer into the milk readily. Venlafaxine is much less plasma protein–bound and will diffuse into milk more easily. Other SRIs are generally reported to pass into the breast milk at low levels, and small studies of infants tend to report that there are no observable behavioral or clinical harmful effects of those SRIs. Carbamazepine is not highly plasma protein–bound, and is found in notable amounts in breast milk, but divalproex is highly plasma protein–bound and is found at low amounts in breast milk. Traditional dopamine blockers are thought to have low amounts of transmission into maternal milk supply; small studies have indicated no observable harmful clinical or behavioral effects in the infant. Similar results have been found with most second-generation dopamine blockers, except for quetiapine, where there are very limited data, and for clozapine, where there is some evidence of accumulation in breast milk and occasional cases of agranulocytosis in the infant.

A key factor in minimizing the infant's exposure in breast milk is pharmacokinetics and timing of dosing the medication. As described elsewhere in this text, it is recommended to take medications once daily as much as possible, often in the evening. If a mother is taking lamotrigine in the evening, it would be preferable to breast-feed the baby before taking the evening dose. Furthermore, she can pump and store breast milk after the evening dose, and feed the baby with milk the next day in the morning or preferably in the afternoon. She can try to pump and store her breast milk long after the half-life of the last dose of the medication. This approach is more effective with drugs with shorter half-lives. In the example just given, for instance, lamotrigine has a half-life of about 29 hours and will remain in the bloodstream even when breast milk is pumped long after an evening dose. Nonetheless, the longer one waits, the lower the amount of the medication in the bloodstream, and the less that will enter the milk supply.

It also is relevant that drug metabolism in the infant is somewhat slow in the first three weeks of life, but then increases and becomes more rapid than in adults by about 12 weeks of life. Hence infants are able to metabolize and excrete psychotropic medications after a few months, and appear to do so even more efficiently than adults.

Categories also exist for lactation risk based on FDA recommendations. These categories are as follows: L1 is safest, meaning that the medication has been taken by a large number of people without observed harmful effects. L2 is safer, meaning it has been studied in a limited number of people without any observed adverse effects. L3 is moderately safe, meaning there are possible or minimal adverse effects noted. New medications tend to be put at this level until they are studied more carefully. L4 is possibly hazardous, meaning that there is evidence of some adverse harm, but the benefits of breast-feeding may outweigh that harm. And L5 is contraindicated, meaning that there is evidence of harm that exceeds benefits of breast-feeding, or there is clear evidence of high risk of damage to the infant. Most benzodiazepines and GABAergic agents are categorized as L3. Among anticonvulsants, lamotrigine is categorized as L3, while carbamazepine and divalproex are categorizes L2, and lithium is listed as L4. Most SRIs and modern antidepressants are listed as L2, except for citalopram, which is listed at L3, as are bupropion, mirtazapine, and venlafaxine. Dopamine blockers are listed as L3 or L4, notably with quetiapine and ziprasidone listed as L4. The only commonly used agents listed as L2 are haloperidol and olanzapine.

POSTPARTUM DEPRESSION

Postpartum depression (PPD), and also premenstrual syndrome (PMS), are analogous in many ways to the concept of seasonal affective illness. As discussed in Chapter 26, seasonal affective depression (SAD) is not a new and separate disease in most people, but rather represents seasonality in affective illness. It involves light as a trigger for mood episodes. It is common, though, in the general population for milder mood effects to occur, so that "winter blues" are experienced, meaning mild sadness but not full-blown depression, in persons without underlying affective illness (bipolar illness or unipolar depression).

Similarly, all women can experience mild mood shifts with monthly menstrual cycles (PMS), but full-blown depression usually occurs in those with underlying affective illness, with the menstrual cycles serving as triggers for mood episodes.

Analogously, all women can experience mild depression after pregnancy, the "baby blues," but those who experience full-blown depressive episodes tend to have underlying affective illness; i.e., genetic and biological susceptibility to full depressive or manic episodes when triggered by certain stressors. Often, they have episodes at other times, not just postpartum. Sometimes, the postpartum mood episode is the index episode of a lifelong recurrent affective illness. So PPD is not a separate "disease" on its own, as is commonly assumed.

PPD is more common in bipolar than in unipolar depression, hence it is a predictor of the former. When it occurs with psychotic features, this is especially the case. These are the cases where tragedies can occur, with suicide of the mother and/or homicide of children.

There are no FDA-indicated treatments specifically for PPD at present, although an agent in development, brexanolone, may come on the market for that purpose. This medication is the main progesterone metabolite, with GABAergic properties so that it has mainly anxiolytic effects. In RCTs, a lower dose produced a 3-point difference versus placebo on the Hamilton Depression Rating Scale (HDRS); a 5-point difference was seen at the higher dose. In a second trial of the lower dose, one month of treatment was not different than placebo, with both groups improving. This agent is given intravenously. These results are similar to the effect sizes seen with SRIs, about 2–3 points on the HDRS, and would not represent a major benefit over the standard monoamine agonists.

More importantly, it would be helpful to begin treatment at delivery to prevent PPD in persons with risk factors; e.g., those already diagnosed with affective illnesses. In some cases, though, as noted, the postpartum depressive episode is the first affective episode of illness.

Some women have the experience of postpartum mania, with or without psychotic features, and sometimes postpartum psychosis occurs without a clear manic or depressive episode. In these cases, pregnancy can be seen as a trigger of mood episodes in a person with bipolar illness, just as many other triggers exist. Since postpartum depression is so common in bipolar illness, it is very important to resume mood stabilizing medications at or around delivery.

PREMENSTRUAL SYNDROME (PMS)

The monthly menstrual cycle can affect mood and anxiety. It is well known that estrogen and progesterone hormones fluctuate around the menstrual cycle. Some have postulated that the rapid reduction of estrogen and progesterone in the late luteal phase, just before ovulation, may be a situation that mimics the rapid fall in estrogen at delivery leading to postpartum depression. In other words, premenstrual syndrome may reflect a mini-postpartum depression every month. Sometimes estrogen fluctuations are experienced as depressed mood, low energy, and low interest, but at other times, the hormonal fluctuations produce clinical effects that involve anxiety primarily, or irritability, instead of depression. In some cases, these various symptoms are all mixed together.

It should be noted that estrogen and progesterone, as well as testosterone, are steroid hormones. These steroid hormones are very psychoactive, as are all steroid hormones. Steroids released into the bloodstream enter the brain freely, and enter neurons without the need for receptor binding; they thus have many neurobehavioral effects. Given the consistent fluctuation of these steroid hormones during the menstrual cycle, it is not surprising that there would be some psychological effects as part of the normal process of menstruation.

This text will use the phrase "premenstrual syndrome" (PMS), rather than the bureaucratic DSM phrase of "premenstrual dysphoric disorder" (PMDD). Despite numerous studies, and the fact that estrogen and progesterone hormones can be measured in the blood, there has been no consistent or replicated association of measurable levels of these steroid hormones in association with PMS. In other words, blood testing has neither predicted nor assisted in the diagnosis or treatment of PMS, based on currently available knowledge. This research is limited by being mostly non-randomized and observational, liable to confounding bias. However there are some randomized studies that do show some benefit with some oral contraceptives in treatment of PMS. One of them, drosperinone, has an FDA indication for treatment of PMDD. There has been some randomized research on supplementation with progesterone, with no benefit for PMS.

In persons with bipolar illness or recurrent unipolar depression, monthly worsening of symptoms to a moderate or greater degree in association with menstrual periods should be interpreted, not as a new illness, but rather as a monthly trigger for the underlying affective illness. These patients do not have bipolar illness plus PMS, but rather perimenstrual worsening of bipolar illness. Perimenstrual symptoms should be seen as symptoms of the underlying effective illness, and the menstrual periods as triggers of episodes or symptoms of the affective illness. If second-messenger modifiers are used to treat bipolar illness, and perimenstrual worsening occurs, then the doses of the second-messenger modifiers should either be increased, or multiple such agents should be combined to provide further mood stabilizing benefit.

In the absence of underlying recurrent unipolar depression or bipolar illness, one can diagnose pure PMS. In these cases, some clinicians report and find benefit with low-dose oral contraceptives to help mood and anxiety symptoms associated with PMS. This benefit is primarily based on observational and not randomized data. Some SRIs have obtained FDA indication for premenstrual symptoms, such as fluoxetine, renamed "Serafem" instead of Prozac, for premenstrual use. Sertraline and controlled-release paroxetine also have indications for PMDD. The use of a new name for fluoxetine, and a new name for PMS, reflects a marketing approach that seeks to convince clinicians and patients that there is something special about this agent for these symptoms. This is not the case. The use of SRIs for PMS is purely symptomatic, since SRIs have a direct anxiolytic effect and thus reduce many of the anxiety and irritability symptoms associated with PMS. These agents also have some symptomatic depression symptom benefit, which can have modest results for PMS. There is no evidence that SRIs are treating the underlying cause of PMS, which probably relates to the steroid hormone fluctuations of the menstrual cycle. The use of SRIs for PMS always produces the long-term dilemma of whether these agents should be used intermittently or continuously. If it is used intermittently, some clinicians recommend beginning the SRI a week or two before menstruation, and then discontinuing it upon menstruation. In this approach, SRIs will be used for about half of each month. Other clinicians prefer continuous use, but this leads to the long-term dilemma of serotonin withdrawal syndrome. When SRIs are used for longer than a year, eventually serotonin withdrawal syndrome will occur if they should be stopped. So, continuous use of SRIs for one year or longer commits the patient to indefinite use, with marked difficulty in ever coming off those agents. For this reason, if SRIs are used for PMS, this textbook prefers intermittent rather than continuous use. Again, such use would not be recommended in individuals with bipolar illness, whose underlying affective illness would be worsened with long-term or even intermittent SRI use.

MENOPAUSE

The average age of menopause in the United States is 51 years. The range is from the early 40s to about 60 years of age. The duration of menopausal symptoms tends to be about five years. In menopause, there is a decline in estrogen and progesterone. Just as with delivery at the end of pregnancy, and the monthly menstrual cycle, this decline in hormones results in emotional effects. Women can have depressive and anxiety symptoms in particular, but also irritability, as with PMS. Unlike PMS, where the changes are monthly and rapid, the changes that occur with female hormones around menopause are more chronic and gradual. The two main periods of concern are perimenopause and post-menopause. As is well known, in the now-classic Women's Health Initiative (WHI) study, a major change has occurred in the treatment of perimenopausal and postmenopausal psychological symptoms. For almost half a century, until about a decade ago, estrogen hormone replacement treatment was standard and common. In some countries, such as Sweden, almost half of women in the perimenopausal and postmenopausal age groups were receiving estrogen hormone replacement treatment into the 2000s. The WHI study demonstrated small but real harmful effects of estrogen hormone replacement for breast cancer risk, as well as some other cancers and cardiovascular morbidity and mortality. No benefits were seen for purported utility in reducing risk of dementia or other harmful medical outcomes. Benefit was seen for psychological symptoms associated with perimenopause, however. The impact of this study was such that physicians moved from prescribing estrogen hormone replacement therapy for the majority of menopausal women, to prescribing it for almost no menopausal women. There has been some criticism that this shift from one extreme to another might have been excessive. It has been pointed out that the WHI study found some benefit for hormone replacement therapy psychologically, although the harms that were discovered generally are seen as outweighing those benefits. The harms in that study were more notable in older women in the postmenopausal age groups, around age 60 and above, whereas it appeared that there were fewer harms for younger women in the perimenopausal age group, meaning around age 50. When deciding whether any estrogen hormone replacement therapy should be given for psychological symptoms of menopause, a risk–benefit calculation should be made, which is not straightforward. Certainly it appears that in postmenopausal age groups of age 60 and above, there is no rationale for long-term estrogen hormone replacement therapy. Harms clearly outweigh any potential benefit. Very short-term use might be defensible if needed as a last resort. In the perimenopausal age group from about age 45–55, in some women, short-term use of estrogen hormone replacement therapy, defined as five years or less, for severe perimenopausal symptoms might provide more benefits than known harms. Very low-dose estrogen treatment should be given, either transdermally or orally. This decision-making would need to be individualized, and should represent a minority of cases, not routine practice.

Regarding psychotropic medications for perimenopausal or postmenopausal psychological symptoms, there continue to be limited options. Gabapentin was shown to be effective for some perimenopausal symptoms, especially hot flashes, in randomized clinical trials. The FDA did not provide an indication for that treatment, because the statistically significant benefits were deemed to be too small and not clinically meaningful. Many clinicians will use the all-purpose SRIs for perimenopausal and postmenopausal mood or anxiety symptoms, and these agents will give symptomatic mild to moderate anxiolytic or depressive symptom benefit. As with their use for PMS, long-term use of these agents always raises the question of whether serotonin withdrawal syndrome would occur eventually. Commitment to long-term use needs to be considered as a potential problem, due to difficulty of coming off these agents. In the postmenopausal age group, where osteoporosis risk increases, the long-term use of SRIs could be problematic, given that these agents are associated with increased risk of osteoporosis, which would lead to fractures. As discussed in Chapter 25, the potential long-term carcinogenicity of SRIs needs to be taken into account as well, especially in older age groups in whom the risk of cancer increases. All in all, the modest symptomatic benefits of SRIs for menopausal symptoms may not outweigh potential long-term harms. Again, very short-term treatment might provide a more beneficial risk–benefit ratio.

These considerations would also apply to the FDA approval of paroxetine for menopausal symptoms, including hot flashes. Again, as with the renaming of Prozac as Serafem for PMS, paroxetine has been renamed "Brisdelle" for marketing purposes in menopause. This medication is the same medication as Paxil for depression, but at a lower dose (7.5 mg/d, versus 20 mg/d for standard initial dosing of Paxil). The benefit scenario was modest, consisting of a decrease in frequency of hot flashes between paroxetine and placebo of one hot flash per day, out of a baseline of six hot flashes per day. It is notable that similar results have been seen with gabapentin in its randomized trials, yet that agent was refused FDA indication.

A consideration that did not appear to be taken into account by the FDA was the problem of serotonin withdrawal syndrome with paroxetine. It is well known that paroxetine has perhaps the worst serotonin withdrawal syndrome of all SRIs, with the exception of venlafaxine. The use of paroxetine for over a year for menopausal symptoms will commit the patient to long-term treatment that will be difficult to discontinue, due to this very severe serotonin withdrawal syndrome. This long-term problem should be taken into account. Furthermore, at higher doses, paroxetine has many drug interactions due to its cytochrome P450 inhibition, and this could be problematic in this age group because of their increasing use of other medications for common medical conditions, such as hypertension or hyperlipidemia. The low doses of paroxetine in the FDA indication for menopause reflect mild selective serotonin reuptake inhibition, which produces a purer anxiolytic effect. It may also have some vasomotor effects, relevant to hot flashes. Again, despite the FDA indication, clinicians and patients should understand that the benefits with paroxetine are symptomatic only, and do not address the underlying process of menopause itself.

The FDA approval of paroxetine for hot flashes during menopause is the first approval given for non-hormonal medications for menopausal symptoms. The FDA advisory committee that reviewed the data on this medication voted strongly against approving it. In the case of gabapentin, this advice led to the rejection of FDA indication. In the case of paroxetine, FDA moved ahead with approval despite the negative judgment of its advisory committee. It appears to have done so because this was the first non-hormonal treatment for menopause. When FDA provides an indication for a new drug mechanism for a condition, and if the condition is very common and otherwise not well treated, FDA has a lower threshold and will provide indications to drugs with less impressive evidence of benefit.

Overall, there appears to be little reason to expect more than minimal benefit with SRIs or other psychotropic drugs for perimenopausal or menopausal symptoms.

DIFFERENTIAL TREATMENT EFFECTS

There is a literature in the treatment of MDD that suggests that there may be differential treatment benefits between men and women with various monoamine agonists. Specifically, some studies suggest that TCAs are more effective in men than in women, and that SRIs are more effective in women than in men. Since MDD is diagnosed more frequently in women, this result would support SRI use in this large population of women with depression. This research is limited and has not been well replicated by different groups of investigators. The infrequent use of TCAs these days limits the relevance of these data as well. Whether SRIs are less effective in men than in women remains an open question.

Among anticonvulsants, there is an important difference in gender effects with divalproex, since that agent is associated with polycystic ovarian syndrome (PCOS) in about 10% of women, versus 1% with lithium. Also, divalproex has anti-androgenic effects biochemically, which probably underlies its propensity to cause PCOS in women. Furthermore, it is teratogenic. For these reasons, many clinicians avoid divalproex entirely in premenopausal women. Nonetheless, except in the setting of very sexually impulsive patients, who may be at high risk of unplanned pregnancy, it should be feasible to use divalproex if needed as a last resort in premenopausal women. Even the PCOS risk can be managed with yearly ultrasound testing, and drug discontinuation if any evidence of PCOS is observed. This approach would not support first-line treatment, but later-line treatment if needed, with divalproex. In this view, there is no absolute, only a relative, contraindication to using divalproex in premenopausal women.

Concerns regarding weight gain as a side effect of psychotropic medications tend to be very common among young women as well. The potential of notable weight gain with divalproex is another factor that leads to its rejection. Indeed, divalproex has more weight gain than lithium, and should not be used as an early-line treatment if other options are available and if weight gain is a major concern. Lithium has less weight gain, but it is not zero, and in some women it can be a problem. Clinicians often lean towards lamotrigine for mood stabilizer treatment in premenopausal women concerned about weight. But lamotrigine is relatively ineffective for treatment of acute manic symptoms or the prevention of manic episodes. In young women who have manic episodes relatively frequently or severely, it is likely that lamotrigine will have limited benefit.

An alternative that is often underappreciated is carbamazepine, which also does not have any weight gain, like lamotrigine, but is effective in prevention of manic episodes to a notable degree, unlike lamotrigine. The main disadvantage of carbamazepine is its multiple drug interactions due to its strong cytochrome P450 induction, but these drug interactions are usually not very relevant for young, healthy premenopausal women, who do not tend to have other medical illnesses or take or need other medications for various medical illnesses. The most common medications used in such women are oral contraceptives; carbamazepine does decrease the efficacy of these agents. The possibility of becoming pregnant should be explained to patients, and they should see their primary care doctors or gynecologists to adjust their oral contraceptive dose upwards with concomitant carbamazepine treatment. If needed, combination treatment with other psychotropic medications can occur with carbamazepine; lithium in particular has no drug interactions with carbamazepine. Blood levels of monoamine agonists and dopamine blockers are decreased with carbamazepine, which reduces their efficacy. An exception applies for paliperidone, where blood levels do not appear to be decreased by carbamazepine.

SELECTED REFERENCES

Armstrong, C. (2008). ACOG guidelines on psychiatric medication use during pregnancy and lactation. *American Family Physician, 78*(6), 772–778.

Berga, S. L., et al. (2007). PMDD spotlight: Diagnosis and treatment. At http://www.medscape.org/viewarticle/563338.

Keers, R., & Aitchison, K. J. (2010). Gender differences in antidepressant drug response. *International Review of Psychiatry, 22*(5), 485–500.

Kohen, D. (2005). Psychotropic medication and breast-feeding. *Advances in Psychiatric Treatment, 11*(5), 371–379.

Orleans, R. J., et al. (2014). FDA approval of paroxetine for menopausal hot flushes. *New England Journal of Medicine, 370*, 1777–1779.

31

Ethnic and Racial Groups

It is a fact that most research on psychotropic medications has been conducted in Western industrialized countries, mostly on Caucasians. It is reasonable to ask about relevance of this research to citizens of the rest of the world, in Asia, Africa, and Latin America, as well as to ethnic and racial minorities in Europe and North America originating in those non-Western countries. Most research on ethnic and racial groups has been conducted on these minorities in Western countries. Specifically, African-Americans, Hispanics, and Asians have been most studied. There is limited research in Africa and the Middle East on the effects of psychotropic medications. In this chapter, available research will be reviewed with a focus on its relevance for clinical treatment as well as on diagnostic aspects.

AFRICAN-AMERICANS

Research in the United States on the African-American population has identified some differences regarding psychotropic medication effects compared to the Caucasian population. Pharmacokinetic metabolism may differ, resulting in higher levels of some medications, like dopamine blockers, at the same doses in the African-American population, compared to Caucasians. These higher levels can then led to more EPS in the African-American population. Intracellular red blood cell levels of lithium, which approximate CSF levels, are higher in African-American than in Caucasian subjects. Some recent research indicates that African-Americans may have genetic polymorphisms such that a subgroup demonstrates slow metabolism of medications through the hepatic cytochrome P450 system.

Regarding diagnosis, African-Americans are more likely to be diagnosed, compared to Caucasians, with psychotic rather than affective illnesses. When they are presenting with delusions, schizophrenia rather than mania is more likely to be diagnosed. These African-American patients will be given dopamine blockers as a consequence more frequently than Caucasians with similar symptoms. Poverty, which is prevalent in the

African-American population in the United States, also has important diagnostic and treatment implications. When treated in underfunded and understaffed government-run clinics, the African-American population often does not receive careful and adequate diagnostic attention. The author of this textbook had the experience of working in a city hospital clinic in Atlanta, Georgia, with predominantly African-American patients. His experience was that almost all patients were treated with antidepressants and antipsychotics. Diagnosis did not matter, as these two treatments could be justified for almost all diagnoses given. When schizophrenia was diagnosed, antipsychotics were given long-term, and antidepressants were added for "negative" symptoms. When schizoaffective illness was diagnosed (it was the most common diagnosis), both antidepressants and antipsychotics were justified. When psychotic depression was diagnosed, as was common, again, both agents were used. Bipolar illness was infrequently diagnosed, and mood stabilizers rarely given. Similarly, nonpsychotic depressive illness was diagnosed less frequently than was the case in another university clinic in the same city frequented by a predominantly Caucasian patient population. This kind of experience is common, and calls for public health attention.

It has been suggested by some African-American psychiatrists that real-world discrimination and dangerous living conditions in poor urban settings may result in a certain level of mild suspiciousness towards others, especially Caucasian medical staff that might be enountered in hospitals. This normal self-protectiveness, given the experience of racial discrimination, can be misinterpreted by Caucasian mental health clinicians as a psychotic-like symptom, or as evidence of some other psychiatric abnormality.

ASIANS

The largest research literature on ethnic subgroups probably exists for Asian populations, studied both in the Far East and among immigrants in Europe and North America. One important finding is that many Asians have a genetic polymorphism that limits their ability to metabolize drugs via the hepatic cytochrome P450 system. Medications would have higher blood levels in this population than in Caucasians. It is estimated that about 20% of Asian populations are poor metabolizers of the cytochrome P450 system, compared to about 1% of the Caucasian population. This effect seems to be genetic, and is present in Asian populations in the Far East as well as Asian-American immigrants. A genetic variation in aldehyde dehydrogenase also exists that produces a flushing effect with alcohol in some Asian populations.

A specific association has been found with a genetic variation, the presence of the HLA-B*1502 allele, which markedly increases the risk of agranulocytosis with carbamazepine. This finding is strong enough that the FDA has added this language to the labeling of carbamazepine.

Regarding diagnosis, an extensive literature in the Far East indicates a very low diagnosable prevalence of MDD, using DSM definitions, based on carefully conducted epidemiological studies. These studies do not reflect clinical practice patterns; they are not based on assessing what clinicians diagnose and practice. Rather, they are based on actual prevalence rates identified by researchers going door to door in the general population, conducting the DSM-based interviews in the language of that population. One interpretation of these results is that the presentation of depression in the Far East is different than in the West. An extensive cross-cultural literature exists on this topic. It indicates a highly somatic presentation and interpretation of the depressive experience in China and other Asian countries. Instead of complaining about sadness and lack of interest, patients will have many physical symptoms, including headaches, chest pain, stomach problems and other physical issues. There also is widespread cultural stigma against the legitimacy of psychiatric diagnosis in many Asian cultures.

In Asia, there is extensive adherence to Eastern medical approaches, dating back to the Middle Ages and ancient times, in which many assumptions of Western medicine do not hold. For instance, the concept of disease applying in the same way to many different individuals is rejected in Eastern medicine. Rather, each individual is felt to have a disease of his or her own. There is no one effective treatment for a specific disease, but many possible effective treatments for each individual person. This approach is hard to quantify and study with standard, accepted, Western scientific methods. Patients in Asia are faced with major cultural differences both in their experience of psychiatric symptoms and in the assumptions behind diagnosis and treatment that guide Western practice.

HISPANIC/LATINO POPULATIONS

There has been limited research on pharmacokinetic or pharmacodynamic variations in Hispanic or Latino populations. Some clinicians believe that patients of this ethnicity are more sensitive to side effects of dopamine blockers and monoamine agonists than Caucasian populations are. The research basis for this clinical opinion is limited.

Regarding diagnosis, some Latin American countries report rather high prevalence rates and epidemiological studies of affective illness, especially MDD, which was found in 25% of the population in Chile, contrasting sharply with around 1% in studies in the Far East. Eating disorders are prevalent in South America, with higher rates of bulimia in Latin America than in European and North American Caucasian populations. Cross-cultural research suggests a common occurrence of somatization as well of depressive or anxiety symptoms. Specific cultural presentations, such as "ataque de nervios," appear to reflect higher prevalence of panic attack symptoms. Although there is much stigma about the legitimacy of psychiatric diagnoses in many Latin American populations, some countries also have a very high rate of use of psychiatric and psychological services. For instance, in Argentina, psychotherapies are utilized in a widespread fashion by the population, and clinical psychologists represent a very high proportion of the population compared to many other non-Western countries.

MIDDLE EASTERN/NORTH AFRICAN POPULATIONS

There are no known clear pharmacokinetic or pharmacodynamic variations in Middle Eastern or North African populations that differ from Western Caucasian populations. This research space is extremely limited, though.

Regarding diagnosis, there are many similarities between the Middle East and the Far East in cultural aspects of the experience of psychiatric symptoms. In many Middle Eastern countries, the prevalence rate of MDD in epidemiological studies is quite low, typically around 1% in the general population. Depression symptom presentation is somatic. There is great cultural stigma against the legitimacy of psychiatric diagnosis. In addition, the tradition of Eastern medicine persists, with a non-Western approach to the concept of disease. Since many countries in the Middle East are highly religious, spiritual explanations of psychiatric symptoms frequently predominate. Despite these highly non-Western aspects to Middle Eastern culture, some countries also mimic Western culture quite closely, with careful teaching and reading of Western textbooks of psychiatry, word for word, in a manner that is uncritical.

Among more Westernized groups, psychotropic medications may be overused for treatment of nonspecific symptoms of anxiety and depressive states. The diagnosis of ADD and treatment with amphetamines has increased markedly in recent years. In this sense, there is a paradoxical coexistence of Western and non-Western attitudes in these populations.

In countries with past colonial histories and strong cultural links to Europe, as in French-speaking North Africa, psychiatric symptoms are identified or experienced in the context of racial and religious conflict and discrimination. French psychiatrists had identified the "North African syndrome" to describe symptoms of apathy, withdrawal, and irritability seen in Algerians and other North Africans who had immigrated to France.

The psychiatrist Franz Fanon described how this syndrome was a projection of racial attitudes of white Frenchmen, and not seen or experienced in the same manner in Algeria itself, or when those same patients were examined by black psychiatrists.

AFRICAN AND CARIBBEAN POPULATIONS

The pharmacokinetic and pharmacodynamic variations in African and Caribbean populations are similar in some ways to those observed in African-American and Latino populations. Again, research is much more limited in Africa and the Caribbean.

In the Caribbean, prevalence of religious traditions that involve African roots such as voodoo influences attitudes toward psychiatric symptoms and treatments. There is great cultural stigma attached to Western notions of psychiatric diagnosis. Culture-specific experiences such as witchcraft exist.

As in the Middle East, there also is acceptance of biological approaches to psychiatry, especially for severe psychiatric conditions such as schizophrenia. Among more

Westernized groups, psychotropic medications again may be overused for treatment of nonspecific symptoms of anxiety and depressive states. Once more, there is an uneasy coexistence of rejection and over-acceptance of Western approaches to psychiatry and psychopharmacology.

SELECTED REFERENCES

Chaudhry, I., et al. (2008). Ethnicity and psychopharmacology. Journal of Psychopharmacology, 22(6), 673–680.

Combs, D. R., et al. (2006). Perceived racism as a predictor of paranoia among African Americans. *The Journal of Black Psychology, 32*(1), 87–104.

Grier, W. H., & Cobbs, P. M. (1968). *Black Rage.* New York: Basic Books.

Kolar, D. R., et al. (2016). Epidemiology of eating disorders in Latin America: A systematic review and meta-analysis. *Current Opinion in Psychiatry, 29*(6), 363–371.

Lin, K.-M. & Poland, R. (1995). Ethnicity, culture and psychopharmacology. In F. E. Bloom & D. J. Kupfer (Eds.), *Neuropsychopharmacology: The 4th generation of progress* (pp. 1907–1917). New York: Raven Press.

Schwartz, R. C., & Blankenship, D. M. (2014). Racial disparities in psychotic disorder diagnosis: A review of empirical literature. *World Journal of Psychiatry, 4*(4), 133–140.

Vohringer, P. A., et al. (2013). Detecting mood disorder in resource-limited primary care settings. *Journal of Medical Screening, 20*(3), 118–124.

32

Psychopharmacology in Medical Illnesses

A VARIETY OF MEDICAL ILLNESSES CAN CAUSE PSYCHIATRIC SYMPTOMS, most commonly depression, anxiety, manic states, and delusions or hallucinations, in that order. Before DSM-III in 1980, psychiatric symptoms caused by medical illnesses were classified as organic mental disorders. DSM-III changed the term "organic" to "secondary to a medical illness." In DSM-5, mania and depression secondary or due to a medical illness were moved to "other mental disorders." These days the terms "organic," "secondary," and "neuropsychiatric" are used interchangeably. As discussed in Chapter 17, the diagnostic hierarchy approach is relevant here. In that view, some diagnostic constructs are subsumed under other diagnoses. The reason for such privileging of one diagnosis over another can be etiological, or it can be for other reasons (e.g., polysymptomatic diagnoses). Thus, if we know that one disease is caused by etiology X, then the symptoms of that disease should not be separately diagnosed as representing other putative diseases. A common example in psychiatry is neurosyphilis, where symptoms of mania, depression, and dementia occur. Such persons should not be diagnosed with neurosyphilis, plus bipolar illness, plus major depressive illness, plus dementia. Rather, one diagnosis excludes the others. Another example is bipolar illness, where mania, depression, distractibility, poor executive function, and delusions can occur. Such persons should not be diagnosed with bipolar illness, plus MDD, plus ADD, plus schizophrenia.

The topic of psychiatric symptoms secondary to medical illnesses is inherently hierarchical, thus one should avoid the DSM-based tendency to interpret such psychiatric states as "comorbidity" of MDD, or bipolar illness, or generalized anxiety disorder (GAD) with the medical illnesses discussed. Rather, those medical illnesses tend to cause the psychiatric states described here. It is worth noting that mood conditions can increase the risk of some medical illnesses, so the opposite causal direction can occur, where psychiatric states can cause some of the medical illnesses described, in which case a more valid comorbidity eventually may occur. This chapter will examine selected neurological and medical conditions that involve psychiatric symptoms, and their treatment.

DIAGNOSTIC CONSIDERATIONS

Traumatic Brain Injury or Chronic Traumatic Encephalopathy

TBI is a disease that is triggered by traumas to the head, which can be single or recurrent, producing mood symptoms like depression or mania, or cognitive symptoms like memory impairment or executive dysfunction, and behavioral changes such as impulsivity or aggression. TBI is a broad category that can include many kinds of injury to the brain. A specific subtype of TBI is CTE, which is a progressive, degenerative disease of the brain found in athletes and soldiers, among others, with a history of repetitive brain trauma, including symptomatic concussions as well as asymptomatic subconcussive hits to the head. Both conditions have important emotional aspects, including aggression, rage, depression, and manic states.

CTE has been known to affect boxers since the 1920s. However, recent reports have been published of neuropathologically confirmed CTE in retired professional football players and other athletes who have a history of repetitive brain trauma. This trauma triggers progressive degeneration of the brain tissue, including the build-up of an abnormal tau protein. These changes in the brain can begin months, years, or even decades after the last brain trauma or the end of active athletic involvement. The brain degeneration is associated with memory loss, confusion, impaired judgment, impulse control problems, aggression, depression, and, eventually, progressive dementia. In one brain autopsy study with 202 deceased football players, CTE was diagnosed in 177 players. Depressive symptoms were found in 67%, and manic symptoms in 22% of patients with CTE. Suicide was the cause of death in 27% of this sample.

Depressive symptoms are most common among persons with TBI. Manic symptoms are less frequent. Lifetime depressive symptoms range from 25–50% in the first year post-TBI, with overall rates of 26–64%. Manic and mixed symptoms affect around 9% of patients with TBI and normally involve right ventral frontal and/or basotemporal injury. Mixed states are important because TBI has a close relationship with suicide ideation, and mixed affective symptoms are important established risk factors for suicide. In one retrospective cohort study in Finland, TBI history was found in 5.5% of a sample that committed suicide, 20% of whom had brain lesions and 80% of whom had concussions.

Movement Disorders

Both Huntington's and Parkinson's diseases are associated with depressive states. In Huntington's disease, depression lifetime prevalence is about 30–40%, with suicide rates 6 to 7 times higher than the general population. Manic syndrome has a lifetime prevalence of 5% to 10% of patients.

Parkinson's disease (PD) involves clinical depression in about 40–50% of patients. The underlying mechanisms of depression in PD remain unknown. The onset of depressive syndromes and their natural history do not parallel the course of motor disturbance. Manic symptoms are more related to dopamine replacement therapy, being reported to occur in up to 16% of patients.

Dementias

Frontotemporal dementia (FTD) is characterized by progressive changes in mood and personality. One meta-analysis found a depression rate in FTD of 33%. Compared with other types of dementia, patients with FTD are twice as likely to be diagnosed with bipolar illness. Vascular dementia is tied to vascular depression and mania, as described previously, often being a later manifestation of the course of vascular illness.

In Alzheimer's dementia (AD), depression, mania, and psychomotor agitation are common. Clinical and epidemiological studies have found that 75–95% of patients experience at least one psychiatric symptom of any severity over the course of the disease, with resulting poor prognosis. Depression is found in 16% of patients in population-based AD studies, and in 44.3% in hospital-based studies. Depression is also a predictor of progression from normal to mild cognitive impairment and then to dementia.

Agitation/mania occur frequently in AD. One case-control study with 19 AD patients and 13 controls reported the following rates: 78.9% with anxiety, 52.6% with irritability, 31.6% with agitation, and 5.2% with elation symptoms. Agitation is associated with structural and functional abnormalities of the brain regions associated with emotional regulation, like the amygdala and hippocampus.

Multiple Sclerosis (MS)

MS is an autoimmune demyelinating disease of the CNS that may lead to severe neurological disability. Clinical depression is the most common neuropsychiatric illness found in MS. Findings from hospital-based clinics reveal that approximately 25–50% of patients with MS develop depression over the course of their lives, two or three times higher than that found in general population. Depression is less common early in MS than in later stages, but fluctuations in mood could correlate with disease relapse. The presence of mania in MS cases is controversial, and often attributed to steroid treatment. It should be distinguished from pseudobulbar affect, which occurs in 10% of patients with MS and involves impulsive laughing and crying, related to cerebellopontine abnormalities.

Epilepsy

Psychiatric symptoms are frequently observed in patients with epilepsy. The prevalence of depressive symptoms is reported to be more than 30% in community-based epilepsy samples and 20–55% in specialist epilepsy clinics. Although epilepsy is a risk factor for depression, recent studies have also revealed that a history of depression is associated with four- to six-fold risk of developing epilepsy. These data suggests a bidirectional relationship. Pre-ictal symptoms of depression typically present as dysphoric mood in which the prodromal symptoms may extend for hours or even days to onset of the seizure. Post-ictal symptoms of depression have been recognized for decades, but only one study has investigated this topic in a systematic manner, reporting 43% prevalence of post-ictal depression. These symptoms occurred after more than 50% of seizures, and their duration ranged from 0.5–108 hours, lasting up to two weeks.

Manic symptoms in epilepsy have been considered less common than depression, with the exception of two specific conditions: post-ictal symptoms, and after epilepsy surgery. Patients and their relatives frequently report post-ictal mania. Manic symptoms are reported in 22% of patients, often with associated psychotic phenomenology. The possible link between temporal lobe epilepsy, seizure activity, and mania is stressed by the high incidence of manic episodes after temporal lobectomies in pharmaco-resistant patients. After surgery, manic episodes occur in around 10% of patients. Patients who undergo right lobectomies carry a higher risk, as do patients with bilateral abnormalities.

Thyroid Dysfunction

The vast majority of patients with depression do not have biochemical evidence of thyroid dysfunction. When thyroid abnormalities do exist, they consist mainly of elevated T4 levels, low T3, and blunted thyroid-stimulating hormone (TSH) response to thyrotropin-releasing hormone. Other studies correlate the level of TSH with the severity of the depression symptoms. Rapid cycling also is associated with hypothyroidism, with a high incidence of 25%. Mania is mostly associated with hyperthyroidism.

Vascular Depression and Mania

As discussed in Chapter 19, the concept of vascular depression was introduced in the 1990s by Alexopoulos, who defined its cardinal features as presence of vascular disease (or vascular risk factors) and late-onset depression (or change in the course of early-onset depression after the onset of vascular disease). The clinical presentation of vascular depression is characterized by psychomotor slowing, lack of initiative, apathy, absence of family history of mood illness, and a medical history of hypertension. Cognitive decline and progression to dementia are common. Treatment resistance to antidepressants and poor prognostic course are common features. The hallmark of MRI-defined vascular depression is the presence of white matter lesions identified as white matter hyperintensities (WMH).

Mania also has been associated with vascular disease, and the term "vascular mania" has been proposed. Its main features are absence of family history of mood illness, mania occurring in the context of clinical and/or neuroimaging evidence of cerebrovascular disease (including white or gray matter hyperintensities), and cognitive impairment.

Cardiovascular Disease

It has long been recognized that mild forms of depression are found in up to two-thirds of patients in the hospital after acute myocardial infarction, with clinical depression generally found in 17–44%. This prevalence is over two to three times that found in the general population. It also is well established that depression, and possibly mania, is an independent risk factor for cardiac illness. Coronary artery disease tends to correlate with general vascular disease, which predisposes patients to vascular depression and vascular mania, reflecting small vessel cerebrovascular disease.

TREATMENT

The treatment of vascular depression was discussed in Chapter 19. The rest of this chapter will examine treatment of psychiatric symptoms in medical illnesses by focusing on two other major medical conditions: vascular depression, treatment of depression in cardiovascular disease, and lithium for behavioral symptoms of neurodegenerative diseases.

Treatment of Depressive States in Cardiovascular Disease

There have been four major RCTs of monoamine agonists in the treatment of depressive states in cardiovascular disease: the Enhancing Recovery in Coronary Heart Disease (ENRICHD) trial, the Sertraline Against Depression and Heart Disease in Chronic Heart Failure (SADHART) trial, the Myocardial Infarction and Depression–Intervention (MIND-IT) trial, and the Canadian Cardiac Randomized Evaluation of Antidepressant and Psychotherapy Efficacy (CREATE) trial.

ENRICHD involved 2,482 patients who had experienced myocardial infarction, randomized to CBT or usual care. If there Hamilton Depression Rating Scale (HDRS) scores were above 24, meaning mild to moderate severity, they received SRIs. The primary outcome was mortality or recurrence of myocardial infarction, with secondary outcomes for depression symptom scores. Overall, there was no benefit with treatment for the primary cardiovascular outcomes in the study, with a mean follow-up of over two years (29 months). There was improvement in depression symptoms of 1.5 points, which is a small effect, compared to the control group.

SADHART involved 469 patients with heart failure randomized to sertraline versus placebo. The primary endpoint was a composite outcome of cardiovascular status at 12 weeks. There was no meaningful improvement in that outcome with sertraline versus placebo. Also, there was very little difference between sertraline and placebo in depression symptom improvement in the three months of treatment. The medication was said to be safe from a cardiovascular perspective, although in a reanalysis conducted for this textbook, it is notable that there was slightly increased overall mortality with sertraline versus placebo (7.7% vs. 6.8%, RR = 1.25, 95% CIs 0.62, 2.33), and greater cardiovascular death rates with sertraline treatment versus placebo (6.8% vs. 4.3%, RR = 1.60, 95% CIs 0.74, 3.47). These differences are not statistically significant, but the study was not large enough to be able to detect statistical significance for these differences. Rather, as discussed in Chapter 8, when assessing studies with low statistical power, effect estimates and confidence intervals are more meaningful. Reanalyzing these data, the relative risk indicates a 60% increase cardiovascular mortality with sertraline, with confidence intervals suggesting that this increase is more likely than not to be a real effect. Other cardiovascular outcomes did not differ appreciably between groups, except for the observation of a small but notable increase in risk of cerebrovascular stroke and sertraline-treated patients versus placebo (4.3% versus 1.7%, RR = 2.51, 95% CIs 0.80, 7.89). In other words, sertraline more than doubled the risk of stroke, with the possibility of even higher risk based on the confidence intervals. Thus, this reanalysis cannot support the conclusion made by the authors and commonly cited from this negative trial that sertraline was shown to be safe in cardiovascular disease. Rather, allowing for infrequent outcomes and low statistical power, the available evidence suggests some increased risk of harmful cardiovascular and cerebrovascular outcomes with sertraline in this heart failure population. A later analysis examined inflammatory markers in the study and reported benefit with sertraline versus placebo in reducing the prevalence of C-reactive protein, Interleukin-6, and fibrinogen.

These two studies are both negative in their outcomes, but they provide some insights that raise some questions regarding the nature of the association between depression and cardiovascular disease. The ENRICHD trial showed some benefit for depressive symptoms, but this benefit did not translate into cardiovascular outcomes, despite long-term follow-up over greater than two years. This finding may mean that depressive symptoms may predispose to cardiovascular disease, but their treatment does not improve cardiovascular outcomes. On the other hand, the improvement seen with the CBT treatment arm in the study was small compared to placebo, so perhaps specific treatment benefits for cardiovascular events would be difficult to observe even with long-term follow-up.

The SADHART study only lasted three months, and an expectation of notable cardiovascular benefits in a short timeframe was probably misplaced. Furthermore, the medication failed to improve depressive symptoms notably in the study, and thus the association between depression improvement and cardiovascular outcomes could not be tested. The failure to have even depressive symptom benefit in this trial also raises the question of whether antidepressants may simply be less effective in treating depressive symptoms in cardiovascular disease. In other words, like vascular depression, it may be that depression in the setting of cardiovascular disease confers poor prognosis and non-response to antidepressants.

The SADHART study results also provide a suggestion that improvement in inflammatory markers may not translate into improved cardiovascular outcomes. In fact, cardiovascular outcomes seemed somewhat worse with sertraline than with placebo, and this especially appeared to be the case for a doubling of risk of cerebrovascular stroke with sertraline treatment.

Turning to the other two randomized trials: MIND-IT was a study of 331 patients with myocardial infarction randomized to mirtazapine or citalopram versus treatment as usual. They were followed for up to18 months. In the primary outcome of depression symptom improvement, there were no notable differences between groups. Cardiac event rates were essentially identical between the two groups as well (14% vs. 13%). It was observed that if patients improved for depression, they had fewer cardiac events. Treatment non-responders for depression had more cardiac events. No differences were seen between the two groups of antidepressant treatment versus treatment as usual.

In the CREATE trial, 284 patients with coronary artery disease were randomized to citalopram versus placebo for 12 weeks of outpatient treatment. Improvement in depression was seen, with a mean difference of 3.3 points on the HDRS, but no improvement in cardiovascular outcomes was seen. No depression symptom benefit was seen with interpersonal psychotherapy versus clinical management. There was a two milliseconds increase in the QTc interval with citalopram versus placebo.

Interpreting these latter two studies: the MIND-IT trial was long and able to assess cardiac outcomes, and confirmed the findings from the ENRICHD trial that no long-term cardiovascular benefits can be seen with antidepressant treatment. The observation that depression symptom improvement in general correlated with better cardiovascular outcomes is important, though, and may be more meaningful than the opposite finding in the much shorter SADHART trial.

The CREATE trial was interesting in that depression symptom improvement was shown, in contradiction to the SADHART trial, but again, cardiovascular benefits were not seen with short-term treatment. The observation of no depression symptom improvement with interpersonal psychotherapy raises the question whether patients with depression and cardiovascular disease may be less responsive to psychotherapies as well. This finding is somewhat consistent with the ENRICHD trial, in which only a small benefit was seen with CBT for depression symptoms.

In sum, these large randomized trials of depression and cardiovascular disease generally suggest limited benefit with either monoamine agonists or psychotherapies, both for depression symptoms and for cardiovascular outcomes. There may be a disconnection between improvement for inflammatory pathophysiology and clinical mood and cardiac outcomes. In fact, there is some evidence that some SRIs, like sertraline, may in fact increase the risk of poor cardiac or cerebrovascular outcomes.

This interpretation of these results complicates standard recommendations regarding the use of SRIs in depression for coronary artery disease. The recommendation of the U.K. National Health Service (NHS) is that sertraline should be a first-line treatment, based on the reported safety results of the SADHART trial. This conclusion is put into some doubt, based on this analysis. Other SRIs tend to be avoided due to drug interactions, in the case of fluoxetine and paroxetine, and because of increased risk of cardiac arrhythmias for citalopram and escitalopram. Venlafaxine should be avoided due to evidence of increased risk of sudden cardiac death in individuals with coronary artery disease and history of cardiac arrhythmias in particular. It also increases coronary risk factors such as high blood pressure. If sertraline also is excluded, based on the poor outcomes for cardiovascular and cerebrovascular safety described here, then almost all SRIs would be avoided in the treatment of depression and coronary artery disease. In the past, bupropion tended to be recommended, due to the absence of drug interactions, but it has the pharmacological properties of the amphetamine class, which are known to increase risk of cardiac arrhythmias. Bupropion has been shown to increase blood pressure. Hence, there may be reason to avoid bupropion in this population as well.

Use of Psychotropic Agents for Neurodegenerative Diseases: Focus on Lithium

A prominent risk factor for dementia is depression, which more than doubles the risk. The most effective long-term preventive treatment proven for depression, especially in its bipolar variety, is lithium. In recent years, it has become clear that lithium also has major neuroprotective effects, far more in extent and human relevance than any other psychotropic agent. Five out of seven epidemiological studies have found an association between standard-dose lithium and low dementia rates.

For instance, one cross-sectional, retrospective study examined 114 elderly patients, selecting subjects older than age 60 who had euthymic bipolar disorder and who had received at least six months of treatment with lithium or other mood stabilizers, and then comparing presence or absence of AD. The researchers found, as has repeatedly been shown, elevated rates of AD of 19% in this sample, versus 7% as the usual rate in a similar-aged population control. This finding represents the usual two to three-fold increased risk of AD with bipolar disorder. Two major factors predicted presence or absence of dementia: age and lithium use. There was a 5% dementia rate in lithium-treated bipolar patients (mean age 68 years) versus 33% in non–lithium treated patients. If these results are valid, lithium reduces the risk of dementia in bipolar disorder to slightly below the population norm, and 86% less than otherwise would occur in bipolar disorder (RR = 0.14; 95% CIs 0.04, 0.44). The lithium-treated group had taken that agent for a mean of 5.93 years; interestingly, in the non-lithium group, the majority (68.8%) had also previously taken lithium (for a mean of 4.5 years) but had been off lithium for a mean of 4.95 years. Thus, if lithium has benefits, these data may suggest that those benefits do not persist once lithium is stopped. Cognitive impairment did not differ between the groups, being 20% in the lithium-treated sample versus 25% in the non-lithium group. Thus, if lithium prevents dementia, it may not inherently prevent milder cognitive decline. Other medication treatments were also reported to have no effect.

These epidemiological studies have been confirmed again with another recent report in Denmark consisting of a nationwide sample of over 800,000 persons with a median age of 80.3 years. Dementia was more common in areas with lower levels of lithium exposure. Dementia rates were similar in association with low lithium exposure in the drinking water, irrespective of the type of dementia, such as AD versus vascular dementia. The amount of lithium associated with these changes was quite low. Compared to low lithium levels of less than 5 mcg/L, if lithium levels were above 15 mcg/L, dementia risk was decreased by 17%. This amount of lithium corresponds to a fraction of the smallest dose of lithium available as a pill (150 mg/d).

All four RCTs of lithium for AD found some clinical or biological benefits versus placebo. These four RCTs range from 6–15 months in duration. An early study was reported as negative in a biological marker of Glycogen Synthase Kinase (GSK)-3 activity, but it actually found improvement in the Alzheimer's Disease Assessment Scale–Cognitive (ADAS-Cog) subscale, with twice as much benefit in lithium-treated as opposed to placebo-treated patients. This benefit was not successfully significant, given the small sample size, but it was present. The other three randomized trials showed benefit both in biological markers and in clinical outcomes. One study used very-low-dose lithium of 300 μg daily in mild AD, showing no further worsening on the Mini-Mental State Examination (MMSE) over 15 months of treatment, compared to notable worsening in the placebo group (RR 2.0, lower CI 0.64, upper CI 6.20).

Lithium has also been studied in other neurodegenerative diseases. In amyotrophic lateral sclerosis (ALS), animal data indicated that lithium delayed progression of ALS in a mouse model. In an initial open randomized study of 44 patients with ALS, in 15 months of follow-up, patients were randomized to lithium versus riluzole. In the riluzole group, there was 29% mortality at 15 months, versus none in the lithium group. Assessing disease progression with pulmonary function, the lithium group declined much less than the riluzole group (15.1% decline versus 33% decline; all differences were statistically significant). A replication study was widely reported as negative, though careful examination of the results suggests otherwise. In that study, researchers used a website program to match 149 lithium-treated patients with ALS to 149 non–lithium-treated ALS controls. At 12 months follow-up, no notable differences in disease progression were seen between the two groups.

Two key points need to be considered: First, this study was not an RCT; it was an observational comparison of two matched groups, which introduces much more confounding bias than is seen in a prospective randomized trial. Also, endpoints were self-reported over the internet, not based on direct clinical evaluation.

A true RCT that again is viewed as a refutation of lithium efficacy in ALS is also mistakenly interpreted because it did not have a non-lithium control arm. Rather, it compared 171 ALS patients randomized to standard-dose lithium (level 0.4–0.8) versus low-dose lithium (0.2–0.4). In all, 117 patients (68.4%) discontinued the study because of death/tracheotomy/severe disability, adverse events (AEs) and serious AEs (SAEs), or lack of efficacy, and the study was stopped prematurely. The investigators concluded that lithium was not well tolerated even at low doses, and that the two doses had similar results in survival, disability, and functional data. Outside of tolerability, one cannot draw conclusions about neuroprotective effects, however, given the absence of a non-lithium control arm. It is important to realize that "therapeutic" lithium levels are only established for mania in people with bipolar disorder. What is therapeutic to mania can hardly be assumed to generalize to a completely different illness like ALS. Thus, the question of what is a therapeutic level for ALS cannot be assumed, and is open.

Given the higher toxicity of lithium in older and medically compromised persons, such as in ALS, the doses and levels of lithium used in such patients should not be the same as in the treatment of mania in younger persons (i.e., 0.6 ng/dl or above). Rather, low doses are safer and may be effective. As discussed in Chapter 27, a recent systematic review reported that nine out of eleven epidemiological studies, using drinking water sources, found an association between trace-dose lithium and low suicide/homicide/mortality rates. These benefits are seen with very low doses of lithium, equivalent to about 25 mg/d of lithium carbonate. Thus, doses prescribed for neurodegenerative diseases, whether for suicidal symptoms or other behavioral problems, could be as low as 150 mg/d or even less. Future research is needed to confirm efficacy of such low doses, as suggested in the recent study of micro-dose lithium (300 micrograms/day) for treatment of early AD.

Besides lithium, other agents studied for dementia include valproate. A large NIMH-sponsored study assessed efficacy of valproate for aggression and clinical progression of AD in 313 patients with moderate dementia, double-blind randomized to valproate or placebo and followed for up to two years. No benefits for agitation were seen, nor for AD progression. Increased cortical atrophy was seen with valproate. Valproate had been chosen because it shared a few second-messenger mechanisms with lithium, such as protein kinase C (PKC) inhibition, and it is much better tolerated in the demented elderly than lithium. The hope was that if valproate overlapped enough in mechanisms with lithium, it would prove an effective alternative for dementia progression. In fact, the evidence for neuroprotection with valproate, though present, is weak and counteracted by evidence in animal studies of neuronal toxicity in standard doses, unlike lithium. Thus these results may not be surprising.

Other agents, like some monoamine agonists and some modern dopamine blockers, have been reported to be neuroprotective in some animal studies and in some human studies. However, negative studies exist also in animals and in humans, thus this literature is much less consistently positive than is the case with lithium. Furthermore, there are no epidemiological or randomized studies that show benefit with monoamine agonists or dopamine blockers in prevention of dementia.

Some epidemiological studies suggest there may be increased risk of dementia with benzodiazepines in humans, but other clinical studies find otherwise, and there are animal data indicating neuroprotective benefits with benzodiazepines.

In sum, among psychotropic drugs, the evidence is strongest and most consistent that lithium has the most neuroprotective effects, and the current literature may support its use in prevention and/or treatment of some neurodegenerative diseases, such as dementias. Even if lithium does not prove effective in treating such conditions, it should not be harmful, given its neuroprotective effects, unlike some other agents such as valproate and some dopamine blockers. Lithium may provide benefits for behavioral treatment of agitation and depression, or in suicide prevention in such subjects, without worsening the underlying neurodegenerative condition.

SELECTED REFERENCES

Berkman, L. F., et al. (2003). Effects of treating depression and low perceived social support on clinical events after myocardial infarction: The Enhancing Recovery in Coronary Heart Disease (ENRICHD) patients randomized trial. *Journal of the American Medical Association, 289,* 3106–3116.

Joost, P. V. M., et al. (2007). Effects of antidepressant treatment following myocardial infarction. *British Journal of Psychiatry, 190,* 460–466.

Kessing, L. V. (2017). Association of lithium in drinking water with the incidence of dementia. *Journal of the American Medical Association: Psychiatry, 74,* 1005–1010.

Lesperance, F., et al. (2007). Effects of citalopram and interpersonal psychotherapy on depression in patients with coronary artery disease: the Canadian Cardiac Randomized Evaluation of Antidepressant and Psychotherapy Efficacy (CREATE) trial. *Journal of the American Medical Association, 297,* 367–379.

Mauer, S., et al. (2014). Standard and trace those lithium: The systematic review of dementia prevention and other behavioral benefits. *Australia and New Zealand Journal of Psychiatry, 48,* 809–818.

O'Connor, C. M., et al. (2010). Safety and efficacy of sertraline for depression in patients with heart failure: Results of the SADHART-CHF trial. *Journal of the American College of Cardiology, 56,* 692–699.

33

Polypharmacy

Presumptions are of vast importance in medicine, as in law. A man is presumed innocent until he is proved guilty. A medicine . . . should always be presumed to be hurtful. It always is directly hurtful; it may sometimes be indirectly beneficial. If this presumption were established . . . we should not so frequently hear . . . that, on the whole, more harm than good is done with medication. Throw out opium, which the Creator himself seems to prescribe, for we often see the scarlet poppy growing in the cornfields, as if it were foreseen that wherever there is hunger to be fed there must also be pain to be soothed; throw out a few specifics which our art did not discover, and is hardly needed to apply; throw out wine, which is a food, and the vapors which produce the miracle of anesthesia, and I firmly believe that if the whole materia medica, as now used, could be sunk to the bottom of the sea, it would be all the better for mankind,—and all the worse for the fishes.

—Oliver Wendell Holmes

THESE WORDS WERE SPOKEN IN 1860 BY A HARVARD PROFESSOR OF anatomy, Oliver Wendell Holmes, in an address to the Massachusetts Medical Society. Holmes' statement has been a favorite of some leaders at the FDA. Holmes felt the profession of medicine, as well as the public, was harmed by use, and overuse, of inadequately proven medications. In 1860, Holmes went after pharmacology in general, which meant polypharmacy.

"Polypharmacy" means the prescription of multiple medications at once. Sometimes this is justified, sometimes not. Some clinicians prefer the term "co-therapy" or something of that ilk to justify the practice. In this chapter, the term "polypharmacy" is retained and evidence for harms as well as benefits are examined.

Medical care before the 1940s often consisted of polypharmacy because physicians usually prescribed multiple medications at once. One major factor might have been, as Holmes claimed, that almost no medications worked, thus physicians tended to use many medications, hoping to elicit benefits that were not present when meds were used singly.

Holmes was sensitive to this problem partly because of his 1843 essay, "The Contagiousness of Puerperal Fever." With epidemiological techniques of observation, Holmes confirmed that puerperal ("childbed") fever, a postpartum infectious disease that led to the deaths of many young mothers, was spread by hand contact from physicians to patients. He showed that by proper handwashing alone, the incidence of puerperal fever could be markedly reduced. This was long before the first microbe was identified, or the germ theory of infection was suggested, much less accepted. Like Ignaz Semmelweis, who made similar observations in Vienna at the same time, Holmes had many opponents, who could not fathom why handwashing might prevent or cure a disease. (Semmelweis ended up in a mental asylum and committed suicide. Holmes, of more sanguine disposition, continued his life as a Harvard professor.) Holmes had discovered that doctors could prevent, rather than treat, diseases by certain methods. In fact, it might be argued that many more diseases have been prevented by epidemiological methods than cured by pharmacological ones.

Take tuberculosis: Antitubercular antibiotics, developed in the last 50 years, have many side effects and are sometimes ineffective. There is little doubt that the prevalence of tuberculosis began to decline long before those antibiotics became available or widely used. The main factor leading to this decline was the discovery that tuberculosis was much more prevalent in unsanitary, crowded living conditions, and, when those conditions were ameliorated, the disease began to abate. Consider poliomyelitis: There still is no cure for this condition. But it almost disappeared after a preventive vaccine was discovered and applied extensively in children.

The major diseases that plagued mankind throughout the 19th century have been mainly prevented by non-pharmacological means, rather than cured by medications, much as Holmes presaged. The result is that 21st century medicine is left with many conditions that are less preventable. The medical profession, having exhausted a great many of its epidemiological tools, is left with its other main tool of pharmacology.

If there is polypharmacy in psychiatry today, it is relevant to appreciate how current attitudes to psychotropic medications might be spurring their overuse. To do so, it is relevant to examine the history of how the psychiatric profession has viewed medications.

Medications were poor cousins to psychotherapies in psychiatry until the last few decades. In fact, medications designed for use in psychiatric illnesses were not systematically studied until the 1950s, and did not begin to enter relatively common use until the 1960s. Yet, from the humble beginnings, it is not much of an exaggeration to assert that the birth of psychopharmacology revolutionized the entire field of psychiatry by the 1970s. In the last two decades, psychopharmacology has so grown in stature that some psychiatrists are worried that the entire field of psychiatry is being reduced to psychopharmacology.

This outcome would have been unthinkable four decades ago. In the 1960s, psychopharmacology was still meekly knocking at the door of mainstream psychiatry, seeking to be given some recognition at the hands of most psychoanalytically oriented leaders in the profession. In that decade, many leading psychiatrists viewed medications as being relevant to practice only to the extent that they fostered the psychoanalytic process during counseling. Other psychoanalysts simply opposed medications *toute suite*, seeing them as useless at best, to the extent that they are superficial and symptomatic in their benefits, and harmful at worst, in that they may remove the anxiety or psychic pain that brings patients to, and keeps patients in, psychoanalytic psychotherapy.

Until the 1970s, so few effective medications and other treatments were available and proven that psychiatric treatment was left to psychoanalysis almost by default. Over time, the development of tolerable effective medications made psychopharmacology an irresistible force on its own, leading to a wholesale reorganization of psychiatric classifications in 1980, the DSM-III. By the 1980s, psychopharmacology was on the ascendant, and when the "decade of the brain" arrived (1990–2000), new generations of antidepressants and antipsychotic agents placed psychopharmacology on a throne of power it had never held before. In the process, medications became used more and more frequently, and in more combinations. Once any kind of medication treatment became acceptable, polypharmacy frequently became the rule.

To understand how the rise of psychopharmacology led to the ubiquity of polypharmacy, the ascendant path taken by psychopharmacology itself must be understood. In general, there are five factors associated with the rise of psychopharmacology that later led to frequent polypharmacy: scientific advances in biochemical research, and the economic (pharmaceutical industry), political (the FDA), cultural (the appetite for medications), and clinical (DSM-III and the revolution in psychiatric nosology) contexts.

The cultural component is large, and is discussed in the following chapter. The role of scientific advances in biochemical research in psychiatry is obvious. The most important factor may be the economic context, which heavily influences clinical nosology. It is a simple fact that, without medications, there would be no pharmacology and no polypharmacy. It is also a basic fact, granted by almost everyone, that many medications are quite helpful to persons with many illnesses, and that private enterprise (capitalism) is necessary to research, develop, and distribute many of those medications. Thus, economic factors drive pharmaceutical companies, which are for-profit industries like almost every industry in a modern capitalist economy. As a result, in a great many instances, economic factors influence the availability and use of medications in medicine, including psychiatry.

It is worth noting that, in the 1950s, when the pharmaceutical industry began to be interested in medications for psychiatric conditions, its interest was limited and inchoate. The psychotropic effects of the first psychiatric medications—chlorpromazine for schizophrenia and imipramine and iproniazid for depression—were first noted as side effects of attempts to use those agents to treat other medical conditions. (The only exception was lithium.) Therefore, it is not true to assert that the pharmaceutical industry was interested in producing psychiatric medications from the start; in fact, the industry was quite reluctant. But the patients were there: thousands and millions of psychotic and depressed and agitated patients who filled many psychiatric hospitals for decades in wards that sometimes were filthy and degrading. And the doctors were there, trained often in psychoanalysis, but realizing that their training helped them little in the treatment of severe mental illness and that it cured practically no one. It was individual psychiatrists, like Nathan Kline and Roland Kuhn, who observed the benefits of the first psychotropic agents and pressured the pharmaceutical companies to pursue more research with those medications. After a while, some pharmaceutical companies took note of the fact that there appeared to be many psychiatric patients diagnosed with schizophrenia in particular, and some with depression, and that these medications might not only help those persons but might also prove profitable. In that era, psychiatrists were diagnosing many patients with schizophrenia, ergo the original focus on that condition as regards medications. With time, clinicians and pharmaceutical companies also began to recognize the importance of depression, and much later, bipolar illness. Lithium, in fact, was not marketed or developed by any pharmaceutical company but rather by academic psychiatric researchers. Lithium is the exception to the rule suggested here: that the first step to the transformation of modern psychiatry was the entry of the pharmaceutical industry into the research and practice of psychiatry.

When chlorpromazine and imipramine were introduced, the pharmaceutical industry participated in funding the education of psychiatrists regarding the conditions of schizophrenia and depression. Conferences were held and books distributed that advanced ideas at odds with standard psychoanalytic thinking and more in line with traditional medical models of psychiatry. The new "psychopharmacologists" harked back to views held by psychiatrists before the rise of psychoanalysis, particularly the observations of Emil Kraepelin, Eugen Bleuler, and their followers, which divided all psychosis into "schizophrenia" and "affective disorders." The fact that the pharmaceutical industry provided such support for different views broke the monopoly of psychoanalytic thinking on psychiatry.

Another factor is political, related to economics, and less well recognized: the regulatory influence of the FDA. The FDA's role is complex and confusing. On the positive side, FDA performs a major service in ensuring, at a minimum, that new medications are safe and effective for the specific circumstances for which they are indicated. The Progressive movement in the United States influenced the public and politicians to recognize the need to regulate food (unclean meat-packing had led to much illness) and drugs (tetanus outbreaks had occurred due to unsanitary preparation of smallpox vaccines). The Food and Drug Act was passed in 1906, but a federal agency to enforce the act was not instituted until 1938, during the New Deal, when the FDA was created. The 1938 amendment specified that the FDA needed to declare a drug safe before it could be marketed, and it asserted FDA control over how a drug was to be advertised (e.g., banning false statements). Prescription-only drugs, introduced as a category before World War I, were made the province of FDA control in a 1951 amendment. Finally, in the major move that completed the evolution of current rules, a 1962 amendment specified that the FDA had to declare a drug effective, and not just safe, before it could be marketed. This last move came on the heels of the thalidomide disaster, when this drug, marked for sedating properties, was given to women during pregnancy, and resulted in limb deformities in exposed fetuses. Thus did the current state of affairs evolve: The federal government established an enforcement agency, the FDA, charged with identifying prescription-only medications, which could not be marketed unless they had proven their safety and efficacy to the FDA.

In 1962, the wording of the amendment was loose enough to leave open the details of what kinds of data would be required to prove a drug effective to the FDA's satisfaction. Over time, these standards have developed, and they somewhat differed among different branches of the FDA. The branch relevant to psychopharmacology, the Neuroscience branch, has evolved its own requirements over time. It appears that in 1962, the main change brought to the private market by the FDA was that drugs should establish efficacy based on randomized controlled trials. The principle of randomization was rather new and important in medicine.

Introduced in the early 1950s in psychiatry with trials of lithium and chlorpromazine, random assignment of patients to either receive or not receive the study medication became the hallmark of a clinical trial, as opposed to clinical observation. The problem with simple clinical observation, as Holmes and others had pointed out in the 19th century, was that it could be biased based on the wishes of the doctor or the patient. Furthermore, a doctor might choose a specific drug preferentially in less ill persons, thus making it seem effective. Randomized assignment to receive a drug or not would appear to take care of those biases. Thus, the randomized clinical trial was born in psychiatry in the 1950s, and codified as a necessary component of psychopharmacological research by the FDA in the 1960s.

Two further steps soon followed: randomized trials might still be biased if the doctor or patient knew who was getting the new, and potentially more effective, drug. The double-blind was introduced, to hide the active treatment from both. Furthermore, simply being in a clinical trial, and knowing that one would receive a potentially exciting new treatment, might lead to a placebo benefit for any medication. The placebo comparison became commonly required. The process of proving the efficacy of a drug and being allowed to market it in the United States went from loose guidelines focusing on a drug's safety to the requirement of randomized, double-blind, placebo-controlled clinical trials.

Another step, equally important, became more prominent in the 1950s and 1960s. With the new FDA amendments, a consensus arose that the FDA was not in the business of providing general approval for medications. Since efficacy was now required, this meant efficacy for diseases. By focusing on diseases rather than symptoms, the FDA was following the tradition of Holmes and Osler; at the same time, in psychiatry, this approach led to a presumption in favor of medical models of diagnosis as opposed to other models (such as the Freudian reluctance to diagnose).

This process—requiring proof of efficacy as well as safety, insisting on RCTs, and wanting a focus on specific diseases—proved rather expensive for pharmaceutical companies. As a result, research data at this level (randomized, double-blind, placebo-controlled) required extensive funding from either pharmaceutical companies or other sources. Other sources were limited, since private foundations were few, and the federal research branches (mainly the NIMH) tended to gear most of its funding to basic animal studies rather than clinical human drug studies, partly reasoning that clinical human studies already had sources of support in the pharmaceutical industry, whereas animal studies had fewer other sources of support. Thus, more clinical drug studies, over the years, have been conducted with private pharmaceutical research funding than with National Institutes of Health (NIH) funding. And, since the pharmaceutical funding is largely geared to FDA requirements, the FDA's rules for regulating the pharmaceutical industry have, de facto, comprised the entire content of most controlled clinical research in psychopharmacology, as well as the rest of medicine. These studies usually involve a single drug being compared to placebo, which is what is needed for FDA registration. A comparison to other drugs is infrequent, because it is not required for FDA approval. The absence of such head-to-head studies, though, leaves a major void in the scientific literature, since clinicians do not have definitive evidence to guide them when choosing among agents.

This brings us to the connection to polypharmacy. Psychiatrists do not know if one medication for an indication—say, depression—is better than another. If one does not work, they have little rigorous evidence that instructs them what to do next. They either switch to another agent by trial-and-error, or they add another agent by trial-and-error. Since the minority of persons respond sufficiently in the real world, in terms of both symptoms and function, to one agent for many conditions, polypharmacy ensues. Part of the reason for this polypharmacy stems from the lack of adequate data to inform clinicians about which specific drugs would be effective in which specific persons in which specific circumstances. Also, polypharmacy, when required, is often haphazard rather than data-based, simply because there are no data, and part of the reason for the lack of data is that research and funding is skewed toward registration studies, with their expensive simple design: double-blind, placebo-controlled, parallel group short-term treatment for a specific indication.

Polypharmacy has some deservedly pejorative connotations. These derive partly from the appropriate influence of medical leaders like Holmes, who led the field of medicine away from random therapeutics toward a more scientific approach to understanding, preventing, and treating disease. A follower of Holmes was William Osler, often credited with being the father of modern medicine. He was eminently likeable, had remarkable oratorical skill with a taste for the classics, and published a general textbook of medicine that went into many editions. Yet his reputation did not rest solely on these factors, nor on any specific experimental discoveries. Osler's main mark was in moving medical education and practice from the old apprenticeship model, which focused on experience and treatment, to a newer scientific model, focused on experiment and understanding disease. Osler, like Holmes before him, felt that his medical colleagues overemphasized drug treatments, which were largely useless, and needed to focus instead on the scientific understanding of diseases. He probably laid out the most accessible version of his philosophy on this subject in a lecture to his colleagues at McGill University in Montreal in 1895, titled "Teaching and Thinking: The Two Functions of a Medical School."

In that lecture, he first laid out the imperative of studying disease for the first two years of the medical curriculum, before any clinical work or contact with treatment.

> A man cannot become a competent surgeon without a full knowledge of human anatomy and physiology, and the physician without physiology and chemistry flounders along in an aimless fashion, never able to gain any accurate conception of disease, practising a sort of popgun pharmacy, hitting now the malady and again the patient, he himself not knowing which. (Osler, p. 197)

These words were still revolutionary in 1895, as they had been when Holmes intoned similar thoughts a generation earlier. Osler, like Holmes, felt that it was a sign of the advance of scientific medicine that fewer medications were being used. Polypharmacy was a characteristic of the pre-scientific era:

> With the diminished reliance upon drugs, there has been a return with profit to the older measures of diet, exercise, baths, and frictions, the remedies with which the Bithynian Asclepiades doctored the Romans so successfully in the first century. Though used less frequently, medicines are now given with infinitely greater skill; we know better their indications and contradictions, and we may safely say (reversing the proportion of fifty years ago) that for one damaged by dosing, one hundred are saved. . . . But know also, man has an inborn craving for medicine. Heroic dosing for several generations has given his tissues a thirst for drugs. As I once before remarked, the desire to take medicine is one feature which distinguishes man, the animal, from his fellow creatures. It is really one of the most serious difficulties with which we have to contend. Even in minor ailments, which would yield to dieting or to simple home remedies, the doctor's visit is not thought to be complete without the prescription. And now that the pharmacists have cloaked even the most nauseous remedies, the temptation is to use medicine on every occasion, and I fear we may return to a state of polypharmacy, the emancipation from which has been the sole gift of Hahnemann and his followers to the race. As the public becomes more enlightened, and as we get more sense, dosing will be recognized as a very minor function in the practice of medicine in comparison with the old measures of Asclepiades. (Osler, pp. 200–201)

To summarize, Oliver Wendell Holmes and William Osler exemplify the movement among leaders of medicine in the 19th century away from polypharmacy and towards more of an emphasis on understanding and preventing diseases.

Meanwhile, the evolution of psychiatry in the 20th century has been characterized by little understanding of the disease processes underlying major mental illnesses, and a plethora of treatments, mostly ineffective or only marginally so. Part of the reason for continued polypharmacy in psychiatry has had to do with the resistance of psychiatric diseases to yielding their secrets to biological research, but also to nosological and socioeconomic factors, including the insufficient scientific validity of the DSM system, as discussed in Chapter 16.

Polypharmacy is a reality in psychiatry, and often it reflects the unscientific nature of many aspects of the field, just as in medicine in general in the 19th century. And, in those cases, where possible, psychiatrists would be likely to benefit from heeding the advice of Holmes and Osler, focus on prevention or nonspecific measures of support, and recognize that "less is more." In other cases, polypharmacy in psychiatry reflects the state of research and knowledge in the field, partly driven by the structure of FDA-mandated rules and pharmaceutical companies' needs. When used in a manner that combines common sense with scientific evidence, polypharmacy can then be useful and effective in treating individual persons with complicated psychiatric syndromes.

SELECTED REFERENCES

Ghaemi, S. N, (Ed.). (2002). *Polypharmacy in psychiatry*. New York: Marcel Dekker.

Holmes, O. (1860; 1911). *Medical essays (1842–1892)* (pp. 173–208). Boston, MA: Houghton Mifflin Company.

Osler, W. (1895; 1951). Teaching and thinking. In G. L. Keynes (Ed.), *A way of life and other selected writings* (pp. 194–204). New York: Dover.

34
Cultural Aspects of Psychopharmacology

Benjamin Rush is generally considered to be the founder of American psychiatry. His likeness is on the seal of the American Psychiatric Association, and most psychiatrists are aware that he not only wrote the first psychiatric text in American medicine, but he also was a signer of the Declaration of Independence. For Oliver Wendell Holmes, Rush exemplified the "can-do" approach of American medicine, its optimism and activism, all of which predisposed Americans in particular to polypharmacy. Given that Rush is the role model of American psychiatry, Holmes' comments are even more relevant to understanding cultural aspects of polypharmacy in American psychiatry:

> There are . . . special American influences which we are bound to take cognizance of. . . . If I wished [a student] to understand the tendencies of the American medical mind, its sanguine enterprise, its self-confidence, its audacious handling of Nature, its impatience with her old-fashioned ways of taking time to get a sick man well, I would make him read the life and writings of Benjamin Rush. . . . Dr. Rush must have been a charming teacher, as he was an admirable man. He was observing, rather than a sound observer; eminently observing, curious, even, about all manner of things. . . . He taught thousands of American students, he gave direction to the medical mind of the country more than any other one man; perhaps he typifies it better than any other. It has clearly tended to extravagance in remedies and trust in remedies, as in everything else. (Holmes, pp. 192–193)

Introducing Rush thus ("the most conspicuous of American physicians"), Holmes leaves no room for doubt that the founder of American psychiatry was also the founder of American medicine. And he connects Rush's activist temperament to the tendency of American physicians to use medications aggressively.

Much of this activist tendency in psychiatric practice has been marked in the United States by a generally pragmatic approach. "Pragmatism" is a term that some DSM-IV leaders in particular emphasized as central to their perspective. Culturally, it has reflected an American willingness to experiment and try different approaches. It focuses on results in practice, and it has a utilitarian edge. In American psychiatry, the pragmatic attitude has manifested itself in two different epochs, the rise of Adolf Meyer's school of thought, and contemporary empirical psychiatry (exemplified in particular by DSM-III).

Meyer was a Swiss psychiatrist who had emigrated to the United States in the late 19th century and would later be chairman of the department of psychiatry at Johns Hopkins University Hospital for decades. Meyer taught and influenced more leaders in American psychiatry than probably any other single academic psychiatrist. Meyer had been thoroughly trained in neuroanatomy; he was also quite familiar with psychoanalysis. Unwilling to give up one or the other approach, Meyer advocated "psychobiology." In practice, Meyerians put much more emphasis on the "psycho-" than on the "-biology," partly because Meyer conceived of psychiatric syndromes as "reactions" to life events, in which a biological susceptibility interacted with environmental events to produce psychopathology. Since the biological aspects of life seemed unchangeable, Meyer, and his pragmatic and optimistic American students, focused on the changeable psychological and environmental aspects: "I am not particularly interested in data concerning which I have to accept the fact that the dice have already been cast and that life is practically nothing but the dance of factors largely settled by heredity and constitution" (Meyer, p. ix). Meyer avoided putting much emphasis on diagnosis and did not see diagnoses simply as diseases, as had Kraepelin and his school. "I put my emphasis on specificity. It is 'the story' that counts in a person" (Meyer, p. x). Meyer's approach is stamped all over the first two handbooks of psychiatric diagnosis, DSM-I (1952) and DSM-II (1968), which spoke of "manic-depressive reactions" rather than disorders or diseases.

Meyer did not write much about somatic treatments in psychiatry, but the gist of his pragmatic philosophy tended toward intervention and treatment. He certainly repeatedly criticized Kraepelin and the German schools for pessimistic resignation and a hands-off attitude to treatment ("therapeutic nihilism").

The proponents of DSM-III sought to make psychiatry more empirical, and much of this drive came from the need to diagnose entities that could be treated with the newly emerging psychotropic drugs. In retrospect, it could be concluded that what happened was that both Meyer and the DSM-III–oriented neo-Kraepelinians implemented an American pragmatic attitude to psychiatry that has tended to both polynosology and polypharmacy. The spirit of pragmatism, introduced to American psychiatry by Meyer, still lives in the world of contemporary psychiatry, and it is not Kraepelinian at all.

Kraepelin believed that the diagnoses he described probably corresponded to disease entities. He did not think that psychiatrists would be able to treat those disease entities until the etiologies were discovered. In this general approach, the reader might note that he was in the tradition of Osler and Holmes, what we might call the tradition of scientific medicine. As a result, as Karl Jaspers later noted, Kraepelin and his school were "therapeutically hopeless but kind." Kraepelin was no pragmatist. Meyer felt that the Kraepelinian emphasis on diagnosis and disease was not useful, and he introduced the pragmatic notion that each case should be examined for its specific characteristics, and action should be taken wherever possible. In Meyer's day, treatment consisted mainly of psychotherapies and rehabilitative services. With the arrival of the psychopharmacological revolution, the proponents of DSM-III combined these two historical sources. They returned to Kraepelin's emphasis on nosology and an implicit belief in disease entities underlying diagnoses, but they also retained Meyer's activist interest in intervening in each case wherever possible. By the 1980s, however, drugs were as easily available as psychotherapies for treatment, and today, insurance or governmental restrictions make drug treatment much easier than psychotherapies. Combining an activist approach to treatment with the easy availability of psychotropic drugs, and with the renewed focus on identifying many diagnoses, American psychiatry has reached a point where psychiatric practice consists of aggressive diagnosing and aggressive treating (mainly with medications).

One can now turn to a larger view of what predisposes American culture to polypharmacy in psychiatry, focusing less on the profession of psychiatry and more on the attitudes of the lay public, those who request and want medications. First, there is the question of "pharmacological Calvinism." This is a phrase that Gerald Klerman coined and that Peter Kramer has popularized. Kramer defines it as "our society's aversion to prescribed medication" (Kramer, p. 274). Klerman defined it as "a general distrust of drugs used for nontherapeutic purposes and a conviction that if a drug 'makes you feel good, it must be morally bad' " (Kramer, p. 274). As discussed in the prior chapter, in the 19th century, the leaders of American medicine worked quite hard at persuading their colleagues and the lay public to adopt a *more* skeptical attitude toward medications. Skepticism towards medications today is the result of the evolution of American medicine from the 19th century pragmatic attitude that fostered polypharmacy, to the 20th century scientific attitude that focused on understanding disease and preventing rather than curing diseases. In this sense, what Klerman identified was not an underlying Calvinistic attitude that is part of America's cultural fabric, but the hard-won evolution of scientific medicine.

Thus there probably is a part of the population that is conservative about taking psychotropic medications for vaguely philosophical reasons, and perhaps an almost Calvinistic guilt about not being in pain has something to do with it. But most Americans are naturally inclined to take medications, to intervene actively if they are ill or suffer from painful symptoms, and this inclination has mainly to do with the inherently pragmatic bent of the American mind.

Perhaps Klerman's point, which is slightly different from Kramer's, may explain the reluctance of some Americans to take medications specifically for mental symptoms. Some persons might be willing to take medications for physical symptoms but not mental ones, which presumably reflects the stigma associated with mental illnesses. In this sense, there may be an influence of a specifically *psychopharmalogical* Calvinism on American culture, rather than a greater distrust of medications per se.

Also, it should be noted that Klerman was referring to the distrust people might feel toward medications that make them feel better, whereas Holmes pointed out that people seemed to have a special inclination to take "noxious" substances that made them feel temporarily worse, in the apparent belief that such harsh medicine would eventually kill off the illness. There is a larger issue here, which has to do with pleasure and pain.

Kramer discussed this point in the context of the belief, prevalent in American schools of psychotherapy, that a certain amount of psychic pain (anxiety, depression) is necessary for psychotherapy to proceed with any benefit. In other words, "affect tolerance," the ability to tolerate some anxiety or depression, is an important part of a healthy personality and a necessary component of psychological growth. This was the skeptical perspective that many psychoanalytic leaders held in the 1960s, when faced with the claims of curative benefits with the new psychotropic drugs.

There is another way of looking at this topic that suggests that Americans might be particularly inclined to *take* at least some psychotropic drugs (like antidepressants and amphetamines). There is a sense in which some persons are inclined to take psychotropic medications that they feel will enhance their normal functioning, even if they do not suffer from a diagnosable illness. Even before the newer antidepressants, amphetamine stimulants were frequently used for this purpose. (This topic is discussed in more detail in the next chapter.)

There are other more straightforward cross-cultural differences in the propensity towards taking psychotropic drugs in the United States and allied Western cultures. In Asian cultures, for instance, pharmacology is more or less identified with polypharmacy. When a patient goes to the doctor, she expects to leave the office with not just one prescription, but three or four, preferably one being for a shot of some kind or other. Asian patients tend to take a "more is better" approach to medications. Also, herbal treatments in Asian culture are usually compounds of many active agents; polypharmacy in one pill. It is also notable that Middle Eastern culture, for one, is characterized by a high degree of somatization, as discussed in Chapter 31. Patients frequently are not able or willing to discuss mental symptoms in mental terms, and even diagnosed depression tends to be associated with more somatic symptoms than in the West. Taken together, these anecdotal observations on Asian and Middle Eastern culture suggest that the lay public in these civilizations prefers polypharmacy, and that it tends to prefer specific medications for symptoms; rather than the preference of Western medicine to avoid polypharmacy and to use medication for disease-complexes rather than symptoms.

At one level, 19th century Western medicine seems quite similar to the basic approaches taken today in Asia and the Middle East. And indeed, the Western lay public still has a tendency to use medications for symptoms, as can be seen with the large symptom-oriented non-prescription and herbal/alternative drug sectors of the economy. So perhaps there are more cultural similarities than differences here. Differences may be less at the level of the culture of the lay public than at the level of the culture of mainstream medicine. In the West, the mainstream medical establishment has evolved along the lines promoted by Holmes and Osler, and it has, to some extent, modified the views of the lay public accordingly. In Asia, this medical evolution has not happened, for better or for worse.

In sum, the cultural aspects of psychopharmacology are varied. The bulk of American medical and cultural history suggests that American culture is predominantly pragmatic and disposed toward taking psychotropic drugs. This natural inclination has been retarded by the evolution of 20th century scientific medicine, which has tended to limit pharmacology, but it has reasserted itself with the psychopharmacology revolution, and the attendant changes in the practice of psychiatry. Making diagnoses has become more important and more central to modern psychiatry, with a frequent implication of a specific pharmacological treatment to follow. The recognition of diagnoses and treatments is partially influenced by economic and political factors. And the pragmatic desire to help, and optimistic attitude toward action, has combined with these other factors to make psychiatrists and patients much more likely to use psychotropic medications than in the past.

SELECTED REFERENCES

Ghaemi, S. N. (Ed.). (2002). *Polypharmacy in psychiatry*. New York: Marcel Dekker.

Holmes, O. W. (1892). Currents and crosscurrents in medical science. In *Medical Essays (1842–1882)*. Boston: Houghton Mifflin, pp 173–208.

Jaspers, K. (1986). An autobiographical account. In E. E. L. Ehrlich & G. B. Pepper (Eds.), *Karl Jaspers: Basic philosophical writings*. Atlantic Highlands, NJ: Humanities Press.

Kramer, P. D. (1993). *Listening to Prozac*. New York: Viking.

Meyer, A. (1948). *The commonsense psychiatry of Dr. Adolf Meyer*. New York: McGraw-Hill.

35

Treatment versus Enhancement

THE CONCEPT OF "TREATMENT" IS BASED ON A "BIOMEDICAL" MODEL OF disease. In this model, illness represents a breakdown of the physical constituents of the body, leading to a functional loss of a capacity to perform typical activities of the organism. Applying the biomedical model, depression, for instance, represents an abnormality of the brain leading to a restriction of the ability of the individual to pursue the activities that will allow the achievement of the individual's goals in life. A proponent of this approach would hold that "treatment" is indicated to heal the brain and allow a resumption of normal functioning as compared to one's peers.

The proponent of the "enhancement" approach to the therapy of depression comes at the problem from other disease models. In one, advocated by the World Health Organization (WHO), an explicit rejection of the biomedical conception occurs: "Health is a state of complete physical, mental, and social well-being, and not merely the absence of disease or infirmity." This approach invokes an equivalence between health and happiness. Another model holds that disease represents some deviation from a statistical norm; for instance, hypertension is defined as a diastolic blood pressure above or equal to 95; thus a person with a diastolic blood pressure of 94 does not have disease. Similarly, depression might be defined as a mood state outside of the usual range of individuals in the relevant society. Another model that seeks to avoid the biomedical approach is a values-oriented or normative approach, wherein one defines disease by certain value-based judgments that rest on moral intuitions or beliefs, and are thus relative to one's ethical theories. Hence, depression may represent a mood state that is deemed unacceptable or harmful from an ethical perspective, because it is thought to interfere with certain accepted virtues or certain necessary ethical criteria for good living. Any of the alternative non-biomedical models imply the conclusion that therapeutic interventions in depression should seek to enhance the functioning of the individual, rather than simply permit redress of loss of functioning.

Traditionally, physicians have supported the "biomedical" model of disease and the consequent "treatment" approach to depression. In their description of the logic of clinical judgment, Pellegrino and Thomasma suggest ideas that could undermine the mainstream biomedically oriented argument. They state that clinical decision-making in medicine consists of three phases: First, there is observation and the collection of information; this is the art of medicine. Second, the collected data are understood on the basis of knowledge about syndromes, diseases, prognosis, and effectiveness of treatments; this is the science of medicine. Third, a treatment decision occurs on the basis of value judgments, made by the patient and the physician, which in turn depend on a number of factors (cultural, economic, interpersonal, ethical, and religious); this is the ethics of medicine. It is this last step, they suggest, that makes medicine what it is and no other activity. What characterizes medicine as opposed to pure science or pure humanities, they hold, is the fact that its goal is not knowledge for knowledge's sake, or art for art's sake, but the right *action* in the interest of the patient. This final end, action, is what characterizes the "ethical" nature of medicine. And it is this last step that could trip up the attempt to apply the treatment/enhancement distinction in depression. The distinction, it could be argued, is one of values, not data; ethics, not science; personal decisions, not health policy. If one were to adjudicate the treatment/enhancement distinction in depression on a case-by-case basis, one could make a good argument for enhancement, as follows: If one is unhappy, one will seek to become happy. If there is a medication that can make one happy, one will take it, as long as the degree of subjective unhappiness one is feeling must seem worse than the possible side effects or risks of medication.

Economic issues do not come up in this argument because it is approached as an individual ethical decision-making process, not as a larger moral decision with social implications. Assuming one can afford the medication, or that insurance will pay for it, the financial aspects do not enter the decision-making process. Moreover, arguments against enhancement that rely on a lack of scientific effectiveness for the proposed treatments hold little weight; if something has not been *proven* to work, it may still work for the individual. Thus, in any individual case, once the values of the participants become part of the decision-making process, enhancement may seem to be a viable therapeutic option.

It might be proposed that these arguments fail to refute each other clearly because they hold incompatible underlying theories of health and disease. The main reason why the treatment/enhancement distinction represents a philosophical dilemma rests on this problem.

This treatment/enhancement dilemma has been raised now only with Prozac and other SRIs for depression, as discussed previously, but increasingly with amphetamines for ADD. As discussed in Appendix IV, the validity of ADD could be questioned, at least in some settings. In adults, for instance, given the absence of any "hyperactivity," the experience of distractibility and executive disorganization is often seen through the lens of the diagnosis of ADD. It also could reflect being at the extreme of the normal trait of inattention. Instead of treating a disease, clinicians may be enhancing a normal trait. The abuse of amphetamines by the normal population would tend to support this hypothesis. College-age students commonly use amphetamine prescriptions given to their friends. Sometimes this use is for pure pleasure, but sometimes it is to help with academic work. Baseball players are diagnosed with ADD in about 10% of the major league professional population. The general population rate in adults is 3%. Thus, either playing baseball predisposes one to developing ADD, or this apparent elevation in "ADD" prevalence reflects an attempt to enhance attention in a sport that involves very advanced eye–hand coordination.

If SRIs and amphetamines were very benign, perhaps there would be no or little concern regarding their use for enhancement of mood or attention. Indeed, many clinicians who extensively prescribe these agents believe them to be benign. This perspective also is common among many patients. As discussed previously in this textbook, though, both SRIs and amphetamines have numerous real and potential risks, ranging from immediate side effects like sexual dysfunction and anxiety, to longer-term problems such as serotonin withdrawal syndrome, to potential long-term harms such as carcinogenicity and neurotoxicity. Though not proven definitively in the latter two concerns, some evidence exists to raise those questions, and safety has not been proven.

In the end, at least in the United States, medication decision-making is an individual choice between a clinician and a patient. Yet, besides important relevant financial and social aspects to such decisions, this chapter seeks to emphasize the need for paying careful attention to the ethical aspects to such decision-making. Clinicians and patients should think about whether they are applying an appropriate model of disease or non-disease, and whether they sufficiently appreciate the real and potential risks of the psychotropic medications used.

In the Hippocratic tradition, as discussed in Chapter 16, treatment of disease alone is supported, as opposed to treatment of symptoms, and certainly as opposed to enhancement of normal variations. The enhancement approach certainly lies outside the Hippocratic tradition. This fact does not mean that enhancement is unethical, only that it is outside of traditional medical practice. Like cosmetic surgery or cosmetic dermatology, individuals have rights to improve themselves physically or psychologically, if feasible. The economic costs of such improvement normally should be borne by the patients themselves, though, not larger society. And the risks of such enhancement need to be appreciated carefully. In surgery, in the hands of ethical physicians, such risks are understood and discussed extensively. In psychiatry, the reality of enhancement has tended to be denied, under a mask of treating diagnoses that may instead reflect enhancement in some cases. As a consequence, clinicians and patients have not had careful and cautious ethical discussion of the risks and benefits of enhancement with psychotropic drugs.

SELECTED REFERENCES

Kramer, P. D. (1993). *Listening to Prozac*. New York: Viking.

Pellegrino, E. D. & Thomasma, D. C. (1981). *A philosophical basis of medical practice*. New York: Oxford University Press.

36

The Pharmaceutical Industry

A TEXTBOOK ON PSYCHOPHARMACOLOGY THAT SEEKS TO BE COMPREHENSIVE should not avoid addressing important economic aspects of this field. Central to the field of psychopharmacology is the existence and role of the pharmaceutical industry. In recent decades, there has been extensive public debate about the role of the pharmaceutical industry in psychiatric and other medical practice. It would seem worthwhile to acknowledge this debate, and to examine some of the claims and counterclaims made, as well as to suggest some potential avenues for contributing to this debate in a constructive manner.

The question at hand is the role the pharmaceutical industry in clinical psychopharmacology. Clearly, a central role is the development and marketing of the medications that compose the field of psychopharmacology. There are both supporters and critics of the pharmaceutical industry in terms of its role at present and in the past. This chapter will examine different views about the pharmaceutical industry and its influence on clinical psychopharmacology, and strengths and weaknesses of those views.

Current views of the pharmaceutical industry might be summarized in four categories:

1. One view holds that it is malevolent, seeking profits at the expense of health. This view is prevalent among many popular books, and is central to what is sometimes called the "anti-psychiatry" movement.
2. The opposite view is that the pharmaceutical industry is benevolent. It produces drugs that save lives, with appropriate safeguards against harm. Whatever negatives exist are the same as with any aspect of a capitalist economic system.
3. The third view is neutral. The pharmaceutical industry, like all corporations, is neither simply benevolent nor malevolent. In a capitalist economic system, it is accepted that private companies can look out for their best interests, and in the big picture, this competition of interests produces the best social outcomes. This is the "free enterprise" argument. In this view, the industry should be regulated as little as possible.

4. A fourth view sees both malevolent and benevolent aspects to the pharmaceutical industry. It produces both helpful and harmful drugs. There are both honorable and dishonorable activities associated with the development and marketing of drugs. Like all companies in the capitalist system, the pharmaceutical industry should pursue its own interests, but because of its important impact on public health, it should be more regulated than most companies.

What follows are analyses of some claims and assumptions made by the first three viewpoints.

Regarding the free-market perspective, important deviations from free-market capitalism occur with large pharmaceutical companies ("Big Pharma"). Because of patent protection laws, government intervention is central to the ability to make profits for the pharmaceutical industry, and prices are fixed during the patent, as opposed to being developed through the economic system of supply and demand. Furthermore, extensive political lobbying of Congress and funding of candidates in elections is a reflection of the dependence of the pharmaceutical industry on a highly regulated market. The pharmaceutical industry has one of the largest political lobbying groups in Washington, D.C.

Proponents of the free market perspective often emphasize that drug development is extremely expensive. The usual figure cited is that it takes about $2 billion to bring a single drug to the market in the United States. This is because about 95% of potential drugs developed and studied in earlier phases of drug development never make it to FDA approval and enter the medical market in the United States. This high expense of drug development is the rationale for the high cost of drugs, according to this view. In most companies, the expense that is put into research and development of new drugs is only somewhat higher than the expense given to the advertising expenses of drugs that reach the market. Hence, it could be argued that the high prices of medications could be reduced if less money were spent on their promotional marketing.

Advocates of the free market approach emphasize that the pharmaceutical industry produces new drugs, not academic researchers. This is true, because the economic resources needed for drug development are not provided to academic researchers by the usual funding sources of federal government. This need not be the case, though, if government did put more money into research for new medications. Such a change in government policy in the United States and Europe is unlikely. The only other possible source for new drug development will continue to be private enterprise. Unfortunately, too often, medications are "me-too" drugs, meaning they repeat the same mechanism of other medications already on the market. They are developed for profit primarily, and have little impact on improving public health compared to medications already available. Sometimes this is not the case, and new drugs can have fewer side effects in various ways that are useful. Frequently, the differences between newer drugs with the same mechanism of older drugs are quite minor, however.

Instead, truly new drugs with novel mechanisms often are developed by small pharmaceutical companies, and then are later bought by large pharmaceutical companies for marketing and distribution. In other words, innovation occurs in the private enterprise setting, but less often in large than small pharmaceutical companies. This situation may be changing, as Big Pharma has reached the end of patent life of many psychotropic drugs that were lucrative in prior decades. This claim also was not true in the 1950s and 1960s, when large pharmaceutical companies were central for developing truly innovative psychiatric medications such as the first antidepressants and antipsychotics. At that time, these drugs were opposed by most academic leaders in psychiatry, who were supporters of psychoanalytic theory and opposed biological treatments such as medications. The pharmaceutical industry was central to helping psychiatry become more open to new ideas about medications, and these medications changed the nature of psychiatry in the late 20th century. This change was driven by the pharmaceutical industry, despite opposition from most psychiatrists in the university setting, at least in the United States. Therefore, while pharmaceutical industry is central for innovative research on new drugs in psychiatry, it has not played that role as extensively in recent years as it did in the middle of the 20th century.

Although promotional marketing can be seen as excessive, as mentioned, critics of the pharmaceutical industry often do not appreciate that another reason for possible overuse of drugs involves demand,; namely, the desire of the public to take medications. As discussed in Chapter 32, this social factor had been known long before modern pharmaceutical companies existed, and was well described by William Osler in the 19th century.

The controversies regarding the pharmaceutical industry therefore are neither simple in nature nor simple in solutions. Some have argued for complete disengagement between academia and the pharmaceutical industry. While such an approach would solve the problem of conflicts of interest, it would impoverish both groups, since the development of new drugs that are truly helpful to people requires both academic expertise and the resources of the pharmaceutical industry. Instead, a collaboration that is ethical is needed. In this respect, a reduction of promotional marketing would make sense, as well as limited to no interaction of a purely promotional fashion between academia and the pharmaceutical industry. Some practices of dubious ethical nature should be stopped, such as "ghost authorship," where academic authors of research papers are not those who actually created and conducted a pharmaceutically sponsored research study.

Furthermore, the almost complete disengagement of government funding agencies from psychopharmacological research should be reversed, and there should be more support from funding sources from the government, as in the NIMH in the United States, so that psychopharmacology researchers would not be dependent solely or primarily on the pharmaceutical industry. There is precedent for this larger role of the NIMH in psychopharmacology research, such as in the classic studies cited throughout this textbook that have proven so important to clinical practice: large multicenter grants given in the 1990s by the NIMH for treatment trials of schizophrenia (CATIE), bipolar illness (STEP-BD), and unipolar depression (STAR*D). The results of these studies are groundbreaking, refuting some common treatment assumptions, and are likely to play out for over a decade in psychiatric practice. Yet there are no follow-ups to these large NIMH-funded clinical studies, if current policy continues, for the next few decades and more. Now, only about 10% of the NIMH budget is used for clinical trials, only a portion of which involves medications. That's at most $100 million yearly, compared to $60 billion yearly in pharmaceutical industry research spending.

Clinicians themselves also need to do what they can to maximize a positive role for the pharmaceutical industry in the practice of clinical psychopharmacology. As discussed throughout this text, and especially in Chapter 16, the status quo clinical psychopharmacology practice too often is simply a matter of giving pills for symptoms. It has been estimated that about 80% of psychiatrist office visits in the United States are associated with the handing over of a prescription. Clinicians practice what Osler called a "penny-in-the-slot" practice, immediately meeting each symptom with a drug. Clinical psychopharmacology practice has not taken the approach recommended in this textbook of focusing on treating diseases, not symptoms. The Hippocratic tradition frowns on symptom management because it causes more harm than good, and it underpins a sensibility that all drugs are harmful, and that they should not be presumed safe until proven harmful, but vice versa. The overuse of medication is not merely a problem of supply, i.e., by the pharmaceutical industry, but also a problem of the demand, from clinicians as well as patients. All sides need to move closer to the practice pattern that is both more conservative but also more scientifically informed.

SELECTED REFERENCES

Ghaemi, S. N. (2013). Postmodern medicine: An analysis of the pharmaceutical industry and its critics. *Perspectives in Biology and Medicine*, *56*, 223–235.

Wootton, D. 2006. *Bad medicine: Doctors doing harm since Hippocrates*. Oxford, UK: Oxford University Press.

37

Drug Discovery

Future Treatments

THE CURRENT RANGE OF MEDICATIONS AVAILABLE FOR THE TREATMENT of psychiatric conditions is more limited in its effectiveness and safety than might be desirable. The "Seventh Truth of Psychopharmacology" is an unfortunate fact: The most effective psychotropic medications available tend to be the oldest ones. Newer medications in the last two decades have not been more effective than prior generations of medications; they have been more tolerable. This improved tolerability is a benefit, but equal or diminished efficacy is a concern.

These points can be examined with each major clinical condition. The most effective treatment for schizophrenia is clozapine, which was introduced to the European market in the 1960s. The most effective treatment for the acute depressive episode is electroconvulsive therapy (ECT), which was developed in the 1930s. The most effective drug treatments for the acute depressive episode are the MAOIs, which were developed in the 1950s. The most effective treatment for bipolar illness is lithium, which was discovered in 1949 and introduced to the U.S. market in 1970.

In short, since the 1970s, psychotropic medications have not been more effective than their predecessors. The important changes seen with newer medications in the 1980s and 1990s have to do with tolerability: second-generation dopamine blockers had fewer EPS than their predecessors, and the SRIs had fewer side effects and overdose risk than their predecessors. These tolerability benefits are important, but it is important to note that these agents were not more effective than their predecessors, and in fact often were less effective.

This observation is important when considering what should be done for the future to produce safer and more effective medications for psychiatric illnesses. This topic is usually called "drug discovery," and it generally is the province of the private pharmaceutical industry. The pros and cons of the role of the pharmaceutical industry in psychopharmacology are discussed in the previous chapter. The focus here will be on the process of drug discovery in academia and the pharmaceutical industry, its current state of affairs, and prospects for the future.

A major distinction that needs to be made regarding any future psychotropic medications has to do with determining whether those agents are disease-modifying or merely symptomatic palliation. While there is always some benefit to be gained from medications that are somewhat more tolerable, the development of more purely symptomatic drugs for psychiatric conditions does not meet any important medical need. Currently there are dozens of symptomatically effective medications for depressive states, manic states, and schizophrenic exacerbations. However, there are very few medications that are disease-modifying for these conditions. It could be argued that there are no medications that are disease-modifying for recurrent unipolar depression and schizophrenia. Lithium and perhaps a few anticonvulsants appeared to be disease-modifying for bipolar illness. Hence the major unmet need in the treatment of these conditions is to develop disease-modifying drugs for all of them.

Since the drug discovery process usually occurs in the private pharmaceutical industry setting, it tends to be heavily influenced by commercial and economic judgments that have to be made by private companies in a capitalist environment. The primary goal of such companies is to obtain profits. If it is easier to obtain profits one way rather than another, the economic motivation will tend in the former direction rather than the latter. It often appears to be the case that the development of symptomatic agents that are similar to other agents already on the market is an easy course of action from a purely commercial perspective. These "me-too" drugs can be developed easily by chemists who work for the firm's industry by making minor adjustments to the chemical structure of already known effective compounds. These minor chemical adjustments can produce some differences in tolerability, but rarely major differences in efficacy.

To develop new agents that are more effective, the pharmaceutical industry would have to shift to identify new disease-modifying drugs, rather than following the pharmacological mechanisms of agents already on the market. The process of identifying disease-modifying medications is complicated and unclear. Current methods can be divided into two large categories: genetic or pathophysiological.

In the genetic approach, researchers examine genes that have been associated with psychiatric illnesses, and then analyze what those genes do, so as to develop drugs that affect the physiological mechanisms produced by those genes. This process would appear to be quite rational, but there are many steps in which it can be unpredictable. The genes associated with serious psychiatric conditions tend to be related to diseases like schizophrenia, bipolar illness, and severe depression. Yet even those highly genetic states are polygenic, which means that many genes of small effect together produce the illness. There are no genes of large effect that can be targeted. Hence, even with the immense amount of money and effort put into genetic research such as the Human Genome Project, the results are not straightforward. Those studies identifying dozens of "SNPs" (single-nucleotide polymorphisms) for schizophrenia and bipolar illness, for instance. Each of those SNPs represents hundreds of specific genes. Also, the SNPs identified, even when replicated, have relatively small effect sizes in association with those diseases. Hence, even with this most well-established and popular research, hundreds of specific genes are identified, and even in the strongest associations, they have mild effects in increasing the risk of those diseases. Drug researchers would have to pick only one of those genes to identify and target in drug development. There is no rational way to choose one out of a hundred such genes. It is basically a guess, and statistically it is highly likely to be wrong. Even after making this guess, the process of drug development would take years and involve extensive funding, despite a low statistical likelihood of success. In short, the probability of effective and successful new drug development based on genetic targeting of psychiatric diseases is quite low.

The second approach is pathophysiological. This method would focus on research that identifies certain pathophysiological patterns with specific psychiatric conditions, and try to develop drugs that would affect those pathophysiologies. An example is the association of circadian rhythm abnormalities with bipolar illness. Specific aspects of the biology of circadian rhythms could be targeted in developing new drugs that might then influence bipolar illness. Another example is the association of elevated inflammatory cytokines with depressive states: anti-inflammatory treatments could be targeted as potentially being disease-modifying for depressive illness. A potential problem with this approach is that a single disease can have multiple pathophysiologies, and the choice of one pathophysiological pattern could be wrong. Another limitation can be the fact that animal models often are needed to identify and test the effects of drugs on biological pathways, but there is some skepticism about the validity of many of the animal models used for psychiatric conditions. For instance, a standard animal model for depression in mice is the swim test. In this model, mice are placed in water, and after swimming for some time, they give up, and swim less. If they swim less than other mice, this behavior is viewed as being akin to depression in humans in the sense that decreased motor activity reflects a loss of motivation. Some researchers criticize this model because they claim that one cannot know that the mice are "sad." This is a mistaken criticism when one understands that mood states, like sadness, are not central to the clinical phenomenon of depression. Rather, as noted elsewhere, depression reflects a slowing down of thinking, movement, and feeling. Decreased motor activity in mice could correlate with clinical depression thus defined. A standard animal model for potential antipsychotic medications is the catalepsy model. In this type of study, medications given to mice will cause stiffness or rigidity. Such agents can then be determined to have antidopamine effects, which tend to translate in humans into benefits for psychotic symptoms. Unfortunately, using such models, all antipsychotic drugs that are developed will have EPS.

Current drug discovery research has moved away from animal models and has become very oriented to genetic studies. An immense amount of funding is being spent both in academia and in private industry on genetic studies. Little work is being done on developing new and better animal models. If this analysis is correct, effective drug development would benefit from more balance in the current distribution of resources.

THE IMPORTANCE OF CLINICAL RESEARCH AND THE OBSTACLE OF THE DSM

Another important aspect to improve drug discovery in the future is a recognition of the importance of clinical research and the role of DSM diagnosis as an impediment to successful drug development. Chapter 16 discusses in detail the limitations of DSM from a scientific perspective, and provides the evidence for the statement that the DSM is not developed primarily from scientific evidence. Therefore, it does not help scientific research. Since it is based primarily on social-constructionist needs of the profession, it does not correlate with biological features of the outside world such as genes or pharmacological mechanisms. Hence a major problem with drug development in the pharmaceutical industry is that the use of DSM constructs will doom certain drugs or drug classes. A great deal of basic neuroscience research can be done to develop a drug with good pharmacological features and even strong pathophysiological effects. If that drug is then given to a group of patients who are defined clinically using scientifically invalid definitions, it probably will not work, since it will not be given to a biologically meaningful clinical sample.

Often it is said that the pharmaceutical industry must use DSM constructs because FDA registration cannot be obtained otherwise for the commercial marketing of medications. This is not the case. The FDA has stated that it is open to non-DSM clinical constructs, as long as there is a scientific consensus in the clinical and academic community about such definitions. The latter issue may be a bigger problem than the FDA. The psychiatric profession has not yet appeared ready to give up DSM constructs, thus academic leaders advise the FDA in a way that will limit the ability to use non-DSM definitions for the marketing of new medications. In the future, a key factor in developing more effective drugs that are disease-modifying will be persuading the academic psychiatric community to become more flexible in its diagnostic thinking outside of DSM restrictions.

Related to this point, it is important to emphasize that the development of more effective drugs in the future will require more funding and effort put into clinical research, as opposed to basic neuroscientific or genetic research. The vast majority of funding of the NIH goes to basic biological and genetic research (which means either research on animals or research on humans that involve biological factors, e.g., neuroimaging or genetics), with little funding given for clinical treatment research in humans (only 10% of the yearly NIMH budget). Similarly, the vast majority of funding in the pharmaceutical industry is directed to basic chemical and neuroscientific research, with little effort put into clinical diagnostic or psychopathological research. Neuroscientific and genetic research is published in the most prominent journals, and is often communicated immediately to the public in press releases. Clinical research on human beings related to symptoms and diagnoses tends to be published in lower-tier journals with little public attention. A bibliometric study of the top psychiatric journals in the United States found that 50% of published articles involve basic biological research (mainly genetics and neuroimaging), and 50% of published studies are related to clinical research on human beings regarding symptoms, diagnosis, or treatment. This result contrasted with the top internal medicine journals, where only 20% of published studies were biological in content, while

80% involved clinical studies of human beings regarding symptoms, diagnosis, or treatment. In other words, the field of internal medicine supports clinical and non-biological research more than mainstream psychiatry.

If the clinical phenotypes of pharmacological research are invalid or poorly studied and little understood, then the best and most subtle neuroscientific research will not be able to match up with those clinical phenotypes in a way that will produce good clinical trials demonstrating effective new medications.

Effective new drug discovery cannot be a one-sided process, focused almost solely on neuroscience and genetics. A large increase in funding and effort needs to be put into research on valid scientific clinical diagnosis and the symptoms of psychopathology, as well as studies of better methods of assessing treatment outcomes in the clinical setting.

In short, contrary to the widespread perception that psychotropic medications in the last few decades have been better than their predecessors, it appears to be the case that psychopharmacology research has stalled since the 1970s in terms of producing more effective medications. It is suggested here that future drug discovery research should focus on developing disease-modifying medications, but such work will not succeed if the field of drug discovery continues with its current approach of emphasizing genetic and neuroscience research almost exclusively. It is recommended that much more attention be given to clinical research in humans on diagnosis and psychopathology, and further, that the DSM definitions, often based on limited or no scientific evidence of validity, should be discarded in the interests of developing truly more effective medications in the future.

SELECTED REFERENCES

Kendler, K. S. (2005). "A gene for . . .": The nature of gene action and psychiatric disorders. *American Journal of Psychiatry, 162,* 1243–1252.

Stone, K., et al. (2012). A comparison of psychiatry and internal medicine: A bibliometric study. *Academic Psychiatry, 36,* 129–132.

SECTION VI

The Art of Psychopharmacology

38

The Diagnostic Interview

THE "FIRST TRUTH OF CLINICAL PSYCHOPHARMACOLOGY" IS THAT TREATMENT is only as good as the diagnosis. Good psychopharmacology practice depends on accurate diagnosis, which in turn depends on an effective clinical interview. This chapter examines how to conduct a diagnostic interview.

PSYCHOPATHOLOGY FIRST, THEN DIAGNOSIS

The basic order in which one should assess a case is psychopathology, then diagnosis, then treatment. One cannot know the diagnoses until the symptoms are established; that's why psychopathology goes first. Experienced clinicians do not begin with diagnoses in mind; they begin with a search for symptoms. Then they later organize their understanding of those symptoms into potential diagnostic groupings. If a diagnosis then fits the psychopathology, they can begin to think about and discuss treatment options. These days, the psychopathology step is usually skipped, as clinicians immediately seek to apply DSM diagnostic groups. The existential tradition in psychiatry always began with trying to understand the patient's experiences, to see if they represent psychopathological symptoms, and only then, in some cases, to proceed to a diagnosis. This diagnostic interview discussion will focus on assessment of mood symptoms, but a similar approach would apply to anxiety or delusional or other symptom groups.

BEFORE THE INTERVIEW: ASK FOR FAMILY AND FRIENDS TO BE PRESENT

Usually, when clinicians go to the waiting room to find their patient, someone else is there, a family member or friend. About half the time, that other person remains seated. Most clinicians don't invite that person to join the interview. They should. Not only that, it is wise to inform patients before their first interview that they should seek to bring a family member or friend along with them. This is for two reasons: first, family members and friends can corroborate the history or, in the case of mania or psychosis, actually provide accurate history; whereas patients, due to lack of insight, often invalidly deny the presence of some features of their personal history, especially manic or hypomanic episodes or delusional experiences. Second, when discussing treatment options, the presence of others in the office improves the likelihood that the treatment plan will be understood and implemented; frequently, patients are depressed and cannot clearly understand the complex treatment options being described—family members can hear and later repeat to the patient what was said. Furthermore, if family members aren't present, the patient will later have to explain what is said to them; it is better for the family to hear what clinicians have to say directly from the clinician, rather than secondhand.

If there are concerns about certain confidential topics (which do not often directly impact on the diagnostic interview anyway), family can be asked to leave the room for a few minutes in the middle of the interview, and then invited to return toward the end when clinicians provide diagnostic impressions and treatment recommendations.

BEGIN WITH DEPRESSION

In the setting of the differential diagnosis of an affective illness, the presenting complaint usually is depression. As the psychotherapeutic saying goes, it is best to "meet patients where they are"; so clinicians should start with the non-controversial and straightforward determination of the presence of clinical depression.

At one level, a clinician simply identifies depression to get beyond it. In other words, it often is easy to know that a patient has a current clinical depression—it may only take five minutes to quickly review current neurovegetative symptoms—but that is not the end of the evaluation, only the beginning. This is because depression is not a diagnosis, but only a constellation of signs and symptoms. Diagnoses are bipolar depression, secondary depression, or unipolar depression—with unipolar depression signifying that the bipolar and secondary diagnoses have been ruled out. Even then these diagnoses are insufficient: further subtyping is needed, into melancholia; mixed states; or vascular, neurotic, or pure depressive subtypes. This process goes beyond simply identifying "depression"; more detail is needed.

After subtyping the depressive states, clinicians need to shift the focus to identifying past mania or hypomania and assessing possible secondary causes (mainly medical). Obviously, an assessment of concurrent psychotic symptoms can be diagnostically and therapeutically relevant, and an evaluation of suicidality is necessary; but soon after identifying depression, the clinician should shift the focus to the more onerous task of looking for past mania or hypomania, and possible secondary causes.

ASSESS THE COURSE OF DEPRESSIVE ILLNESS

Before doing so, however, it is important to emphasize something that is rarely done: *evaluate the course of the depressive illness.* The reader will recall that the course of depression, unlike the details of current depressive symptoms, *can* differentiate between bipolar and unipolar conditions, as well as help identify secondary depression. Too often, clinicians simply say "The patient has major depression," as if that were enough to make a diagnosis. They have no idea when the depressive episodes began, how many there have been, how long they have lasted, precipitating factors, inter-episode symptoms, and so on.

The course of depressive illness is important diagnostically: age of onset, number of episodes, duration of major depressive episodes, and inter-episode status. Clinicians should ask patients how far back they can remember having depression for the first time, refreshing their memory as to the definition of a full depressive episode (daily depressed mood or anhedonia with multiple neurovegetative symptoms; day in and day out; most of the day; nearly every day; for weeks on end or more).

Then clinicians should ask how long depressive episodes have lasted in the past. Here patients usually throw up their hands and claim ignorance, but patients' guesses are better than those of clinicians. Patients need to be persuaded to make their best estimates about the course of the illness. Usually they can give an average duration for depressive episodes; it need not be precise—and if they are especially exasperated, clinicians can offer some options, like a multiple-choice test: Did the depressive episodes last more than a month, less than a month, about six months, over a year? These are the time-frames that are diagnostically relevant, since unipolar depression lasts six months to a year or longer, while bipolar depression is shorter, usually three to six months or less. Also, clinicians should ideally assess the durations in untreated periods to understand the natural unmedicated history, but if a patient has been non-responsive to medications, then treated periods can reflect the natural history of the illness.

Next clinicians should ask how many episodes the patient has had: "How many times in your life have you felt very depressed like that?" Usually, if currently depressed, patients overestimate their past depression: "Forever," is the common desperate answer. "Really?" one could reply, "All your life, every day, day in and day out, without ever having one day of being different, forever?" Usually, they back off at that point. "So how many times?" "I don't know, Doc." Again one can offer multiple-choice answers: "Just once? A few times? More than five times? More than 10 or 20 times?" Sometimes it is obvious in the history that the patient has had many episodes, more than 10 or 20; in that case, the exact number matters little. What does matter diagnostically is that if a patient has had one or two or three episodes, this is common in unipolar depression and uncommon in bipolar disorder. Having many episodes is more common in bipolar illness, especially if they are brief (less than three months in duration).

Finally, once you have identified the ballpark number of episodes, clinicians should determine if there were periods of wellness between episodes. This is usually not difficult; either patients will claim they are always depressed, which may reflect inter-episode dysthymia or subclinical depression, or they have periods of euthymia, which they or their family can clearly describe: "Were there ever times when you were not depressed and were your normal self, or normal like everyone else, in your mood energy, for weeks or months on end or longer?"

These periods of relative wellness also are an opportunity to delve into the important task of identifying affective temperaments. Frequently, patients will say they have "always" been depressed, or manic, or both. They tend to mean that they always have some mood *symptoms*, which is not the same as always having mood *episodes*. Outside of the full episodes, in those cases, mood symptoms may be present all the time as part of the affective temperaments of dysthymia, cyclothymia, or hyperthymia. The self-report TEMPS scale (Temperament Scale of Memphis, Pisa and San Diego) can be an invaluable aid at this point in the evaluation (preferably short versions such as the 50-item scale).

SPEND MORE TIME ASSESSING PAST MANIA OR HYPOMANIA

In the typical interview, it might have taken 10 minutes to establish that the patient has a current clinical depressive episode, and to subtype its specific nature. Another 5 minutes can assess baseline affective temperament. Another 10 minutes should establish the depressive course of illness. At this point, one has gone about halfway through a 50-minute interview. Next, one should take as much time as needed (up to 15 minutes or more) to examine the ins and outs of possible past mania or hypomania. Unfortunately, this part of the interview is often conducted with only a single question or hurriedly. The clinician should take his or her time, and come at the question slowly and in a roundabout fashion, so as to avoid patients' natural defensiveness about the stigma of bipolar illness. As important, family members who are present should be queried separately from the patient. If all questions are clearly denied by family and the patient, then this part of the interview may not need to be extensive. Often, though, the matter is complex, and more time and effort are needed to assess possible past manic or hypomanic episodes.

It is helpful to begin with an open-ended question, especially if clinicians have established a period of normal or euthymic mood in the past in the assessment of the course of depressive illness: "Did you ever feel the opposite of depressed, where you were not sad and down and depressed, but you also weren't just your normal self?" With equivocal responses, one might get more specific: "Did you ever have times where you were more energetic than normal, compared to when you were not depressed, or more energetic than most people around you, so that you were doing lots of things or not sleeping much and not feeling tired?" Or perhaps: "Did you ever have periods where you were angry and irritable but not depressed, and full of energy, doing lots of things?"

When examining a change from baseline, it is important to have established the presence or absence of an affective temperament already. For instance, if someone has hyperthymia, they will deny any change in baseline for manic episodes, because they always experience manic symptoms. In such cases, the questioning should begin with the manic baseline, and ask about further worsening beyond that state. Similarly, if someone always has dysthymia, depressive episodes should not be diagnosed unless they are clear worsening periods different from the depressed baseline.

If a somewhat positive response is elicited, or if the patient comes to the appointment with possible past mania as a clinical question, clinicians can ask an open-ended question, so as not to direct the patient toward manic criteria, but seeking to get their own words about it: "Tell me about how you felt, and how you behaved, or what people told you about how you were, during that time (when you felt hyper or more energetic than usual or where you or your doctor or others said you might be manic or hypomanic)?"

Then, importantly, clinicians should *write down what the patient says verbatim.* It is very important to do this. Bipolar illness is such a controversial topic, with patients getting different opinions from different doctors, that it is important to avoid miscommunication by letting the patients speak for themselves. Consider if clinicians write: "The patient had elevated mood, with decreased need for sleeping, flight of ideas, distractibility, and increased goal-directed activity for five days." The patient may disagree and go to another clinician, who is skeptical about the bipolar diagnosis, and that clinician might simply disbelieve the first clinician's interpretation of what the patient had said. But no one could deny mania if clinicians write: "The patient stated that he would feel 'hyped up and like I could do anything, I was a tyrant, felt I was smarter than everyone else, like there was nothing I couldn't do, I didn't need to sleep for days on end yet I was full of energy, I was giddy at times, my thoughts were all over the place, I couldn't keep up with them, I would wake up in the middle of the night and clean the house five times over, then the next day I would paint the house inside and outside even though it was perfectly fine, and a week later I would do it again with a different paint color."

Once a manic or hypomanic episode is identified, the diagnostic process is over: the diagnosis of bipolar illness has been made. If mania or hypomania cannot be identified, the interview is still not over; then the absence of mania/hypomania needs to be confirmed by third parties. This is done most efficiently if family or friends are present at the interview; if they are not present, the clinician should call, or ask the family to call, to quickly review mania criteria over the phone. Sometimes clinicians can make this phone call during the patient interview; sometimes later.

EXAMINE CAUSES OF SECONDARY DEPRESSION

These causes are most often medical, though they can also be psychosocial. It is important to distinguish between a trigger and a cause. A trigger is the final event that leads to the episode, but it is not the sole or even the main cause of the episode. This is similar to what Aristotle called "the efficient cause." Sometimes there is a certain trigger, sometimes another trigger, and sometimes no trigger. Clinicians should not focus on triggers, though they may be somewhat relevant later, especially in psychotherapy; they are irrelevant diagnostically.

Unfortunately, most patients, and many clinicians, focus on the most recent psychosocial triggers as if they were absolute causes of episodes. This is a big mistake. The best way to think about this problem is to recognize that the brain is a rationalizing machine. The classic split-brain experiments in epilepsy show how: In patients with intractable seizures requiring corpus callosotomy (severing the two hemispheres of the brain from each other), one creates a circumstance where the right hemisphere might note something and yet not be able to transfer that information to the left hemisphere, where verbal control is located. Since the left visual field is transmitted to the right hemisphere, researchers can place the right visual field behind a blindfold, and show pictures in the left visual field, such as violent and anxiety-provoking images. The right hemisphere sees these pictures, and the patient feels scared and nervous. When asked why, the patient says: "Well, my neighbor had a car accident last week and I was thinking about that?" or "I was thinking about the recent war in the Middle East." In other words, the patient cannot verbalize why he suddenly feels anxious or scared, yet he comes up with an explanation, any explanation, as long as it is plausible, even though it is wrong. People do this all the time: so when patients say they are depressed because of x, y, and z happening in their lives—they may be right, and they may be wrong: clinicians cannot take those explanations at face value as true.

True psychosocial causation—secondary depression due to a psychosocial cause—should be obvious and should be placed in the context of a non-recurrent course of illness: The patient may have one episode after a horrible psychosocial trauma, or maybe two episodes after two horrible psychosocial traumas; but most people, fortunately, do not have many isolated psychosocial traumas (or if they are the victim of recurrent abuse, they usually experience prominent post-traumatic symptoms rather than simply major depressive episodes alternating with euthymia). If recurrent major depressive episodes occur, the psychosocial factors should be seen as triggers, not causes.

The role of substance abuse should be seen in the same way as a psychosocial stressor. If a patient never had mania, then takes cocaine for the first time in her life, and then has a manic episode, one can call that condition cocaine-induced mania. But if she has experienced many manic episodes and many periods of cocaine use, it would seem difficult to demonstrate a one-to-one correlation so as to justify the diagnosis of mood disorder secondary to cocaine use. Often the situation is the reverse: cocaine use frequently occurs in those settings as the result, rather than the cause, of manic episodes.

The same is the case with medical factors. One might have no past depression, then have a stroke, and then experience a major depressive episode. That is post-stroke depression. Most individuals do not experience repeated strokes (since most persons get treated) followed by depressive episodes after every stroke. On the other hand, mild hypothyroidism may be a factor in contributing to recurrent depressive episodes.

Unlike the previous scenarios, there is a kind of secondary depression that, when present, is *sui generis*. Perhaps the most important secondary cause of clinical depression is "vascular" depression. As discussed in Chapter 19, this condition consists of small microvascular cerebral infarcts, visible on MRI, usually the consequence of hypertension and/or diabetes. This type of depression is common in middle and older age, and has a poor prognosis.

TREATMENT HISTORY

The rest of the history involves obtaining treatment history, family history, and other aspects of a standard medical evaluation. This chapter will not examine these topics in detail except to say that treatment history and family history should be examined in more detail than is commonly the case. For treatment history, for instance, the relevant factors needed are not only the names of the medications, but the durations of treatment, doses if available, and concomitant medications used. For each medication, one should assess efficacy and side effects and the reason for discontinuation. Whatever the patient can recall should be documented as well as possible.

At times, patients claim they cannot remember details and are often over-concerned with being exact. For instance, when clinicians ask how long they took a certain drug, they become exasperated because they cannot remember if it was 2 months, 3.5 months, or 4.25 months. Since they can't be precise, they will just say they don't remember. Clinicians can then give them multiple-choice options: "Was it less than one month, more than one month, more than one year, more than ten years?" Obviously this forces them to say something, and clinicians can get some valuable data, such as the idea that they took the drug for somewhere between one and six months.

However long it was used, clinicians should ask about whether other medications were taken with a drug. Often patients can say that other medications were taken, but they do not remember which ones. It is just as important to know that they did *not* have monotherapy trials, especially with mood stabilizers in bipolar disorder, than to know the details of the other medications they received. Clinicians can then ask whether they thought the medication trial was effective or not, and whether they had side effects. People usually remember side effects more clearly than efficacy, though sometimes they can be clear when a drug was either definitely not effective or definitely extremely effective. It is still useful clinically to see if one can elicit either extreme response marked "efficacy" or marked "inefficacy," or the absence of ever having had such clear good or bad effects. Sometimes, if a patient has taken many drugs from the same class (such as ten different antidepressants), clinicians can simplify the efficacy assessment by asking, "Was there any one of these that worked very well for you, that stands out as especially effective?" Also, if efficacy is reported, one should ask about whether the drug maintained its benefits if used long-term (to assess tolerance or "poop-out").

FINAL STEPS

When a diagnosis is made, clinicians should describe their rationale for that diagnosis, based on symptoms, course, genetics, and treatment response—the four classic validators of diagnosis. Then treatment options can be discussed. It is important, respectful, and humane to explicitly state the diagnosis to the patient before discussing treatments in any way, and further to elicit a two-way dialogue about the patient's feelings about the diagnosis.

The clinician should keep in mind, and the patient should be told, that working diagnoses are just that—working; so they are liable to change, and in fact should not uncommonly change, in the course of months to years of follow-up. In psychiatry, the course of the illness is the final arbiter of diagnosis (Box 38.1). Time will tell; both clinicians and patients need to be open-minded and revisit the diagnosis over time. A major mistake, often seen in public mental health settings, is that a diagnosis (often schizophrenia or "depression") is parroted over a course of years, often from clinician to clinician, without ever being reevaluated, even though the course of illness often clearly proves it wrong.

BOX 38.1
STEPS IN THE DIAGNOSTIC INTERVIEW OF MOOD CONDITIONS

Identify a current clinical depressive episode and establish its subtype (10 minutes).

Assess the course of depressive illness (10 minutes).

Identify affective temperament (5–10 minutes).

Assess past mania or hypomania (5–15 minutes).

Examine causes of secondary depression (5 minutes).

Obtain past treatment history (5–15 minutes).

Discuss the rationale for the diagnosis (5–10 minutes).

Discuss treatment options (5–10 minutes).

**Suggested times will vary based on the complexity of a patient's history. In a newly diagnosed patient, no time is needed for past treatment history, and more time can be spent on course of illness, secondary triggers, and discussion of diagnostic rationale. In a patient with extensive past treatment, the other sections might be somewhat briefer to allow for more extensive examination of past treatment history.*

BOTTOM LINE

- In the diagnostic interview, don't forget to assess course of illness.
- Assess manic symptoms more extensively and more indirectly than depressive symptoms.
- Obtain past treatment history in detail.
- Always discuss the rationale for diagnosis.

39

The "Med Check"

A MAJOR MYTH IN CONTEMPORARY PSYCHIATRY, REPEATED BY PSYCHIATRY residency directors and their residents, is the cliché "'Psychopharm' is easy; psychotherapy is hard." Many psychiatry residencies pride themselves in the extensive didactic time given over to teaching psychotherapies; in contrast, little formal didactic time is given to psychopharmacology teaching. "The residents will learn psychopharmacology in practice (in the clinic, which is often a hit-or-miss experience)," one hears. Of course, one learns a lot in practice, but not enough, and often not the right things.

The truth is that learning psychopharmacology is as hard as learning psychotherapy, perhaps harder, because it entails not only knowledge about medications, but knowledge and skill about diagnosis, about interviewing, and about relating to the patient. Those latter skills overlap with formal psychotherapy, thus what is hard about psychotherapy is also hard about psychopharmacology. This dismissal of psychopharmacology teaching as important is one factor that feeds into the clinical reality of "med check" psychopharmacology, for which a synonym is "poor psychopharmacology." Psychopharmacology needs to be taught as assiduously as psychotherapies are taught.

SOME UGLY FACTS

It is one of the ugly facts of clinical practice that about one-half of patients do not return for treatment. They may leave after the first, second, or fifth visit, but they "drop out." Despite much research on this problem of "treatment adherence," as it is politely called, little major impact appears to happen in real-world clinical practice. At best, clinicians have the long-term opportunity to treat and improve only half of their patients.

Another fact, not ugly but certainly difficult, is the reality that, although our medications usually always help, they are only partially effective for most patients, depending on the condition and the treatment—somewhat more for some conditions, somewhat less for most psychotic conditions. Half of one-half becomes "one-quarter of our patients achieve full remission."

Good clinicians are able to make about one out of every four patient completely better with our treatments. This may seem like a small number, a baseball batting average of .250, but it is consistent with the statistical concept of the "number needed to treat" (NNT), where a one-in-five or better frequency of efficacy is considered a large effect size (NNT = 5), but one in 6–10 is considered a small amount of benefit, and less than one in 10 is considered a very small effect size.

The reality of clinical practice is that we do not, and cannot, give most patients complete remission. This, of course, is exactly like the rest of medical practice for chronic medical illness. If clinicians manage one in four, they are good clinicians. If they manage better, like one in three, they are excellent clinicians. Clinicians cannot expect to improve most of their patients, given the constraints of treatment adherence and medication efficacy.

To improve outcomes, most research effort in psychopharmacology is put into the question of medication efficacy. Equal effort could be put into the problem of treatment adherence, or more generally, the problem of relating to the patient (and their significant others).

This is why psychopharmacology is not about, and cannot be about, "facts about pills." It is equally about the science of diagnosis, and equally about psychotherapeutic aspects of relating to patients.

"MED CHECKS"

Mental health professionals who are not psychiatrists sometimes disparage the "med check" as a rapid-fire superficial accounting of symptoms and side effects, which, when repeated four times per hour, serves a primary purpose of providing income for the clinic or the prescriber. This drug-for-symptom practice has been likened to being a "Volkswagen mechanic," on the analogy of fixing something that is easy to fix. In fact, psychiatric diseases are complex conditions, difficult to identify at times, and harder to treat, especially in the long-term, where they are chronic or recurrent, much like medical conditions like hypertension, diabetes mellitus, or autoimmune disease. The Volkswagen turns out to be a Porsche, and the drug-for-symptom psychiatrist turns out to be a very ineffective physician.

The "med check," practiced superficially, is indeed harmful, as its pejorative connotations imply. The practice of psychopharmacology, in a manner that is both scientific and humanistic, is much more complicated—and necessary.

THE FIRST THIRD OF THE PSYCHOPHARMACOLOGY VISIT: LISTENING

Patients must feel heard before they will listen, the psychoanalyst Leston Havens used to teach. So the first step in an interview is to listen, not talk. The clinician who asks lots of questions will put patients on the defensive and will get misleading answers. Instead, if the clinician just asks the patient to tell her story, in her own words, then many of the questions that might have been asked will be answered without being asked. The first third of the visit can be conducted this way.

In this way, the approach to a psychopharmacology visit would be the same as the approach to a psychotherapy session. Ever since Freud, psychotherapists have learned the importance of letting patients speak their minds freely; in fact, this was the primary rule of Freud's "free association" method. This technique can be taken too far, and has been. But, there is wisdom in it, too: people will tell you what you want to know, if you just let them talk.

For most purposes, the psychopharmacology visit can begin, and move into its middle stages in much the same way as a psychotherapy session begins and evolves: patients speak freely, and clinicians listen or interact in such a way as to help patients feel comfortable speaking about their experiences since the last visit.

This approach has the key impact of strengthening the therapeutic alliance. By listening, the clinician sends the message to patients that they deserve respect. It almost doesn't matter what is said; patients experience that they are being heard; that's what matters. Immediately, the patient will be more prone to listen when the clinician finally speaks. Also, by waiting to hear what patients have to say, clinicians open the way for discussion of difficult or embarrassing subjects, such as sex. If patients feel heard and understood, they are more likely to bring forward such topics. When asked questions, without a strong therapeutic alliance, they will be defensive on those topics.

Listening is the method to establish a relationship with a patient that is human to human, not superior to inferior. Even if the doctor will play a professional role, and make a diagnosis based on specialized knowledge, the provision of diagnoses and treatments will be more effective when given on the basis of an underlying human-to-human relationship.

Of course, psychopharmacologists have to do things that psychotherapists do not: The clinician who prescribes medications has to have a clear diagnosis, has to measure symptoms, and has to monitor side effects. These are important practical tasks, but they have to be added to, not replace, psychotherapeutic interactions.

THE FALLACY OF "TARGET" SYMPTOMS

The "med check" promotes a symptom-based approach to psychopharmacology practice. If time is limited, it is easiest to just identify symptoms and treat them, rather than to do the hard, slow work-up of a differential diagnosis of possible underlying diseases. To simplify matters further, many advocate picking a few symptoms to treat, usually those that are most severe or most bothersome to patients: "target" symptoms.

As discussed in Chapter 16, this practice contrasts with the Hippocratic tradition, which rejects treating symptoms as the main method of medical practice. Instead, the Hippocratic tradition emphasizes treating the underlying disease, which will resolve symptoms more effectively. This is much harder work for the physician, though. Identifying symptoms is easy; uncovering the disease can be difficult.

Current psychopharmacology practice takes the non-Hippocratic approach one step further. Not only should clinicians treat symptoms, they should focus on "target" symptoms. So patients with "depression" receive sedating antidepressants because of insomnia, or "stimulants" for their low energy, or drugs with benefits for anxiety symptoms because they are worried and tense. Sometimes clinicians ask patients to identify which symptom bothers them the most, and then a drug is selected for that target symptom.

This approach is medically and biologically unsound. There are many medical conditions in which the most severe symptom is not important diagnostically or therapeutically. A high fever in pneumonia is a target symptom that can be treated with acetaminophen, but such an approach, without a focus on treating the underlying infection, would be poor medical practice. Some diseases, like many cancers, have no symptoms at all. There are no symptoms, and yet early treatment of the underlying disease is imperative.

So, too, in psychiatry: A manic patient may not complain of many symptoms—in fact, one-half of patients deny having any illness at all—yet treatment is needed for the manic syndrome. A depressed patient may complain bitterly of poor attention and insomnia, but those symptoms will not improve until the underlying depression is treated. And a patient with repeated manic and depressive episodes, presenting in a severe depression, will be tortured by sadness and despair, but will not improve with an "antidepressant." Such a patient will need a second-messenger modifier (mood stabilizer) like lithium or valproate to treat and prevent such episodes of bipolar depression.

Of course, as in all of medicine, some attention to alleviating symptoms is needed, but this symptom-oriented approach should not be the main, and certainly not the sole, focus of medication-decision making. More attention should be given to identifying the underlying disease, and treating it.

This perspective is the main rationale for a need for medical training in the practice psychopharmacology, as opposed to lay prescribing by psychologists or others. No medical training is needed to identify and treat symptoms. A few months of basic factual knowledge education would be sufficient to allow non-physicians to learn to use drugs for symptoms in psychopharmacology. Years of study in medical school are devoted to understanding diseases with the goal of translating that knowledge to the bedside in clinical practice, translating patients' symptoms into diseases that should be treated. The target symptom approach is the exact opposite of this medically and scientifically sound tradition.

EXISTENTIAL PSYCHOPHARMACOLOGY

Psychiatrists who were trained in the 1980s or earlier, when psychoanalytical approaches predominated, had more experience with psychotherapeutic methods. This was the first generation of psychopharmacologists, and they effectively interwove psychotherapeutic techniques into their clinical care.

In the experience of the author of this text, one of the prime examples of this generation of clinicians was the Washington, D.C., psychiatrist Jacob Katzow. His method was natural to him, but it was also a reflection of his unique amalgam of his psychoanalytical training and his pharmacological approach. He would sit down with patients and just talk to them; they'd talk about whatever they wanted, for about 20–30 minutes, and in the course of the session, he would make judgments about symptoms and medications, and, after they left, he would jot down a few lines for his chart. His clinical notes were clear and told the reader what he needed to know about symptoms and improvement and drugs. What was not recorded was the half hour of getting to know the person behind the patient. He always began with his patients as "human beings," not as an "illness," and would find out what he needed to know about their illnesses by and by.

Katzow was practicing a kind of existential psychopharmacology. He was, with his patients, human being to human being—that's the existential part. But he also was evaluating his patients for diseases, and knew how to treat them correctly, if found, with drugs—that's the psychopharmacology part. Too many people who profess an attachment to humanistic attitudes, or even identify themselves as existentially oriented, refuse to accept the reality of disease, and view all biological talk as "bad" biological talk. Diseases parade in front of these self-proclaimed humanists, and they see nothing. They think they see clearly only because they refuse to change their focus beyond one line of sight. In contrast, as is well known, many biological reductionists just treat every symptom with a drug and never get to know the person whose brain they are manipulating.

Too often, mental health professionals seem to believe that psychopharmacology is about nothing but biology and pharmacology, while psychotherapy is about the mind—that is, human beings as persons. The former is not humanistic, it follows, while the latter is humanistic. In reality, if someone has a disease, it is anti-humanistic to fail to diagnose and treat that disease. Furthermore, in the course of diagnosing and treating a disease, it is a poorly trained physician who ignores and cares little for the feelings of the human being who has that disease.

In short, clinicians cannot be humanistic unless they are also scientific, even biological. And they cannot be medically effective in their biological interventions unless they are also humanistic. Science and humanism need each other.

MAKING DECISIONS

The concept of a "treatment plan" is central to psychopharmacology practice. What is a treatment plan?

The perspective suggested here is that the treatment plan should reflect the intersection of patients' preferences and clinicians' recommendations. The two aspects need not be identical. Too often, clinicians tailor their recommendations to patients' preferences. If patients want a certain kind of medication, or refuse to take another kind, they get what they want. The opposite scenario also is problematic: patients just follow whatever recommendations they are given by clinicians.

The two extremes are wrong for the following reasons:

If clinicians simply do what patients want, then clinicians are not bringing any specialized knowledge to the interaction. Why, then, do clinicians have prescribing privileges? In such an approach, the patients might as well be able to choose their own medications over-the-counter, without a prescriber. Obviously there is a benefit to taking into account patients' preferences, in the interest of adherence; but such respect for patient preferences need not result in capitulation of the clinician's expertise.

If patients simply do what clinicians want, then patients are at the mercy of the expertise of their clinicians, and not all clinicians are equally expert. Some are more expert than others, depending on the problem. If patients are in the hands of competent and careful clinicians, they will do well; but sometimes this is not the case. Patients should draw on the expert knowledge of clinicians, but they should check this knowledge against the expertise of other clinicians (second opinions), or otherwise look into what is being recommended themselves, by studying legitimate sources of medical knowledge on the topic. Patients should trust, but verify, their clinicians' recommendations. These days, with the internet, this process is much easier than in the past, as long as patients can steer clear of illegitimate or one-sided opinions on the internet.

In short, a good treatment plan depends on intersecting circles, not complete overlap. Clinicians should take into account patient preferences, but not accede to all or even most of them. Patients should rely on clinicians' expert recommendations, but they should confirm and verify whether those recommendations are well-founded.

It is fine if patients reject some legitimate clinician recommendations, and it is fine if clinicians reject certain patient preferences. All that is needed is some overlap; then those decisions can be accepted by both clinicians and patients, and treatment can begin.

There are no easy decisions. Patients often seem to seek medications that will be effective for their problems, but that will not harm them. There is no such drug. If a drug can help, it will also harm. This is because an effective drug has to be active biologically; if so, it affects physiological processes, and not just one, but many. Some of those processes may be the benefits for which the drug was developed; other processes will have occurred without being intended, causing some harm. If a drug has no harm, then it will not be active biologically, and hence have no benefit.

Hence, all effective medications will cause harm, and thus all medication decisions involve weighing risks and benefits. The question is whether to start on the risk, or the benefit, side of the ledger, as discussed in Chapter 34.

One should start with benefits. The menu of options for treatment does not include all the drugs in the world, but only effective drugs. There is no point in taking ineffective drugs. Now some drugs are proven ineffective, and others have not been studied, thus their efficacy is not known. Many clinicians will feel justified in using agents that are not proven effective, but that also are not proven ineffective. They *might* work, so why not try? With this approach, many apparently benign drugs are tried, with little benefit if they do not work. One might call this the "gabapentin syndrome," in honor of this anticonvulsant with relatively limited side effects. It became popular in psychiatric practice for a wide range of potential uses, even though it was not effective for more than a handful (epilepsy, pain, anxiety; but not depression or mania). Or "oxcarbazepine syndrome," the anticonvulsant analogue to carbamazepine, which is not proven effective for bipolar illness, yet is commonly used. In the meantime, when benign ineffective drugs are used, other proven effective drugs are ignored. In the case of gabapentin or oxcarbazepine, many patients are treated for years without benefit, while lithium is not tried at all.

In medicine, clear right or wrong answers are infrequent. There are probabilities of risk and harm, and the art of medicine is the art of balancing those probabilities, as Osler said. An analogy can be made with stock investing. It's not right or wrong to be conservative, and invest only in bonds and large, stable companies, or to be aggressive, investing in new, small companies with volatile prices. Even a "balanced" portfolio is not always the best decision. Sometimes, one can take a risk; other times, it might be wiser to be cautious. Some people are risk-averse; others are risk-takers. Neither is right or wrong; they are just different. So, too, with medication decisions. Some patients are very cautious; others take risks; some clinicians are very conservative; others aggressive. These are personality types, not moral facts.

The important point is that clinicians should expose patients to the whole spectrum of decision-making, from cautious to aggressive, with in-between options. Probabilities of benefits and risks should be given for each approach, then patients should be allowed to assert their preferences, within the constraints of the spectrum of recommendations that clinicians consider to be sound scientifically.

SUMMARY

The psychopharmacology visit needs to more than a superficial symptom-oriented brief "med check." At its best, it should consist of a listening-oriented approach to the first part of the visit. It should produce an agreed-upon treatment plan based on involvement of patients in decision-making, while at the same time using psychoeducation to direct patients towards decisions based on scientific evidence.

If clinicians take this approach to focusing on diagnosis and relating to the patient, they can capture perhaps some of the half of patients who never return for treatment, and improve a proportion of them who would not have been helped otherwise. They'll also get further with those patients who remain in their care, as the therapeutic alliance combines with scientific expertise to produce the best results in clinical psychopharmacology.

SELECTED REFERENCES

Fava, G. A., Cosci, F., Offidani, E., et al. (2016). Behavioral toxicity revisited: Iatrogenic comorbidity in psychiatric evaluation and treatment. *Journal of Clinical Psychopharmacology, 36*, 550–553.

Ghaemi, S. N. (2011). Volkswagen psychopharmacology. *Psychiatric Times*. June 1, 2011 issue. Accessed at http://www.psychiatrictimes.com/psychopharmacology/volkswagen-psychopharmacology (accessed 15/09/17).

Ghaemi, S. N., Glick, I. D., & Ellison, J. M. (2018). A Commentary on Existential Psychopharmacologic Clinical Practice: Advocating a Humanistic Approach to the "Med Check". *Journal of Clinical Psychiatry, 79*, 18ac12177.

Hanrahan, M., & Glick, I. D. (1996). Improving outpatient treatment for severely mentally ill persons: Doing the right thing. *Administration Policy in Mental Health, 23*, 459–463.

40

The Placebo Effect

UNTIL THE 1960S, PHYSICIANS IN THE UNITED STATES COULD LEGALLY PRESCRIBE "placebo" on a prescription pad and handed to a patient. It was not unethical to do so. Placebo had long been known to be an effective treatment for various medical conditions. For millennia, physicians new that many of their treatments were ineffective and that many conditions could not be treated. Instead of giving treatments that have some pharmacological properties, which meant they would have some side effects and be harmful in some way, it was viewed as more ethical to give an inert pill, a placebo, which would cause no direct pharmacological harm. The view was that the patient might get some psychological benefit from the apparent treatment. None of this was blinded, meaning that the patient saw that the prescription was written for placebo. The whole procedure was aboveboard. A patient recalled, as a child in the 1950s, that her physician was a family friend. He was older and had thick eyebrows. She had much difficulty sleeping, which years later would turn out to be part of a severe manic depressive illness. No available sleeping pills helped her. Her family doctor looked at her from under his bushy eyebrows and handed her a prescription on which he wrote: "Placebo." Before he gave it to her, he stared at her intently and said in a deep and low voice: "This is the strongest medication that you have ever taken. Use it very carefully." She recalled decades later that she slept well that night, better than she had with any prior treatment.

In the 1960s, after the first randomized clinical trials had been conducted in the prior decade, the FDA decided to require proof of clinical efficacy with randomized clinical trials (RCTs) for future drugs. These RCTs often used placebo as a comparator arm. Once placebo began to be used as part of proof of efficacy research studies, where it was the ineffective control arm, it was then seen as unethical to prescribe an agent in clinical practice that was defined as being ineffective. At that point, the FDA removed placebos from the clinical marketplace. Ever since then, and increasingly in the last few decades, researchers and clinicians have begun to speculate more about the placebo effect, especially since many medications fail to do much better, or indeed any better, than placebo.

In these discussions in psychiatry, there are two common assumptions:

First, it often is held that the placebo effect simply reflects psychological expectation. In this assumption, the relationship between clinician and patient is seen as the main mechanism of the placebo effect. The psychological skills of the clinician are presumed to be important. The wishes of the patient are also seen as impactful. In this interpretation of the placebo effect, any benefits seen relate to what would occur in the psychotherapy setting as well. Clinicians conclude that placebo effects provide support for psychotherapy treatment.

Second, many believe that placebo effects are specific to certain conditions. It is claimed, for instance, that the placebo effect in schizophrenia is low, and in depression or anxiety, it is higher. It is believed that placebo effects will be the same for the same condition in different studies.

These assumptions deserve some analysis. It is true that placebo effects can involve psychological expectation and reflect the clinician–patient relationship. It is not true that they always do so. In fact, studies of the placebo effect suggest that the role of psychological expectation depends on the illness being studied. For instance, in terminal medical illnesses, such as end-stage cancer, there is very little placebo effect. Psychological expectation does not change the course of such a terminal illness. Similarly, few effects of psychological expectation are seen in placebo studies of hypertension. Yet notable placebo effects occur in studies of pain rather consistently. Among psychiatric conditions, placebo effects tend to be very high in studies of anxiety, but lower in studies of mania or severe psychotic states. In other words, both assumptions are partially true in that psychological expectation is sometimes relevant, but it is so for conditions that are more subjective in nature, such as pain and anxiety. Where more objective outcomes are being examined, such as death, psychological expectation has little effect. Furthermore, it may be added that even when placebo effects are present for a subjective condition, there is a general consistency to the observation that placebo effects decline with severity and time. Placebo effects are strongest early in treatment, and decline over time. They also are stronger for mild symptoms, and weaker for more severe symptoms. These general observations apply across a wide range of psychiatric and medical conditions.

These considerations bring us to a second major aspect of the placebo effect, besides psychological expectation: the natural course of the illness (Figure 40.1). This is the

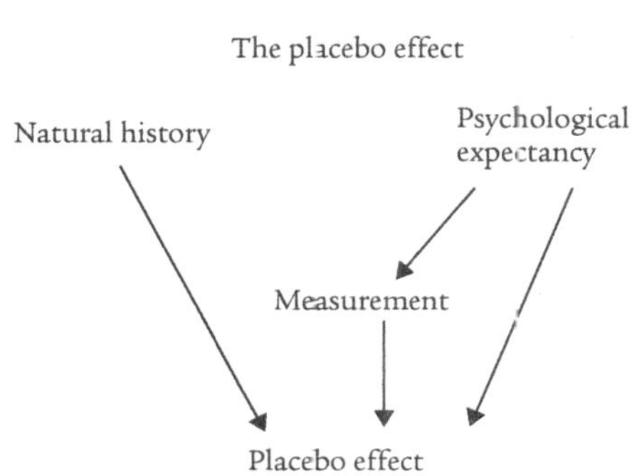

FIGURE 40.1 *The placebo effect.*

major aspect of the placebo effect that is important from a research perspective. It is relevant to conditions in which there is at least short-term spontaneous recovery by natural history. For example, in manic-depressive illness, mood episodes occur. By definition, episodes have a beginning and an end. Therefore they will always end. Therefore there will always be spontaneous recovery at some point, given the natural history of illness. In the case of depression happening in bipolar illness, the average duration of the natural untreated episode is about three to six months. For unipolar depression, it is longer, about six to twelve months. If placebo is given in a randomized clinical trial of acute bipolar depression for three to six months, there will be a very high placebo effect. Almost all patients will recover on placebo. This is not because bipolar depression is inherently placebo-responsive, nor is it because of the psychological skill of the researchers. Rather, it is simply a reflection of the natural history of the illness, meaning that if drug efficacy is to be shown, the duration of the clinical trial should be less than three to six months.

Where an illness is chronic or consistently deteriorating, and not episodic, there is no spontaneous recovery. In principle, there will be no placebo effect due to natural history. In such settings, one could justify not using placebo at all. For example, in the very first randomized clinical trial in human history, which occurred in 1948 in England in a study of streptomycin for miliary tuberculosis, patients were randomized to receive streptomycin or not. There was no need to give them an inert pill, since miliary tuberculosis had a natural history of absolute mortality.

Other factors that could affect the placebo response, as shown in Figure 40.1, include measurement factors, such as expectation effects for raters of rating scales, as well as for subjects in studies. If researchers are highly devoted to a certain result, they may rate patient symptoms with a bias in one direction or another. Similarly, if patients are motivated for a certain result, they may report their symptoms in a research study more in one direction or another. These measurement factors may be relevant to the observation in the last decade or two in pharmaceutical industry–sponsored clinical trials that the placebo effect appears to be rising. This rising placebo effect is occurring in pharmaceutical trials of different kinds of drug classes in different conditions. It appears to be nonspecific, happening with antidepressants and antipsychotics alike, in schizophrenia, bipolar illness, unipolar depression, or anxiety diagnoses. The pharmaceutical industry has focused a great deal of effort on trying to minimize the placebo response in these studies. A number of hypotheses have been raised. One observation that appears to be consistent is that the placebo effect correlates with the number of research centers in a clinical trial. The more research groups in a study, the higher the placebo effects, irrespective of drug or diagnosis. This observation seems to reflect an important measurement factor; namely, that each center will have very few patients, and those patients will be seen as having a very high motivation to stay in a research trial as long as possible, to its completion. There often is an economic motivation for researchers as well as patients, who are paid per visit. Instead of dropping out of a clinical trial, patients may report, or clinicians may rate, fewer symptoms so as to keep patients in a study. Of course, treatment is double-blinded, so if a patient happens to be randomized to placebo, such higher scores will appear to be a stronger placebo effect.

The phenomenon of regression to the mean also is relevant; this is a statistical phenomenon where extreme measurement on one occasion usually is followed with a more average measurement on the next occasion. Such natural tendencies automatically will minimize differences between active drugs and placebo.

In short, psychological expectation is only one possible aspect of the placebo response. Other aspects are the natural history of the illness, which is perhaps the most important factor, and measurement factors, including the economics of pharmaceutical industry–sponsored clinical trials. For clinicians, the most important point probably is that the natural history of the illness always is relevant, and if there is natural recovery, then it will be reflected in a placebo effect.

IMPACT IN CURRENT CLINICAL PRACTICE

It was noted that clinicians today no longer can prescribe placebo overtly. They still do so covertly, though, with about one-half of US internists reporting in a 2006 confidential survey that they prescribe vitamins or over the counter analgesics as placebo-equivalents. Placebo effects are observed and measured only in research studies. Yet everyone knows that they in fact do occur in clinical practice; they just are not observed or measured. Clinicians should take this fact into account as they make judgments about their clinical experience regarding the effectiveness of psychotropic medications.

Two common clinical scenarios will illustrate the importance of this matter. One involves pharmaceutical industry–sponsored studies of antidepressants for MDD. The other involves randomized clinical trials of antidepressants for acute bipolar depression. In the MDD studies, as discussed in Chapter 19 and shown again in Figure 40.2, there has been a great deal of controversy about the efficacy of antidepressants over placebo in the FDA database of randomized clinical trials. It was shown that

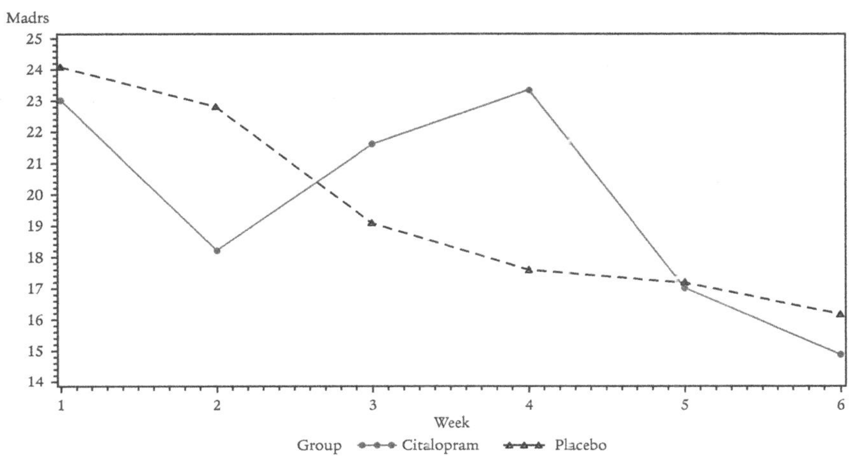

FIGURE 40.2 *Citalopram in bipolar depression: A double-blind, placebo-controlled acute and maintenance study.*

antidepressants are only slightly more effective than placebo, with a mean benefit of about two points on the HDRS. As Figure 40.2 shows, though, this mean score is somewhat misleading, since more benefit was seen in severe depression. Yet, certainly in mild depression, there was no appreciable benefit of antidepressant over placebo. As noted, the antidepressant benefit was consistent in mild, moderate, or severe depression. It was not that antidepressants were more effective in severe depression; rather, placebo was less effective. Placebo was more effective in mild depression, and less effective with increasing severity of depression. As noted, this is a common and consistent finding with placebo effects in various conditions. In clinical practice, though, clinicians only experience the antidepressant effect shown in Figure 40.2. They do not see or experience the placebo effect, because they do not prescribe placebo explicitly. Since placebo can no longer be prescribed clinically, clinicians must rely on such RCTs to inform their clinical practice, not just for the drug efficacy shown, but also for the placebo efficacy shown. In other words, clinicians should look at Figure 40.2 and conclude that when they give antidepressants in mild depression, they observe improvement, but not because of the pharmacological effects of the antidepressants. Clinicians have made this judgment, understandably, because they appear to observe a cause-and-effect relationship in which patients improve after receiving antidepressants. They could not know that those patients would have improved after receiving an inert pill as well. These RCTs teach clinicians that this is the case, and they now can conclude that antidepressants are not necessary in such cases of mild depression. In that case, no treatment at all, or possibly psychotherapy intervention, would appear appropriate.

A similar judgment could be made regarding clinical experience with antidepressants in acute bipolar depression. Despite repeated studies showing that antidepressants are not more effective than placebo in acute bipolar depression, most clinicians continue to prescribe these agents, and many experts also continue to support this practice. There is no scientific basis for supporting a treatment that is proven to be no more effective than placebo. Yet clinicians insist that their clinical experience supports benefit with these medications. Again, they are inferring a cause-and-effect relationship by giving a treatment and observing the beneficial outcome. As in chapter 19 Figure 19.6 shows, studies of antidepressants in bipolar depression show no difference with placebo, not because neither treatment works, but because both treatments do. In other words, patients improve with antidepressants, and they also improve equally with placebo. In clinical practice, again, clinicians would not see the placebo line. Their clinical experience would simply be that antidepressants are given, and the patient improves. They could not know that this benefit is not due to the pharmacological effects of the antidepressants. The scientific practice of psychopharmacology would require that clinicians should incorporate these RCT data into their clinical experience, not because they are focused solely on drug efficacy, but because they should pay also attention to placebo efficacy. If they did so, they would conclude that their clinical experience of benefit with antidepressants for bipolar depression was due to the natural history of the illness, not the pharmacological benefit of the supposed "antidepressant."

PSYCHOTHERAPY AND PLACEBO

It is important to distinguish between the placebo effect and the judgment of psychotherapy efficacy. The role of natural history is the primary competing explanation for placebo benefit. How can one distinguish between these two factors? One way to do so would be to look at studies that compare placebo treatment with no treatment at all. These studies would give drug versus an inert pill versus nothing at all. The completely no-treatment arm often reflects a waiting list, where subjects are not entered into a research study but are followed for their outcomes. One review paper assessed antidepressant efficacy in acute depression studies in MDD, examining the kinds of RCTs where a no-treatment arm existed. Ten studies were identified, and the overall benefit of no-treatment versus placebo was a Cohen's d effect size of 0.50, which is larger than the effect size of benefit with antidepressant over placebo in the FDA database of RCTs (d = 0.32). In other words, antidepressants were mildly better than placebo overall, but no treatment at all (meaning natural history of the illness) was even more beneficial than placebo overall.

The point of this analysis is to throw some doubt on the assumption that the placebo effect should translate to a recommendation of psychotherapy treatment. The natural history of depressive illness in particular should not be underestimated. The milder the symptoms, the more likely it is that the condition will resolve, at least for the short term. The larger question becomes not how to treat acute symptoms, which often improve well by themselves, but how to address either long-term recurrence of such symptoms, or long-term chronicity of mild symptoms. Some psychotherapies like CBT are much more proven short-term than long-term, and are more effective for acute episodes than for chronic conditions.

Given these natural history findings, one might conclude that the concept of the placebo effect in psychiatry often is exaggerated. In fact, one might ask, as did a classic meta-analysis of this topic: "Is the placebo was powerless?" As explained in this chapter, it may be that the placebo effect is not entirely powerless in terms of its psychological aspects, but it indeed may be powerless when it is a stand-in for the natural history of the illness. When the natural history of illness is respected, then clinicians can return to the wisdom of Hippocrates and his followers, who argued that most conditions improve by themselves, and the role of the physician is to stay out of the way. Sometimes this is not the case, such as when a disease exists and a treatment is proven effective; in that case, and in that case only, physicians should intervene. The art and science of medicine are about knowing when to do the former, and when to do the latter.

SELECTED REFERENCES

Hróbjartsson, A., & Gøtzsche, P. C. (2001). Is the placebo powerless?—An analysis of clinical trials comparing placebo with no treatment. *New England Journal of Medicine, 344*, 1594–1602.

Kirsch, I., et al. (2008). Initial severity and antidepressant benefits: A meta-analysis of data submitted to the Food and Drug Administration. *PLOS Medicine, 5*(2), e45.

Rutherford, B. R., & Roose, S. (2013). A model of placebo response in antidepressant clinical trials. American Journal of Psychiatry, *170*(7), 723–733.

Rutherford, B. R., et al. (2012). Contribution of spontaneous improvement to placebo response in depression: A meta-analytic review. *Journal of Psychiatric Research*, *46*(6), 697–702.

Tiburt, J. C., et al. (2008). Prescribing "placebo treatments": results of national survey of US internists and rheumatologists. *BMJ*, 337, a1938.

41

Legal Aspects of Psychopharmacology Practice

LEGAL ASPECTS IN THE PRACTICE OF PSYCHOPHARMACOLOGY INCLUDE informed consent, defensive medicine, important side effects, off-label prescribing, cost-containment and economic factors, and psychological aspects of the doctor–patient relationship.

Informed consent is a central aspect of the practice of psychopharmacology: clinician and patient must assess the risk–benefit ratio of every clinical decision. This means that in each decision, not only should benefits be assessed, but also harms. The concept of informed consent has been addressed in the setting of research, where it must be written down explicitly and approved by an ethics review committee. In the setting of clinical practice, though, informed consent tends to be verbal, and there is no formalization of a written consent under most circumstances. This fact does not preclude the obtaining of written consent, as often happens before some kind of physical procedure. Yet it is not required in writing in the dispensation of medications. The verbal discussion of informed consent is expected, though, and it is best if some form of documentation of that verbal discussion exists in the patient's medical chart. Specific problems that can arise in psychiatry involve the competency of patients to provide consent when they are severely symptomatic, such as with delusions or hallucinations, but also in manic states or other states of impaired insight. Sometimes patients are paranoid, and the psychological state of paranoia can interfere with their ability to rationally assess risk–benefit aspects of medication decision-making. Other times patients are extremely agitated or highly anxious, and although they are not technically incompetent from legal perspective, their thinking is impaired in such a way that they may have difficulty fully engaging in a risk–benefit analysis. In such cases, the question sometimes arises whether clinicians should provide extensive discussion of potential side effects to an anxious patient, given that their anxiety may increase when thinking about such side effects. It is relevant that such patients will always be anxious, whether they receive such information or not, and it is important that the most important side effects always be discussed.

When discussing side effects, there is no reason to go through every single one that might be found on the Internet or in the labeling of the medication by the FDA. It is the clinician's job to provide the patient with a metabolized summary of the most important side effects. One way of approaching the discussion of side effects would be to divide them into a few major groups: medically important side effects, common nuisance side effects, and infrequent nuisance side effects. The first two groups should be discussed under most circumstances, and at the very least, a discussion of the first group of medically important side effects should be documented in the chart. For example, with lamotrigine, the chart should always document a discussion of serious rash or Stevens-Johnson syndrome (SJS) as a potential medically serious side effect. A list of infrequent nuisance side effects need not be documented, nor even discussed in most cases. It is important to note that a handout of side effects is not sufficient to protect against potential legal problems, if there is no documentation in the chart of a discussion of that handout.

Turning to serious side effects that are of legal importance, the example of SJS with lamotrigine was just given. Other examples include tardive dyskinesia (TD) with traditional dopamine blockers, agranulocytosis with clozapine, and long-term kidney impairment with lithium. These types of standard serious medical risks should be documented in the chart, in most cases when these medications are begun. If the patient develops any of these problems in the future, that initial documentation will protect the clinician in most cases.

Regarding the use of medications in FDA non-approved indications, it is important to realize that the FDA explicitly allows for physicians to use medications outside of FDA indications. What is not allowed is for pharmaceutical companies to *market* such use to physicians. However, physicians can discuss such use among themselves, study those uses, publish those uses, and hold conferences that are not promotional in nature about non-FDA-indicated uses of medications. In other words, it is an accepted part of standard medical practice that clinicians are the individuals who have the right to decide how and for whom to use medications. FDA indications are meant primarily to regulate marketing by the pharmaceutical industry, not to regulate clinical practice. Where specific problems arise in medical practice that are brought to the attention of the FDA, the FDA will bring that information to clinicians in alterations of language regarding specific medications. For instance, a serious side effect will be included in a "black box warning," which would be added to the labeling of some medications. These recommendations are in the form of advice, not strict regulations, and certainly not legally bound judgments. Nonetheless, in the setting of malpractice cases or other legal complaints, patients and their lawyers often use FDA labeling to criticize clinicians and to argue that poor treatment occurred. Many clinicians are sensitive to this aspect of practice, and are loath to use medications outside of FDA labeling. It is true that the use of medications within FDA labeling gives legal protection to clinicians; it also is true that good medical practice requires treatment with medications outside of FDA labeling, as discussed further later.

Economic factors also are important in influencing legal aspects of psychopharmacology. These factors include limitations placed by insurance companies and pharmaceutical companies on the availability of drugs, and their cost. The availability of generic compounds certainly helps in decision-making, but with new medications it is frequently the case that generic compounds are not available, and costs are high in the early phases of patent life. Insurance companies respond by putting high barriers to approval of medication in their first years on the market. Clinicians are left in a quandary in deciding whether and how to give such medications to patients. The short-term use of samples of medications is insufficient due to the need for longer-term treatment if patients should respond.

Given these economic restrictions, clinicians can be faced with an ethical problem in that they may feel that the best treatments are new but not allowed to be given to patients. They may provide older, cheaper agents, which may cause harms or prove ineffective, with later possible legal consequences. It is wise to document the clinician's preferred treatment choices, irrespective of cost and availability, and then to document insurance or government restrictions as limiting the clinician's options.

ADMINISTRATIVE ASPECTS OF PRACTICE

Besides these general issues in relation to legal aspects of psychopharmacology, there are some specific administrative and clinical matters that deserve attention. The administrative issues involve providing sufficient time for patient appointments, chart documentation, and awareness of the risks involved with complaints to state medical boards as opposed to traditional malpractice lawsuits. The clinical issues involve legal risks that are specific to different clinical conditions, such as antidepressant-induced mania in bipolar illness, suicide, and specific medication harms. A few of these clinical scenarios will be examined here.

Regarding administrative matters, a key issue involves brevity of appointments. The "med check" visit, often 10–15 minutes in duration, can lead to misunderstanding on the part of both patient and clinician. Insufficient time to explain the rationale for treatment, or to explore diagnosis, can lead to the feeling that decisions are being made too quickly or unscientifically. Brevity of clinical appointments also impairs the ability of clinician and patient to connect interpersonally.

The problem of the psychological "transference" is always present in psychiatric care. This problem is exacerbated when appointments are brief and relationships are established in a setting where many misinterpretations can occur. This matter will be explored further in the following chapter, but for now, it is worth mentioning that legal problems arise when clinician–patient relationships are strained, and a simple factor relevant to that problem is the amount of time given to the appointment.

Another key administrative feature that is well known is the matter of chart documentation. The classic teaching is that if it isn't documented, it didn't happen. As far as the state medical boards or lawyers are concerned, as soon as any complaint arises, they will ask for the chart. The clinician can write a letter at that time explaining what may or may not have happened, but such explanations generally are disregarded or are interpreted skeptically. What is written in the chart counts for much more, because it predated the complaint. It is for this reason that one cannot overstate the importance of adequate chart documentation for legal purposes. By stating that this documentation needs to be intended for legal purposes, what is meant here is that clinicians need to learn that chart documentation is not for themselves, nor for other clinicians, but really should be aimed at future potential legal evaluation. In short, clinicians should write as if lawyers or state board staff would read the chart, not as if other clinicians would read the chart. Obviously, the original intention of medical charts was for communication between clinicians, and this remains the case to some extent. It is fair to say, though, that these days, the legal use of medical charts is their most important use. Clinicians should adjust their documentation accordingly. The chart is not meant primarily to provide medical information to other clinicians, but rather to demonstrate that the treating clinician is providing adequate care. This demonstration requires some expression of the rationale for decision-making regarding treatments, and consideration of alternative treatments and alternative aspects for diagnostic judgments. Any potentially serious side effects should be documented in some way, even if briefly.

STATE MEDICAL BOARD COMPLAINTS AND MALPRACTICE

A third important administrative aspect to the legal nature of psychopharmacology practice, at least in the United States, is the relevance of state medical boards. Many clinicians imagine that the main risk has to do with malpractice lawsuits. In fact, malpractice lawsuits are uncommon, and in the vast majority of cases are won by clinicians. It is true that if they occur, they are extremely time-consuming and even when acquitted, they cause damage to the clinician, in time, money, and stress. Nonetheless, in the United States, malpractice lawsuits are limited by the fact that they require that the prosecuting attorney conclude that a jury trial would probably lead to a judgment against the clinician. Since prosecuting attorneys usually take such cases on commission, meaning they are not paid unless they win, the main limiting factor to such cases involves the prosecuting attorney's judgment about the likelihood of success. This is not the case in other countries with other legal systems, but in the United States, because of an adversarial legal system that is tilted in favor of accusers, malpractice risks are higher than in other countries.

For these reasons, although malpractice lawsuits are important risks, they are not the most important legal risk in the practice of psychopharmacology in the United States. The most common and important legal risk in the United States involves complaints to state medical boards. These boards consist not only of physicians, but also of lawyers and patient advocates. State medical boards are set up as consumer-advocacy groups, and do not need to follow traditional legal guidelines set up for criminal cases. When clinicians are accused in a state medical board, they are not innocent until proven guilty, but rather guilty until proven innocent. The burden of proof is not on the accuser, but on the accused. It is not a formal legal setting, so the legal safeguards set up for criminal cases do not apply. There is an explicit and intended bias in favor of patients, and against clinician defendants. Oftentimes, clearly false complaints may be made, perhaps in the setting of a psychotic state during hospitalization. In those cases, complaints can be dismissed immediately by the state boards. But when complaints are made by patients who are not psychotic, those complaints are accepted and investigated in almost all cases by state medical boards. These investigations usually take about a year or so to occur. The recommendation here is that clinicians obtain legal counsel in explaining their perspective during these cases, because if they lose, the state medical board complaint can lead to a larger malpractice suit. Many times, clinicians do not retain legal counsel since the state medical board complaint is not itself a formal legal process. This is a risky decision to make, especially in the litigious setting of medical practice in the United States. In the best-case scenario, after a year of evaluation, complaints are dropped. In that case, there is no public documentation of complaints. If a complaint is not dropped, and the board decides against a clinician, that judgment is made public and can be identified easily via Internet search. Even if the clinician is allowed to practice, such a judgment against the clinician can influence patients to avoid seeking care, thereby possibly affecting the clinician's livelihood. If a judgment is made against the clinician, and it is more severe, the punishment can include suspension of practice for a number of years, or permanently. In these cases, the clinician essentially is deprived of the ability to earn a livelihood. Even if the judgment is not followed by a malpractice lawsuit, the loss of one's livelihood, or its impairment, is a major blow that a state medical board can easily apply to any clinician. Since it is not a fair and equally balanced assessment, but rather one biased in favor of patients, such state medical board complaints should be taken very seriously. Furthermore, there is no restriction, unlike in malpractice lawsuits, for patients to make a complaint regarding a clinician to a state medical board. The decision merely requires filling out a short form, easily completed on the Internet. Unlike malpractice lawsuits, where the prosecuting attorney often decides against pursuing the case due to its long-term costs, a complaint to a state medical board has no cost, and can be completed by a patient without any legal advice within a few hours. In short, there is a very low threshold for patients to make complaints to state medical boards, and there are very high risks to clinicians of such complaints.

Given these realities, what should clinicians do? Most mental health clinicians know that they have entered this profession primarily with the motivation to help others. Clinicians tend to be quite sympathetic to the suffering of others with psychiatric conditions. Feeling this empathy, clinicians often believe that their primary role is to put a patient's interests first. This approach to practice is taught in training programs. It is repeated in discussions of the ethics of practice: Put the patient first. This has been the tradition of medical practice going back millennia. But state medical boards and malpractice lawsuits did not exist in the Hippocratic era. It is an unfortunate reality that clinicians cannot practice solely with the patient's interest in mind. Clinicians need to preserve some space for their own self-interest. In the end, this self-preservation can be seen as being in the interests of patients as a whole, because if clinicians are sued or receive negative state medical board judgments and no longer can practice, they certainly cannot help other patients any longer.

One learns these lessons in psychiatric residency programs when exposed to the reality of the need to set limits in clinical settings, as with patients diagnosed with borderline personality, antisocial personality, substance abuse, or delusional states. The teaching that many trainees need to receive, painful as it is, was reflected in the motto of the

Massachusetts General Hospital psychiatric consultation program: "No good deed goes unpunished." This concept should not be exaggerated, but neither can it be denied entirely. It is true that one can try too hard, and try to do too much, and even with the best of intentions, such good efforts can rebound to cause harm to the clinician. Clinicians need to learn to set limits not only on patients, but on themselves. These limits involve not just the standard aspects of malpractice, such as not having sex with patients, but also accepting that one should put a limit to one's attempts to help a patient. For instance, in a non-emergency setting, a clinician is under no ethical, legal, or moral obligation to treat a particular patient. In the first interview, a clinician may have a feeling that the treatment with that patient will not go well, or that there is a problematic transference. For these reasons, or for any other reason, it is perfectly legitimate for the clinician to decline to treat the patient. After the first appointment, if a patient's treatment has begun, there are limitations to what clinicians can do due to the legal inability to abandon patients. But before a patient–doctor relationship has been established, either via prescription of medications or a formal agreement to treat, a clinician can decide not to treat a patient. Furthermore, even after treatment has begun, a clinician may decide to transfer the patient to the care of another treater after some failed treatment trials, or a clinician may ask a patient to agree to termination of treatment. All these limitations are reasonable, based on a clinician's taking into account not only the patient's interests, but the clinician's own interest in providing care to others in a way that will not lead to legal complaints. Some of these ideas can be referred to as "defensive medicine" in a pejorative manner, and it is true that one can practice over-defensively. The point here is that some level of attention to legal risks and to self-preservation is reasonable in clinical practice.

OFF-LABEL TREATMENT

It is worth pointing out one way in which there is excessive attention to legal aspects of medical practice. This approach, common in outpatient clinical practice in the United States, is to focus on staying within the guidelines of the FDA on diagnosis and treatment. In this approach, clinicians give medications mainly when they have FDA indications for specific diagnosis, and rarely, if ever, make diagnoses in any other way than the method accepted by the FDA. Drugs are rarely prescribed off-label. The problem with this approach is that it limits practice, at least in contemporary psychiatry, solely to features that are promulgated by the pharmaceutical industry. This outcome is the case because FDA labeling is intended primarily for the purposes of pharmaceutical marketing. Put another way, FDA indications exist only because some pharmaceutical companies make the economic judgment that it would make sense to conduct certain studies on certain indications and then to market those treatments to clinicians. These comments are not intended to deny that such indications or treatments might be valid, but rather to suggest that if practice is limited primarily to those treatments and indications, then clinical practice would be limited to whatever the pharmaceutical industry felt was worthwhile. Since those judgments are primarily economic rather than clinical, such clinical practice would ignore many aspects of care that have no economic value, such as the use of generic treatments, or the use of diagnoses for which no treatment has yet been developed, or the application of creativity in clinical practice leading to innovation that may produce future FDA indications for treatments originally developed for other purposes.

Clinicians can go too far in the direction of innovation, using medications in ways that are idiosyncratic, but this danger is no worse than slavishly following FDA indications. Many clinicians take to the super-conservative FDA-indication approach to treatment on the grounds that they will be protected legally. Any legal complaints against them will be weak if they can show that they simply followed FDA guidelines. This is true generally, but this approach veers too far in the direction of defensive medicine in a pejorative sense, and puts too little emphasis on the need to provide the best care possible to patients.

In short, there needs to be a balance between self-preservation and the patient's best interest. Clinicians should not ignore their own self-preservation, and they should take steps to protect themselves, including refusing to treat certain patients or terminating care. At the same time, they should not go too far in the direction of excessive defensive medicine, and should not practice solely based on FDA labeling and guidelines. Some level of clinical creativity and innovation is justifiable, within the constraints not only of FDA labeling, but also of current scientific knowledge, as well as with attention to staying sufficiently near the standard of care so as to protect oneself legally.

CASE EXAMPLES

The final section of this chapter will provide a few clinical examples of legal issues and psychopharmacology practice. These clinical examples will vary based on the conditions and drugs used; here the examples provided relate primarily to treatment of depression and bipolar illness.

In general, the most important clinical issue from a legal perspective in psychiatry is suicide. This outcome certainly raises legal risks. It is known that in about 90% of cases, clinical depression is present at the time of suicide. Hence, this risk is most present in the setting of treatment of mood conditions. Suicide is somewhat more common in mixed states than in pure depression. There have been a number of high-profile lawsuits regarding antidepressant-related suicides. As discussed in Chapter 27, the relationship between antidepressants and suicidality appears to be a real one, especially in young adults and adolescents. Furthermore, as discussed in Chapter 19, it is well known that antidepressants can cause mania, at least in some of their drug classes and at higher doses. Frequently, antidepressant-induced mania occurs in monotherapy, when mood stabilizers are not given. This scenario is most common when bipolar illness is misdiagnosed as unipolar depression. Among modern antidepressants, the agent with the highest risk of mania is venlafaxine. A number of legal cases exist where venlafaxine was given for apparent MDD, followed by mixed manic states, and ensuing suicide. Even though venlafaxine is an FDA-indicated treatment for MDD, the misdiagnosis of that condition when bipolar depression was diagnosable puts the clinician at legal risk. This is one example where careful diagnosis is important not only for good patient outcomes, but for avoidance of harmful legal outcomes.

Another common scenario with legal problems in psychopharmacology practice has to do with serious side effects. In the past, TD was a major concern legally. Given the very low frequency of that side effect with modern dopamine blockers, that issue is much less prominent these days. Other medications can have serious effects, even if rare, and adequate documentation, as well as adequate rationale for use of those agents, is essential. The example of lamotrigine and SJS was given earlier. Legal cases exist of malpractice suits against clinicians who prescribed lamotrigine with the occurrence of SJS as a consequence. If clinicians did not document in the chart that the patient was warned about SJS, and if it was not documented that SJS is potentially fatal or very harmful, then patients can claim that they never knew of such harms, and clinicians would be at legal risk. If clinicians prescribed lamotrigine outside of FDA indication, and outside of defensible scientific evidence, then the use of that agent with potential serious harm would put clinicians at legal risk. This risk would be increased if clinicians did not document that they either discussed or offered alternative treatments for whatever diagnosis was being treated. For instance, lamotrigine has FDA indication for prevention of mood episodes in type I bipolar illness, but not for acute treatment of a clinical depressive episode. Imagine a case where lamotrigine was given for treatment of an acute depression in bipolar illness, even though it has no indication for that treatment and in fact is proven equivalent to placebo. Suppose further that there is no documentation of alternative options, such as some of the FDA-indicated dopamine blockers. In that scenario, clinicians would be at legal risk if SJS occurred. This example is provided to point out that clinicians can protect themselves if they develop the habit of adding a line every time they prescribe certain medications, such as lamotrigine, to the effect of "potentially fatal SJS discussed." Or, they could write, "alternative treatments like lithium discussed, and patient prefers to try lamotrigine," so as to show that a discussion of treatment rationales and options occurred. This kind of documentation would demonstrate that the patient was involved in the decision-making process. This factor is very important if patients later make legal claims regarding harms or inadequate care. The involvement of the patient, documented in the chart, is central to combating such claims.

In conclusion, clinicians practice in the real world, And there are some unfortunate realities in the real world, including the fact that some patients will seek to make complaints or seek to pursue legal cases when such complaints or cases are not justified. Obviously, sometimes such complaints and cases are justified, and patients have legal rights as well. Given this reality, clinicians who are practicing ethically and who are making their best efforts to help patients need to realize that they still could be the recipient of such complaints or lawsuits, despite all their best intentions. Attention needs to be given to protecting themselves at some level, without interfering with providing excellent clinical care to their patients.

SELECTED REFERENCE

Appelbaum, P. S., & Gutheil, T. G. (Eds.). (2006). *Clinical handbook of psychiatry and the law, 4th edition.* Philadelphia, PA: Lippincott Williams & Wilkins.

42
Psychology of Psychopharmacology

THE PRACTICE OF PSYCHOPHARMACOLOGY HAS IMPORTANT PSYCHOLOGical aspects. The placebo effect is perhaps the most discussed phenomenon in relation to the psychological component of practice. This matter has been discussed in Chapter 40. Other aspects of the psychology of psychopharmacology involve transference and countertransference, secondary gain, the meaning of pill-taking, the social role of clinicians, and cultural setting of clinical treatment. Many of the cultural aspects of psychopharmacology practice are discussed in Chapter 34. In this chapter, the other topics mentioned here will be examined.

TRANSFERENCE AND COUNTERTRANSFERENCE

The psychoanalytic concepts of transference and countertransference were meant to relate to unconscious feelings that a patient and therapist may have for each other. Traditionally, these unconscious feelings were thought to be either sexual or aggressive in nature, and involved association to childhood relationships with one's parents. While this traditional psychoanalytic notion may be valid, a simpler interpretation of the relevance of transference and countertransference for psychopharmacology may be to acknowledge that a patient and clinician will have feelings about each other. These feelings may be beneficial or harmful in their impact on the clinical treatment. Psychopharmacology practice is more than just the clinical act of giving and taking a medication. Patients have feelings about the process of giving and taking medications, and these feelings include their personal relationship to the treating clinician. As in psychotherapy, the clinician should pay attention to evidence in the treatment about the patient's feelings towards the clinician. Such attention need not necessarily result in any change in clinical treatment, but it may do so. For instance, psychotherapy training emphasizes the importance of the concept of limits and boundaries in professional treatment. Especially in the psychotherapy setting, where there often is both verbal intimacy and close physical proximity, risks of inappropriate behavior, whether sexual or otherwise, exist. Attention to limits and boundaries in treatment is necessary to avoid and minimize such risks. The same process holds in psychopharmacology practice, although to a different degree. Attention should be given to the possibility of an inappropriate erotic transference or countertransference in the treatment. A patient may have sexual transference feelings for a clinician, and a clinician may have sexual countertransference feelings. In both cases, the clinician needs to pay attention to these feelings, and either discuss them with the patient, or seek clinical supervision with peers so as to determine what course of action to take. Sometimes termination of treatment is necessary. The opposite can be the case, where feelings of hate may exist between clinician and patient, either in the transference or countertransference, and similarly, the topic should either be discussed directly or via external clinical supervision. In either case, if the relationship between clinician and patient is either too close or too distant, decisions regarding whether and which medications should be given, and whether they are taken, will be less objectively made, and will be less effective. In short, the practice of psychopharmacology requires attention to transference and countertransference in a way that is similar to the practice of psychotherapy.

SECONDARY GAIN

As in other psychiatric settings, patients either come to treatment, or avoid it, because of reasons or factors that may have nothing to do with the actual treatment itself. Such external factors, referred to as "secondary gain," can be either conscious or unconscious. Secondary gain need not be conceived necessarily as a manipulative process on the part of the patient. It could be unconscious, and simply related to needs or wishes that the patient may possess. For instance, a female patient who has low self-esteem and almost masochistic tendencies towards dependency may seek a male clinician and be extremely compliant with any treatment recommendation. In contrast, a rebellious patient may sometimes attend appointments but frequently may be non-adherent to appointments and treatment decisions. Clinicians need to pay attention to both extremes and other types of behavior in the clinical setting that may reflect outside influences or habits. Such behavior should be discussed with the patient in the clinical setting, as well as perhaps with family members and friends of the patient and/or collaborating psychotherapists.

THE MEANING OF PILL-TAKING

There is a selection bias in the clinical setting of practice. Since most clinicians tend to prescribe medications somewhat freely, at least in the United States, patients who come for clinical care tend to be willing to take medications, and sometimes aggressively seek medications. The patients who are opposed to taking medications tend to avoid going to physicians or clinicians, and often seek help in the large alternative medicine marketplace. In the standard clinical setting, where patients often seek medications, clinicians may feel somewhat pressured to prescribe medications either more frequently or longer or at higher doses than they might otherwise prefer. Sometimes clinicians may try to advise patients to stop a medication or not take a certain drug class, and there will be resistance on the part of the patient. Patients might feel disappointed, or even angry. In this setting, it sometimes is the case that the refusal to give medications can have a certain psychological meaning for patients—the feeling that the clinician does not care about the patient. In other words, the meaning of giving a pill may seem to such patients equivalent to the statement "I care about you." Conversely, refusing to give a medication can seem like saying to the patient "I don't care about you." It is important to counteract such interpretations, which may occur at an unconscious level, by focusing on developing the therapeutic alliance with the patient. The patient needs to feel that the clinician cares, regardless of whether medication is prescribed. To achieve this goal, in the practice of psychopharmacology, a great deal of care needs to be given to interpersonal relationship with the patient, much as occurs in the practice of psychotherapy.

THE SOCIAL ROLE OF CLINICAL PRACTICE

A practicing clinician who prescribes medications for psychiatric conditions is placed in a specific role in a social structure. People come to clinicians with problems. Much of the time, these problems do not reflect diseases. They may be social problems, such as sexual trauma or poverty. They may reflect cultural issues, such as social expectations regarding beauty, leading to eating disorders. They may reflect even spiritual dilemmas, such as a sense of loneliness in large cities where one might live far from one's family. In the past, people with personal problems unrelated to diseases often went to priests or other religious guides. Currently, in the industrialized West, fewer people follow those traditions, and many instead seek the help of mental health professionals. Often they go to psychotherapists, and sometimes they come to clinicians seeking medications. Although medications can have symptomatic benefits for a range of expressions of unhappiness, as discussed in Chapter 16, such symptomatic use of medications tends to produce more harm than good in the long run and for society as a whole. Problems that arise at a social level are best addressed at a social level as well; i.e., as problems of public health, as opposed to individual clinical problems to be addressed by face-to-face treatment with a clinician. Public health solutions come from governments and organizations, not clinical offices. Clinicians need to be aware of the limitations of their ability to help patients whose problems cannot be solved in a one-to-one setting. This is not to say that clinicians should not seek to help such patients, but that such help is limited, and clinicians should be cautious about the use of medications, at least long-term, in such settings.

In conclusion, there are important psychological aspects to the treatment of patients with psychotropic medications, and these psychological features of the clinical setting require careful attention from clinicians so as to provide the best treatment possible.

SELECTED REFERENCE

Mintz, D. L, & Flynn, D. F. (2012). How (not what) to prescribe: Nonpharmacologic aspects of psychopharmacology. *Psychiatric Clinics of North America*, 35, 143–163.

43

Innovation in Clinical Practice

Almost everyone can and should do research . . . because almost everyone has a unique observational opportunity at some time in his life which he has an obligation to record. . . . If one considers the fundamental operations or methods of research, one immediately realizes that most people do research at some time or another, except that they do not call their activity by that name. There are seven operations. . . . In simple language they are counting, sorting, measuring, comparing, nature-study, guess testing, and reappraisal. . . . Guess testing is of course what most people think of when the word research is mentioned; except that it is bad manners to call a guess a guess. It should be called an hypothesis. Let me make one plea. Guessing becomes merely a game unless it is also a plan for action. It is a waste of time elaborating untestable hypotheses.

—John Cade

EVERY NEW CLASS OF AGENTS IN PSYCHOPHARMACOLOGY HAS BEGUN WITH clinical innovation and novel observations at the outset. This has been the case with reserpine, which was observed to be associated with depression, and led to the development of MAOIs. Phenothiazines were used as anesthesia and observed to have major tranquilizing effects, and later examined clinically in psychosis with benefit. TCAs were developed for schizophrenia as chemical products of phenothiazines, yet they were observed to improve depression. Lithium was discovered by John Cade, who used it in a small group of selected manic patients (see following). And carbamazepine was initially extended to bipolar illness based on innovative observation of evidence of benefit for mood in epilepsy. In every case, when there has been a fundamental new departure in psychopharmacology, it always began with clinical innovation. It never began in a research protocol with well-thought out methodologies, hypotheses, outcome measures, and guidelines for ethical conduct.

This history is not unique to psychopharmacology. Antibiotics famously began in the serendipitous work of Alexander Fleming. Antihypertensives also were discovered based on unexpected observations. Clinical innovation is the fount of research discoveries for all of medicine, and psychiatry is no different.

Clinical innovation occurs, by definition, outside of formal research protocols. There is a risk that treatment guidelines of any kind, however well-intentioned, will impede clinical innovation unnecessarily. On the other hand, there are limits to acceptable innovation, and in some cases, one can imagine cases of innovation that would appear to be unethical.

The issue at hand is the contrast between "research," bound by strict rules and conducted by "scientists," as opposed to "treatment," conducted by clinicians. In this chapter, it will be held that the two activities have much in common, and that good clinicians should do "research"; i.e., innovate based on their experience. Furthermore, good research needs to be connected to experience from clinical practice.

BACKGROUND

Part of the problem is that the academic bioethics community has sought to cleanly and completely separate clinical practice from research. In the *Belmont Report of The National Commission for the Protection of Human Subjects*, for instance, an attempt was made to separate "practice," where "interventions are designed solely to enhance the wellbeing of an individual patient or client and that have a reasonable expectation of success" (*Belmont Report*, p. 3), from "research," defined as "an activity designed to test an hypothesis, permit conclusions to be drawn, and thereby to develop or contribute to generalizable knowledge" (*Belmont Report*, p. 3). In fact, the clinician/researcher engaging in clinical innovation is not acting with solely one set of interests in mind, but two. On one hand, the clinician/researcher wants to help the individual patient; on the other, the clinician/researcher wants to gain some experience or knowledge from his observation.

Some in the bioethics community set up this scenario as a necessary conflict. They seem to think that a choice must be made: either the clinician must choose to seek only to make the patient better, without learning anything in the process; or the clinician must seek to learn something, without any intention at all to improve the patient's lot. As with so much in life, there are in fact multiple interests here, and there is no need to insist that those interests do not overlap at all. First and foremost in any clinical encounter is the clinician's responsibility to the individual welfare of the patient. Any innovative treatment, observation, or hypothesis cannot be allowed to lead to complete lack of regard for the patient's welfare. Unfortunately, the *Belmont Report* and much of the mainstream bioethics literature presumes complete and unavoidable conflict of these interests:

> When a clinician departs in a significant way from standard or accepted practice, the innovation does not, in and of itself, constitute research. The fact that a procedure is "experimental," in the sense of new, untested, or different, does not automatically place it in the category of research. . . . [but] the general rule is that if there is any element of research in an activity, that activity should undergo review for the protection of human subjects. (*Belmont Report*, p. 4)

This approach leads, it could be argued, to both uncontrolled clinical innovation and over-regulated formal research. The ultimate rationale for clinical innovation is evidence from the history of psychopharmacology that such innovation is essential to the research process. Furthermore, since such innovation, by definition, occurs outside of formal research protocols, if it is granted legitimacy, then clinicians will need to think about how to provide an ethical framework to support it. Two case scenarios may help clarify the subject.

Case Scenarios

Dr. X primarily treats mood disorders and is interested in new drugs because many of his patients have failed treatment with "standard" medications. Many new medications become available to practitioners after being approved by the FDA for disorders other than depression (e.g., epilepsy). Dr. X begins to give these medications to some of his patients with mood disorders, and soon most of his patients are taking various combinations of them. Dr. X never publishes his experience, which is unfortunate because initially studies of those medications for mood disorders are sparse. The studies that do appear are quite preliminary of necessity (uncontrolled, non-randomized, small case series). When asked, Dr. X strongly asserts his beliefs regarding the benefits of certain medications he uses and the lack of utility of others.

Here is another scenario: Dr. Y also likes to use new drugs, similarly for mood disorders, although the medications are FDA-indicated only for other conditions. After using these agents in 5–10 patients, she usually publishes her experience. Sometimes, she then becomes involved in obtaining funding for more rigorous studies of the medications that appear potentially useful based on her publications. In some cases, her early experience is confirmed by randomized studies (and occasionally new FDA indications), and sometimes they are not confirmed.

Neither Dr. X nor Dr. Y prepares a protocol or obtain Institutional Review Board (IRB) approval or a research-based informed consent for their clinical use of any of these medications. Are these doctors practicing ethically?

The classic bioethics approach would be that neither doctor is practicing ethically, because they are not obtaining IRB approval for non-standard practice. One could claim, contrast that Dr. Y is practicing ethically, because she at least is testing her hypotheses, while Dr. X is veering too far from scientifically proven treatments, and is practicing solely based on his personal beliefs.

THE STORY OF LITHIUM

The history of psychopharmacology, such as the story of lithium, may provide a model for understanding how to promote effective innovation in clinical practice. John Cade was an Australian psychiatrist who decided to test a hypothesis he had developed while interned in a Japanese prisoner-of-war camp during the Second World War: that mania and depression represented abnormalities of nitrogen metabolism (excess or deficiency states). After collecting urine samples from patients with mania, depression, and schizophrenia, and normal controls, he injected them into guinea pigs, all of whom died. He concluded that the nitrogenous product, urea, was probably acting as a poison, but a similar dose of pure laboratory urea (equivalent to the urea concentrations in urine) did not have the same effect. Thus Cade began to search for modifying factors in the urine of these patients (such as uric acid) that might be enhancing the toxicity of urea. As part of his effort to study uric acid, he noted that lithium urate, which he chose to study simply because it was the most soluble form of uric acid, actually reduced the toxicity of urea. Although he initially assumed that this protective effect was due to the uric acid, he included a different lithium salt (lithium chloride) just to be certain. To his great surprise, he found that the chloride salt of lithium also provided the same protection from urea toxicity, and, even more to his surprise, the guinea pigs were calm when he handled them, rather than showing the usual agitation triggered by handling. Cade had just witnessed the psychotropic effect of lithium. Cade worked in an era before the existence of mechanisms for formal review of research protocols. Yet his experimental subjects were protected by his own Hippocratic ethic that led him to first try lithium himself before giving it to a patient: "How to proceed? *Primum non nocere*. . . . There is always the number one experimental animal, oneself." Thus Cade was able to detail the signs of lithium toxicity, along with its benefits, in his first report in 1949. In fact, his first patient, W. B., whose case Cade regarded initially as the most successful, developed many side effects, and Cade repeatedly took him off lithium only to feel forced to resume it due to W. B.'s severe chronic mania. A year later, during an admission for severe mania, Cade resumed lithium at apparently therapeutic levels, but W.B., who probably had an infection, suffered a number of seizures, lapsed into coma, and died. Cade was quite concerned and abandoned using lithium further due to its toxicity. It was for other researchers to follow up on his discovery and determine how lithium might safely be used to treat mania. In fact, the first randomized clinical trials in psychiatry were conducted in the early 1950s as follow-up assessments of Cade's original report of six cases.

Would we have lithium if Cade were working today? It is unlikely. If Cade worked in a hospital today, he probably would not have been able to obtain enough animal data to justify using lithium in humans, and he probably would not have been allowed to experiment on himself. Most IRBs would not have allowed Cade to give lithium to acutely manic patients, given the state of his knowledge of the drug.

As noted in the introductory quote to this chapter, drawn from a presidential address given to the Australian and New Zealand College of Psychiatry near the end of his life, Cade identified "guess testing," comparable to the concept of clinical innovation, as essential to psychopharmacological research. And the most essential aspect of innovation, according to Cade, is that there should be hypothesis testing. Innovative use of medications should not be random; it should be driven by legitimate hypotheses, and therefore provable or disprovable. Indeed, Pasteur's famous maxim about chance favoring the prepared mind can be interpreted as involving the combination of serendipity and hypothesis testing. If one has hypotheses, and one is actively seeking to test them, then one is more likely to come across "chance" findings that others may either not observe or not experience.

It also is important to emphasize, nonetheless, that chance findings can be noticed by an alert physician, even if no prior hypothesis exists. For instance, no hypothesis of antidepressant effect preceded the observation that the use of reserpine led to depression, or that imipramine used in schizophrenia improved depression. These two innovative observations, not initially driven by hypotheses, set the ball in motion that ultimately led to a Nobel prize given for the unraveling the biochemical mechanisms of these agents. All this work started with clinical observation without hypothesis. Much clinical innovation begins with the use of a drug for an indication not used before, which then leads to novel observations that lead to a new hypothesis that can then be tested.

One major path of clinical innovation is the path described by Cade, where one possesses an hypothesis, and one is experimentally interested in testing the hypothesis, and new findings occur as a result. Another path of clinical innovation occurs when alert clinicians watch for unexpected effects when using a drug for legitimate purposes. Without having an initial hypothesis, these clinicians find something they didn't expect. This truly serendipitous finding leads to hypotheses that can then lead to further clinical innovation and eventually more organized research.

So innovation begins in clinical practice without proof, and then gets proven in research protocols, returning to wider clinical practice after it is proven. Conceived in terms used by evidence-based medicine (EBM), innovation in psychopharmacology more commonly proceeds bottom-up, rather than top-down. Innovation proceeds usually from low-level case reports, through middle-level naturalistic and non-randomized studies, to high-level randomized studies. Less frequently does it go in the other direction, from initial randomized studies to clinical experience.

Let's illustrate these issues with our two scenarios. Dr. X uses all kinds of medications without attempting to organize, quantify, or publish his experience. Furthermore, he holds strong beliefs about the benefits and risks of medications based almost solely on his clinical experience. Dr. Y uses the same medications, but reports her experience to the scientific community, and is involved in research protocols based on her pilot uncontrolled experience.

What did Cade do? Cade used lithium with a research hypothesis in mind. He further tried it on animals before humans, given the absence of any prior human use. He even tried it on himself before using it with other patients. He reported his experience immediately to the scientific community. And when he experienced a bad outcome, he reported it also and curtailed his use of the medication. Other researchers were able to conduct rigorous research protocols based on Cade's early reports. Cade and Dr. Y have much in common, which we think helps us identify the ideal characteristics of ethical innovation.

THE ETHICS OF CLINICAL RESEARCH

A commonly cited means by which clinical innovation may differ from formal research has to do with the clinician's intention. At one level, it often seems to be assumed that if the intention of the clinician is primarily to treat the individual patient, then it is not research; but if the intention is primarily to advance knowledge, then it is research. This dichotomy is set up to a great extent by the Helsinki Declaration, which seemed to state that research by definition is not primarily concerned with the individual patient's welfare.

Psychopharmacology researchers know that, in many cases, a research study both advances knowledge and is directly beneficial to the patient in equal degrees. This is especially the case with open-label studies. How one can differentiate such research from clinical innovation becomes somewhat unclear. What if the actions in two cases are the same, such as giving unproven drug X openly, but in one setting as part of a research protocol, and in the other as part of daily clinical activity? Is the primary motivation of the doctor the sole difference that would make the activity research in one case, and therefore requiring informed consent and IRB review, whereas it is clinical innovation in another case, which proceeds without oversight?

One could argue that clinical innovation does not require this kind of oversight, though it is, as Cade stated, part of research. The either/or dichotomy derived from the Helsinki Declaration often does not help us in understanding the research process in psychopharmacology.

The only sensible reading of the historical record in psychopharmacology is that there is a factual link between clinical innovation and progress in formal clinical research. Clinical innovation is a legitimate activity, because it often serves as a source of ideas and observations that later lead to classical research conducted in the formal manner of protocols, IRB reviews, and rigorous designs. Sometimes clinical practice can yield important knowledge beyond what can be gleaned from randomized clinical trial protocols. This chapter has reviewed some historical examples, such as John Cade's discovery of lithium. Thus, clinical innovation is a legitimate and important activity.

Does this approach conflict with federal standards, such as the *Belmont Report,* which has been identified by the NIH Office of Human Subjects Research as the philosophical foundation for its ethical regulations? As mentioned before, the *Report* leaves itself open to a strict interpretation when it asserts that "any element of research" requires formal review. Yet even the NIH notes that the *Report* is

> not a set of rules that can be applied rigidly to make determinations of whether a proposed research activity is ethically "right" or "wrong." Rather, these regulations provide a framework in which investigators and others can ensure that serious efforts have been made to protect the rights and welfare of research subjects. (NIH, 1993, p. 4)

In conclusion, it is suggested here that the best clinical research is conducted by active clinicians, and that the best clinical work is conducted by active researchers. The strict wall separating pure research from pure clinical practice is at best a fiction, and at worst a dumbing down of both activities. Clinical innovation is the kind of activity that bridges this gap. Clinical innovation should be legitimized, accepted, and even encouraged within the framework of ethical guidelines, such as those suggested here, so as to avoid the alternative extremes of indiscriminate practice on one hand and over-regulation of all research on the other.

SELECTED REFERENCES

The Belmont Report. Ethical Principles and Guidelines for the Protection of Human Subjects of Research: The National Commission for the Protection of Human Subjects of Biomedical and Behavioral Research, 1979. https://www.hhs.gov/ohrp/sites/default/files/the-belmont-report-508c_FINAL.pdf, accessed August 6, 2018.

Ghaemi, S. N., & Goodwin, F. K. (2007). The ethics of clinical innovation in psychopharmacology. *Philosophy, Ethics, and Humanities in Medicine*, 2, 26.

NIH, 1993, Guidelines for the Conduct of Research Involving Human Subjects at the National Institutes of Health. Washington DC: U.S. Department of Health and Human Services, Public Health Service.

44
Clinical Cases

CASE 1: "TREATMENT-RESISTANT DEPRESSION" AS MISDIAGNOSED BIPOLAR DEPRESSION

An 80-year-old male seeks consultation for severe treatment-refractory depression. He had been depressed for 7 months, without improvement, despite treatment with venlafaxine (Effexor) 150 mg/d for 6 weeks, which was then changed to citalopram (Celexa) 50 mg/d for 9 weeks, which made him more depressed and suicidal. Then olanzapine (Zyprexa) was added to citalopram, up to 15 mg/d, without benefit. Fluoxetine was increased up to 80 mg/d plus olanzapine, and valproate (Depakote, Epival) was added at the same time at 500 mg/d; these last changes made him feel even worse, and valproate was switched to risperidone. At consultation, he was taking fluoxetine (Prozac) 80 mg/d, olanzapine 15 mg/d, and risperidone 3 mg/d, along with multiple cardiological medications.

He complained greatly about anxiety and indecision. "I have a lot of regrets; they bother me a lot. My worry has a basis, but it is overblown." He had a great deal of nihilistic thinking; family reported: "He worries about the least likely thing that could happen." He couldn't function at work. He had clear discrete depressive episodes in 1968 (his first episode, received ECT), 1975 (recovered in 3–4 months), 1996 (recovered in 3–6 months), 2001 (lasted longer, about 8–9 months, saw a consultant, who diagnosed bipolar illness but didn't stop antidepressants), and the current episode (2013). Unlike prior episodes, there wasn't a major psychosocial trigger for his last episode. In between episodes, his family reported that he was "perfectly normal: very social, very gregarious" and functional as a prominent lawyer. No prior psychiatrist except for one consultant had observed that each of the depressive episodes described here had been preceded by a phase of 5–6 months of elevation. According to family: "He was a bit high, even more outgoing, would go and visit so many relatives when he went out for an errand that he'd get distracted, would sleep little, and would read furiously about all different kinds of topics that have nothing to do with his field. He had a lot of energy, would get up very early, and would be very active." He had no past suicide attempts or psychiatric hospitalizations, had a medical history of hypertension and coronary artery disease, and a normal head

MRI. He had no drug allergies and no substance abuse history. He had no history of trauma or abuse, had been married for 55 years, had four adult children, and worked as a lawyer. Medication trials included multiple antidepressants (most of the SRIs), multiple neuroleptics, but only one mood stabilizer (recent treatment with low-dose valproate). In family history, his brother was diagnosed with "schizophrenia" 40 years ago: "He was quite lively, became obsessed with reading all medical books," and was treated with antipsychotics. This brother also had severe depressive episodes with marked loss of appetite and a catatonic state. Bipolar disorder was diagnosed in two second cousins, treated with lithium. A niece committed suicide.

The consultant's diagnosis was bipolar disorder, type II, currently depressed. The diagnosis of bipolar illness is clear, as previously noted by another consultant. Unfortunately, this diagnosis had not been taken seriously, and thus had not been treated with the appropriate treatment; namely, an adequate dose of a mood stabilizer *without antidepressants, which destabilize bipolar illness and counteract the benefits of mood stabilizers.* Prior evaluations missed the fact that each depressive episode is preceded by a clear hypomanic episode that lasts months. These hypomanic episodes are not questionable and are not brief. They exist, yet he has been treated as if they didn't exist. Prior psychiatrists either didn't make the bipolar diagnosis, or saw it as therapeutically unimportant. The consultant who had diagnosed bipolar illness made no effort to stop antidepressants or recommend mood stabilizers. He even focused instead on psychosocial explanations, such as Erikson's stage of "generativity versus despair" in old age. (How this explanation would explain the patient's depressive episodes in his 20s, 30s, and 40s was left unexplained.)

Prior treatment had focused on treating each acute depressive episode with antidepressant and antipsychotic combinations, rather than trying to prevent those depressive episodes with mood stabilizers. Divalproex had been used recently for his acute bipolar depression, but at a subtherapeutic dose of 500 mg/d, added to very high-dose fluoxetine. If antidepressants counteracted the benefits of mood stabilizers, that trial would not have been effective. This case is a good example of how antidepressants simply can be ineffective for acute bipolar depression, as found in the largest randomized clinical trials. Hence the mistaken label of "treatment-refractory depression": *the depression isn't refractory when antidepressants have been proven ineffective for it.*

When the patient improved in the past, it probably was not because of antidepressant treatment, but rather as part of the natural course of bipolar illness; namely, that each depressive episode tends to last a certain amount of time (usually about 3–6 months) and then resolves on its own. When ineffective treatments are multiplied (such as combining olanzapine and risperidone) and increased to maximal doses (such as 80 mg/d of fluoxetine) in an 80-year-old person with coronary artery disease, then the likelihood of harm is magnified. These doses are meant for non-elderly adults. In elderly persons, it is a maxim that doses should be halved, because decreased renal excretion over time leads to lengthening of drug half-lives. Thus 80 mg/d of fluoxetine in a nearly 80-year-old gentleman is quite excessive, and likely to be causing important physical harm. It is especially notable that fluoxetine is a very potent inhibitor of drug metabolism in the liver. Thus, this very high dose is also markedly increasing doses of almost all other medications, including olanzapine and risperidone, which would notably increase their side effects, including Parkinsonian tremor and rigidity, akathisia, and—perhaps most importantly—diabetes and cardiovascular risks (hyperlipidemia and hypertension).

For all these reasons, the patient's medications were ineffective, and at the very high doses given, they posed major medical risks to him, and were probably causing, or would soon cause, serious medical harm. Fluoxetine has the advantage of less serotonin withdrawal than other SRIs. It was tapered off over 2 weeks (40 mg/d for 1 week, then 20 mg/d for 1 week, then stopped). The patient had no SRI withdrawal. Risperidone was discontinued immediately, and olanzapine was tapered off. One week after the initial visit, a titration of lamotrigine was initiated, reaching a target dose of 100 mg/d over another month (25 mg/d for 1 week, then 50 mg/d for 1 week, then 75 mg/d for 1 week, then 100 mg/d). Lorazepam 1 mg twice daily was given for anxiety and SRI withdrawal. Two months later, the patient had improved moderately on lamotrigine 100 mg/d, and lorazepam 1 mg twice daily. Depressive and anxiety symptoms were still present, but somewhat less than previously.

Bottom Line

- This apparent treatment-resistant depression was really mistreated bipolar depression—a common scenario.
- Very high-dose fluoxetine with high-dose olanzapine plus risperidone proved ineffective, and was no better than lamotrigine alone.
- At least we were able to get the patient off medically harmful drugs, like olanzapine, and drugs with major drug interactions (fluoxetine).
- Lamotrigine is now in place to help prevent future depressive episodes, with minimal long-term medical risks in this older gentleman with coronary artery disease.
- Erikson's stages are irrelevant if you get the diagnosis and/or treatment wrong.
- This type of case illustrates the adage: *Your treatment is only as good as your diagnosis.*

CASE 2: TREATING ANXIETY IN PTSD

A 25-year-old female seeks treatment for anxiety and depression. She experienced repeated childhood sexual abuse by her father at ages 8–10. In the last few years, she had constant depression, with periods of worsening related to life stresses. She is also constantly anxious, with panic attacks at times, and flashbacks and nightmares that occur in waves (i.e., a week or two of multiple flashbacks/nightmares, followed by 2–3 weeks without them). She doesn't abuse substances, is a single mother with two children, and lives on disability income. She reports anxiety and depression in family members but they mostly avoid psychiatrists, so most are not diagnosed. Five years ago, she received fluoxetine, later sertraline and duloxetine, each with mild benefit. In the past year, she took venlafaxine, which helped her anxiety moderately at 150 mg/d, but then she began to worsen again in the past few months. Her psychiatrist tried to switch venlafaxine to citalopram, but she experienced marked serotonin withdrawal. Current medications are Effexor 75 mg/d, clonazepam 1 mg twice daily, and quetiapine 50 mg for sleep.

The consultant's diagnosis was PTSD, based on available information. PTSD improves only moderately, at best, with medications. Her history with SRIs was consistent with this scientific evidence. Thus, the consultant felt that there was not much benefit to be gained by medications. Modest symptom benefits on one hand were weighed against non-negligible side effects, the most important now being serotonin withdrawal syndrome. Another reason to minimize medications like SRIs is that it sends the message to the patient that the main treatment is not SRIs but psychotherapies. More time and effort should be focused on the latter, not the former.

Since fluoxetine, with its very long half-life of about one week, has the least serotonin withdrawal, the consultant's recommendation was to cross-taper venlafaxine with fluoxetine. (Add 20 mg of fluoxetine, reduce venlafaxine to 37. 5 mg/d for 2 weeks, then stop venlafaxine. Then reduce fluoxetine one month later to 10 mg/d for one month, then stop it.) Clonazepam was changed to lorazepam 1 mg twice daily as needed for more immediate symptom benefit. In weeks where the patients' flashbacks and nightmares were worse, she was instructed to take lorazepam in standing dose twice daily. When PTSD symptoms remitted, lorazepam was reduced to "as needed." In the year following these changes, the patient's anxiety symptoms were similar to prior years with SRIs; she wasn't better, but she wasn't worse either. She continued to engage in weekly psychotherapy, with gradual improvement in severity/frequency of PTSD exacerbations.

Bottom Line

- SRI benefit for PTSD is limited.
- As-needed benzodiazepine use provided similar benefit to more extensive SRI use, with less medication usage and thus fewer overall harms.
- Psychotherapy, not medication, is the main effective long-term treatment in this case.

CASE 3: SUICIDALITY AND ANTIDEPRESSANTS IN BORDERLINE PERSONALITY

A 25-year-old adopted Asian female is treated with bupropion 300 mg/d and atomoxetine 60 mg/d. She reports chronic and constant suicidal ideation for the past 10 years. She has abused alcohol and marijuana regularly for years, and cocaine as well more recently. She was hospitalized once at age 14, has had many overdoses and some cutting behavior. She also has bulimia at times. She was adopted, so biological family information is not available. She grew up in a wealthy, white, upper-class suburb. Her mother accompanied her, and the family appears very supportive of her. She went to excellent schools and never experienced any trauma of any kind. She has never married, has no children, graduated from college, and lives alone while working for a retail store.

She describes past manic symptoms as follows: "I'm always rushing around, racing thoughts, pretty hyper, I can get so much shit done." This is associated with talkativeness and distractibility: "I'm always confident." She has impulsive behavior of all kinds: sexual, spending, reckless driving. "I've always been nocturnal, I like to stay up at night." Normally, she goes to sleep at 4:00 AM and wakes up at 8:00 AM, without being tired. When she's depressed, she has very low energy and sleeps over 13 hours nightly. There are no definable episodes of mania above this baseline.

She was diagnosed with borderline personality disorder plus MDD at age 15 and has received weekly psychotherapy for 10 years; she also has taken antidepressants for the past 5 years. She briefly received lithium at age 15, added to citalopram, without benefit. Her course of illness was rapid-cycling: 3 months earlier, she had a depressive episode for 1 month; followed by her hyperthymic baseline.

The consultation diagnosis is hyperthymic temperament. As reviewed in the text, mood temperaments exist, but DSM only recognizes dysthymia and cyclothymia. Hyperthymia was also described a century ago by Kretschmer, who formalized the definitions of dysthymia and cyclothymia as well. As a state of constant mild manic symptoms as part of one's personality, hyperthymic temperament can produce unstable interpersonal relationships and constant irritability, which may be mistaken for borderline personality. In the absence of sexual trauma and self-cutting, the approach recommended here is that borderline personality shouldn't be diagnosed mainly based on less specific features such as unstable interpersonal relationships, anger, and suicidality.

The consultation recommendation was to discontinue antidepressants. Her chronic suicidal ideation, persistent for ten years, completely resolved immediately. In 6-month follow up, she refused mood stabilizer treatment but was much better off antidepressants without psychotherapy than she had been previously.

Bottom Line

- Antidepressants caused long-term suicidality in a young adult with hyperthymic temperament misdiagnosed as borderline personality.
- Even without lithium, suicidality resolved once antidepressants were stopped.

CASE 4: LOW-DOSE DIVALPROEX FOR MISDIAGNOSED NARCISSISTIC PERSONALITY DISORDER

A 45-year-old male is diagnosed with narcissistic personality disorder (NPD) comorbid with generalized anxiety disorder (GAD) and MDD. He has been treated with long-term psychodynamic psychotherapy on multiple occasions for 6 months to 2 years at a time. He has taken escitalopram 20 mg/d for 10 years. Sometimes, he has brief periods of depression lasting a few weeks at a time. He has had occasional suicidal ideation for the past 10 years. He has abused alcohol in the past, but has been sober for 5 years. He has never been hospitalized, overdosed, nor engaged in cutting behavior. His first cousin was diagnosed with bipolar disorder and did well on lithium. He was raised by an intact supportive family, became a lawyer, divorced twice, now lives alone, and never had childhood trauma.

He was seen as narcissistic because he has very high self-confidence, generally thinks he is smarter than others, and devalues his ex-wives. When asked about his failed marriages, he says, "They didn't appreciate me enough." At work, colleagues see him as arrogant, and although he is productive, interpersonal tensions and disrespect for authority have limited his promotion in a corporate law firm.

On evaluation, when asked about his energy, sleep, mood, and activities, he reports constant mood swings, on an hourly basis, sometimes very happy for hours and sometimes irritable and down for hours. He usually only needs 4 hours of sleep nightly, and has a high energy and activity level compared to peers', and a very high libido all the time. He reports feeling anxious and having "nervous energy" most of the time. He is an active rock climber, bikes 20 miles each morning before going to work, and sees himself as a "workaholic."

The consultation diagnosis is cyclothymic temperament. He also is high on the personality trait of neuroticism. The constant shifting of his moods, with frequent manic symptoms, was misinterpreted as "narcissism" because the grandiosity of manic symptoms was interpreted in the psychoanalytic paradigm of narcissism, within the DSM categorization of personality disorders.

The patient was treated with low-dose Depakote, 250 mg/d for 1 month, then increased to 500 mg/d. Cyclothymic mood symptoms improved moderately, including inflated self-esteem as part of the manic component. His co-workers noticed that he seemed more responsive to interpersonal cues, interpreted as being less "arrogant." His libido and energy were lower, but still higher than most people's. He remained productive, but had improved interpersonal relations.

Bottom Line

- Manic symptoms of inflated self-esteem were misdiagnosed as narcissistic personality disorder.
- Low-dose divalproex was more effective than long-term psychodynamic psychotherapy.

CASE 5: CARBAMAZEPINE TO THE RESCUE

A 38-year-old female is diagnosed with anxiety and depression. She has had depressive episodes repeatedly, usually lasting a few months at a time. She has also had manic and hypomanic episodes in the past; in college, she said, she "slept with way too many people." These periods of sexual overactivity contrasted with months of decreased libido when she was depressed. During those hypomanic periods, she also had increased overall activity, talked rapidly, and had fast thoughts. Those periods lasted days to weeks. In recent years, her elevated moods were associated with overspending, which led to major financial problems. Depressive periods were characterized by low energy, decreased interest, sadness, insomnia, and high anxiety. Her mood swings were such that she was never able to maintain a long-term stable relationship. She's never been married and has no children. She works in an insurance company. She had no childhood trauma and has never cut or harmed herself. She is pleasant and cooperative in the interview. She has no past substance abuse.

After she failed to improve on paroxetine, sertraline, venlafaxine, or bupropion, her doctor added divalproex to bupropion. She had a moderate improvement in anxiety and depressive symptoms, and fewer manic symptoms, though she still has some hypomanic episodes. She experienced marked hair loss with divalproex, however, with no benefit with mineral supplements. A trial of lithium also caused hair loss. Current medications are divalproex 500 mg twice daily and bupropion SR 300 mg daily. She wants an alternative mood stabilizer that won't cause hair loss.

The consultation diagnosis is bipolar illness type I. Some clinicians would diagnose borderline personality based on the broad DSM criteria of mood swings, unstable interpersonal relationships, and sexual impulsivity. The consultation view was that the absence of childhood sexual trauma and parasuicidal self-harm argues strongly against the borderline label. In contrast, clear manic, hypomanic, and depressive episodes exist.

The two remaining standard mood stabilizers are carbamazepine and lamotrigine, neither of which cause hair loss (nor weight gain). Since she has had notable manic morbidity (financial impairment excludes hypomania), the consultant recommended carbamazepine rather than lamotrigine. Furthermore, since bupropion is a mild amphetamine, which has been proven ineffective in bipolar depression (equivalent to placebo in the STEP-BD study), the view of this text is that it is useless at best, harmful at worst. Since all monoamine agonists (antidepressants) can cause more mood cycling, bupropion could be destabilizing her mood, worsening her continued depressive and hypomanic episodes.

The consultation recommendation was to taper off bupropion (150 mg/d for 2 weeks, then stop) and to replace divalproex with carbamazepine ER 300 mg twice daily. Three months later, her mood had improved markedly, with resolution of hair loss, and no other side effects. Mild anxiety persisted, which responded to lorazepam 1 mg daily.

Bottom Line

- Use carbamazepine rather than lamotrigine when a patient's history involves notable manic episodes with functional impairment.
- Remember to stop monoamine agonists long-term: there is no benefit, only possible harm.

CASE 6: LIFE EVENTS, NOT TRAUMA

A 25-year-old female is diagnosed with anxiety, depression, and PTSD. As a child, she was raised in a supportive family with no known sexual or physical abuse. When she went to school, though, she experienced bullying and had conflicts with some female peers. In college, she felt out of place and had a clinical depressive episode at age 18. She met a young man whom she married and who has been very supportive. In the last few years, she has experienced continued anxiety and depression, although no definable flashbacks or nightmares. Her most recent period of worsening of symptoms relates to the passing of an aunt, to whom she was very close. Also, her husband recently lost his job, which caused her to be worried about their finances. Their family is helping to support them.

Her family genetics involve severe depression in multiple family members going back a few generations, including one person who received ECT and was put into a state hospital for decades. Staying with the course of her illness, she has had definable clinical depressive episodes since age 18, usually lasting about 2–3 months. In between those episodes she always was mildly depressed in mood, but didn't meet full clinical depressive episode definitions. She had not cut herself or made any suicide attempts. She has had no dissociative experiences.

Her clinician saw her as having "complex PTSD" with these multiple life stressors causing her anxiety and depressive symptoms. Multiple SRIs and amphetamines and benzodiazepines produced limited benefit. Her current medications were citalopram 20 mg/d and Adderall.

The consultation diagnosis is recurrent unipolar depressive illness (also known as manic-depressive illness [MDI]). The family genetics of severe mood disease reflects the original concept of MDI. Recurrent severe depressive episodes beginning early in life, around age 18, and being short in duration (2–3 months) reflect the course of illness of what is now called bipolar illness (a variety of manic-depressive disease). Baseline mood symptoms seem to represent dysthymia, a mood temperament that occurs in persons or families with manic-depression. She has no specific features of PTSD as classically described; i.e., no identifiable trauma and no dissociative symptoms. Even if she had PTSD, she was not receiving adequate psychotherapy for it, but rather extensive medication treatment, which is not very effective for that condition.

The consultant's recommendation was to taper off citalopram and Adderall and to replace them with whatever mood-stabilizing agent she could tolerate or was willing to take. She was willing to take lamotrigine, and a fluoxetine cross-titration was instituted to help with SRI withdrawal (since she had been on those agents for years). Since she had no drug allergies, lamotrigine was deemed acceptably safe if dosed very slowly (25 mg every 2 weeks). Over 3–6 months, her mood improved more than it had in the past.

Bottom Line

- This case provides an example of the misinterpretation of life events as traumata.
- Genetics and course of illness provide the definitive diagnostic evidence.

CASE 7: "PREMENSTRUAL MOOD DYSPHORIC DISORDER" OR RAPID-CYCLING BIPOLAR ILLNESS?

A 26-year-old female without prior psychiatric history presents for a consultation upon the recommendation of primary care. Both primary care and gynecology have diagnosed premenstrual dysphoric disorder (PMDD). In 2014, primary care prescribed Sarafem (fluoxetine) for several months, "but it didn't do anything." Primary care also recommended this consultation for an ADHD evaluation. The patient had taken a friend's ADHD medication (Adderall 5–10 mg) and "it brings me up to par. It just really helps with the lows and the attention." The patient describes a long history, since teenage years, of alternating mood cycles. She only became aware of them in 2012 when she experienced several months of continuous depressive symptoms after a family death. She reports that about 14 days before menses she develops significant depressive symptoms, especially very low energy ("it just completely dives"), poor motivation ("don't even want to get out of bed"), no desire to socialize, and very low mood. At the same time, attention and thinking are poor ("I feel like there is this film over my brain, a hard time thinking and articulating things"). In contrast, the other two weeks of the month (at menses and onward), she experiences the opposite: "I'm just motivated, doing a lot better. It's the way I should be feeling all month long." She reports being productive at work, bright and optimistic, "but I think my mood is usually optimistic." The patient reports chronic sleep impairment and racing thoughts since teenage years: "I have always been a night owl. . . . My brain is incredibly more active at night time. I have a hard time shutting my mind off in the evenings." There are periods where sleep is worse and she averages 6 hours at night, (1:00 AM–7:30 AM), but she still has good energy. She denies past manic episodes. In reference to the 2 weeks of elevated mood, energy, and thinking, she denies these as above her baseline: "I feel like this is how I should be. I just feel more organized. I have more motivation to do the small things like working out or doing chores." She recently had another consultation with a psychiatrist who agreed with the PMDD diagnosis but referred her back to her gynecologist. "He said there is nothing behaviorally he could do for me. He said what was happening was a chemical process and I should go back to gynecology." Past medical history is notable for past ovarian cysts. She has taken several oral contraceptives, but each caused more depression.

Family history is as follows: Maternal aunt: was "treated for some depression throughout her life." Father "is like me in a lot of ways, hyperfocused sometimes and stays up late." Brother is diagnosed with ADHD and uses stimulants, "but I think he just uses it for a high stress job." She had no behavioral or academic problems. She was active with many hobbies, including tennis, soccer, and softball. Mother has told patient that she has suspected patient was periodically depressed in high school.

She denies any physical symptoms associated with menses—no bowel changes, cramping, bloating, heavy bleeding, or headaches. Extensive laboratory testing for thyroid stimulating hormone (TSH), follicular stimulating hormone (FSH), prolactin, and cortisol are all within normal limits. During the consultation, her mental status examination was notable for: hyperactivity (restless, fast and quick movements); pressured speech but interruptible; mood "pretty great!"; mildly euphoric affect—very animated, gregarious; and mild tangentiality requiring some redirection.

The consultant's evaluation was that the case reflects a long history of mood cycles, which probably have less to do with her menses than with bipolar illness. Premenstrual dysphoric disorder is unlikely here because of

1. severity of symptoms between pre- and post-menses cycles;
2. lack of any physiological symptoms associated with menses (no bloating or cramping);
3. chronic symptoms of insomnia and racing thoughts (which have nothing to do with PMDD but are a frequent feature of untreated bipolar);
4. family history being suspicious for mood cycling, probably in father;
5. lack of response to Prozac; and
6. oral contraceptives–induced depression.

Timing of cycles may not be as clear-cut around menses as the patient believes, but hormonal exacerbations are probably happening.

There certainly are premenstrual symptoms of mood/anxiety/hot flashes/bloating and so on. These symptoms can be caused by other conditions—like MDI—or they can occur by themselves as part of the normal process of menstruation. The key issue is to differentiate those two circumstances; in other words, to apply the concept of diagnostic hierarchy: Does the patient have anything else that could cause premenstrual symptoms? Mood cycles in bipolar illness often are triggered by stressors, not just psychosocial ones, but also biological ones, and hormonal changes around menstrual periods are common biological triggers of mood cycles in bipolar illness. Since they occur monthly, PMS-related mood episodes are rapid-cycling by definition (>4 mood episodes yearly).

Again applying the diagnostic hierarchy concept, ADD isn't present since distractibility is a consequence of the mood episodes, not a separate "disorder," just as "fever disorder" isn't present during pneumonia. Benefit with Adderall isn't diagnostic of ADD because attention improves in everyone with amphetamines. This would be like saying decreased anxiety with benzodiazepines, which occurs in all human beings, means that everyone has an "anxiety disorder."

Regarding the diagnosis of bipolar illness, the question is whether her 2 non-depressed weeks per month represent normal happiness or hypomanic episodes. One hint is that hypomania is recurrent, happiness is not (a favorite quote of Dr. Hagop Akiskal). Six hours nightly of sleep with good energy is biologically abnormal (sleep studies indicate that about 9 hours of sleep is the biological norm, although culturally most of us don't get it). This is decreased need for sleep, a manic symptom; it is not normal. This symptom, along with increased activities and racing thoughts, supports the higher probability of hypomania rather than normal happiness. The biology of this condition is supported further by her father's apparently similar symptoms.

If one can agree on the bipolar diagnosis, with a rapid-cycling course and type II subtype, then the consultant's recommendation was straightforward, like that for any other person with bipolar illness: Use mood stabilizers. Since this is a rapid-cycling course, multiple mood stabilizers will probably be needed, and lamotrigine in particular has been shown to be ineffective in rapid-cycling. Since many patients are concerned about weight gain, the consultant recommended carbamazepine ER first, because it doesn't have weight gain. If a second agent is needed, lithium at low doses may be sufficient. Dopamine blockers don't combine well with carbamazepine because the latter reduces blood levels of the former, rendering them less effective. Another approach would be to start with lamotrigine, see how much benefit is gained, and then add lithium or dopamine blockers that don't have weight gain, like aripiprazole or ziprasidone or lurasidone, at low doses, preferably.

This patient was reluctant to accept these recommendations. The consultant recommended talking to the patient about the concept of a diagnostic hierarchy, using unimpeachable medical examples such as pneumonia and fever. One could make it a pragmatic decision also: If it doesn't work, she can see someone else to take other approaches. For many people, this pragmatic rationale can be persuasive.

CASE 8: NOT ADD, NOT "DEPRESSION," NOT CHRONIC FATIGUE

A 23-year-old female seeks consultation for unremitting depression and ADD. She had been first diagnosed at age 15 with chronic fatigue syndrome. A medical workup for possible causes of exhaustion was negative. Eventually her doctors decided to treat her with amphetamine stimulants to give her energy. Since age 16, she has taken one amphetamine or another, beginning with methylphenidate, later Concerta, and later Adderall.

In the past year, she began to see psychiatrists, who changed her diagnosis from chronic fatigue syndrome to MDD. They continued Adderall and added various SRIs (duloxetine, fluoxetine, sertraline) without success. She was changed eventually to bupropion. On evaluation, she was taking Adderall 20 mg twice daily, plus bupropion SR 150 mg twice daily.

Besides exhaustion, her parents report that she has marked insomnia and notable cognitive impairment. Her sleep is quite poor: she stays up very late, and has multiple awakenings in the night, followed by tiredness during the day. Her cognition is poor also, with very impaired working and verbal and short-term memory. She has been slowed down in her college studies to the point that despite 5 years of college, she has only completed her sophomore year. She has a great deal of trouble organizing herself for her college work, paying attention in class, and in memorizing material for tests.

Adderall gives her "30-minute glimpses of normality." After she takes the medication, she reports that she feels "like myself" for about half an hour, with improved concentration, energy, and mood, but then she goes back into her usual depressed, low energy, poor concentration state.

She has these depressive symptoms continually, but 2–3 times per week, she has about 1–2 hours of spontaneous high energy states: "I feel elated, happy, like I can convince anyone to do anything. I try to do things, but it doesn't last long enough for me to do anything. My thoughts go fast, I talk a lot, I feel super smart briefly, and then I'm back to my usual unhappy slowed down state."

She reports repeated suicidal thoughts and wishes she was dead, but she has not tried to harm herself. She and her family deny past manic or hypomanic episodes lasting 4 days or longer.

One psychiatrist suggested that she had type II bipolar illness, but he continued Adderall and added lithium 900 mg/d immediately. She stopped lithium after two days due to heart palpitations.

Family history provides evidence for a paternal aunt with severe depression that required ECT. All other illness is denied.

Medical history is otherwise normal, and she has no drug allergies, nor does she abuse alcohol or drugs. She has no trauma history. She has had no psychiatric hospitalizations, suicide attempts, self-harm, dissociative or psychotic states, and no eating disorder symptoms.

The consultation diagnosis is that she is experiencing current mixed depressive states. The broader diagnosis is MDI, or one might use the term "bipolar spectrum illness." These diagnoses reflect brief manic states that occur as part of recurrent depressive episodes. The illness is not pure depression, since manic symptoms are present, nor does it represent classic bipolar illness, since full manic or hypomanic episodes are not present. Hence the concept of bipolar spectrum illness can be used to reflect being in the middle of the spectrum between pure depression and full manic or hypomanic episodes.

The consultant's recommendation was to taper off Adderall and bupropion and to resume lithium again, this time in slow titration and in the absence of any antidepressants/amphetamines. This recommendation is explained thus:

Readers should keep in mind that all amphetamines are antidepressants. They were introduced as the first class of antidepressants in the 1930s. Thus, like all antidepressants, they can have negative effects in bipolar illness of causing/worsening mania, or causing/worsening long-term rapid-cycling. In the case of mixed depression antidepressants seem to worsen mixed states, thus causing more depressive and manic symptoms. They especially seem to worsen suicidality and impulsivity. In an analysis of mixed depression using Koukopoulos' criteria, antidepressants caused three times more suicide attempts in person with mixed depression when compared with those treated without antidepressants.

Furthermore, as mood-destabilizing agents, amphetamines and antidepressants counteract the benefits of mood stabilizers, like lithium. Thus, it is not enough to just add lithium. Adderall and bupropion need to be stopped also. Also, readers will recall that bupropion is an amphetamine in its pharmacological structure—all the more reason to stop it.

This patient's apparent "adult ADD" had not improved with amphetamines because it was driven by her mixed depression. Until the mixed depression improves, the "ADD" will not improve. Since amphetamines worsen mixed depression, cognitive ADD-like symptoms persist.

Lithium is the best agent to choose partly because of its direct suicide prevention benefit, given that this patient has clear suicidal ideation and is at notable risk for suicide.

Specific consultant recommendations were as follows:

Reduce Adderall to 20 mg daily for 2 weeks, then 20 mg every other day for 2 weeks, then stop. Reduce bupropion to 150 mg daily for 2 weeks, then stop. At the same time, begin lithium at 300 mg at night for 1 week, then 600 mg at night for one week, then 900 mg at night, seeking a level close to 0.8. The expectation would be that the patient would get worse before getting better, with amphetamine withdrawal leading to worsened energy and concentration and possible clinical depression. This could be the course for a few months, but then the patient would be expected to improve gradually on lithium alone, possibly with later combination with dopamine blockers and/or other mood-stabilizing anticonvulsants such as lamotrigine.

CASE 9: CHILDHOOD ADD WORSENED BY AMPHETAMINES

A 10-year-old male is brought by his mother for consultation. He has been treated with Focalin, Concerta, Adderall, methylphenidate, and Dexedrine. He also has received aripiprazole and olanzapine, added to the preceding agents. His main problems involved not being able to pay attention in school, and being aggressive and agitated toward other children. In two years of treatment, he had not improved, and was forced to change schools multiple times. At one point, while at a restaurant with his parents, he bolted out the door and tried to run down the street. On other occasions, he tried to open the car door on the highway. His parents were concerned about these impulsive behaviors, which had not improved with multiple amphetamines.

He was markedly anxious and had marked insomnia, but his family denied increased or a high level of energy. They also denied any observable depressive symptoms such as suicidality or noticeable sadness or anhedonia. He was adopted and his biological family history was unknown. He lived in an intact and loving family with two parents and an older adopted sister, who had no psychiatric problems and was very successful in school and social life.

He was observed to be very short for his age, and very thin.

On mental status examination, he was polite but played mostly with a video game, answering questions briefly. He was frustrated about his poor social and academic skills and how it harmed his friendships with his peers. He expressed this frustration appropriately and rationally during the interview. He said he wanted to come off his current medications of methylphenidate 60 mg/d and aripiprazole 5 mg/d.

The consultation diagnosis was that anxiety symptoms were present, which could explain all of his attentional impairment, which could further explain his school-related agitation. The worsened impulsivity was attributed to the harmful manic-like effects of amphetamines. The recommendation made was to stop both methylphenidate and aripiprazole. Since the latter has some dopamine agonist effects, it could be contributing to the worsening impulsivity. Two treatment options were given for symptomatic purposes: very low-dose SRI for anxiety, or low-dose risperidone for pure anti-dopamine effects to target impulsivity. The diagnosis was unknown since family history was unknown and because of his young age. It is typical for anxiety symptoms to be the earliest manifestation of other psychopathology, such as later depressive or bipolar illness.

The recommended approach in children is to use medications minimally for symptoms, provide as many behavioral interventions as possible at school and home to improve function, and then to observe the evolution of the illness until a more definitive diagnosis can be made.

Within weeks of stopping methylphenidate, his parents reported that he was much calmer, less anxious, and less agitated. He began to eat more and was putting on needed weight. A few months later, he became somewhat anxious, and the family chose to start SRI treatment. The consultant recommendation was 10 mg fluoxetine given twice weekly. This is because fluoxetine has a very long half-life of one week, so it can be dosed weekly. This approach would give the lowest amount of SRI feasible, and also the child would not see himself as being medicated daily. Within weeks, his anxiety resolved and his behavior improved notably.

At one year follow-up, taking only fluoxetine 10 mg 1–2 times weekly and no other medications, he had grown a number of inches and was closer in stature to his peers, which markedly improved his self-esteem. He had gained weight and was normal in his body mass index. He was doing very well in a private school with sufficient attention to providing behavioral assistance for executive dysfunction. His peer and family relationships had improved markedly.

CASE 10: HYPERTHYMIA MISDIAGNOSED AS TREATMENT-RESISTANT DEPRESSION

A 50-year-old woman presented with refractory anxiety and depression that had failed multiple antidepressants and dopamine blocker trials. She had experienced decades of anxiety and depressive symptoms, which were more or less constant. Brief periods of worsened depression probably met full criteria for a clinical depressive episode many times in the past, with durations of weeks to months. Her anxiety was generalized, with occasional panic attacks. Benzodiazepines had limited benefit, as did six different SRIs.

In consultation, her family history was mostly unknown, and medical history was uninformative. She had no prior trauma, self-cutting, suicide attempts, psychiatric hospitalizations, or psychosis, and no past manic/hypomanic episodes. She was an active lawyer, with a family of three adult children, and marriage of 24 years' duration. Despite being functional, she was very distressed and felt unable to function as well as she could with less anxiety and depression.

In review of her basic personality traits, she described herself as highly extroverted, sociable, fun-loving, and energetic. She normally slept about 6 hours nightly and was not tired most of the time. The neuroticism/extraversion/openness to experience (NEO) scale confirmed that description, with high scores on neuroticism, extroversion, and openness to experience. She met criteria for over 75% of items of hyperthymia on the TEMPS scale.

The consultation diagnosis was hyperthymic temperament. The treatment recommended was low-dose divalproex, since it has anxiolytic effects directly, unlike lithium or other anticonvulsants. In one month, with 500 mg/d of divalproex, she reported marked improvement, sustained for over one year of follow-up, without notable weight gain or other side effects.

CASE 11: WHEN BENZODIAZEPINES ARE PREFERABLE TO SRIS FOR ANXIETY

A 29-year-old woman presents with a diagnosis of panic disorder and generalized anxiety disorder (GAD), for which she is treated with paroxetine for 6 months. She seeks consultation because she reports "not feeling myself" in recent months. She saw her primary care doctor a year ago for panic attacks, which occurred about once monthly. The primary care doctor was reluctant to give her benzodiazepines, and prescribed paroxetine 20 mg/d. This dose produced tremor, which improved at 15 mg/d. Her panic symptoms completely resolved for 6 months, and her function at work improved. However, about 3 months ago, she began to feel less interested in social activities and less interested in her work. She denied low energy or other depressive symptoms. She had one depressive episode 4 years ago, after a break-up, which improved a year later without medication treatment.

She has no other mood episodes in the past, and denies any manic or hypomanic episodes. Manic symptom denial was confirmed in a phone call by the consultant to the patient's mother. She denies any other past psychiatric symptoms, has no medical illnesses, no drug allergies, and no past trauma. She is single and in a long-standing relationship, and has been productive and functioning well at her work in a publishing company for 5 years. She has no current or past history of alcohol or drug abuse of any kind.

The consultant's impression was that she was experiencing the side effect of apathy syndrome from SRIs. The use of benzodiazepines, like lorazepam, initially on an as-needed basis, and if needed on a regular basis, was recommended. Specifically, it was recommended that paroxetine be stopped and replaced with a benzodiazepine. Since she has no substance abuse history, her risk of benzodiazepine abuse or addiction is very low, probably less than 5% based on some research. She has a troublesome SRI side effect, and long-term SRI treatment itself will be associated with tolerance and major withdrawal symptoms. Her panic symptoms are not very frequent, only once monthly, and she has no need for SRI treatment for any other recurrent mood condition. Thus, the consultant was impressed by the limited nature of her panic symptoms, and the troublesome nature of her SRI side effects, along with absence of a need for constant, long-term treatment of any medication. This clinical picture, along with absence of substance abuse, would support the prescription of benzodiazepines instead of SRI agents.

CASE 12: PTSD OR BIPOLAR ILLNESS?

A 21-year-old woman presented with a new diagnosis of bipolar disorder in the setting of a recent sexual trauma 2 months earlier. She had gone to the emergency room after the trauma, and had experienced anxiety and panic attacks in the week following it. She went back to the emergency room due to the latter symptoms, along with some suicidal ideation, which led to one-week psychiatric hospitalization.

In the psychiatric hospital, clinicians noted that the patient had a family history of bipolar illness in her maternal aunt and maternal grandmother. On history-taking from the patient as well as both of her parents, it was reported that the patient had not experienced past depressive episodes, nor had she experienced past manic or hypomanic episodes. This denial was confirmed with multiple family members.

Until the recent event, she had never been treated with any psychotropic medications, nor had she ever received counseling. She had no prior psychiatric hospitalizations and no self-cutting or prior suicidality.

She and her family denied any prior physical or sexual abuse. Her medical history was normal; she took no medications and had no allergies.

She had many friends in college, and was sociable. She was sexually active, but interview with her and her family suggested that her sexual activity was within the normal range of her peers. She had prior sexual relationships that were not fleeting or inherently unstable, but lasted sometimes 6 months or longer.

In the psychiatric hospital, she was treated with lithium and risperidone. Upon discharge, she stopped risperidone. A few weeks later, her anxiety symptoms had improved notably. She had avoidant behavior about the recent sexual trauma and was teary about it, but denied other depressive neurovegetative symptoms. She denied flashbacks or nightmares related to the trauma, but she reported being anxious when sleeping alone. She was still taking lithium 300 mg/d, reduced from higher doses due to cognitive side effects, but had not started psychotherapy. The family wanted to know if she had bipolar illness and what medication treatments were recommended.

On consultation, the diagnosis of bipolar illness was not confirmed, given her history. It was recommended that lithium be stopped since she was not suicidal, nor did she have any mood episodes currently or in the past. The bipolar genetics were noted, and the family was informed that if mood episodes should begin in the future, then the bipolar diagnosis might be valid at that time, and lithium treatment could be restarted.

Instead, the consultant's view was to recommend individual psychotherapy to help her cope with the acute stress reaction of recent sexual trauma. The patient and family were informed that acute stress reactions to trauma occur in almost everyone, while PTSD is defined as happening 6 months to a year after the traumatic episode. Further PTSD only occurs in about 10–20% of persons who experience trauma. Thus, the importance of psychotherapy is to help the patient cope with the natural acute stress reaction, as well as hopefully to decrease the likelihood of future PTSD. Furthermore, if there are aspects of the history that are unclear, or mild manic symptoms that might be difficult to observe, ongoing psychotherapy may be a place to make such subtle diagnostic observations.

CASE 13: PRE-ADOLESCENT DEPRESSION VERSUS BIPOLAR ILLNESS

A 12-year-old female has experienced depression for three years. During this time, she has had extensive periods of being very sad, low in her energy, and socially reclusive. She also has spurts lasting 3–4 days at a time of high excitability, along with impulsivity, like jumping on a sand castle at a party and ruining it. During these impulsive times, she talks rapidly, and she is very irritating to others. Afterwards, she becomes unhappy, because others have been bothered by her, and she has suicidal thoughts of not wanting to live.

She is also a dancer, and has lost weight extensively. She has been hospitalized repeatedly for anorexia, and has received a feeding tube at times. She has been diagnosed with OCD, because she focuses on her weight and food and is constantly worrying about what others think about her.

She has no history of sexual trauma and has never cut herself. She has made no suicide attempts. She has no substance abuse or other medical history. No known drug allergies.

In her multiple hospitalizations, she has been treated with multiple SRIs. Recently she was tried on venlafaxine, and later switched to duloxetine. She did not improve on any of these medications, and eventually aripiprazole was added.

Her family history is questionable, because she was adopted. Her biological mother reports that her biological father, who is now dead, had been diagnosed with bipolar illness and also had substance abuse.

Consultation was obtained with a child psychiatry expert in mood disorders. The expert believed that the diagnosis was MDD, along with anorexia nervosa. When asked about a possible bipolar diagnosis, the child psychiatry expert opined that a bipolar diagnosis is unlikely for multiple reasons. First, she does not meet full criteria for a DSM-defined manic episode. Second, the possible bipolar diagnosis in her family is questionable, and frequently people get over-diagnosed with bipolar illness. Third, even if her father has bipolar illness, the majority of children of bipolar parents do not develop bipolar illness; rather, MDD is the most common diagnosis in such children. Further use of antidepressants and more extensive psychotherapies were recommended by this expert.

This kind of case is extremely common in children and adolescents. One might divide the world of child psychiatry into pro- and anti-bipolar groups, with the latter being much larger. The anti-bipolar perspective is mainstream and follows DSM to the letter. This case is a good example of the approach. One problem with it is that it provides no hope of any better or improved outcomes beyond the repeated use of already failed medication classes such as antidepressants in this case. The anti-bipolar perspective does not subject itself to refutation based on treatment outcomes. Rather, this perspective is held based on a specific approach to diagnosis, without ever testing the diagnosis by its therapeutic results.

There are several fallacies in the anti-bipolar viewpoint expressed by the child psychiatry expert in this case. First, the child psychiatry expert refuses to view manic symptoms as being relevant at all to diagnosis or treatment if those symptoms are briefer than the DSM duration cutoffs. This approach ignores the fact that the DSM duration cutoffs have no scientific basis in research studies that prove that those cutoffs differentiate bipolar illness from non-bipolar illness. In fact, good scientific studies show the reverse. In other words, manic symptoms lasting a few days or less are important diagnostically and therapeutically, predicting bipolar genetics and poor antidepressant outcomes.

Second, the child psychiatry expert was skeptical about the bipolar diagnosis in the patient's biological father. There is no way to confirm in this case since there is no access to the father. However, on the general issue of bipolar illness being over-diagnosed in adults, there is reason to be cautious. The usual studies cited do not in fact show over-diagnosis of bipolar illness in adults; in fact, they show under-diagnosis. They appear to be misinterpreted by those researchers who want to support the concept of over-diagnosis. This matter has been reviewed in articles in which opposing views have been debated. Furthermore, there are other studies that indicate under-diagnosis, not over-diagnosis, of bipolar illness in adults.

Third, the claim that children of bipolar parents are unlikely to have bipolar illness is a misunderstanding of the nature of psychiatric genetics. Psychiatric illnesses, when genetic, are not Mendelian: they are not autosomal dominant or recessive. It's not a matter of 50% or more relatives having a disease. Rather they are non-Mendelian genetic, which means that many genes are needed for an illness to occur. This is a quantitative risk. The two most genetic psychiatric diseases are schizophrenia and bipolar illness; they are almost completely genetic. In the case of bipolar illness, the baseline risk in the general population is about 1%. In family members of a proband with bipolar illness, the observed risk is about 10–20%. This is a much higher risk than in the general population, about 10–20-fold higher, which is a huge effect size, equivalent to the risk of getting lung cancer by smoking cigarettes. But the absolute numbers could be emphasized rather than the relative risk: it could be claimed that 80–90% of children of a parent with bipolar illness will *not* develop bipolar illness (the most common diagnosis being "MDD"). The claim that bipolar illness is "unlikely," as if one doesn't need to worry about it much, is not rational for a non-Mendelian disease.

Here is an analogy: Lung cancer as a result of cigarette smoking is also non-Mendelian in its risk. There is a genetic component; some people smoke and develop lung cancer, while others smoke and do not. The absolute risk rates are low, in fact: even after 50 years of very high smoking rates, only 20% of smokers would develop lung cancer; 80% do not. These figures are the same as the risk of bipolar illness in children in bipolar parents. Should we then say that cigarette smoking doesn't matter? Why should 80% of the population be restricted and discouraged from smoking for the sake of a minority 20%? (This is actually one of the arguments made by pro-cigarette civil rights groups.) The reality is that relative risks matter, not just absolute risks. And 20% is a lot of people in the general population; if they are worsened by antidepressant treatment for misdiagnosed bipolar illness, it matters.

A final point that the child psychiatry expert didn't address: Even the concept that children of parents with bipolar illness "only" have MDD is an illogical concept, since the whole concept of "MDD" is based on the notion that it is genetically different from bipolar illness—i.e., that it should not happen, or very infrequently, in families of persons with bipolar illness. Thus, the claim that most children of parents with bipolar illness have MDD, or unipolar depression, only argues against the concept that unipolar depression is a different disease than bipolar illness. It argues for the old MDI concept; namely, that unipolar and bipolar subtypes are part of the same disease.

If one thinks about these factors, whether this child has bipolar illness of some variety or MDI, then it would not be reasonable to continue to go down the path of antidepressants, and refuse to use lithium or mood stabilizers. Furthermore, if we are able to take bipolar or MDI concepts more seriously, we could take the step that most child psychiatry clinicians refuse to take in cases like this one; namely, to stop duloxetine and all antidepressants altogether, and to use lithium or mood stabilizers without any antidepressants.

The consultant's recommendation in this case was to switch duloxetine to fluoxetine 20 mg/d, and then to taper the latter over 3 months, while starting lithium for the mixed depressive state along with suicidality, as well as to add aripiprazole 2 mg/d for the acute mixed states. The patient began to improve when lithium was added and aripiprazole was not needed. The patient eventually tapered off fluoxetine and all SRIs, and was maintained on lithium alone 450 mg/d with notable improvement and no side effects. Higher doses were not given since clinical benefit was sufficient at that dose.

CASE 14: FIRST DEPRESSION IN A YOUNG ADULT

An 18-year-old male has a first depressive episode. For the last two months, he reports decreased interest, energy, concentration, and appetite. Two weeks ago, his parents took him to his primary care doctor, who diagnosed depression, and began treatment with fluoxetine. The patient had no prior psychological problems or treatment, and has done quite well in school. A few days after starting fluoxetine, the patient reported some suicidal ideation, but denied any intent or plan. He also admitted to drinking some alcohol with friends. He has no other medical problems, no allergies, and is taking no other medications. There is no history of trauma, and he was raised in an intact and supportive family. He has multiple family members with depression, and one aunt diagnosed and treated for bipolar illness.

In consultation, the observation was made that the course of illness and genetics of this case are more consistent with bipolar illness than MDD. The occurrence of suicidal ideation after treatment with fluoxetine was noted and a causal relationship implied. It was observed that the whole concept of MDD was associated with a lack of bipolar genetics and an age of onset around 30, as opposed to bipolar illness, which began around age 19 and had bipolar genetics. The concern was raised that this depression may be the first episode of bipolar illness (with future mania), or at least cannot be the first depressive episode of MDD, given bipolar genetics and course of illness. The consultant's recommendation was to discontinue fluoxetine and begin lithium.

The patient saw a psychiatric nurse practitioner who concurred with the diagnostic and historical assessment, but concluded that lithium was a "third-line" treatment for more severe illness than this patient possesses. In contrast, fluoxetine was a less intensive and more conservative treatment. Fluoxetine treatment was continued, with a plan to consider lithium later.

Fluoxetine is not a more conservative treatment than lithium in this case. Fluoxetine increases suicidal ideation and suicide attempts by about 70%, whereas lithium reduces completed suicides by about 90%. Thus lithium is a more conservative treatment than fluoxetine from the perspective of suicide risk. Since this patient has suicidality, this issue is important. Furthermore, the increased risk of suicidality with fluoxetine specifically occurs in patients in this young adult age group. Finally, the bipolar genetics of this patient raises the possibility that the patient may have bipolar illness, or at least does not have straightforward "MDD." Lithium is proven effective for both unipolar depression and bipolar illness, and is the only drug proven to reduce suicide risk. The psychiatric nurse practitioner's concern may have had to do with the perception that there are many more side effects with lithium than with fluoxetine, especially medical risks like kidney impairment. But, as discussed previously, lithium's kidney risk occurs in a 20-year time frame, and is irrelevant to treatment for an acute depressive episode. Also, even though lithium has a long list of side effects, most patients don't experience any of them, and they are dose-related. Fluoxetine has its own list of concerning side effects as well, besides suicidality (which is bad enough), including severe sexual dysfunction and serious long-term serotonin withdrawal syndrome risk.

CASE 15: STOPPING ANTIDEPRESSANTS FOR "DEPRESSION"

A 30-year-old female has been diagnosed with MDD since age 21. She initially was treated with sertraline, which helped, and then she got worse again about a year later. Bupropion was added, which also helped, and then she stayed well for three years on both agents. She finished college and got a job. She then relapsed into another depressive episode around age 25, and the doses of sertraline and bupropion were increased. She improved, got married, and now has just had another depressive episode that began about 2 months ago. She has remained on sertraline and bupropion this entire time. She has been treated by her primary care doctor, although she had a psychiatric consult when she started bupropion.

Her family history is significant for bipolar illness in a sibling and in a cousin.

She has no medical illness, no allergies, no substance abuse, and works as a podiatrist. She is happy in her marriage and has many friends.

There is no past trauma of any kind.

There was no major trigger for her current depression, although she has more anxiety at work when she is depressed because she feels less capable of functioning. She has managed to continue to work despite her current depressive episode. Her symptoms involve decreased sleep and interest and energy and concentration, but no suicidal ideation. She has never had manic or psychotic episodes.

She describes her baseline personality as "bubbly, high energy, very active." She exercises a lot, and is very extroverted.

The consultation diagnosis was recurrent unipolar depressive episodes with bipolar genetics and hyperthymic temperament. This clinical presentation is typical for the classic diagnosis of MDI, which means both recurrent unipolar depression and bipolar illness. Bipolar genetics was supposed to be absent in unipolar depression, as a rationale for the legitimacy of unipolar depression as being a valid independent diagnosis separate from bipolar illness. Otherwise, they both are part of the same illness—MDI.

In this scenario, the patient is a squared circle, an illogical and supposedly rare phenomenon: unipolar depression with bipolar genetics almost never should occur. The consultant states: There are only two alternatives; either the textbooks are wrong, or you don't exist. Since the patient exists, the textbooks are wrong.

The consultant concluded that sertraline and bupropion may have had acute efficacy, but the history repeatedly showed that they do not have maintenance efficacy in prevention of future depressive episodes.

The consultant recommended that the patient taper off both agents, with cross-taper of fluoxetine for sertraline to manage serotonin withdrawal syndrome. Lithium or lamotrigine were recommended for maintenance prevention of future depressive episodes. Hyperthymic temperament puts the patient at some risk for future depressive episodes, and low-dose lithium and valproate appear to help it, but lamotrigine probably does not help hyperthymia since this agent has no acute antimanic effect. Thus, low-dose lithium (300–600 mg/d) was the consultant's recommendation.

The patient went to her primary care doctor, whose reaction was: "You have depression. There's no way I'm taking you off antidepressants!" Similarly, the primary care doctor might have said, after penicillin failed repeatedly: "You have an infection. There's no way I'm taking you off antibiotics." The mistake is to view the drug class as equivalent: antidepressants are not "antidepressants," because they don't work for all kinds of depression. Similarly, not all infections respond to antibiotics.

The patient went to a psychiatric nurse practitioner, who agreed to implement the recommended changes, with gradual improvement over months.

CASE 16: ANTIDEPRESSANT PLUS ANTIPSYCHOTIC DO NOT EQUAL MOOD STABILIZER

A 43-year-old male has been diagnosed with psychotic depression, schizoaffective disorder, and OCD. He had a first episode of depression with acute catatonia and psychosis at age 25. He was treated with paroxetine and risperidone and subsequently attempted suicide by drowning, leading to a one-week hospitalization where he was treated with paroxetine, olanzapine, and ziprasidone. He eventually tapered off olanzapine a few months later, and then paroxetine 6 months later. He had a relapse of psychotic depression treated with olanzapine and paroxetine, and again went off both agents about 6 months later. Between episodes, he demonstrates hyperthymic temperament. His OCD symptoms mainly occur when he is depressed.

He is a gifted musician, teaches as a mathematician, and is generally outgoing and creative, sometimes taking on more projects than his wife feels he can cope with. He is happy with his current medications, paroxetine and olanzapine, and feels he is doing very well. His last depressive episode occurred a year ago.

Family history is relevant for the fact that his paternal aunt committed suicide. Diagnoses in siblings include severe depression, treated with medications, and anorexia nervosa.

He had never been treated with any mood stabilizer. He was referred for consultation with the following questions: Is the diagnosis bipolar illness? Should he be treated with a mood stabilizer?

The consultant concluded that this is a classic case of using the "poor man's mood stabilizer"; namely, an "antidepressant" plus an "antimanic" agent. Clinicians and patients believe that the combination is mood-stabilizing because one moves your mood up and the other moves your mood down, stabilizing you in the middle. These metaphors have no scientific basis to them. It's not about "stabilizing in the middle," and it's not about moving your mood up or down. This patient has repeated depressive episodes; they go away and come back; they recur. This is classic Kraepelinian recurrent affective illness. The main treatment is prophylaxis: a medication that prevents the recurrence of future depressive episodes. If we wanted to use the word "mood stabilizer," that's what it should mean, not moving the mood up or down. The question is whether the combination of an SRI like paroxetine along with an antimanic agent like olanzapine has ever been shown to prevent mood episodes in recurrent unipolar depression. The answer obviously is no. There never have been such data on the combination; it's never even been studied.

What has been proven? Lithium has been proven to prevent depressive episodes in unipolar depression. One might argue that SRIs alone have been shown to do so, but the problem of the invalidity of enriched maintenance designs throws doubt on such claims, as discussed before. Olanzapine alone only has such data in bipolar illness, with the same problem of the likely invalidity of the enriched maintenance designs upon which such efficacy claims are based. So, purely from a scientific perspective, the claim of efficacy with this combination was not supported by valid evidence.

The consultant turned to two other aspects of the case: (1) the patient's preference, and (2) the likely diagnosis and recommended treatment.

Regarding the patient's preference: the patient was happy with his treatment, probably because he is in a phase of remission. The medications now probably were not keeping the patient well. They were neutral, probably ineffective. Nature, by giving this illness phases of remission, keeps the patient well, and the patient is crediting the medications. Since the patient has hyperthymia, it could be also that the constant SRI use feels good to the patient, that it makes him a little more manic, which he enjoys. These aspects of the case could be explained to the patient. It could be explained that hyperthymia puts the patient at increased risk of future depressive episodes, and that the current medications, especially the paroxetine, do not decrease that risk, but actually increase it by potentially worsening manic symptoms of hyperthymia. Patients with manic symptoms often lack insight into those symptoms. This seems to be worse, paradoxically, the milder the manic symptoms. Thus, there is lack of insight in about one-half of patients with severe manic episodes, but it is higher in mild hypomanic episodes, where about 2/3 of patients lack insight into their hypomanic states. It probably is even worse in hyperthymia, since the manic symptoms are mild and constant, thus patients generally do not see them as abnormal because they have no normality with which to compare their experiences. It may be difficult, but if the patient can receive some psychoeducation on these matters, he may begin to understand the nature of his condition.

Regarding the diagnosis and treatment, the patient has MDI, defined as recurrent depressive episodes along with hyperthymic temperament. The fact that his depressive episodes have psychotic features makes it more likely that he has MDI, because psychotic depression is much more common in bipolar illness than in unipolar depression. The "diagnosis" of psychotic depression is meaningless, even though it is in the DSM, because this is clinical acute state, like an acute depressive episode. This is not a longitudinal diagnosis, but a cross-sectional picture. There is no such thing as "psychotic depression" as a diagnosis, just as "severe fever" is not a diagnosis. The patient has recurrent depressive episodes, with psychotic features, which is the diagnosis of recurrent unipolar depression. In between these episodes, he has constant manic symptoms, which is the diagnosis of hyperthymic temperament. Put together, that's a common presentation of MDI. Family history of suicide confirms the genetics of a severe mood disease, which is what MDI is.

The consultant's recommendation was to taper off paroxetine, which has severe serotonin withdrawal syndrome, by replacing it with fluoxetine and then gradually tapering over 6 months. Olanzapine could be stopped. The main treatment for hyperthymia is low-dose lithium or divalproex, increasing doses if needed for breakthrough mood episodes. The consultant recommended starting with lithium since he has genetics for suicide, at a dose of 300–600 mg/d, to see if it agreed with him. If it was sufficient, that dose could continue. If unhelpful standard doses and levels of about 0.8 could be used. If not tolerated, then Depakote could be used, but very low-dose lithium (150–300 mg/d or less) would still be recommended for suicide prevention and for long-term cognitive benefits of dementia prevention.

With these agents, it would be possible that he would not need other treatments, but if needed, other, safer, dopamine blockers could be used, without risk of worsening heart disease risk, like risperidone, aripiprazole, asenapine, or lurasidone.

After consultation, the patient agreed to phasing off SRIs and was able to taper off fluoxetine over 6 months. In the meantime, low-dose lithium agreed with him at 600 mg/d and provided sufficient benefit so that he did not need other agents. He continued to experience long periods of remission, without any depression or OCD symptoms, on long-term lithium treatment.

CASE 17: SEASONALITY IN AFFECTIVE ILLNESS

A 40-year-old man has had repeated depressive episodes throughout his life, more often in the fall and winter, but sometimes in other months. He has been treated with multiple SRIs for a depressive episode that began in October. He was switched to nortriptyline in March, and improved in May. He relapsed into another depressive episode the following October. On consultation, it was determined that the apparent improvement with nortriptyline probably represented a seasonal natural remission, as reflected in his relapse into depression a few months later despite continuing nortriptyline. On further interview, it was found that the patient had heightened energy and decreased sleep most years in the springtime, in April and May. These manic symptoms lasted weeks and were associated with elevated mood and rapid thinking. Hypomanic episodes were diagnosed and the diagnosis changed from seasonal affective disorder to bipolar illness with seasonal features. Lithium was used in place of nortriptyline with good benefit. The following year, the patient relapsed into a milder depressive episode in November. The consultant recommended raising the bedroom shades, and the patient did not experience fall depressive episodes in future years.

45

Curbside Consults

Questions and Answers

QUESTION: A PATIENT FELT DEPERSONALIZED MOST OF HIS LIFE, alienated from himself, "spaced out." Years of psychotherapy had had no impact. A consultant said that he had "depersonalization disorder" and that marijuana could help. It did for a few hours after each use. Should he request medical marijuana?

Answer: The most common cause of depersonalization is anxiety, such as panic attacks. If this person's anxiety is lifelong, and it isn't solely related to depressive episodes or panic attacks, for instance, then the anxiety can be conceived of as a personality trait, like a high amount of neuroticism. In that case, a low dose of a benzodiazepine (like 0.5–1 mg/d of lorazepam) can move the person's neuroticism up on the normal curve somewhat closer to the middle range. This reduced anxiety would then be accompanied by reduced feelings of depersonalization. Marijuana has strong anxiolytic effects, so the benefit this person had with that agent is probably a reflection of anxiety as the cause of the depersonalization symptoms.

The DSM approach of adding "disorder" to every symptom is not scientifically correct or clinically helpful. Rather, the question should be: What is causing the symptoms? In this case, anxiety as a personality trait seems most likely. Keep in mind that any intervention for personality will have modest symptomatic benefit at best: personality traits aren't completely removed, like diseases; they are increased or decreased. So the patient should have modest symptom-benefit expectations. Furthermore, long-term treatment will be needed, and benzodiazepines are most useful short-term. Low-dose SRIs could be used if the patient doesn't have any variety of bipolar illness.

Question: **Do benzodiazepines increase the risk for dementia?**

Answer: The potential association between benzodiazepine use and dementia was highlighted by a recent large epidemiological study (Billioti de Gage et al., *BMJ*, Sept 2014). That report was prominently published, and has had a good deal of attention.

These non-randomized epidemiological studies always suffer from some confounding bias. This is why readers should never take the results of such epidemiological reports at face-value.

The best way to reduce confounding bias in such non-randomized studies is to use regression modeling. This means that some potential confounding factors—which could influence the results—are measured and "adjusted for" in the statistical model. In this case, the question was whether benzodiazepines increase the risk of dementia. Many things increase the risk of dementia, like age, diabetes, depression, anxiety, substance abuse, hypertension, and other factors. The problem with large epidemiological studies is that people are impressed with largeness, rather than quality. But the larger the study, the more common it is that confounding factors aren't measured or adequately adjusted. In other words, huge samples have the advantage of hugeness, but the disadvantage of not characterizing clinical features in much detail.

All that being said, this epidemiological study was adjusted for some important confounding factors. Besides the usual easily measurable factors of age and gender, a regression model adjusted for some medical illnesses (like diabetes and hypertension) and for depression, defined as the diagnosis of "major depressive disorder" in medical charts. This is better than nothing, but whether or not the study adequately adjusts for the presence and severity of depressive illness fully relies on whether the treating clinicians in this large sample had accurately and adequately identified and documented depressive symptoms. Given that clinical charts aren't fully accurate for research purposes, there is some room for doubt as to whether the study adequately adjusted for depression, at least. Furthermore, one might ask a question that has to do with "confounding by indication." Benzodiazepines are frequently used for anxiety. Anxiety increases adrenal hormone activity, which increases the risk for dementia. How do we know that the association between benzodiazepine use and dementia wasn't a classic case of confounding bias, where the third factor of anxiety, associated with benzodiazepine use, directly causes dementia?

One can't rule out this possibility from this analysis because anxiety diagnoses or symptoms weren't adjusted in the regression model, simply because the data weren't collected as part of the routine clinical practice that was the basis for the data used in the study.

Randomized studies would be much more definitive, but they haven't been done. In the meantime, it's worthwhile noting that some animal studies show that benzodiazepines are neuroprotective, keep neurons alive, in human and animal studies of stroke (Huang et al., *Psychiatry Clin Neurosci*, 2014; *68*, 255–262). Thus, there are some biological data to counter this clinical hypothesis that benzodiazepines might increase dementia risk. There are other clinical studies that also don't find increased risk of dementia with benzodiazepines. As with many medical topics, the question remains to be answered with reasonable confidence. But we can say these data, as they stand, don't prove the claim that benzodiazepines hasten dementia.

***Question:* What do you think of extended-release (ER, XR) formulations of drugs?**

Answer: There's no general answer to this question. Sometimes extended-release formulations are useful; sometimes they're not. Some examples: Lithium ER, which is now generic, probably is preferable to standard-release (SR) generic lithium because the initial peak of a single dose is reduced, which may cause fewer renal effects or fewer cognitive or gastrointestinal effects. Carbamazepine ER, also generic, has fewer nuisance side effects (dizziness, ataxia, diplopia) than standard carbamazepine. Divalproex delayed release (Depakote DR) has much weaker gastrointestinal side effects than generic valproic acid. But Divalproex extended release (Depakote ER) produces no further appreciable reduction in side effects. Venlafaxine XR and Bupropion SR have less side effects than their immediate-release versions, but Bupropion XL produces no further reduction in side effects. Quetiapine XR has less sedation than immediate-release, but no other appreciable benefit. An important point: slow-release formulations don't necessarily extend the half-life of a drug. For instance, Depakote ER hardly increases the half-life of Depakote immediate release (18 hours for ER versus 12–16 hours for immediate release); lithium and carbamazepine ER don't appreciably lengthen half-lives versus immediate-release alternatives. The most common benefit, when present, involves possible reduction in some specific side effects, but this isn't always the case

***Question:* What are your thoughts on the common combination of amphetamines and benzodiazepines? This is so very common and even worse in patients with substance abuse.**

Answer: This common combination makes sense, in a rather absurd way. Amphetamines cause anxiety, which is then treated with benzodiazepines. Another relevant reason for the combination is that anxiety states, as discussed previously, often cause impaired concentration. Such patients then get mistakenly diagnosed with adult ADD, and treated with amphetamines, which worsen the underlying anxiety that caused the inattention to begin with, hence the addition of benzodiazepines. In short, the effect is mistaken for the cause, and inattention is treated with amphetamines, which worsen the causal anxiety, leading to further treatment with benzodiazepines.

Both classes of agents are addictive potentially, but at least in animal models, amphetamines appear to produce more addictive behavior than benzodiazepines. Certainly the former have more evidence of neurotoxicity harm than the latter.

Thus, the perspective of this text is that if a patient has an anxiety condition, which is not due to some other diagnosis like a mood illness, then it is reasonable to treat that anxiety condition with benzodiazepines. If such anxiety states cause poor concentration, then those inattention symptoms should improve with benzodiazepines alone, without the need to add amphetamines. The use of amphetamines in persons with anxiety conditions is self-defeating, as is the case with using those agents in bipolar illness. Amphetamines worsen anxiety and manic states, hence they worsen anxiety and bipolar illnesses. The only condition they do not worsen is pure depression, where they had been used for years as primary antidepressants.

As reviewed in Appendix III, it is reasonable to conclude that most apparent cases of adult ADD in fact represent inattention symptoms caused by other diseases; most commonly bipolar illness, but also anxiety conditions. Thus, if anxiety diagnoses are made, the recommendation here is that adult ADD should not be diagnosed, and the anxiety condition be treated, with benzodiazepines or in some cases with SRIs. In most cases, attentional symptoms then resolve with treatment of the underlying cause, without ever needing to use amphetamines.

***Question:* Are the newer dopamine blockers safer from a cardiac perspective than other agents? You said that they cause less cardiovascular disease because of metabolic syndrome effects. Does this mean they also have less QT effects?**

Answer: No. The QT effects of dopamine blockers are a separate issue from the insulin resistance effects of some agents (clozapine, olanzapine, quetiapine) that cause or worsen diabetes and coronary artery disease. Of modern dopamine blockers, only ziprasidone has notable worsening of QTc duration. Other agents have little to no effect on QTc interval duration.

***Question:* Do you have a preferred antidepressant for major depressive disorder? Do you endorse the approach of choosing the agent by symptom subtype?**

Answer: The approach of this text is to apply the subtyping of depressive experiences based on mixed states, versus melancholia, versus neurotic depression, as explained in Chapter 19. Antidepressants would be avoided in mixed states altogether. The bipolar/unipolar distinction is less important than these three basic depressive subtypes. This subtyping is not symptomatic alone, but takes into account genetics and course of illness to separate manic-depressive illness (MDI) (e.g., mixed states and recurrent melancholia) from other depressive states (e.g., neurotic depression). Since MDD is not a clinically valid disease, as explained in Chapter 19, this text does not recommend simply using "antidepressants" (monoamine agonists) for depressive episodes. If used, the interpretation here of the scientific literature is that it indicates no notable differences in efficacy among modern monoamine agonists. Thus, if they are used, decisions would be based mostly on side effects.

***Question:* I have not found lamotrigine to be helpful in treating hyperthymic or cyclothymic temperaments. What is your experience?**

Answer: To put it briefly, readers are familiar with dysthymia, or mild depressive symptoms. But they probably are not familiar with the opposite state of mild manic symptoms, called hyperthymia. Cyclothymia represents the alternation between the two. In the classic German literature, especially in the work of Ernst Kretschmer in the early 20th century, these temperaments were seen as variants of MDI. They were biologically and genetically related to that disease. They were not different conditions, as DSM sets it up, nor were they diseases in themselves. They were personality constructs, a constellation of traits seen in a certain way in persons with MDI, *in between their episodes*. These affective temperaments also were seen in relatives of persons with MDI.

With that basic definition, the rationale for this textbook's approach to treating affective temperaments may be understandable: the use of low doses of mood stabilizers. The treatment type is the same as in MDI; namely, mood stabilizers, but since affective temperaments are the mildest shade of MDI, then lower doses can be effective for them. There is some evidence to support this hypothesis in an observational study with divalproex in cyclothymia, and in some research with dysthymia, but so far there are no published treatment studies of hyperthymia.

Lamotrigine has been proven to be ineffective for acute mania. It does not work for manic symptoms directly. It also is less effective in prevention of manic than depressive episodes. Thus, of the four major mood stabilizers (lithium, divalproex, carbamazepine, and lamotrigine), the one agent that has a major weak spot, in the case of mostly manic presentations, is lamotrigine. If this is the case, then this agent is not likely to be effective for hyperthymic temperament, which is a purely manic condition. Nor is it likely to be as effective in cyclothymia, where manic symptoms are frequent, as opposed to the three other alternative mood stabilizers.

No studies yet exist on this topic, but your experience is consistent with available clinical experience among those with expertise in affective temperaments, thus the approach of this textbook is not to recommend lamotrigine as the primary treatment for hyperthymic or cyclothymic temperaments. Instead, low-dose divalproex or lithium seem most effective for those conditions.

***Question:* Does quetiapine have any of the antidepressants' risks (for manic activation or rapid cycling) if used in the context of bipolar disorder, given its serotonin and other receptor profile?**

Answer: One way of answering this question is to infer that any medication that can elevate mood; that is, improve depression, should also have some risk of causing mania, or cycling back-and-forth between mood episodes in the long term. It appears that some of the dopamine blockers that treat bipolar depression can cause mania, but less frequently and less severely so than with monoamine agonists. Specific agents that have some evidence in this regard are aripiprazole and ziprasidone. There are hardly any reports of mania being caused by quetiapine. Even though quetiapine is FDA-indicated for bipolar depression, the biochemical rationale for its efficacy is unclear. In contrast to aripiprazole, which is a dopamine agonist, and ziprasidone, which is a powerful serotonin and norepinephrine reuptake inhibitor, quetiapine has very small monoamine agonist properties, with only mild partial agonism at the 5HT1A receptor. It's an extremely sedating medication due to very high antihistamine potency, though, and some have suggested that the large effect size seen in placebo-controlled trials of acute bipolar depression may be due partly to the inability to truly "blind" patients who receive quetiapine versus placebo, because of the immense sedating properties of the former. So the apparent "antidepressant" effects of quetiapine may not be as large as suggested by the RCTs of bipolar depression. If this is the case, the relative absence of apparent manic induction would be consistent with less of an antidepressant effect than is commonly believed.

***Question:* How long would you use Symbyax (olanzapine/fluoxetine) for bipolar depression?**

Answer: That medication is proven effective in an eight-week trial, as with most acute depression studies. Thus it is proven for two months, not longer. It has not been studied in maintenance prophylaxis designs, and the olanzapine maintenance studies do not include fluoxetine (besides having the preceding limitations). Thus, you cannot and should not assume maintenance efficacy based on acute efficacy. Otherwise, everyone who receives penicillin should take it forever. For that reason, this text recommends use of Symbyax, if given, for the acute phase only, not long term.

Question: **What do you think about current practice in use of benztropine (Cogentin)?**

Answer: That medication is an anticholinergic drug given by many clinicians to treat or prevent Parkinsonian side effects of neuroleptic agents. It has some benefit, and may be useful in some extreme cases of severe schizophrenia. There is reason for concern regarding the extensive use of this medication as a preventive treatment, co-administered along with neuroleptics, even before patients experience any Parkinsonian side effects. This is unnecessary because many patients will not experience Parkinsonian side effects with different neuroleptics, or not severe ones. In any case, tremor and rigidity are not life-threatening in almost all cases, and are not usually a major cause for drug discontinuation. Rather, akathisia is the major EPS that both leads to drug discontinuation and can be life-threatening, by leading to suicide. Yet anticholinergic agents do not have much if any benefit for akathisia, which is best treated or prevented with beta-blockers such as propanolol. Thus, using benztropine for prevention does not prevent the most important EPS, akathisia, and may not be necessary for the less important Parkinsonian side effects that can occur. One should add that such preventive treatment also adds potentially unnecessary cognitive side effects, which occur routinely with anticholinergic drugs, among other harms (constipation, potential delirium in older persons).

In sum, the view of this textbook is that this medication is overprescribed and should not be given routinely as prophylaxis of EPS.

Question: **I use lithium on a regular basis, not only for manic or hypomanic conditions, but also at lower doses in treating depression. Over the years that I have used it, side effects have been rare. I regularly monitor kidney and thyroid function. Rarely have I had to discontinue because of decreased kidney function. Fairly recently, a male patient of mine on both topiramate and lithium started developing increased creatinine and decreased** glomeular filtration rate (**GFR**). **Both can have adverse effects on kidney and I decided to stop both. Kidney function is now normal. The decision to stop was based on several serial kidney panels. He is doing fairly well, but did better on lithium. Levels were about 0.6. I am wondering whether or not to restart the lithium and closely monitor kidney function.**

Answer: It's common to note that when lithium is stopped for renal reasons, many patients don't do as well with other agents, such as valproate or lamotrigine, as they did with lithium. After trying other agents, you could have a full informed-consent discussion with the patient about the merits of resuming lithium, despite the renal side effects that the patient has experienced. Perhaps it could be used at slightly lower levels, and/or with nephrology consultation as well. All of medicine is about weighing risks and benefits; and even if the risks are more than mild, if the benefits are equally higher than other options, the tradeoff may be acceptable to the patient. In the end, it's the patient's decision, though, with the clinician's role being to provide the information the patient needs for a fully informed decision.

Question: **How neuroprotective is lithium? And if this is the case, should it be given in low doses to other individuals or in general?**

Answer: There's no definitive answer to this question yet, but one could justify the view, based on the available research evidence, that it is reasonable to consider giving very low-dose lithium (equivalent to about 5 mg/d elemental lithium) to individuals who are not diagnosed with mood conditions, if they have other risk factors for dementia, such as a strong family history. Lithium is strongly neuroprotective, much more so than any other psychotropic agent. Unlike other agents, the neuroprotective effect of lithium is repeatedly proven in many different animal species and in humans. This effect is very robust neurobiologically in vitro and in vivo, including in the clinical human studies.

***Question:* A type of depressive syndrome is chronic, low-grade depression that in my opinion is related to chronic systemic inflammation caused by multiple medical problems. I work with a lot of patients who have several chronic conditions such as diabetes, hypertension, or heart disease. They tend to present with a low-grade type of depression characterized by low energy and motivation, fatigue, anhedonia, low mood, poor sleep, and isolation. They don't seem to have anything in their presentation or history that would trigger me to think of bipolar, melancholia, or neurotic depression. There is some evidence looking at the role of chronic inflammation in mood issues. I haven't found them to respond very well to "traditional" depression treatments such as SRIs or CBT. Often they come to me already on duloxetine (Cymbalta) for chronic pain issues or may have been started on citalopram, sertraline, or other SRIs by primary care. If the mechanism is more inflammatory, it may not be a surprise that their depressive symptoms aren't responding to these medications. Sometimes I use bupropion for the stimulant-like effects, but I haven't found a good solution for most of them. What are your thoughts in these patients?**

Answer: The question of depression and inflammation is a popular research topic. As you note, there may be kinds of depressive syndromes that are based in medical causes that are unrelated to MDI (bipolar or unipolar depression), and unrelated to specific subtypes of depression such as mixed depression, melancholia, or neurotic depression. All of these depressive presentations are part of what might be called "primary" depressive illnesses, or, for want of a better word, "psychiatric" causes of depression. Medical illnesses can cause "secondary" depression in persons who do not have the "primary" psychiatric causation of family genetics. In those medical cases, the depressive syndromes are caused by various factors. Perhaps the most common is so-called vascular depression, which involves brain micro-infarcts leading to white matter abnormalities. This condition is highly associated with diabetes and/or hypertension, and monoamine agonists (antidepressants) are less effective in these vascular depressive conditions, as opposed to primary depressive conditions.

Another major medical cause of depression is known inflammatory disease. Some would argue that all depression involves inflammation, which is present in the pathophysiology of depressive states. Cytokine activity is increased, natural killer cell activity is decreased, and various changes are present in the kynurenine system, which many think relate to the link between inflammation and depression. Many monoamine agonists have anti-inflammatory effects in persons with depressive syndromes; in other words, when their depression improves, their inflammatory states normalize with monoamine agonists.

However, the reverse doesn't seem to be the case: anti-inflammatory agents that are not monoamine agonists (like NSAIDs) have been studied in acute depressive episodes and generally are found to be ineffective. Steroids, which are potent anti-inflammatory agents, actually cause or worsen depression in many persons (and cause mania in others). So the relationship between depression and inflammation is complex.

The observation that monoamine agonists are less effective in depressive conditions related to medical or inflammatory diseases would be consistent with the general observation that this is the case with most medically caused secondary depressive conditions. Traditionally, as in post-stroke depression, mainstream psychiatry has recommended amphetamine stimulants, like bupropion. Of course, those agents have some risk of sudden cardiac death and/or arrhythmias, which should give us pause in using them, in addition to the animal studies indicating neurotoxicity of the more potent amphetamines such as methylphenidate.

One could justify using the monoamine agonists that are available in such cases, but the risks of amphetamine stimulants could be interpreted as sufficient reason to avoid those agents. Perhaps bupropion is the least risky of that class.

One idea to consider is minocycline, an antibiotic that has been studied and found to be effective in some randomized trials, both for depressive syndromes as well as for psychotic symptoms of schizophrenia. Typically dosed at 150 mg/d, the proposed mechanism of benefit is inflammatory, involving the kynurenine system. Still, the general prognosis of these patients is likely to remain worse than for primary depressive syndromes.

***Question:* Is the adjunctive use of buspirone for obsessive-compulsive disorder (OCD) effective?**

Answer: Buspirone has a reputation for having mild benefits in whatever use, whether anxiety or depression. There was some surprise that it showed more benefit than expected for refractory depression in the Sequenced Treatment Alternatives for Depression (STAR*D) study. In that study, it was similar in benefit, when added to citalopram, to switching to a different antidepressant, such as venlafaxine. Its use in generalized anxiety has been limited, with mild benefit in general. It also has had limited benefit if any in OCD. Buspirone is a complex drug, with essentially mild 5HT1A agonistic properties. The mild clinical benefits are consistent with its limited biological effects. On the other hand, it also has few side effects. Thus, in general, one could conclude that buspirone isn't a particularly effective treatment for any condition, including OCD.

***Question:* What do you think of medical marijuana?**

Answer: The potency of tetrahydrocannabinol (THC) in the legalized marijuana appears to be much higher than the potency in the illegal plant used in past decades. This high-potency marijuana appears to be causing some cases of paranoia or even possibly onset of depressive or delusional states. Furthermore, its addictiveness is heightened if used in high-potency form.

One observation that is important is that some younger people in particular appear to be confusing "legalization" with "safety." Alcohol is a legal substance, but it is not safe. Amphetamines are legal substances, with a prescription, but are not safe in many settings, or at certain doses. The viewpoint here is that it is important to discuss with patients that there is a difference between legalization and safety. There are known risks of marijuana in animal studies in terms of harmful effects on the brain, just as is the case with alcohol. This in itself is not a reason to criminalize it, but it also remains a fact, even if the substance is legalized.

As with all substances, harms should be understood well and consented to if used recreationally or medically. As with alcohol and amphetamines, whether in recreational or medical use, harms should never be ignored.

The history of amphetamines suggests a possible repetition. Those agents were available freely without prescription in post–World War II Japan, and a huge addiction problem arose. They were available in post–World War II United States with a prescription, but there was no FDA control upon them. Most prescribed amphetamines were diverted to illegal use. Both in Japan and the United States, those agents remained legal, but only in medical use, and with strict controlled-substance regulation.

In contrast, alcohol was widely used recreationally, then prohibited disastrously, and then returned to recreational use. It has never been given for medical purposes primarily. And it remains the most widely abused class of substance in the United States, leading to attention primarily by law enforcement, as with strict drunk driving punishments in most states.

Time will tell what the future holds for marijuana use in the United States, whether it follows the pattern of amphetamines or alcohol, or a mixture of both. One thing is clear: it is a substance of abuse, and legalization does not imply safety.

***Question:* What do you think about** divalproex **(Depakote) and depression in bipolar illness? I've heard it causes it?**

Answer: This is a common misconception. In fact, there are multiple randomized placebo-controlled trials (RCTs) that show that divalproex is effective in acute bipolar depression. These multiple studies were meta-analyzed some years ago. Added up, they provide much more convincing data of efficacy than anything that can be mustered for monoamine agonists ("antidepressants") in bipolar depression, as reviewed in Chapter 19, even though those agents are so commonly used for that condition. The divalproex RCTs are also much more consistent and effective than the multiple lamotrigine RCTs in acute bipolar depression, which show that agent to be ineffective, contrary to popular opinion. In short, ignore the false clinical lore and look at the science: Divalproex doesn't cause bipolar depression; it treats it.

***Question:* What do you think of bupropion (Wellbutrin) for bipolar depression?**

Answer: Like all antidepressants, bupropion is ineffective in bipolar depression, proven to be equivalent to placebo. Agents that are ineffective generally should not be used. It is popular because it has been shown to have a low manic switch rate. This is probably because it is given at low dosages. But even if it doesn't cause mania, it is ineffective, thus there is no point in using it.

It should be noted that bupropion is an amphetamine in its structure. Hence it isn't surprising that it causes weight loss, enhances sexual libido, and causes anxiety. All amphetamines can cause mania and destabilize bipolar illness, as shown in some studies. Bupropion may be less potent than other amphetamines, and thus may be less likely to have those harmful effects in bipolar illness, especially at low doses. But if it is dosed high enough, it will cause mania and it will destabilize bipolar illness.

***Question:* Is there a good scale to assess affective temperaments?**

Answer: The most proven scale is the TEMPS (Temperament Evaluation scale of Memphis Pisa San Diego). It is very well-validated and studied to assess hyperthymia, cyclothymia, and dysthymia. Conveniently, 39-item and 50-item self-report versions are available via the internet.

***Question:* Is there sufficient evidence to recommend lithium, divalproex, carbamazepine, or a dopamine blocker as the first drug of choice in a particular bipolar patient? For example, divalproex/ziprasidone over lithium for a mixed, dysphoric bipolar depression or lithium for the MDI pattern (mania, M, followed by depression, D, followed by a normal interval, I) patient with euphoric mania?**

Answer: In general, the view of this textbook is that if we were to generalize to the average patient with bipolar illness with the most common types of symptoms, all other things being equal (i.e., proneness to side effects, medical illnesses), lithium is the most proven and most effective second-messenger modifier overall.

All other things being equal, lithium is the "drug of choice" for bipolar illness.

The reasons for this general preference for lithium are as follows: Lithium is the most proven agent for prophylaxis, both for depression and mania. No agent is proven more effective than lithium for prevention of either pole, including lamotrigine for depression (see Chapter 19). Unlike other second-messenger modifiers, lithium has the added benefit of being the only agent proven to prevent completed suicide. Furthermore, unlike other agents in this class, lithium is the only agent with notable evidence of dementia prevention and of biological neuroprotection benefits in animals and humans in replicated studies. Lithium also is the only agent proven to reduce overall mortality, extending the average lifespan in bipolar illness by a decade (due to reduced cardiovascular mortality as well as suicide prevention). Many of these lithium benefits occur at low doses, and thus low-dose lithium (300 mg/d or less) can be considered for all patients with bipolar or unipolar mood illness, for these proven or likely mortality reduction and dementia prevention benefits.

However, there are some provisos to this general recommendation, and there are some specific situations where other agents might be preferred to lithium. In the acute mixed manic episode, divalproex and carbamazepine are proven more effective than lithium. In rapid-cycling bipolar illness, lithium alone is proven ineffective (as is divalproex alone and lamotrigine alone), but lithium should be combined with divalproex or carbamazepine. Regarding other patterns of course of illness (mania followed by depression, or depression followed by mania), that literature is mostly observational, and one should not draw strong conclusions. With active severe substance abuse comorbidity, divalproex has somewhat more evidence of benefit than lithium.

Perhaps the most important issue with lithium is its long-term renal impairment. The risk is about 1% at 20 years of treatment, as reviewed in Chapter 11. This risk can be lowered by giving lithium once daily, which reduces constant renal exposure to lithium levels, and by keeping the overall level as low as possible. Many people, especially with non–type I bipolar illness, will respond to levels below 0.6. That said, in choosing to use lithium, another factor to take into account is when to start the clock, so to speak, on its renal effects. In a 50-year-old, 1% at 20 years is not as much of a concern, as opposed to a 20-year-old, who will only be 40 years old with potential renal impairment, and who will have more likelihood of renal impairment by his/her 60s, when they still will have many years of life ahead of them in most cases. Thus, this author's preference is to use lithium less, all other things being equal, in adolescents and "twenty-somethings," and to use it more in middle age. Obviously, there is also higher risk of toxicity with lithium in the elderly, especially at standard levels. Very low doses of lithium, specifically for suicide prevention in the young (300 mg/d or less), or for dementia prevention in the elderly (150 mg/d or less), would still be feasible and recommended where either suicide risk or dementia risk was notable. But, as the primary "mood stabilizer" for prevention of full mood episodes, if all other things were equal, it would be reasonable to lean away from lithium in adolescents and young adults, and toward lamotrigine or carbamazepine (neither of which causes weight gain) or divalproex (in males, due to PCOS risks in young women). Similarly, in those above age 70, it would be reasonable to lean away from standard-dose lithium and towards lamotrigine preferably, and divalproex secondarily (if manic states are more prominent). Divalproex is secondary in the elderly because it has been shown to cause cortical atrophy in that age group. Carbamazepine should be avoided in this age group due to notable hepatitis risk, as well as the many unavoidable drug interactions in most persons at this age who will need medications for other common medical conditions.

***Question:* A 34-year-old woman with severe bipolar illness is prescribed lithium 900 mg/d, aripiprazole 20 mg/d, and hydroxyzine 50 mg BID for anxiety. She stopped taking aripiprazole for a month or so and then reported increasing anxiety. Her sleep is good when her family (child age three and husband) are away, but impaired when they are home. How should her anxiety be managed?**

Answer: Aripiprazole is a complicated medication. It is more effective for depressive symptoms at lower doses (<10 mg/d) and for manic symptoms at higher doses (>15 mg/d). In this case, it isn't clear what her current or recent mood symptoms have been. If she has been mostly depressed recently, then it would be reasonable to reduce aripiprazole to 5–10 mg/d to see if she is willing to take it, assuming she doesn't have akathisia or some other important reason why she can't take it. If she has had akathisia, or was recently or currently manic, then it probably makes sense to replace aripiprazole with a different dopamine blocker, like asenapine or risperidone. Despite her current anxiety, quetiapine would have the disadvantage of weight gain and metabolic syndrome, unlike asenapine. Another option could be to add divalproex to lithium, since divalproex has direct anxiolytic effects. It can cause weight gain, but it doesn't cause metabolic syndrome.

***Question:* When and how should clinicians treat the painful symptoms of grief with medication when there is no prior history of depressive episode?**

Answer: One approach is to differentiate grief from depressive illness by the course of illness. If there are past depressive episodes, then this recurrent condition would be seen as an illness. The setting of grief could be seen then as a trigger, not a cause, of the current depressive episode.

The question seems to be whether, and how, and when one might consider medication treatment when grief is diagnosed, not recurrent depressive illness. In other words, the patient never had a prior depressive episode, but is currently experiencing severe grief.

Should such patients receive medications, like SRIs? In such settings, the use of medication would be symptom-based, not disease-based. Symptom-based treatment is discouraged in this textbook, but this is a matter of emphasis, not prohibition. One should prescribe medications less frequently, at lower doses, and for shorter durations, when such treatment is purely symptomatic.

So in this case of pure grief that is severe, a clinician might decide that some medication could be given if the patient refuses psychotherapy, or if the latter is not available, or if psychotherapy is not helpful enough. Any SRI could be used, such as citalopram, fluoxetine, or sertraline, but it would be reasonable to use as low a dose as possible, for as short a time as feasible. Thus, one might give sertraline 25 mg/d, and if the patient remained symptomatic, increase to 50 mg/d. If there was sufficient benefit, it might be continued for three to six months, and then stopped.

Cultural considerations are relevant. In Muslim countries, for instance, grief is valued, even when severe. However, the clinician should keep an eye on patients so that suffering doesn't become extreme. Suicidality, if present, could be treated with low-dose lithium 150-300 mg/d.

***Question:* Sometimes patients have severe anxiety all their lives, which persists even when the bipolar illness is under control and offending agents like amphetamine stimulants are discontinued. I've seen a person who was a complete nervous wreck all her life until Viibryd 40 mg was added. Lithium, Viibryd, Latuda 120 mg, and Ativan 1 mg bid have gotten rid of 90% of her anxiety. If successfully treating the bipolar disorder still leaves severe anxiety, do you think sometimes it is okay to use SSRI medicines in that the pros and cons lean towards the pros of using SSRIs and then there will be cases where it will not destabilize the person's mood? I usually use 1/4 of the depression dose of the SSRIs to treat the anxiety so as not to destabilize mood. My go-to medicine now for severe anxiety is 20 or 40 of** vilazodone, **and** many people say it is helpful.

Answer: Chapter 20 describes how anxiety is a symptom, not usually a disease or "disorder" itself. If someone has bipolar illness, and they are adequately treated such that they no longer have definable mood episodes of any notable severity, then the continued presence of anxiety would rule out the idea that the bipolar illness itself caused the anxiety. However, two other options exist.

One possibility is that the anxiety is part of the personality trait of neuroticism; the person just is highly anxious as part of her personality, just as some people are tall or short, and some people are introverted or extroverted. That's not a disease that can be taken away with medication. It's not an illness to improve. However, you could make the argument that such personality traits can be modified modestly with medications, and that one can "take the edge off" the anxiety as part of the personality trait, and that some benefit would ensue functionally or subjectively. Another possibility, which is often ignored, is that the mood episodes may not be causing anxiety, but the person may have an affective temperament that could be causing the anxiety.

Affective temperaments are quite common, occurring in about 50% of persons with bipolar illness or unipolar depressive illness, and in many of their relatives. In other words, in between mood episodes, these persons have constant mild mood symptoms.

They are either always manic (hyperthymia), always depressed (dysthymia), or always both (cyclothymia). Especially in the cases of the manic temperaments (hyperthymia and cyclothymia), it is common to have a good deal of anxiety (and often distractibility), leading to misdiagnoses of GAD or adult ADD.

These possibilities need not be mere speculations. Affective temperaments can be measured using the 50-item TEMPS scale. The cut-off recommended by some research is that if 75% or more of the items are endorsed, then an affective temperament is present. Sometimes, 50% or more of items may be sufficient given the clinical history. If someone has cyclothymia or hyperthymia, then those temperaments could explain constant anxiety, even if full mood episodes are managed with the standard mood stabilizers. In that case, low-dose SRIs would not be recommended, since those agents can worsen the manic symptoms of hyperthymia or the mood lability of cyclothymia.

If the TEMPS scale is negative, the neuroticism/extraversion/openness to experience (NEO) scale can be used to measure neuroticism. If the score is high, then it may be that the person has the personality trait of high neuroticism. Low-dose SRIs can "take the edge off" anxiety in that case. Such low doses may not destabilize bipolar illness in terms of causing mood episodes, especially if the personality is otherwise normothymic (i.e., no affective temperaments). In that case, such judgments as our colleague makes here may be relevant. However, even there, one is committing the patient to lifelong treatment without the option of coming off SRIs, due to severe serotonin withdrawal syndrome. One wonders whether low-dose benzodiazepine might not be a better alternative. There is withdrawal there, too, but usually not as severely as with SRIs. There is tolerance and a very small addiction risk, of course, which is higher in persons with substance abuse. Either way, whether with SRIs or benzodiazepines, the treatment of neuroticism with medications is a low-risk, low-yield proposition. Such symptomatic treatment has modest benefit at best, so even with small risks, the benefit–risk ratio is questionable, especially in the long term. As described in Chapter 16 on Hippocratic psychopharmacology, such symptom-oriented treatment was discouraged since in the long run, more harm than good occurs.

46

Key Research Studies in Clinical Psychopharmacology

DIAGNOSTIC VALIDATORS IN PSYCHIATRY: BEYOND SYMPTOMS FOR DIAGNOSIS

Eli Robins and Samuel Guze, Establishment of Diagnostic Validity in Psychiatric Illness: Its Application to Schizophrenia. American Journal of Psychiatry, Volume 126, Issue 7, January 1970, pp. 983–987.

As discussed in Chapter 17, a scientific approach to clinical diagnoses in psychiatry rests on the use of diagnostic validators beyond symptoms. Symptoms vary between illnesses and often overlap; they are not sufficient by themselves to pick out valid diagnoses. Other lines of evidence are needed—like course of illness and genetics—to differentiate illnesses from each other. In medicine, pathology is the gold standard. In psychiatry, there is no gold standard, so multiple lines of evidence have been identified that could differentiate diagnoses from each other.

This paper is the classic article that lays out this way of thinking, with schizophrenia as its main example. The general idea is over a century old, though, and has its roots in the classic approach to medical diagnosis that evolved in the 19th century with the rise of pathology at autopsy as a means of confirming or disconfirming clinical diagnoses.

Here again is the background: A patient has pneumonia with cough and headache. Another patient has pneumonia without a cough and headache. Are these two different "disorders"? A patient has depression with mania. Another has depression without mania. Are these two different "disorders"? Mania has a different set of symptoms than depression, but cough and headache are different symptoms, which do not represent a different disease. That's the intuition behind the concept of diagnostic validators.

One cannot define diagnoses based on symptoms and use as justification the fact that they involve different symptoms. This is mere tautology. Some different line of evidence, separate from symptoms, is needed. For pneumonia, pathology is relevant: tests can show evidence of inflammation in the lung. In psychiatry, there is no access to pathology. This article addresses what alternative independent lines of evidence can be used instead.

This classic article revolutionized psychiatry. Eli Robins was influenced by Kraepelin, who taught that "diagnosis is prognosis," that the course of illness tells you which symptoms represent different diseases. Robins trained a series of researchers who produced the change in U.S. psychiatry that led to the third edition of DSM (DSM-III) in 1980—a change that has hardened into the new credo of DSM-IV and DSM-5. With his colleague Samuel Guze, Robins articulated four other diagnostic validators that, along with symptoms, should be used to identify if groups of patients differ from each other enough to justify seeing them as having different diagnoses. Those validators are:

- Symptoms
- Course of illness
- Genetics
- Treatment effects
- Laboratory tests or biological markers

As noted in Chapter 17, the most important diagnostic validator is course of illness, Kraepelin's key criterion. Some conditions are chronic, others episodic. Some begin earlier in life, others later. Not all conditions are genetic, so the next validator, family history, is relevant sometimes, but not always. Laboratory tests are not usually available for routine practice, though sometimes they can be relevant for treatment as opposed to diagnosis (e.g., pharmacogenetic testing for rapid versus slow metabolism). MRI is relevant directly for the diagnosis of vascular depression. Robins and Guze also referred to "delimitation from other disorders," which meant that symptoms were specific to one condition rather than another. This is not always the case, since many symptoms, like anxiety, can occur in many conditions. Since that classic study, instead of delimitation, the diagnostic validator of treatment effects has been used, although it is the weakest validator, since many drugs are non-specific in effect, and some, like amphetamines, are even effective in normal individuals. Treatment effects are thought of as a proxy for biological markers, but this is the case only if treatment effects are specific to an illness (like antidepressant-induced mania).

As noted in Chapter 17, these diagnostic validators were used initially by Robins and Guze and their colleagues at the Washington University of St. Louis to support certain diagnostic definitions that were included in DSM-III in 1980. However, even though these validators were used to define those diagnoses for inclusion in DSM-III and later, the validators themselves were not included in DSM criteria. In other words, genetics and course of illness were important to define some DSM diagnoses, but they were excluded from DSM criteria for those diagnoses, which were limited to symptoms alone. Borderline personality disorder is a clear example of this approach, where sexual abuse was excluded from the diagnostic definitions, even though this course criterion was central to the whole concept of borderline personality.

The importance of the concept of diagnostic validators in clinical practice is that it helps clarify many diagnostic controversies that are worsened by the DSM reliance on symptoms alone. Is the attentional problem ADD or bipolar illness? Is the sexual impulsivity mania, a paraphilia, or borderline personality? These debates will never end as long as they are conducted on the single dimension of symptoms.

This classic paper reminds us that symptoms only go so far: as with cough and fever, clinicians need to look elsewhere to know which symptoms matter diagnostically and which do not. They need to look to course of illness, genetics, and treatment effects.

Bottom Line

- In a diagnostic dilemma, stop assessing symptoms and turn to the other three diagnostic validators: course of illness, then genetics, then treatment effects.
- Look where those other validators direct you; they matter as much as, if not more than, symptoms to clarify the real diagnosis.

A MAINTENANCE RCT OF OLANZAPINE IN BIPOLAR ILLNESS: A DEMONSTRATION OF THE INVALIDITY OF THE "ENRICHED" MAINTENANCE RESEARCH DESIGN IN PSYCHIATRY

M. Tohen et al., Randomized, Placebo-Controlled Trial of Olanzapine as Maintenance Therapy in Patients with Bipolar I Disorder Responding to Acute Treatment with Olanzapine. American Journal of Psychiatry, 2006, Volume 183, pp. 247–256.

The first dopamine blocker to receive a maintenance indication for bipolar illness, which occurred in 2004, was olanzapine. That indication was based on multiple maintenance trials, all of which were enriched. One study involved the addition of olanzapine to standard mood stabilizers (lithium or divalproex); another, which is presented here, involved monotherapy with olanzapine versus placebo. Besides these studies, other maintenance RCTs also were conducted, in which olanzapine was compared to lithium in one study, and compared to divalproex in another study. This analysis focuses mainly on the monotherapy study, which was the basis for the FDA indication. This study was organized and conducted by Eli Lilly specifically to obtain FDA indication.

Read simply, as presented in the abstract, the results are that 225 patients received olanzapine compared to 136 patients who received placebo, for up to 48 weeks. After recovery from an acute manic episode with olanzapine, those who stayed on it had much more benefit than if they came off. The main outcome was time to a mood episode relapse, which was much shorter with placebo (median of only 22 days) versus olanzapine (median of 174 days). The overall relapse frequency was 80% with placebo, versus 47% with olanzapine.

This basic description of the study results seems stunning. Olanzapine is incredibly effective. There is twice as much relapse if you don't take it than if you take it.

But even with this simple description, the results should raise a question in the mind of the reader. Note that placebo-treated patients relapsed, on average, only 22 days into the study. That means that when the randomized study began, and patients were given a double-blind pill and they didn't know what they were receiving, the placebo patients relapsed massively in just three weeks. Why was that the case? If you start a research study designed to assess long-term relapse in one year of follow-up, why would all the patients in one arm suddenly relapse within weeks of starting the study?

This brings us to a central demonstration of the invalidity of the enriched design: acute withdrawal effects. In the case of this study, acute withdrawal relapse with placebo is obvious.

Let's set the stage. Before the maintenance study began, patients were recruited with an acute manic episode, and they were treated with olanzapine. This was not double-blind or placebo-controlled. It was open-label and unblinded, which means that the patients and doctors were engaged in standard clinical treatment, like you would conduct outside of research. The point was not to show that olanzapine was effective in acute mania; this was already proven. The point was to select out olanzapine responders and make them better so that you could then put them into the maintenance trial to see how long they would stay well. Thus, at the beginning of the maintenance trial, everyone was well. But a few months earlier, they were all in acute manic episodes, and responded to olanzapine.

The preselection process is the central place where the enriched design can become invalid. Let's review who was treated with olanzapine *before* the maintenance study began, and what happened to them.

In the acute mania phase, before the maintenance trial began, 731 patients were recruited and treated with olanzapine. On average they had had two mood episodes in the prior year, one manic and one depressed. They had been in their current manic episode for about one month on average (median, 31 days). As noted, 361 patients entered the study, which means that about one-half of the sample (49.4%, 361/731) did not respond to or tolerate olanzapine for the acute manic episode.

Hence the maintenance trial of 225 olanzapine and 136 placebo patients is actually a study in which twice as many patients were included originally, but half of them were excluded because they didn't do well with olanzapine. This is a preselected group of olanzapine responders, representing only about one-half of patients who have manic episodes. Then, if they improved with olanzapine, they were put into the randomized trial after two to four weeks of staying well. The average amount of time before entering the maintenance trial was two weeks (median 15.9 days for olanzapine, 16.7 days for placebo).

To restate it in clinical terms: Suppose clinicians had patients with acute mania, lasting for one month. They then treat them with olanzapine, and some improve and get well. Two weeks later, clinicians stop olanzapine. What would happen? This expensive randomized trial provides a definitive answer: They would relapse in three weeks (median 22 days).

Has it been proven that olanzapine is effective as a maintenance treatment for prevention of new mood episodes one year or longer in the long-term treatment of bipolar illness? Is it proven that olanzapine is a "mood stabilizer?" No. All that is shown is that if patients improve with olanzapine for an acute manic episode, they should not stop the dopamine blocker two weeks later. That doesn't mean they should stay on it for two years or 20 years. What is shown is only an acute discontinuation effect during the manic episode, not a prevention effect for new mood episodes.

Figure 46.1 tells the story. All patients are well initially; this means that they're in the half of the original acutely manic sample that responded to olanzapine. The *y*-axis represents their relapse rate, starting with 1.0, meaning that 100% are well. The *x*-axis is days to relapse. Looking at the placebo arm, you'll notice a steep fall as soon as the study begins, with half relapsing in 22 days, and about 80% relapsing by about 90 days. From three months onward, the placebo line is basically flat, as is the olanzapine line. In other words, all the action is in the first three months; namely, massive relapse rates with placebo, and less so with olanzapine. After three months, nothing seems to be happening.

Figure 46.1 supports visually what was described previously conceptually and quantitatively. This study is not really a study of long-term relapse at six months to one year of new mood episodes, but rather of short-term discontinuation relapse in three months or less back into the acute manic episode that existed only a few weeks before the maintenance study began. It doesn't, therefore, provide evidence of long-term maintenance prophylaxis of new mood episodes in bipolar illness.

If all this is true, readers might be wondering why the FDA didn't figure it out. If this study is so invalid, why did the FDA give a maintenance indication for olanzapine based on this design?

The answer is complex, but we can begin with the fact that the FDA accepts the enriched design as valid; FDA statisticians do not accept the critiques made here about the invalidity of the preselection process. And indeed, there are ways in which the enriched design can be seen as potentially valid, if conducted in a different way than presented here, but that is a larger story (it relates to other topics, like oncology).

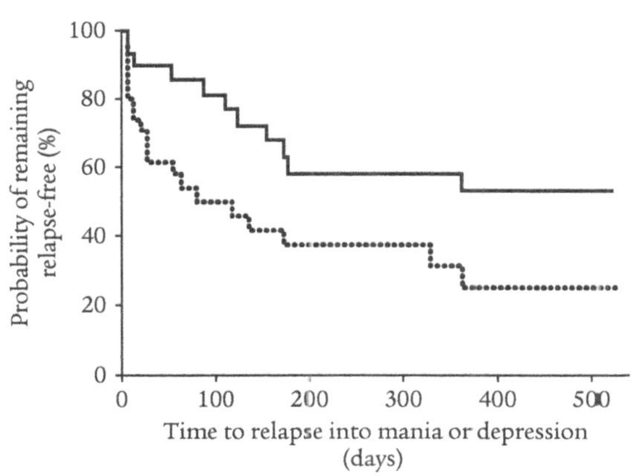

FIGURE 46.1 *Rapid withdrawal relapse, not maintenance efficacy: Olanzapine in bipolar illness.* SOURCE: *Reprinted with permission of Cambridge University Press. Tohen et al. Relapse prevention in bipolar I disorder: 18-month comparison of olanzapine plus mood stabiliser v. mood stabiliser alone. British Journal of Psychiatry 2006;184:337–345.*

The FDA approved olanzapine with a low threshold of scientific evidence, partly because there were no prior dopamine blockers with indications for maintenance treatment for bipolar illness. When there are no or few proven treatments, the FDA is somewhat more liberal in approving new treatments. But after the approval, and during the peer review process for publication, important questions were raised about this study. The author of this textbook will disclose here, as he has in public lectures previously, that he was one of the peer reviewers for this study when it was submitted to the *Archives of General Psychiatry*, the highest ranking general psychiatry journal. In that anonymous peer review, the author made the critiques described previously, especially the massive acute withdrawal relapse rates with placebo. Based on that peer review and those of other reviewers, that journal rejected this study for publication. Thus, this study was good enough for FDA indication, and thus approved for general medical practice, but it wasn't good enough for publication in the *Archives of General Psychiatry*. (Readers will note that it was eventually published in a different journal two years after the same study passed FDA review for an indication.) The questions that were raised in the scientific community by some researchers influenced the FDA to some extent in that, in October 2005, about a year after giving approval, the FDA held an advisory committee meeting in which it wanted to get advice on the question of whether and how the olanzapine-style trial could be improved to be made more valid. The main focus was on the two- to four-week period of remission from acute mania required before the study began. The FDA wanted to suggest a six-month or longer period of remission before entry into a maintenance trial. This suggestion was reasonable because it is consistent with the natural history of bipolar illness, as described in Chapter 6. It takes up to six months to get out of the acute phase for manic or depressive episodes, so if you want to be certain you are preventing new mood episodes in the maintenance phase, not just relapsing back into the same acute mood episode that you had before the randomized maintenance study started, then six months or longer is a wise time frame.

FDA meetings are publicly available, so readers can read, if they like, the minutes of the 2005 meeting online (https://www.fda.gov/ohrms/dockets/ac/05/minutes/2005-4186M1.pdf). A few academic experts, who claimed to be present on their "own dime," joined pharmaceutical industry representatives and some patient advocates, in opposing the FDA suggestion. The opposition from the pharmaceutical industry was obvious: to require six months or longer of treatment, even before the maintenance study officially begins, would be very expensive for them, and difficult to complete. Perhaps they knew that if half the patients drop out with just a few weeks of treatment, as happened in this olanzapine study, very few patients would remain in treatment six months later, and thus their maintenance trials would have tiny samples and would fail. The academic experts and patient advocates took the view that the FDA request was an example of "stigma," putting too high of a standard on psychiatric research, beyond what is the case with other medical conditions. They didn't appear to realize that the enriched design is, in fact, a very low standard of scientific proof. In fact, there is no other medical discipline in which the FDA approves long-term maintenance treatments based on enriched randomized discontinuation designs. All other medical specialties have a higher standard: you cannot preselect your patients at all for treatment response. Thus, the academic experts in particular were uninformed in their attack on the FDA suggestion, and the upshot, as can be read in the minutes, was that the FDA advisory committee decided against the idea of having a long period of remission before enriched maintenance trials in psychiatry. All agreed, though, that two to four weeks was much too short, and a new standard was set of two to four months of remission, which has become the way other dopamine blockers have been assessed since that time (like aripiprazole, quetiapine, and lurasidone). Two to four months is better than two to four weeks, but it still isn't long enough to avoid bias against placebo due to acute withdrawal relapse, and it still does not address the basic problem that preselection for drug responses biases the results in favor of the drug.

Even if one took these results at face value, and believed that they are valid, one still should ask an important question: not how good was olanzapine compared to placebo, but how good was olanzapine, period? The benefits suggested in the olanzapine group may not be as great as they seem, when you switch your focus from the relative effect of comparison to placebo and instead look at the absolute effect of overall benefit.

Recall that these patients were preselected to respond to olanzapine already. Recall also that the natural history of bipolar illness is that the average patient has one episode per year. In this study, patients were manic just before the study began, and they were required to have had at least two other manic episodes in the prior six years of treatment, thus their natural history was selected such that they were likely to relapse in one year of follow-up, and definitely would relapse within two years.

How did olanzapine do in these patients? About one-half (47%) relapsed during the study, and they did so, on average, by about six months (median 174 days).

So, in a patient population selected to relapse by natural history once in one to two years, one-half of them relapsed within six months, despite being preselected to respond to olanzapine and *staying on* olanzapine after getting better from an acute manic episode. This relapse rate doesn't bode well. At that pace, everyone would have relapsed in one to two years of follow-up, just as would be expected if they were completely untreated. (Remember the placebo group isn't a valid assessment of non-treatment in this study because of the invalidity of the enriched design, leading to massive placebo relapse just three weeks into the study due to acute withdrawal effects, as described previously.)

Bottom Line

- The olanzapine trial does not show long-term efficacy in prevention of mood episodes in bipolar illness, despite its FDA indication.
- It mainly reflects massive and immediate placebo relapse due to an acute withdrawal effect after recovering from acute mania a few weeks earlier with olanzapine.

- Even if taken at face-value, half of olanzapine-treated patients relapsed in six months, a pace that is consistent with the natural history of recurrence of mood episodes.
- The FDA sought to correct some of the research design problems involving rapid acute withdrawal, but it was resisted.

SYSTEMATIC TREATMENT ENHANCEMENT PROGRAM FOR BIPOLAR DISORDER (STEP-BD)—ANTIDEPRESSANTS ARE INEFFECTIVE FOR BIPOLAR DEPRESSION

G. S. Sachs et al., Effectiveness of Adjunctive Antidepressant Treatment for Bipolar Depression. New England Journal of Medicine, 2007, Volume 356, Issue 17, pp. 711–722.

In the late 1990s, three classic NIMH-sponsored studies of clinical treatment were conducted, one each in MDD (STAR*D), bipolar illness (STEP-BD), and schizophrenia (CATIE). STEP-BD was mostly an observational cohort study, but one large randomized trial was conducted with over 300 subjects to test the hypothesis that antidepressants are effective for acute bipolar depression. This was a randomized trial of paroxetine or bupropion versus placebo, added to mood stabilizers for the acute depressive episode. The main result was that both antidepressants were equal to placebo for acute efficacy. The two groups were also similar for acute mania induction.

The straightforward interpretation is that paroxetine and bupropion were not effective in the treatment of acute bipolar depression. However, experts often interpret this study by emphasizing the lack of difference in mania induction as well, thus concluding that antidepressants were neither harmful nor helpful for bipolar depression.

The lack of mania induction was unsurprising, given the fact that these two antidepressants were specifically chosen based on prior studies indicating that they had the least risk of acute mania compared to other antidepressants. When they were given with mood stabilizers or neuroleptics, of course, this risk would be even lower. It would be incorrect to infer from lack of acute mania with the agents that are at least risk of it that no medication in the antidepressant class can cause acute mania.

The larger finding, often underemphasized, is that the antidepressants did not work pharmacologically. Patients improved, but not because of the effects of paroxetine or bupropion; they also improved on placebo, which reflects either natural history or the impact of mood stabilizers alone. In any case, in this study, which is the largest and most definitive RCT of this question, antidepressants were found to be ineffective in the treatment of acute bipolar depression.

Bottom Line

- STEP-BD demonstrated that antidepressants were not effective in acute bipolar depression when combined standard mood stabilizers.

- STEP-BD also found that paroxetine and bupropion were not more likely than placebo to cause acute mania, when combined with standard mood stabilizers or neuroleptics.

BALANCE: THE BEST MODERN MAINTENANCE STUDY OF BIPOLAR ILLNESS

J. R. Geddes et al., Lithium plus Valproate Combination Therapy versus Monotherapy for Relapse Prevention in Bipolar I Disorder (BALANCE): a Randomised Open-Label Trial. Lancet, 2010, Volume 375, pp. 85–95.

The most important feature of this study is that it is a throwback to the old prophylaxis study design in bipolar illness. It is not a relapse prevention study. Patients did not have to respond to lithium or valproate to enter it. They only had to tolerate those agents for a brief time (four to eight weeks), after which they entered the maintenance study. There was no requirement for a recent acute episode of mania or depression either. BALANCE is as close as we have to a classic prophylaxis study, similar to some of the original designs used with lithium in the 1960s and 1970s. By abjuring a relapse-prevention preselection of drug responders, it sets a far higher standard for maintenance efficacy than the relapse-prevention designs in the pharmaceutical company–sponsored trials of neuroleptics and lamotrigine.

The BALANCE researchers designed the study to be practical, large, and simple; hence the lack of blinding and the absence of placebo. One benefit of this simple approach, besides generalizability, is that only 60% of the sample completed the two-year study, while in most bipolar maintenance trials, 90% of the samples have dropped out by the end of one-year studies. This allowed them to recruit 330 patients, though they still needed over 40 sites in six years to do so. BALANCE was headquartered at the University of Oxford, part foundation-funded and part pharmaceutically funded (without, however, any corporate input on design or implementation). This kind of research—conducted by academic researchers, with primarily government or foundation funding—is uncommon.

Patients entered the study stable and in remission. They were randomized to receiving lithium alone, or divalproex alone, or the combination of both in up to two years of follow-up. The outcome was either hospitalization or the need for new medication intervention for worsening symptoms. Overall, the combination of lithium plus valproate was more effective than either agent alone. Subgroup analyses found that this effect was driven mainly in mania prevention. For depressive episode prevention, though, lithium alone was as effective as the combination, and more effective than divalproex alone.

This result indicates that lithium is effective to a high degree in prevention of depressive episode relapse in bipolar illness, contrary to mistaken judgments made from the lamotrigine studies, which were enriched and preselected for lamotrigine responders, and thus were biased against lithium. The BALANCE study, which was not preselected for lithium responders, proves that lithium has excellent benefit in depressive episode prophylaxis. It also proves, with the largest available randomized sample, that the strategy of combining mood stabilizers is more effective than either alone, after failure of mood stabilizer monotherapy.

Bottom Line

- Lithium has excellent benefit in depression episode prophylaxis in bipolar illness.
- The combination of lithium plus divalproex is more effective than either alone.

BRIDGE—HALF OF "MAJOR DEPRESSIVE EPISODES" ARE MIXED STATES

J. Angst et al., Prevalence and Characteristics of Undiagnosed Bipolar Disorders in Patients with a Major Depressive Episode: the BRIDGE Study. Archives of General Psychiatry, August 2011, Volume 68, Issue 8, pp. 91–98.

This study was a large, international cross-sectional evaluation of DSM-IV-defined major depressive episodes in 5,635 patients around the world. Only 14% were found to meet criteria for bipolar disorder (past manic or hypomanic episodes), thus 86% were diagnosable with DSM-defined MDD.

The main outcome examined was the presence of multiple manic symptoms irrespective of duration, called the "bipolarity specifier." In other words, the DSM-based cut-off of four days for hypomania was ignored. The question was: Do depressed patients experience multiple manic symptoms at all? The researchers did not simply accept the DSM edict to ignore all manic symptoms if they last less than four days. They were doing what researchers should do: they tested that hypothesis to see if it was valid.

Their main result was that 47% of the sample was diagnosable with the "bipolarity specifier." In effect, they disproved the DSM-based duration cut-off criterion for manic symptoms. If DSM was correct, then there should be very few patients who have manic symptoms that last less than four days. In fact, about half of all depressed patients have this experience.

Furthermore, the presence of these manic symptoms during depressive episodes—which defines mixed states—was confirmed as being diagnostically important because it correlated with standard validators of diagnosis, like genetics and treatment effects. Patients who had the bipolarity specifier were about four times more likely to have family genetic history of bipolar illness (odds ratio 3.8) and almost ten times more likely to experience mania with antidepressants (odds ratio 9.6). In both of these associations, the bipolarity specifier had a much larger effect than even the official DSM-defined bipolar diagnosis.

Another relevant point is that the primary author of this paper, Jules Angst, is the same researcher whose work in the 1960s and 1970s was used by the makers of DSM-III in 1980 to make the radical distinction between bipolar disorder and MDD. In other words, Angst's work back then found that bipolar and unipolar definitions differed in diagnostic validators of symptoms, genetics, course, and treatment effects.

Half a century later, the same researcher now finds the reverse: much of DSM-defined MDD is *not* different from DSM-defined bipolar disorder in symptoms, genetics, course, and treatment effects. Science is about falsifying hypotheses. This study provides data that falsify the DSM distinction between bipolar disorder and MDD.

Bottom Line

- Half of all major depressive episodes, whether unipolar or bipolar, are mixed states because they include multiple manic symptoms.
- Such patients are at high risk of mania with antidepressants, and have strong bipolar genetic loading in family history.

BRAIN EFFECTS OF DOPAMINE BLOCKERS—A REVIEW FINDS THAT MEDICATIONS CAUSE CORTICAL ATROPHY

P. Fusar-Poli et al., Progressive Brain Changes in Schizophrenia Related to Antipsychotic Treatment? A Meta-analysis of Longitudinal MRI Studies. Neuroscience and Biobehavioral Reviews, 2013, Volume 37, pp. 680–1691.

There has been some debate for some time whether antipsychotic medications cause or worsen cortical atrophy in the brain in patients with schizophrenia. It has been known from a range of studies that schizophrenia itself is associated with brain changes. Hippocampal atrophy has been reported, and ventricular enlargement (which reflects atrophy of midbrain structures such as the caudate and putamen) is a well-replicated finding in middle and later stages of schizophrenia in particular.

The question has then arisen as to the effects of using dopamine blockers for long-term treatment of schizophrenia, in a setting of possible underlying neurodegeneration that occurs as part of the disease. Are dopamine blockers protective in any? Are they neutral? Or do they hasten or worsen the degenerative process in the brain in schizophrenia?

Until recent decades, these questions couldn't be answered, partly due to insufficient duration of treatment to assess long-term effects, partly due to the inherent expense and difficulty of conducting such long-term studies, and partly due to inadequate technology to measure brain structure and function. Beginning with some studies in the 1990s, MRI studies have been conducted. This review paper is a systematic review and meta-analysis of this topic.

Thirty longitudinal MRI studies were identified, 1,046 patients with schizophrenia versus 780 controls. They were followed for an average of about 1.5 years (72 weeks).

Brain volumes before and after antipsychotic treatment were examined. Duration of exposure to treatment was recorded as a primary predictor. Researchers also assessed duration of illness, as well as a measure of severity of illness, along with other clinical and demographic variables included in the 30 studies.

Baseline evaluation, *before* treatment with antipsychotic medications, showed that the patients with schizophrenia had smaller whole-brain volumes and enlarged lateral ventricles, compared to controls. This finding confirms the general view, dating back to Kraepelin, that schizophrenia involves a neurodegenerative process such that there is loss of neurons in various parts of the brain. Overall gray and white matter volume did not differ between schizophrenia and controls. Most of the baseline changes were probably driven by smaller midbrain structures.

After treatment with antipsychotic agents, there was new reduction in gray matter volume, and the lateral ventricular enlargements also worsened. These results were observed in patients with schizophrenia, but not in controls. These worsened outcomes correlated inversely with duration of antipsychotic exposure. The longer antipsychotic treatment was given, the worse the neurodegenerative outcomes of gray matter volume reduction and ventricular enlargement.

When other possible factors were examined, such as severity of illness or duration of illness, these other illness factors did not influence the finding of greater gray matter cortical atrophy and further ventricular enlargement. The worsened neurodegenerative results seemed to be associated with dopamine blocker treatment, and could not be accounted for by severity of illness or duration of illness.

In short, schizophrenia itself is a neurodegenerative disease, mainly with midbrain cortical atrophy producing lateral ventricular enlargement. Over time, antipsychotic treatment appears to worsen this midbrain atrophy, and it also seems to be related to causing or worsening generalized gray matter cortical atrophy.

These results could be interpreted as providing evidence that antipsychotics do not have beneficial disease-modifying effects long-term in schizophrenia. This conclusion does not take away from their symptomatic benefits short-term for acute exacerbations of schizophrenia.

Other studies report that cognitive function improves in schizophrenia clinically with dopamine blocker treatment. This clinical benefit would make sense since the harmful cognitive effects of delusions and hallucinations would be ameliorated. This clinical benefit does not change the fact, as shown in this review, that the underlying neurobiological impact of those agents does not appear to be benign or beneficial.

Bottom Line

- Dopamine blockers (antipsychotics) appear to worsen the neurodegenerative process in schizophrenia in long-term treatment.
- Their main benefit is for symptomatic improvement of acute psychotic exacerbations.

DO ANTIDEPRESSANTS PREVENT DEPRESSION? AN FDA REVIEW OF ALL ITS AVAILABLE DATA

A Borges et al., Review of Maintenance Trials for Major Depressive Disorder: A 25-Year Perspective from the Food and Drug Administration. Journal of Clinical Psychiatry, 2014, Volume 75, pp. 205–214.

There has been a great deal of controversy in recent years regarding the efficacy of antidepressants in acute depression. As a result of some of that public debate, the FDA conducted an internal review of a related but different question: the long-term maintenance efficacy of antidepressants. The issue of long-term efficacy has been discussed in research circles for some years in relation to a question of methodological bias. The FDA review sought to address some of those concerns.

The research design question for maintenance studies is important to understand. These studies are called "enriched" because patients are preselected to respond to the drug being studied.

Think of it this way: To do a maintenance trial, a study to prove long-term prevention, patients have to be well, not ill, when they enter the study. Then one sees whether new episodes of illness happen in the future.

So patients needed to be recruited into the maintenance studies who were well. But most well persons aren't motivated to go into randomized placebo-controlled trials. Usually, instead, they come for treatment or research when they are ill or symptomatic. In the case of depression, patients would be recruited when depressed, and treated with an antidepressant until they became well, and then they would enter the randomized maintenance trial to see if they stayed well.

In other words, in these studies, patients are treated before they enter the research study, so that prevention can be tested. But what should they be treated with? Any antidepressant? Or the antidepressant being studied for prevention?

Since these studies usually are designed by pharmaceutical companies, they tend to use their own medication for the initial acute treatment, to get patients well, before they enter the maintenance prevention trial. Thus, the study of prevention is conducted in patients who have responded already to the drug being studied. Does this bias the study?

The claim could be made that since acute treatment efficacy may not be the same as maintenance or prevention efficacy, then the design isn't biased necessarily. Two different kinds of outcomes are being assessed.

In unipolar depression, there is consensus that the acute phase of depression lasts three to six months, and that the maintenance phase of prevention of new episodes begins 9–12 months or longer after the acute phase. Thus, the question of whether new episodes are being prevented has to do with whether outcomes are being assessed one year or longer after the acute depressive episode.

Do the maintenance randomized trials of antidepressants show such benefit? The FDA decided to review its data to help answer this question. Pharmaceutical companies are required by law to give all their data to the FDA when they seek indications for marketing. These data are patent-protected, so they remain confidential within the control of the FDA. Pharmaceutical companies are under no obligation to publish those data, and the FDA is under an obligation to keep them confidential. But the FDA can analyze and publish those data without identifying features, and researchers can access anonymized data using the Freedom of Information act. This paper represents an internal FDA review of all the data it possessed for the past 25 years on this topic, which consisted of 15 studies.

The FDA found that all 15 studies showed antidepressant efficacy for maintenance prevention. That's 100% success! In contrast, the FDA database has been studied repeatedly, and it has been found that about 50% of acute depression studies in MDD show efficacy of antidepressants, but about 50% show inefficacy.

So what is the case? Are antidepressants incredibly effective in long-term prevention, but only so-so for acute treatment? Or is there something wrong with the "enriched" design for long-term prevention?

The FDA addressed a main concern regarding the enriched design, which is that there can be withdrawal effects. This means that since patients are being treated with the antidepressant being studied, before the study begins, and then the responders enter the maintenance study, those who get switched to placebo have a rapid-withdrawal relapse. The FDA defined "withdrawal" as two weeks or less after randomization, but only 6% of patients had such relapse. Thus, the FDA concluded that there was not much withdrawal relapse.

The FDA was very impressed that the studies were consistently positive and concluded that antidepressants are very effective in prevention of MDD. But there are some legitimate concerns regarding the FDA's rosy interpretation.

The concept of withdrawal relapse isn't limited to two weeks. The idea is that if only drug responders are included in a study, the study is inherently biased because it is testing what was already proven. The only way it could work would be if the maintenance drug response was a different outcome than the acute drug response. Maintenance is defined as one year or longer, not two weeks. The FDA review didn't assess outcomes after one year versus before one year, or even after six months versus before six months.

In fact, the FDA review included a figure, shown in Figure 6.1, which depicts how almost all the benefit seen with antidepressant over placebo in the "maintenance" trials occurred in the first six months of follow-up, which is not the maintenance phase of treatment, but is still part of what is called the "continuation" phase, meaning that the acute episode has not yet resolved naturally. Any relapses seen in that time frame are back into the same episode that was active a few months earlier, and cannot be assumed to represent new and different mood episodes.

After six months, there was no further benefit with antidepressants over placebo. The FDA review shows this figure, but it doesn't acknowledge its relevance to the question of whether the enriched maintenance study design is biased. Thus, it could be concluded that because it doesn't assess or prove benefit six months or longer after the acute phase ended, the FDA review doesn't really answer the question of whether there was inherent bias in the design.

There is another sign that the FDA review didn't solve the problem of bias of the enriched maintenance design: the absolute 100% success rate. It doesn't make sense that the same drug class would fail to be effective half the time in acute two-month studies, and then succeed 100% of the time in one-year maintenance studies. At the very least, the question can be raised that the enriched maintenance design may succeed 100% of the time because it is biased; that's the whole point. It never fails because it isn't fairly testing anything.

Even if this critique of the enriched design is granted, it doesn't prove that antidepressants are *ineffective* in prevention of depressive episodes in unipolar depression. It only means that they aren't *proven* effective, despite the apparent efficacy of these 15 studies.

The same concern regarding this enriched design applies to other drugs and other maintenance studies, such as dopamine blockers in bipolar illness, as discussed in Chapter 6.

Bottom Line

- Antidepressants are proven effective for maintenance prevention of depressive episodes in 15/15 MDD studies in the possession of the FDA.
- Either antidepressants are incredibly effective agents in long-term prevention of depressive episodes, or the enriched maintenance design is too biased to prove or disprove such efficacy. This text leans toward the latter interpretation.

PAROXETINE IN DEPRESSION—A REANALYSIS 14 YEARS LATER INDICATES SRI WITHDRAWAL CAUSES SUICIDALITY

J. Le Noury et al., Restoring Study 329: Efficacy and Harms of Paroxetine and Imipramine in Treatment of Major Depression in Adolescence. British Medical Journal, 2015, Volume 351, h4320.

It took over 100,000 hours of work to get access to the actual data from a research study from 2001, conducted by SmithKline Beecham (SKB) on paroxetine for major depressive disorder (MDD) in children. That published study reported benefit. Over a decade later, a reanalysis with the same data reports no benefit.

The difference partly is about what we mean by "benefit." There was about a 2 point improvement with paroxetine over placebo. This is a small "benefit," but the original paper made a big deal about it because it was "statistically significant." This is a mistake, because a benefit that is very small is still very small, even if it's real. Yet it wasn't even statistically significant, we now know, after 100,000 hours of digging: The original statistical analyses that were planned before the study began showed that it wasn't statistically significant. Yet the authors of the first paper went on to use other statistical comparisons that found statistical significance in some weeks of the study, and they emphasized those outcomes. They also emphasized four outcomes that were statistically significant, even though they weren't part of the original study plan. Called "post-hoc," those outcomes could have occurred by chance at a higher likelihood than the study ever acknowledged.

In the original paper, the authors worked hard to show positive results with their statistics in the interests of the study drug. The original study was ghostwritten by a company hired by the manufacturer, not by the academic "authors," who only revised it. Furthermore, the original paper reported low rates of worsened suicidality (increased ideation or attempts or self-harm) and dismissed those results because they weren't "statistically significant," which again is wrong since the study wasn't designed to assess those outcomes, and thus was "underpowered" (didn't have enough subjects) to test for statistical significance (which means the effect of chance on a result that is sufficiently powered to assess that outcome). The reanalysis reexamined the actual patient charts in part of the sample and found that there were twice as many cases of worsened suicidality as originally reported (11/93, 11.8%, vs. 5/93, 5.4%), and this was much more than placebo (2/93, 2.2%). Part of the reason for more cases of suicidality in the reanalysis has to do with patients who became more suicidal when they were in paroxetine withdrawal—i.e., as they were switched from paroxetine to placebo. The original study didn't count these patients as having effects related to paroxetine. This is important, though, because we know that SRI withdrawal is a major clinical problem, that patients often do and sometimes should stop their SRIs, and that agents like paroxetine produce withdrawal-related marked agitation, anxiety, impulsivity, and now we can add, even suicidality.

In short, SRI withdrawal produced more suicidality.

The author of this textbook has conducted a further analysis, using the same data previously but not presented in the current *British Medical Journal* analysis. Converting those raw numbers to relative risks, we find the following: The relative risk (RR) of worsened suicidality with paroxetine versus placebo in the new reanalysis is 5.50 (95% CIs 1.25, 24.1). This compares to RR using the original 1994 publication of 5.00 (95% CIs 0.59, 42.0).

The basic effect of this reexamination of this new *British Medical Journal* reanalysis is the same as in the original 2001 paper. There was a relative risk of about 5 in both analyses, meaning about a five-fold increased risk of suicidality with paroxetine over placebo. But, in the 2001 paper, SKB and its authors dismissed the result because it was "statistically nonsignificant," meaning that it could have occurred by chance more than 5% of the time. As mentioned, this isn't legitimate statistically since the study wasn't designed to assess suicidality, thus one could have results that don't meet statistical significance in those equations because there aren't enough people in the study to assess an infrequent outcome (i.e., suicidality in 5–10% of the sample). With the new *British Medical Journal* reanalysis where the number of suicidal outcomes is doubled in the paroxetine group (and doubled in the placebo group), we have the same relative risk of five-fold increase, but now the increase in frequency of outcomes produces confidence intervals that do not include the null value of one. What this means is that the results are statistically significant with the new analysis, if we care about statistical significance.

The clinical bottom line is the same as the FDA black box warning: SRIs can worsen suicidality in some children. The scientific bottom line is the same as we knew, but this analysis proves with the same database as previously published by SKB: pharmaceutical industry clinical trials are ghostwritten in such a way that they overstate drug benefits and minimize drug harms. There needs to be independent scientific analysis of those data before we can understand them fully.

Bottom Line

- The original paroxetine study misrepresented a small clinical benefit as more important than it was, by emphasizing statistical significance in ways that weren't legitimate.
- The original study didn't report the full extent of suicidal side effects, downplaying this harm by relying on statistical non-significance when it shouldn't have.
- SRI withdrawal can cause suicidality.
- Clinicians shouldn't rely on ghost-authored studies by the pharmaceutical industry in which databases are never accessible publicly for verification by independent researchers.

THE NATURAL HISTORY OF TREATED DEPRESSION TODAY—FEW PEOPLE WITH "MDD" RETURN FOR TREATMENT

K. L. Musliner et al., Heterogeneity in 10-Year Course Trajectories of Moderate to Severe Major Depressive Disorder: a Danish National Register–Based Study. JAMA Psychiatry, 2016, Volume 73, pp. 46–353.

In Scandinavia, medical treatment is provided and recorded in a national health care system for all people. One of the benefits of this system is that researchers can access data on medical treatment for all people in those countries. This Danish study uses the national medical database to look at the course of treatment for depressive conditions, as diagnosed by clinicians as similar to the DSM-5 definition of "major depressive disorder" (MDD).

The sample identified consisted of 11,640 persons in Denmark who were diagnosed with MDD and for whom researchers had medical data for 10 years in prospective follow-up. They were diagnosed in the 1995–2002 time period. A majority were women (64%), as is typical of depression studies. The main outcome measure was whether or not they continued to be seen for MDD treatment in each year of follow-up.

Four patterns of outcome were observed:

- In the majority—77% of the sample—their contact for follow-up treatment was not extensive and was limited to two years or less.
- The next-largest group—13% of the sample—was far smaller, but it was this group that had extensive contact for up to five years, with less contact afterwards.
- A third small group—7% of the sample—had continued contact in the second half of the 10 years of follow-up (the second five-year period).

- The smallest group—only 3%—had consistent and persistent contact for treatment of MDD in the entire 10-year period.

The first thing to notice is that the vast majority of patients just didn't need much attention. It isn't clear whether this is good or bad news.

The rosiest interpretation would be that they all were cured with their prescription of an antidepressant, and they didn't need much further contact for a decade. This optimism is unwarranted, though, with the low one-year response rates in the STAR*D study. (In that large randomized trial, overall one-year response was present in about one-third of the sample.)

The less rosy interpretation would be that most patients either didn't respond to, or didn't tolerate, treatment, or simply changed their mind for psychological reasons, such as denial or stigma. There is a huge literature supporting the impact of these factors on clinical outcomes.

An important piece of context is that many studies of compliance in outpatient psychiatric treatment of non-psychotic conditions indicate that about one-half of patients drop out of treatment within the first few months to one year. In other words, the baseline for any psychiatric diagnosis (excluding severe psychoses like schizophrenia) is that about one-half of patients will not return for adequate treatment.

So the 75% low-treatment rate in the Danish study should be compared to a 50% baseline. It may not be as terrible as it seems, but it still is worse than what is seen in other settings or other studies. What explained the 25% or so of extra failure to follow up on treatment?

One idea is that this added failure may be due partly to a failure in the concept of MDD. When many different kinds of depression are mixed into a single broad category, including many persons with "neurotic depression" who have mild constant depressive/anxiety symptoms, it may not be surprising that they don't change much with some SRI treatment, and thus they don't return for more of the same. Another possibility is that our drugs may just not work well in real life.

In contrast to the previous comments, the authors of the paper focused instead, not on the majority of patients who didn't come back, but rather on the minority who remained in treatment. They had good medical chart data on some, but not most, important clinical features of practice. Thus, they had information of family history of other psychiatric conditions, and they had chart data on severity of symptoms.

They found that the 3% group with the most treatment had the most severe symptoms and were more than twice as likely to have family history of schizophrenia. Since "MDD" is not associated with a genetics of schizophrenia, this observation raises some questions about accuracy of the MDD diagnosis. Only 4% of the sample had schizophrenia genetics, and only 2% had recorded bipolar family histories. Of course, these assessments also could be inaccurate, with some under-reporting, given that this was a national clinical database of real-world treatment, not a research study in which patients were recruited and analyzed with a specific research protocol of interviews.

The authors' main conclusion was that MDD is "heterogeneous" in its outcomes. Since the course of illness is a diagnostic validator, this study is another new replication that throws doubt on the scientific validity of the MDD concept. This is so despite the fact that the profession has refused to change the basic structure of the MDD concept one iota, including in DSM-5, since its initial formulation in 1980 with DSM-III.

Bottom Line

- The course of MDD in this study was heterogenous, throwing doubt on the validity of the MDD diagnosis.
- The vast majority of patients appear to have dropped out of treatment, or simply did not need much treatment.

ADULT ADD: A PROSPECTIVE STUDY—MOST CASES DON'T INVOLVE CHILDHOOD ADD

A. Cayet et al., Attention-Deficit/Hyperactivity Disorder Trajectories from Childhood to Young Adulthood. JAMA Psychiatry, 2016, Volume 73, pp. 705–712.

In Brazil, a birth cohort study was started in 1993 of 5,249 persons who were followed from birth throughout childhood and up to age 18. About 80% of the total cohort was successfully followed. At age 11, they received an ADD screen that was repeated at age 18.

Overall, 8.9% of the sample met ADD criteria at age 11. This prevalence increased to 12.2% at age 18. This observation would seem to support the view that ADD persists into adulthood in all patients; in fact, some new cases are picked up.

This study used the concept of a diagnostic hierarchy, however, unlike almost all prior studies of adult ADD. It didn't ignore other diagnoses. Thus, it assessed whether ADD was present in adulthood only in the setting of other diagnoses that can cause inattention, specifically mood (bipolar and MDD) and anxiety (GAD and social anxiety) conditions. When those other diagnoses were ruled out, and researchers assessed the presence of only ADD itself, without any other potential diagnostic causes, the adult prevalence rate fell by about one-half, from 12.2% to 6.3%.

Thus, to review, about 9% of children met ADD criteria. This rose to 12% of young adults at age 18. But this fell again to about 6% if ADD was defined as meeting ADD criteria and not having other psychiatric diagnoses that can cause inattention.

At first glance, even with this complex analysis, it would still seem that about two-thirds of children who had ADD persisted into adulthood: 9% at age 11 versus 6% at age 18. However, this wasn't the case, because they weren't the same people.

Of children at age 11 who met ADD criteria, only 17% continued to meet those criteria at age 18. In other words, ADD went away in 83% of children by adulthood. This finding is consistent with over half a dozen course studies conducted prior to the introduction of medications for adult ADD. In that literature, up to about the year 2000, the overall finding was that about 90% of children with ADD no longer met criteria by around age 20. This Brazilian study confirms that earlier literature. It also throws some light on current debates about adult ADD, however, in that it still found a good number of young adults met ADD criteria, even though they didn't have ADD as a child.

Thus, the second important observation here was that only 12.6% of the adult ADD cohort also had been identified as having ADD as children in this prospective study where they had been assessed previously for ADD. In other words, 87.4% of adults who met DSM criteria for ADD as adults had not experienced it as a child.

How believable are these results, and what do they mean? The authors refer to a recent meta-analysis of adult persistence of childhood ADD that fully agreed with their findings: adult persistence was less than 20% overall. They also refer to another large recent study that found only 5% persistence of childhood ADD when followed further into middle-age adulthood.

The observation that about 5% of adults have impaired attention, which cannot be attributed to ADD or to other psychiatric conditions like mood and anxiety syndromes, is important. It's important to emphasize that these persons do not have "ADD" because this study proves that their inattention is not persistence of childhood ADD. So what do they have?

One possibility is that they experience "normal" inattention, in the sense that they are at the extreme of a normal curve for inattention. Since selective attention is a normal psychological trait, what we might appreciate is that attention exists on a normal curve, with most of us at the middle, near the 50th percentile. But two standard deviations to either side will represent about 5% of the general population, who are either overly focused (which is consistent with obsessional or manic thinking) or under-focused (which is frequently labeled "ADD"). This perspective, about normal variations in attention, has been described in Appendix III, and this study result can be interpreted as supportive of that interpretation. It should be noted that these persons did have some clinical consequences of their inattention, such as increased criminal behavior, incarceration, and suicide attempts.

Importantly, personality conditions were not assessed, so the possibility that some of them had mood temperaments would also be present. Furthermore, prior research suggests that a subgroup of patients with childhood ADD later are diagnosable with antisocial personality, which could correlate with some of the findings in this study.

Bottom Line

- ADD does not persist into adulthood in about 80% or more of children.
- About one-half of apparent adult ADD may be caused by mood and anxiety conditions.
- About 5% of adults in this sample met ADD criteria but did not have adult ADD, since they did not have prior childhood ADD.
- The presence of inattention in 5% or less of the general population is due to causes other than ADD, which could include mood temperaments or normal variation on the psychological trait of attention.

TREATMENT RESPONSE IN FIRST-EPISODE DEPRESSION—ALL TREATMENTS ARE SIMILAR

B. W. Dunlop et al., Effects of Patient Preferences on Outcomes in the Predictors of Remission in Depression to Individual and Combined Treatments (PReDICT) Study. American Journal of Psychiatry, 2017, Volume 174, pp. 46–556.

The Holy Grail has long been sought: Prove that one treatment for depression is better than another. The STAR*D trial was funded by NIMH in large multi-center style to prove that one drug is better than another, or that a combination of antidepressants might be more effective than a single agent. STAR*D found they were similar.

This PReDICT trial reluctantly reaches the same conclusion. In this NIMH-sponsored study, the special feature was supposed to be that all patients would be treatment-naive having never been treated for depression before, and most would be in their first depressive episode. In practice, it's quite difficult to identify and treat the actual first depressive episode of many patients, since most people don't seek treatment immediately. Rather, such "first episode" studies really reflect "first treated episodes." In this study of the first treated episodes, in fact about one-half of patients were in their first depressive episode. The other half had had one or more prior depressive episodes.

This study is unique in that there are few if any prior first-episode depression studies (in contrast to numerous first-episode mania studies in bipolar illness and first episode psychosis studies in schizophrenia). To find first-episode subjects, the researchers, based in Atlanta at Emory University, had to resort to advertising for subjects. They also recruited from a large inner-city public institution, Grady Hospital, at a Spanish-speaking clinic where subjects were identified who hadn't been previously engaged by the healthcare system.

A reasonably large sample of 344 patients was obtained, blindly randomized for 12 weeks of acute depression outcome to one of three arms: a pure SRI (escitalopram), an SNRI (duloxetine), and cognitive behavioral therapy (CBT). There was no placebo control, which is an unfortunate weakness. (One should prove, not assume, that these treatment-naïve patients wouldn't have improved by natural history or based on nonspecific psychological factors.)

The main outcome was the Hamilton Depression Rating Scale (HDRS) score, which reduced similarly in all groups (10.2 improvement with CBT, 11.1 with escitalopram, 11.2 with duloxetine). The 1-point difference between CBT and medications was clinically small and not statistically significant. However, at each week-by-week visit, CBT was slightly less effective than the medication options. Despite the vaunted marketing of "dual-action" on norepinephrine reuptake as well as serotonin, duloxetine was exactly the same in efficacy as escitalopram. This result contradicts the neuromythology that affecting two neurotransmitter systems produces more efficacy than affecting one.

The researchers had wanted to find means to support "personalized medicine," a popular phrase these days. But they found nothing, or very little. In effect, it didn't matter if patients received a pure SRI, an SNRI, or CBT: the result was more or less the same.

In an accompanying paper, the same researchers report neuroimaging results that differentiate the antidepressant medication response groups from the CBT response groups. These distinctions involve the subcallosal cingulate cortex (SCC) connectivity to other areas of the brain. These findings may be important, but they were not the primary hypotheses of the study, and could reflect post-hoc false-positive statistical findings. Nonetheless, they are interesting, suggesting that different regions of the brain may predict CBT versus medication response. However, again, no distinctions were found in comparing one kind of antidepressant medication to another.

Another aspect to understanding this study is the overall response rates, defined as 50% or more improvement in depression symptoms. Those response rates were 42% for CBT, 47% for escitalopram, and 55% for duloxetine. These response rates do tend to support somewhat increasing efficacy in moving from psychotherapy to single neurotransmitter effects to multi-neurotransmitter effects. But again, the effect sizes are relatively small, and not statistically significant.

Lastly, overall, as with STAR*D, only about one-third of patients had remission, meaning the resolution of almost all depression symptoms. This is the same result as STAR*D, where most patients had recurrent episodes and prior treatment. Here in the PReDICT study, we have half the sample in its first episode, and none ever treated previously. And still the results of this treatment-naïve sample are the same as in STAR*D. In other words, the poor results in STAR*D didn't reflect a treatment-refractory sample.

These results aren't terrible. Half the patients improved short-term. But they aren't overwhelming either. Furthermore, for those who interpret the limited benefits of antidepressant medications as implying a need to use more psychotherapy, the CBT results in this study indicate that psychotherapy isn't any better.

Perhaps because the treatment efficacy results weren't very exciting, this primary paper for this study emphasizes in its title the question of whether patient preferences for randomization influenced outcome. Before randomization, patients were asked whether they preferred one of the three options; they were randomized irrespective of their preferences. The Hispanic subgroup had a preference against medication, while the African-American subgroup had a preference for CBT, and the white subgroup had no overall preference. These stated preferences didn't predict any differences in treatment outcomes, though. Instead, a mismatch of preference to randomized treatment (i.e., getting medication if you preferred CBT) predicted less treatment adherence, as expected.

Bottom Line

- Antidepressant response in a treatment-naïve, partly first-episode depression population was not better than in the treatment-refractory STAR*D study.
- Duloxetine was only slightly more effective than escitalopram, if at all.
- Except for neuroimaging possibly, predictors of treatment response couldn't be identified.

ANTIDEPRESSANTS WORK!?—THE MOST RECENT AND LARGEST META-ANALYSIS CLAIMS EFFICACY, BUT STILL FINDS LITTLE CLINICALLY MEANINGFUL BENEFIT

A. Cipriani et al., Comparative Efficacy and Acceptability of 21 Antidepressant Drugs for the Acute Treatment of Adults with Major Depressive Disorder: a Systematic Review and Network Meta-analysis. Lancet, 2018, Volume 391, pp. 357–1366.

A recent highly touted meta-analysis has been seen as showing definitively, as one media article reported, "Confirmed: Antidepressants work!" The latest defense comes from one of the most prestigious medical journals, the *Lancet*.

The basic finding of the meta-analysis, as reported in the published paper, is that antidepressants work because they are all better than placebo. What is not clarified in the published paper, but was shown in the details of the online appendix, is that they are hardly any better than placebo, and not in any way that is clinically meaningful for most agents. The only drug with clinically meaningful benefits is one that is used rarely today, amitriptyline, a tricyclic antidepressant.

Context is important: As discussed in Chapter 19, multiple other meta-analyses in the past decade have looked at the same topic, antidepressant randomized clinical trials for MDD, usually conducted by pharmaceutical companies for government registration. Those studies have found, repeatedly, that antidepressants either are no more effective than placebo, or they are slightly more effective, with an effect size that does not translate into clinically meaningful benefit. The effect sizes seen are about a 2-point improvement versus placebo on the HDRS, which is lower than the minimum threshold of 3-point improvement for clinically meaningful benefit set by the U.K. NICE criteria.

Another way of looking at it is via Cohen's d standardized effect size. This statistic is reported as a standardized mean difference, which means that the actual scores are divided by standard deviation. This allows studies with different scales to be compared directly. This "Cohen's d" effect size a simple way to compare the absolute benefit seen. A general rule of thumb with Cohen's d is that a score of 0.0 to 0.25 is small to no effect, 0.25–0.50 is a mild benefit, 0.5–1.0 is a moderate to large benefit, and above 1.0 is a huge benefit. It is a convention that a Cohen's d of 0.5 or larger is a standard threshold for clinically meaningful benefit. The meta-analyses conducted over the past decade find an overall modern antidepressant effect size of about 0.31–0.32, which is small and below clinically meaningful benefit.

This study claims in its published form to be finding something different; that is, that antidepressants are effective. In fact, its results are basically the same as these prior analyses', confirming that almost all antidepressants are ineffective, or at least not clinically meaningfully effective, when examined as a whole compared to placebo.

In other words, the only thing this study confirms is that prior studies were right when they reported that antidepressants "don't work." How can this be?

It is common these days for the most prestigious medical journals, like the *Lancet*, to publish huge "network" meta-analyses, with resulting high levels of attention to the publication. This article is produced by the Oxford University psychiatry department's very active meta-analysis research group. That group of researchers has published many meta-analyses, and the entire research activity of a central core of those researchers is devoted to meta-analysis.

The key feature to analyzing this study is to understand the concept of meta-analysis. The authors looked at 522 antidepressant versus placebo randomized clinical trials in MDD. Altogether, 21 drugs were examined, and the overall sample exceeded 100,000 patients. Overall, all antidepressants were more effective than placebo, and in the "network" analysis, the authors report the lowest direct efficacy, with an odds ratio (OR) of 1.36, for reboxetine, and the highest efficacy, with an OR of 2.13, for the TCA amitriptyline.

If these results were accepted at face-value, we would conclude that clinicians should feel confident that all antidepressants are effective in MDD in general, and they would lean towards the agents listed previously that were "more" effective, and against those that were "less" effective. Unfortunately, these results are not true as stated.

On the positive side, the authors included much unpublished data (52% of all the studies), and their results are not limited to or mostly influenced by, the published literature, which is known to be markedly biased in favor of antidepressant drug efficacy (this is because pharmaceutical companies usually have not published negative studies of antidepressants).

On the negative side: Nowhere in this dense and detailed paper did the authors report the absolute effect size of benefit with antidepressants on the depression rating scales used. They provide odds ratios, which are relative effect sizes over placebo. So a drug might be 50% better (an OR of 1.50), but this could be a difference between 2 points with drug and 3 points with placebo on a depression rating scale (a tiny and clinically meaningless effect), or it could be a difference between 20 points with drug and 30 points with drug on the scale (a huge and clinically meaningful effect). In other words, how much better did patients get?

The real truth in this study is nowhere in the published paper, but rather in a busy table on page 142 of the online appendix. There the authors report what we want to know: what was the actual difference between drugs and placebo, before and after treatment, on the depression rating scales?

On page 142 of the online appendix, readers can find that the Cohen's d standardized mean difference effect sizes range from a low of 0.19 to a high of 0.62 with amitriptyline. Thus amitriptyline exceeds the clinically meaningful threshold of 0.50, with a traditional meta-analytic method. No other drug does so, with the closest second place being fluvoxamine with a *p*-value of 0.44.

Looking at all the agents, 10 drugs have *p*-values that are less than 0.30, thus very small and clinically meaningless. Four agents have effect sizes from 0.30–0.34. Thus 74% (14/19) of antidepressants clearly have little or no clinically important benefit in this analysis (for some reason, no data are provided in this table of traditional meta-analysis with two drugs). Four drugs have effects sizes of 0.37–0.44, and as noted, one agent exceeds the 0.50 threshold (amitriptyline).

Perhaps a clearer conclusion than anything else is the old well-proven fact that the TCAs are more effective than newer agents. (There were no MAOIs in this meta-analysis.)

The main point to conclude from the previous description is that almost all antidepressants had small, clinically meaningless benefits. And *only one agent* exceeds the threshold of a Cohen's d effect size of 0.50 or greater, which can be considered clinically meaningful benefit.

In short, one has to go to page 142 of the appendix to find the real result of all this effort: *This meta-analysis confirms the results of prior meta-analyses that find that antidepressants have small overall effects in "MDD," and do not provide major clinical benefit in general.*

This conclusion puts aside the more important issue of the scientific validity of the MDD concept itself, which the authors ignore completely. Maybe the problem is with "MDD," which is a heterogenous clinical syndrome that is not valid scientifically as a single diagnosis rather than with antidepressants. In other words, these drugs do something biologically, but maybe we aren't giving them to the right clinical group of patients to see benefits.

The only clear take-away from this analysis—besides confirming the prior analyses that antidepressants are not very effective—is that amitriptyline is the most effective antidepressant tested, and apparently the only one with clinically meaningful benefit.

Bottom Line

- Modern antidepressants are better than placebo, but they do not provide clinically meaningful improvement overall.
- The only antidepressant with clinically meaningful improvement in this meta-analysis was amitriptyline.

47

Historical Insights in Psychopharmacology

IN THIS CHAPTER, HISTORICAL INSIGHTS IN PSYCHOPHARMACOLOGY ARE provided with excerpts from writings of two thinkers in this field, Emil Kraepelin and Aubrey Lewis.

Kraepelin was the famed great late 19th-century psychiatric leader from Germany who identified the basic distinction between schizophrenia (dementia praecox) and manic-depressive illness. He laid the foundations of much of psychiatric diagnosis that remains relevant today, as discussed repeatedly in this book, and he was a committed defender of the biological approach to psychiatry, although he was conservative with the use of drugs, which were ineffective in his day. The excerpt is drawn from his reflections near the end of his career, in 1917. He looks back at the prior 100 years of psychiatry. Compare his observations with the next 100 years, ending almost exactly with the publication date of this textbook.

Lewis (1900–1975) was the most prominent figure in British psychiatry through most of the 20th century. He was the leader of the Institute of Psychiatry at the Maudsley Hospital for much of the middle of the 20th century. That institution in London was the most influential educational center for psychiatry in the nation. Through his leadership there, Lewis was extremely influential. He tended to be skeptical about the use of psychotropic medications, and emphasized social aspects of psychiatric illness. In the 1958 essay cited here, Lewis addresses the general question of the extent to which psychiatrists know anything. This article, published in the *Lancet*, was directed toward a medical audience that was skeptical about the professional credibility of psychiatry. There Lewis looks at the nature of psychiatric knowledge in 1958, and makes some observations, which are still relevant today, about psychopharmacology in its early modern period.

EMIL KRAEPELIN, 1917

If we compare the situation of mental patients today with the circumstances that prevailed a century ago, the revolution that has been accomplished comes into clear focus. . . . One by one prejudices have been overcome, abuses and cruel practices eliminated, new means found to alleviate mental diseases. Spearheading this advance was the growing body of scientific knowledge relating to the nature and etiology of insanity and deriving from study of data in different fields of investigation and from overall progress of the science of medicine. Unrelenting effort on the part of a large number of alienists gradually transformed the sad lot of the mentally ill, with the result that today we are actually nearing the end of our struggle. To be sure there are still many defects to be remedied and improvements to be made, but we are not being presumptuous in stating that we have discovered the approach to be followed henceforth in psychiatry.

Our satisfaction over the progress already made is tinged with regret. When we consider the extraordinary sacrifices made by those responsible for the evolution of psychiatry, we are constrained to lament the fact that all the hopes tied to it can never be fulfilled. We must openly admit that the vast majority of patients placed in our institutions are according to what we know forever lost, that even the best of care can never restore them to perfect health. Our treatment probably makes life endurable for a vast number of mental cripples whose plight would otherwise be intolerable, but only rarely does it effect a cure. . . .

We must therefore ask if there are other, more promising, approaches. The answer is a resounding yes. Most promising is the prevention of insanity. . . . The nature of most mental disorders is now obscured. But no one will deny that further research will uncover new facts in so young a science as ours; in this respect the diseases produced by syphilis are an object lesson. It is logical to assume that we shall succeed in uncovering the causes of many other types of insanity that can be prevented—perhaps even cured—though at present we have not the slightest clue; a case in point was cretinism before the discovery of the thyroid treatment. . . .

The great war in which we are now engaged has compelled us to recognize the fact that science can forge for us a host of effective weapons for use against a hostile world. Should it be otherwise if we are fighting an internal enemy seeking to destroy the very fabric of our existence?

AUBREY LEWIS, 1958

It is the common state of reflective and inquiring minds to be somewhere between untrammeled guesswork and certainty. . . . We [psychiatrists] are, however, sometimes suspected of luxuriant speculation and of invincible faith in our tenets: and I propose to explain how this reputation has arisen.

More than most branches of medicine, psychiatry can be regarded as an art. One of its distinctive procedures—psychotherapy—manifestly depends on subtle relationships and incommunicable qualities of personality. . . . Psychiatry in this is like the rest of medicine, combining moral and personal principles of action with those arrived at by the methods of science, and depending on the last for any increase in its power to prevent and control disease. . . .

It would be easy to pile up instances showing that psychiatry is not the only branch of medicine—or of knowledge—to be pilloried for lax thinking and complacent dogmatism. It has, however, troubles which seem peculiar to itself, and some ministrants who seem peculiarly indifferent to the scientific method as understood by the rest of the world. . . .

The aims of medical treatment are ordinarily to remove or lessen disabilities and pain, to put an end to morbid changes in the patient's body of which he may not be aware but which must sooner or later cause disability, and thirdly, to enable him to live as satisfying a life as possible, in spite of persistent disability and morbid process. Applied to mental illness, all this becomes equivocal. The patient will often be unaware of disturbances very plain to others; he may not complain of his symptoms; he may even cherish them. He may lead a less satisfying life when his symptoms have been got rid of than when he had them. The morbid process often has no physical substrate that we know of: and the psychopathology may be obscure and inaccessible. The criteria of recovery are therefore hard to specify, and like the criteria of improvement, depend on an assessment of the patient's happiness, competence, and well-being which involves moral and social values as well as plainly medical ones. . . .

A rather silly but often repeated truism says that the aim of psychiatric treatment is to promote mental health. It is hard to tell what the latter phrase means. Mental health is an invincibly obscure concept. . . . [It] is an abstraction which is very loosely interpreted. . . . *[Lewis goes on to criticize our ability to know whether our treatments work, whether they be physical, like insulin coma or drugs, or psychotherapeutic.]*

. . . [T]he medley of "tranquilizing" drugs may pass . . . into the like chiaroscuro of approval and rejection. But the doubts which attend physical methods of treatment are dwarfish alongside the giant misgivings and disputes which envelop psychotherapy in dust and fog. The trouble is of long standing, and has divided psychiatrists bitterly. . . . Psychotherapists are seldom skeptical or, as one might say, ambivalent about the treatment they give, and "philosophic doubt" is not in keeping with their métier. . . . Here then is a great domain of psychiatric practice in which there has been an excessive proportion of guesswork and rather a lot of subjective certainty. . . .

There are some awful warnings of what a craving for certainty can lead to. You may remember the philosopher Cratylus who, as Aristotle tells us, decided never to say anything but what was certainly true, and so he ceased to talk at all and confined himself to wagging his finger. Psychiatry suffers much from hopeful illusions and clichés used as incantations, just as a few decades ago it suffered, even more, from pessimistic and resigned inertia. . . . It is easy to lay failings like those at the door of psychiatrists, blaming their lack of scientific training, their loose habits of thought, their incuriosity, their passion for psychoanalysis or for physical methods of treatment, their preoccupation with the fascinating art of understanding other people. To think this seems to me facile and unjust. More important than the deficiencies of doctors [is] the inherent complexity of the problems. . . .

I have not enlarged on the attainments of psychiatry, its solid groundwork of detailed, minute, and orderly observations, its empirical successes, its accretions thorough application of the basic medical sciences to clinical problems. . . .

Clearly we are a long way from certainty, and when we meet anyone who is sure that he knows how to tackle the problems of mental disorder and to remedy the failings of psychiatrists and psychologists, we may recall Lord Landsdowne's remark: "I wish I could be as sure of anything as Tom Macaulay is of everything." Guessing, too, has its perils and is arduous: it takes unkindly to the discipline which is good for it. Yet between those who are nearly certain and those who guess much there is the bond which Isaac Newton spoke of: "I doubt not we have one common design: a sincere endeavor after knowledge, without valuing uncertain speculations for their subtleties, or despising certainties for their plainness."

SELECTED REFERENCES

Kraepelin, E. (1962). *One hundred years of psychiatry*. New York: Citadel Press, pp. 150–152.
Lewis, A. (1958). Between guesswork and certainty in psychiatry. *Lancet, 1*, 171–175; 227–230.

48

Reflections on the Art of Psychopharmacology

"In the future, we will have new medications in the future. Our challenge will be in teaching doctors how to use them. Otherwise it would like giving a driver's license to someone who can't drive."

—Frank J. Ayd, Jr., MD

"Irrationally held truths are more harmful than reasoned errors."

—Thomas Huxley

"All who drink of this remedy recover in a short time, except those whom it does not help, who all die. Therefore it is obvious that it fails only in incurable cases."

—Galen

"All drugs are toxic; only the dosing and the indication makes them therapeutic."

—William Osler

"All substances are poisonous; the dose differentiates a remedy from a poison."

—Paracelsus

"The prime object of the physician in the whole art of medicine should be to cure that which is diseased....Whenever the illness is too strong for the available remedies, the physician surely must not expect that it can be overcome by medicine. To attempt futile treatment is to display an ignorance that is allied to madness."

—Hippocrates

"The chemical industry of our days produces various substances for which no market can yet be found. . . .We know that a great number of physicians, without rhyme or reason, go after every new remedy that is recommended to them. If an industrialist is but shrewd enough to advertise sufficiently, he usually succeeds in increasing the sale of his product – for some time at least – and thus enriching himself."

—R. Buchheim, on the wish to use medications and the role of pharmaceutical marketing, in Germany, circa 1876,

Uber die Aufgaben und die Stellung der Pharmakologie an den deutschen Hoschshulen,

—Arch Exp Pathol Pharmakol 5: 261, 1876.

Our knowledge is just enough to obscure our ignorance."

—quoted by William Gowers, MD

"I believe we may safely affirm, that the inexperienced and presumptuous band of medical tyros, let loose upon the world, destroys more of human life in one year, than all the Robinhoods, Cartouches and Mcheaths do in a century. . . I wish to see a reform, an abandonment of hypothesis for sober facts, the first degree of value set on clinical observation, and the lowest on visionary theories."

—Thomas Jefferson, letter to Dr. Caspar Wistar, 1807

"Nearly all men die of their treatments, not their diseases."

—Moliere, 1673

"The young physician starts life with twenty drugs for each disease, and the old physician ends life with one drug for twenty diseases."

—William Osler

"Psychiatry is neurology without physical signs, and calls for diagnostic virtuosity of the highest order."

—Henry George Miller, MD, 1970

"We do go about curing a substantial number of ailments...But there is another part of the mystique. It's the great secret of doctors, known only to their wives, but still hidden from the public. Most things get better by themselves; most things, in fact, are better in the morning."

—Lewis Thomas, MD

"To say the truth, every physician almost hath his favourite disease, to which he ascribes all the victories obtained over human nature."

—Henry Fielding, 1749

"Philosophical insight requires that we be content with what is possible for us. We have to operate within limits wherein realization through us is possible. If we want more than we know and are able to do, our thinking becomes deceptive and ruinous at the same time."

—Karl Jaspers

"All successful medical diagnosis is the precise and intelligent recognition and appreciation of minor differences."

—Joseph Bell, MD, teacher of Arthur Conan Doyle, MD, who wrote *Sherlock Holmes*

"The first principle of science is that you must not fool yourself, and you are the easiest person to fool."

—Richard Feynman, physicist

"It's easier to fool people than to convince them that they've been fooled."

—Mark Twain

William Osler's Three Rules for Medical Practice

1. Consume your own smoke. Don't complain about the inevitable trifles of the day's routine. Things cannot always go your way.
2. The practice of medicine is an art, not a trade; a calling, not a business. We are not here to get all we can out of life for ourselves, but to help others become happier.
3. The hardest of all—Love, charity, requires not only beneficent acts, but an end to hard thoughts.

—William Osler

"Science and opinion are different. Science is the father of knowledge, while opinion breeds ignorance."

—Hippocrates

"Disease has a plurality of forms and a plurality of cures."

—Hippocrates

"Psychiatry is the part of medicine furthest away from settled maturity, as strong as any in observation (perhaps even the richest, considering that social observations are much better accepted in psychiatry than in most of medicine), and weakest in correlations and calculations. It is like an adolescent, disputatious, alternately arrogant and humble, strong, full of promise, inconsistent, able to see what others can't, even preoccupied with sex."

—Leston Havens, *A Safe Place*

"Therapeutic effort has prospered at the expense of therapeutic discrimination . . . "

—Aubrey Lewis, *Education of Psychiatrists*

"A thousand contradictions crowd together, but they are found in nature."

—Voltaire

"The sciences cannot be without charlantry. People wish to have their opinions accepted."

—Voltaire

49

Ten Fallacies and Ten Truths of Psychopharmacology—Explained

TEN FALLACIES OF PSYCHOPHARMACOLOGY

1. More is better

The first fallacy of psychopharmacology has to do with a belief that is logical, but needs to be proven in clinical practice. Examples abound of useful and effective medications that are harmful at too high of a dose. Aspirin at very low doses prevents heart attacks and strokes, but at average to high doses it has no further preventive benefit, and instead causes gastrointestinal bleeding. In low to average doses, lithium is very effective for manic episodes, but at higher doses, it is toxic and can cause kidney failure. Tricyclic antidepressants at average doses are effective for depression, but at higher doses cause cardiac arrhythmias. One could multiply examples for almost every drug class.

The disadvantage of high doses is not always related to toxicity. Some medications are less effective at higher doses. For instance, aripiprazole is more effective for treatment of the acute depressive episode at less than 10 mg per day compared to more than 10 mg per day. It is frequently the case that higher doses lead to a plateau of effects. For example, haloperidol does not produce more benefit above 10 mg per day than below 10 mg per day. Lithium does not produce more benefit above a level of 1.0 than below that level. Steroids do not produce more benefit for autoimmune diseases above low to average levels.

Certainly more benefit can be obtained with somewhat higher doses in the effective dose ranges of certain medications, but those dose ranges need to be established. It is not a rule in a general sense that increasing doses routinely will lead to more benefit. In fact, it is a much more general rule that after a certain dose range, increasing doses will lead to a plateau of effects, with usually more side effects, toxicity, or harm.

2. What gets you well keeps you well

This is the "happily ever after" fallacy. The idea is that if medications are helpful acutely, then they should be continued, and the patient will continue to do well, and live happily ever after. Again, this belief is consistent with common sense, but unfortunately, common sense is not consistent always with scientific truth. There are many examples of drugs that work acutely, not preventively, and vice versa. For example, sumatriptan is effective acutely for migraine, but does not prevent it. In contrast, propanolol is effective for prevention of migraine, but does not treat it acutely. Penicillin and other antibiotics are generally effective acutely for various infections, but do not prevent infections if continued long-term. Steroids are generally effective acutely for autoimmune disease exacerbations, such as lupus, but continuation of steroids does not effectively prevent future exacerbations.

In short, there is no scientific or biological reason to believe that what gets you well keeps you well. In psychiatry, this is one of the most common and harmful fallacies. SRIs are given acutely for depressive and anxiety symptoms, with some benefit, and then continued forever, for years and decades, with no exit plan, and with the eventual occurrence of very severe withdrawal syndrome if any attempt is made to come off them. Dopamine blockers are continued long-term for schizophrenia, based on short-term benefits, even though their maintenance benefits are limited, and there is evidence now that they cause cerebral atrophy long-term.

3. Treat to remission

This fallacy has become the mantra of many psychopharmacology researchers. Clinicians and researchers have been justifiably bothered by the limited benefit obtained with psychotropic drugs in recent years. The early excitement about psychotropic drugs in the 1960s to 1980s has not been sustained. It has been replaced by an inability to obtain equally impressive outcomes compared to those early years. The joke has become that one should hurry up and use a new medication before it stops working. The reaction of many clinicians and researchers has been to increase the dose of medications, as in the first fallacy, and then to combine medications from the same or different classes, as in this fallacy. The view is that if patients are not improving sufficiently, it is simply because clinicians are not trying hard enough. If we use more medications and at higher doses, we will be able to achieve more benefit. In the absence of new and different medications developed by the pharmaceutical industry, clinicians and researchers have focused on the same classes of medications that have been available for the last few decades, but just use them more aggressively. The problem of "residual" symptoms is to be fixed by more and more medications of the same kind. These clinicians and researchers sometimes don't appreciate that the problem may be that the wrong kinds of medications are being used for the wrong kinds of diagnoses. Or, as a related problem, the diagnoses, often based on the DSM, may not be biologically valid enough to improve markedly with certain drug classes. In other words, the underlying assumption behind this fallacy is that our diagnostic system is legitimate and we just need to get better treatments for those diagnoses. This assumption itself is questionable.

A related topic is that even if we have valid diagnoses, and effective treatments for those diagnoses, there may be some benefit to allowing for the occurrence of mild symptoms. Or, it may be that the balance of harms and benefits with medications may be such that lower doses that lead to mild symptoms may be preferable to higher doses that may lead to zero symptoms. For example, mild symptoms of depression are associated with the positive traits of empathy and realism, and mild symptoms of mania are associated with the positive traits of creativity and resilience. The occurrence of mild manic or depressive symptoms is associated with being more functional in many cases, and with success in the creative arts as well as in politics and leadership. It may not be necessary or even desirable to completely remove all manic and depressive symptoms in such persons, even if complete remission were feasible.

4. Polypharmacy is good

Even if remission is not set as the goal, there is the belief that multiple medications will be more effective than any single medication. This approach, called polypharmacy, has been criticized in medical tradition going back to the 19th century, but in recent years, it has seen a resurgence in psychiatry. An effort is made to legitimize this approach by changing the name, to terms such as "polytherapy," or "combination pharmacotherapy." These changes in language cannot hide the basic idea, which is related to the first and third fallacies; namely, the view that more medication should produce more benefit. Sometimes medications in the same class are combined, and sometimes medications in different classes are combined. In either case, one cannot assume that combinations of medications are more effective than monotherapy. Sometimes they are, but sometimes they are not, and the adjudication has to rely on clinical research that proves the matter one way or the other. For example, it has been shown that about one-third of persons with bipolar illness have complete resolution of almost all of their symptoms with lithium monotherapy. Two-thirds may need other medications in combination treatment, but one-third do not. The view that almost everyone should be on combination medications for bipolar illness, which is held commonly, leads to over-medication of one-third of that population, who would do well with just one very effective medication such as lithium. Furthermore, in the STAR*D study, it was shown that combination treatment with multiple antidepressants was not more effective than switching to a different antidepressant (see Chapter 19). Thus, in general, it cannot be claimed that combination treatments are more effective than a single medication. This is an empirical question, not a logical one.

5. Make one change at a time

Sometimes clinicians will say that they like to make one change at a time, because they want to know what is causing what. Although laudable in principle, this approach can lead to an overly slow process of finding the right medication or medication combination in an individual. One can go too fast or too slowly in practice. The rationale for making one change at a time is not really a clinical rationale. One wants to know what is causing what, but this is only a secondary concern to wanting to get the patient better. The primary purpose of clinical practice is to improve the patient's clinical state, not to obtain knowledge. The latter is a goal for research. Knowing what is doing what is a knowledge question and really belongs to the world of research. Getting patients better is the first goal of the clinician. Even if two changes are made at the same time, or three, what really matters is whether patients improve. How can clinicians know which change led to improvement? Later, when patients are doing well, clinicians can remove one medication from the mix to see if improvement persists. Then clinicians can tell whether a first or second medication led to the change. It is better to make these changes when patients are well, rather than ill. The main goal when patients are ill is to get them well. Once they are well, clinicians can begin a slow process of obtaining knowledge about which medication is doing what. But to go slowly when patients still are sick, on the grounds that one wants to have adequate knowledge about the effects of medications, is to let patients suffer excessively, and in a way that is not justifiable given the primary goal of clinical practice.

6. Four to eight weeks is a sufficient trial of a drug

The opposite problem to the fifth fallacy is the problem of going too fast. This is the case when multiple medications are tried, one after the other, for one to two months in duration. This belief that one to two months is the timeframe for a medication trial is based on clinical research studies, often for depressive episodes, where acute efficacy is being studied. Many of these research projects are conducted by the pharmaceutical industry, and the eight-week acute efficacy design is based on what is required by the FDA for a marketing indication. This timeframe is not necessarily relevant to clinical practice, depending on what is being treated. Acute indications are emphasized by the pharmaceutical industry because they are cheaper and quicker to obtain than long-term indications. Clinical practice, in contrast, typically involves long-term treatment, not just treatment for one to two months. Almost always, then, what is relevant for clinical practice is long-term maintenance prevention of symptoms or episodes of illness, not just its acute treatment. As discussed in the second fallacy, one cannot presume that there will be long-term maintenance prevention benefit with a drug that is only been proven effective for acute short-term symptoms. The duration of the trial that is sufficient to prove long-term benefit depends on the illness being studied, but it typically involves six months to one year of treatment or longer for the classic conditions in outpatient psychiatric treatment, like affective illness or schizophrenia. This does not mean that clinicians should wait one to two years with each trial of every medication, because then they would be going too slowly, as in the fifth fallacy. But one to two months is probably too fast. For example, in a trial of a monoamine agonist for depressive illness, or a mood stabilizer for a bipolar or depressive illness, or even a dopamine blocker for schizophrenia, it probably makes sense to try new medications for about three to six months, depending on the severity of symptoms and the need to go more quickly or more slowly based on that severity.

7. Dose low, go slow

This fallacy again relates to going too slow. The first part of this belief has to do with the idea of starting a low dose with every patient. This is not reasonable, because many patients present with severe acute symptoms that require medium to higher doses for immediate symptom control. For instance, in a severe outpatient acute manic state, medium to high doses of a dopamine blocker should be given quickly to prevent possible hospitalization. If risperidone is used, it should be given at 2–3 mg per day for that purpose. If given at 0.5–1.0 g per day, it will be better tolerated, but the patient may end up being hospitalized. Going slowly, which is the second part of this fallacy, is not necessarily rational either. In some cases, one may start with a low dose to assess and ensure tolerability, but a relatively rapid increase in dose may be needed for a more severe condition. For instance, divalproex might be started at 250 mg per night, but in a patient with moderate manic symptoms, it should be increased to at least 750 mg per day relatively quickly, meaning three- to seven-day intervals between doses, but no longer.

8. Always taper a drug

The view that medication should always be tapered is restrictive to an excessive degree. There are many medications that do not have withdrawal syndromes, nor any known, clear, common risks from discontinuation, such that tapering is unnecessary. For instance, bupropion has no withdrawal syndrome, and the claim of rebound risk of seizures is not based on any clear empirical evidence. Unlike SRIs, bupropion can be stopped without the need for a slow taper. Especially when one is making more than one change at the same time, as discussed before in relation to the fifth fallacy, it is important not to engage in unnecessary drawing out of those changes, such as with slow tapers of medications that do not have serious discontinuation syndromes. Another example is divalproex, which has no withdrawal syndrome and can be stopped when needed. This fact contrasts with lithium, which has a withdrawal syndrome, and should be tapered in a one-month time frame or longer. Again, there is no general logical rule here, but rather a need to ask for empirical evidence and then to decide one way or the other.

9. Treat the most severe symptom

It is common for clinicians to rely on the concept of "target symptoms." Frequently, the target symptom is the most severe symptom that a patient experiences. This fallacy comes back to the problem of taking a symptom-oriented approach to treatment, as opposed to a disease-oriented approach. It would be like focusing on fever as the most severe symptom of an infection, rather than trying to treat the underlying disease. One could give the patient plenty of Tylenol, but only modest symptomatic benefit would be achieved without an antibiotic. This scenario may be similar when multiple or higher doses of monoamine agonists are given for anxiety or depressive symptoms, but the underlying affective illness is not treated. It is the case with medical diseases that the most severe symptoms are not related directly to the underlying disease. Many medical diseases have no symptoms at all, such as hypertension or cancer. The severity of symptoms therefore does not correlate at all with the disease, nor does it accurately direct which kind of drug should be selected.

10. Always incorporate the patient's preference

In contemporary medicine, it is no longer acceptable to be paternalistic with one's patients, at least in the United States. This laudable approach to practice, which is consistent with the American emphasis on individual and civil rights, runs into a problem when a clinical profession is supposed to possess specialized knowledge that is unavailable to the general population. In the case of clinical psychiatry and the mental health professions, clinicians are presumed to possess such specialized knowledge, and they are held accountable for the application of that knowledge both ethically and legally. They can be subject to state board complaints or lawsuits based on the fact that they have specific obligations to know certain things and to apply that knowledge in practice. Hence, the view that the patient's opinion is as important as that of the clinician needs to be balanced by the reality that the clinician is held to a higher standard than the patient. In short, clinicians need to be aware that they are expected to have knowledge that is not possessed by the patient, and they need to determine how they can apply that knowledge in a way that is respectful of the patient's individual liberties, but without equalizing their relationship in a way that is neither factually true nor legally protected.

In psychiatry, one also faces the special problems of stigma and lack of insight. Because of stigma, many patients have culturally influenced attitudes about certain psychiatric diagnoses or medications. Those attitudes are based on insufficient or incorrect knowledge, and it is not appropriate for the clinician to allow such opinions, based on stigma, to hold equal weight to other opinions that are based on more adequate knowledge. In such settings, patients are free to have their own opinions; clinicians are also free, and in fact obligated, to educate patients as best as possible. In the case of lack of insight, clinicians face the problem that it is the nature of some diseases, such as mania or schizophrenia, that patients will not be aware that they have those illnesses. In such cases, it is not a matter of education or knowledge, rather it is part of the disease that patients will have viewpoints that may not be correct. In the United States, the clinician's role is to provide the best possible advice and knowledge to patients, and then to leave it to patients to decide what to do, within the constraints of the legal system. When symptoms are very severe, and there are risks of self-harm or harm to others that is imminent, legal aspects come into play that may require clinicians to intervene, at least short-term, to prevent physical harm either for the patient or for others, if feasible. Outside of that extreme setting, though, patients are free to make their own decisions; it is important also to realize that clinicians are not obligated to accept or follow decisions of patients that may be mistaken, based either on stigma, lack of insight, or inadequate knowledge.

TEN TRUTHS OF PSYCHOPHARMACOLOGY

1. Your treatment is as good as your diagnosis

This concept flows out of the general Hippocratic perspective that we should treat diseases not symptoms (Chapter 16). So if the disease is unknown or not diagnosed, the treatment of symptoms will only have partial benefit at best, often counteracted by many side effects. One of the problems in contemporary psychiatry is that it doesn't pay much attention to diagnosis; many clinicians just treat symptoms. Another way it works is that diagnoses are made using the DSM system, which is mostly invalid, as discussed in Chapters 16–18. In that case, if the diagnosis is invalid, the treatment will be ineffective. This axiom was told to the author by Dr. Edwin Cassem, former chairman of the department of psychiatry at Massachusetts General Hospital, and also a Jesuit priest.

2. Treat diseases, not symptoms

As said previously, the Hippocratic principle is that we should treat diseases, not their symptoms. William Osler stated this perspective most clearly at the turn of the 20th century. When a disease is treatable, then effective treatments will manage all symptoms, and even notable side effects will be outweighed by benefits for the overall disease. When a disease is unknown, untreatable, or invalidly defined, then treatment of its symptoms may occur to a partial or modest extent, but it will never be complete. Furthermore, since all drugs have side effects, as in the following principle, those side effects often outweigh partial or modest benefits. As an example, Tylenol will never completely get rid of fever, but penicillin will. This is the case, even though penicillin has no direct anti-fever effect, and Tylenol does. Similarly, in psychiatry, so-called antidepressants will never completely rid patients of depressive symptoms, but a medication to treat the underlying disease that causes depressive episodes, such as lithium, can and will.

3. All drugs are guilty until proven innocent

This is the principle that relates to the Hippocratic tradition that can be called "Holmes's rule," given its historical basis in the teachings of Oliver Wendell Holmes, Sr. In this perspective, all medications have side effects, therefore they should not be used, because side effects are always harmful. However, if medications are proven effective, and a disease is improved or cured, then those medications can be used since those benefits will outweigh side effects in most cases. This approach relates to the classic risk–benefit analysis of medical treatment. Clinicians know that all treatment involves the weighing of risks and benefits.

4. All drugs are toxic; dosing and indication make them therapeutic

This is a classic teaching derived from Paracelsus. It builds on the last few truths just cited. All medications have side effects and harms, thus in a sense they are all toxic. But side effects and toxicities vary with dose. Many times a medication can be quite harmful at high doses but quite safe at low doses. So dosing is an important aspect of making judgments about the risks and harms of medications. Indication for treatment relates to efficacy and benefits of medications. If a medication is proven effective, as discussed before, for a certain diagnosis or disease or indication, then it can be used even if it has many side effects or toxicities. So the judgment that a medication is harmful or toxic should never be made in isolation. For instance, one often hears that lithium is a "strong" medication, or that it is toxic. But lithium is not toxic at all at very low doses, and its side effects and harms are greatly outweighed by its many benefits for bipolar illness, unipolar depression, and possibly other conditions like dementia.

It is quite important to be clear and explicit about whether one starts on the risk side of the ledger or the benefit side. Many clinicians start on the risk side: they first ask themselves whether a certain medication is harmful or has many side effects. Or, when considering a class of medications, they asked themselves which are the safest ones to use, or which are the ones with the fewest and mildest side effects. Then they begin to assess potential benefits among those medications that they deem safest or most benign. Often, the search for efficacy is quite limited or even ignored, and medications are simply used because they are apparently benign. It is important to always remember that no medication is truly benign. All medications have harms, therefore this approach of using medications that might be ineffective based on the belief that they are safe is itself a dangerous approach. It is well established that, over time, apparently safe medications turn out to have been harmful. The medical profession has had this experience with hormone replacement therapy recently, and with other medications in the past such as aspirin in children or diethylstilbestrol (DES) during pregnancy.

The alternative approach is to start, not with risks, but with benefits. Before thinking about which medications to use, clinicians should focus first on what medications are proven effective, or are deemed to be most effective. Then with that winnowed list, clinicians can assess which ones are safest or have the fewest side effects. Start with efficacy, then assess side effects, not vice versa. This is a truth taught by Holmes in the 19th century, still as true now as ever.

5. Always have an exit strategy

When patients get better with medications for current symptoms, clinicians and patients should not then conclude that those medications should be continued indefinitely. This is not the case in general medicine. One does not go to one's general practitioner with pain, then receive medication that improves the pain, and then decide to stay on that medication for the next few decades of one's life. It is the case in psychiatry, however, that patients routinely come to clinicians with symptoms of anxiety or depression, for instance, receive symptomatic treatments for anxiety or depression, and then improve over the course of a few weeks to a few months. Often those medications tend to be continued indefinitely, not infrequently for decades. There is no medical or biological rationale for this approach. It can make sense in some cases, where there are recurrent mood episodes, and some medications are proven to prevent those mood episodes. Those medications often are the so-called mood stabilizers, which have less acute benefit for the mood symptoms than so-called antidepressants.

In other words, treating patients in some ways is similar to deciding to go to war. A general should have an exit strategy. Before prescribing the first medication, you should have in mind how long you would continue that medication if it works. Clinicians should tell patients how long that duration of treatment would be, as opposed to waiting to address that decision later. One problem with waiting is that patients are unwilling to stop medications after they have improved. They have a fear that their symptoms or illness will return, a fear that is not medically or biologically sound if the analogy with Tylenol for fever is correct. Patients should be told ahead of time that they will need to come off their medications in three months, six months, or one year, however long is judged prudent by the clinician. Otherwise clinicians will have a hard time persuading many patients to come off medications later.

Another reason to discuss how long medication treatment will continue at the beginning is that it may enhance patient compliance among those who are skeptical or nervous about taking medications. If they are told that medication treatment will continue for no more than one year, for instance, they may be more willing to begin medication trials and stick with them for that timeframe. This is important because research shows that by six months of treatment with antidepressants, the vast majority of patients have stopped taking their medications. Another aspect that is important to the exit-strategy approach is the problem of long-term withdrawal syndromes. It is now clear that SRIs have very serious withdrawal syndromes after one year of treatment. In the long run, those withdrawal syndromes can cause much more harm than any benefits that were achieved symptomatically in the shorter term. It is important to avoid such withdrawal syndromes, unless absolutely necessary, and an approach of emphasizing treatment for one year or less with SRIs would make sense in many cases.

6. Most current psychotropic drugs have some dramatic benefits but are not disease-modifying. The clearest exception is lithium

Many clinicians who have come to the mental health professions in the last four decades entered a field that widely accepted the efficacy of most medications. It is important to realize that when the modern classes of psychotropic medications came into existence in the 1950s and 1960s, a major factor in the excitement about these agents was the belief that they were not purely symptomatic. For over a century beforehand, physicians and clinicians had had access to many medications with symptomatic benefits, such as sedating agents or tranquilizers. It was believed that the antidepressants were special because they actually removed the whole clinical condition of depression, and not simply because they improved some of its symptoms. It was believed that antipsychotics were special because they removed the whole clinical syndrome of a psychotic episode, taking it away completely, and not just because antipsychotics had some symptom benefits for delusions or hallucinations. It was held that anti-anxiety agents could completely remove anxiety conditions like obsessions. In other words, by the 1980s, it was believed, implicitly or explicitly, that psychotropic medications cured the overall clinical syndromes of depression, mania, psychosis, and anxiety states. In short, it was held that they modified diseases causing those symptoms, and were not purely symptomatic treatments. They were held to be more like antibiotics than like Tylenol.

Almost half a century later, we have enough clinical and scientific experience to say that these beliefs do not appear to have been confirmed. The majority of psychotropic drugs are symptomatic in their effects, and do not alter or improve the underlying disease process that might be causing those symptoms. This has been proven to be the case with antipsychotics in schizophrenia, which do not improve the course of the illness. It appears to be the case with antidepressants in unipolar depression, where long-term maintenance efficacy is questionable, as discussed in Chapter 19. It appears to be the case with most anxiety states, where symptom benefits with SRIs are seen, but long-term removal of anxiety symptoms is less apparent. An exception to the prior statement may involve SRI efficacy in OCD. Another exception to this overall rule is that mood stabilizers like lithium do alter the course of bipolar illness and unipolar depression, and prevent mood episodes in a way that is often curative.

7. Older drugs are more effective than newer drugs

It is the case that the most effective medications in psychiatry are its oldest medications. The most effective treatment for depression is ECT, which was discovered in the 1930s. The most effective medication class for depression is the MAOI class, which was developed and discovered in the 1950s. The next-oldest class of antidepressants, the TCAs, is more effective than the newest class of antidepressants, the SRIs. The most effective treatment for mania is achieved by neuroleptic medications, without any increased benefit with new agents versus older ones. The most effective treatment for bipolar illness overall is still lithium, which is the oldest agent. The most effective treatment for schizophrenia is clozapine, which was developed in the 1960s and 1970s. In short, since the 1970s, the wide variety of new psychotropic medications has not produced a single medication that is more effective than medications in prior generations.

8. Newer drugs are more tolerable than older drugs

The flipside of the prior truth is that the newer generation of medications in the past few decades has been developed to have fewer side effects than older medications. This is the case with second-generation antipsychotics versus older antipsychotics, and with SRIs versus TCAs. It also is the case with some anticonvulsants compared to lithium. However, it should be clear that these medications have become popular and widespread in use primarily because of their increased tolerability and fewer side effects, not because they are more effective than older medications. In many cases, they are less effective than older medications, but still effective enough to be used clinically, and with their lower side effect burden, they are more feasible to use. The point is not that clinicians and patients should never use older drugs, nor that they should be satisfied with newer drugs, but merely that they should realize that any benefit with the newer drugs that has been achieved in the last few decades is really related primarily to tolerability rather than efficacy.

9. Treatment "resistance" usually reflects either misdiagnosis or an invalid diagnosis

The current attention to treatment resistance in psychiatry is a reflection of the acceptance of the current diagnostic system as valid, while looking for better treatments for those diagnoses. If the current DSM diagnostic system is only partially valid, then insufficient benefit with medications could reflect the fact that the clinical phenotypes being treated are not real enough to produce notable benefits with treatments that affect biological mechanisms. In addition, a different issue may be that the diagnosis is simply wrong, and that other valid diagnoses have been missed. For instance, bipolar depression is misdiagnosed as unipolar depression, followed by use of antidepressants that are ineffective in the underlying bipolar depression, unbeknownst to the patient or clinician (see Chapter 19). This kind of misdiagnosis is still common and quite problematic. However, a larger problem is that even if clinicians do apply diagnostic criteria correctly, and use current knowledge as they have been taught, poor treatment results would follow because the current diagnostic system is simply wrong.

10. Course, not symptoms, reveals the diagnosis

This is an axiom of psychiatric diagnosis based on the tradition of Kraepelin. The DSM system takes an opposite approach, using symptoms to make diagnoses in almost all cases, without reference to the course of the illness. Since many different illnesses can have many different symptoms, often overlapping, this symptomatic approach leads to diagnostic complexity that is both unnecessary and harmful. Many illnesses reveal themselves over time by their course, even if they overlap in symptoms to a great extent. This was the classic insight of Kraepelin into the differentiation of schizophrenia from manic-depressive illness. It holds just as well for differentiating mood conditions from anxiety conditions, from personality states, or from cognitive conditions. In general, clinicians focus too much on current symptoms, as DSM teaches them, and do not carefully assess the prior long-term course of illness in making a diagnosis, nor do they carefully assess the prospective long-term course of illness in either confirming or changing their initial diagnostic impressions. Pay attention to the course of illness: it is equivalent to pathology for psychiatry. It tells you which symptoms reflect which diseases, as opposed to assuming that each symptom is its own disease.

APPENDICES

Diagnostic Controversies

In the main body of this textbook, certain diagnostic concepts were discussed that are relatively unknown in contemporary psychiatry, despite having a long history and extensive research about them. To provide further detail regarding those ideas, this diagnostic appendix has been added regarding the concepts of "mixed states" in affective illness, the bipolar illness versus borderline personality debate, adult ADD, and schizoaffective illness.

Appendix I

Mixed States

A key issue to understanding the phenomenon of depression is knowing how it contrasts with mania. One approach is the DSM approach: compare this number of criteria versus that number of criteria for this or that amount of time. This is how most clinicians are taught. What they don't realize is that the DSM definitions are based on very broad concepts of depression and very narrow concepts of mania.

Let us turn to the classic psychopathology literature and ask the question, decades and centuries before DMS-III in 1980: How did the great thinkers of medicine and psychiatry define depression versus mania?

The answer is simple: Depression meant a slowing down of one's thinking, feeling, and moving. Mania meant a speeding up of one's thinking, feeling, and moving. Translated to current terms, depression was equivalent to psychomotor slowing and mania was equivalent to psychomotor excitation.

Readers will note that in this classic psychopathology, mood is not central to the definitions of depression or mania. Psychomotor slowing can come with sad mood, or it can come with normal mood. One sees this kind of depression in the classical seasonal depression of the fall/winter: patients describe loss of motivation and anhedonia but not sadness of mood. Similarly, psychomotor excitation can come with euphoric mood, or it can come with irritable mood, or with sad mood, or with anxious mood, or with none of the above.

The term "mood disorders" is false in both words. The term "disorder" is a DSM term that is applied to all conditions so as to produce a purposeful vagueness (in an effort to be "atheoretical"). The use of "mood" implies that a mood change is central to these conditions, whereas in fact, psychomotor activity appears to be central and primary; the mood experience is epiphenomenal and secondary. Perhaps the older term "affective" would be preferable, as it implies a larger and more complex construct than the subjective mood experience.

This distinction is important in understanding mixed states. A systematic review that provides the empirical evidence in support of this classic psychopathology found that psychomotor excitation or activation is central to the phenomenon of mania. If mania is thus understood, as opposed to solely accepting the DSM criteria, then some major changes follow in our understanding of affective states like depression.

THE PRIMACY OF MANIA HYPOTHESIS

Athanasios Koukopoulos was a Greek psychiatrist who practiced most of his life in Rome. He passed away a few years ago, after about 50 years of active clinical practice in a prestigious private practice. He published some of his observations and ideas over the years, and, in his last decade, he summarized his central thinking in the theory of the "primacy of mania." In this theory, depression is the effect of mania. Mania is the cause, the primary driver, of depression. This idea turns traditional psychiatric thinking upside down in at least two ways. It has been taught for a century that mania is a "flight from depression," that manic states are superficial reactions to not being able to acknowledge and experience the painful state of depression. As with most psychoanalytic thinking, there has never been any empirical scientific proof of this hypothesis. In current DSM-based thinking, depression (MDD) and mania (bipolar disorder) are viewed as two distinct and separate conditions. They overlap in symptoms of depression, but they are different "disorders" and are assumed by most clinicians to be different illnesses. As discussed in Chapter 19, this DSM belief contrasts with the older Kraepelinian theory of manic-depressive illness (MDI), which held that all depressive episodes and manic episodes were part of the same illness, MDI. In other words, unipolar depressive illness was the same disease as bipolar illness. Koukopoulos adds a twist to this Kraepelinian idea. He holds that depressive episodes do not happen unless they are preceded by or caused by manic episodes or symptoms.

MANIA IS THE FIRE, DEPRESSION IS THE ASH

Another large category of persons with depressive episodes have manic episodes during the depressive episodes; i.e., mixed states. This group of patients was of most interest to Koukopoulos. These mixed states can be defined in different ways, outside of DSM constraints. The simplest approach is the "bipolarity specifier" described by Benazzi; in this definition, a mixed state would be defined by a clinical depressive episode in which three or more DSM-defined manic symptoms occurred for any amount of time (not limited to the four days or longer DSM criterion of duration for hypomania, or one week or longer for mania). Using this definition, Angst and colleagues found that 47% of a large sample of 5,635 outpatients with depressive episodes met the mixed state definition. One could also use Koukopoulos's own definition of "mixed depression," which is even broader than the bipolarity specifier because it goes beyond DSM criteria. In Koukopoulos's definition, as described in more detail later, mixed depression involves the presence of a clinical depressive episode along with psychomotor excitation, which can be limited to psychomotor agitation and/or marked rage. Using Koukopoulos's definition of mixed depression, in his own Rome clinic, 51% of 435 consecutive patients with clinical depressive episodes had mixed depressive states.

If we combine the approach of Angst and Benazzi on one hand and Koukopoulos on the other, we can conservatively estimate that about 50% of all depressive episodes are mixed with manic symptoms, and thus are mixed states, not pure depression. The theory of the primacy of mania would apply if we accept the notion that these mixed states are driven by their manic components; in other words, one cannot separate the depressive from the manic symptoms—they come from the same pathophysiological source. Without the manic symptoms, the depressive symptoms would not occur.

So here are another 50% of depressive episodes, the largest chunk, which would not happen without mania. Combined with the 15% of classic manic-depressive cycles in bipolar illness, we account for the majority, 65%, of depressive episodes so far, meeting the definition of the primacy of mania.

What about the remaining 35%? Are they purely depressive cases, so-called unipolar depression? Now we turn to the concept of affective temperaments. The idea was that mild mood symptoms could occur in persons with mood illnesses, in between the severe episodes, and these mild symptoms were present all the time, as part of one's temperament. These conditions were defined as dysthymia, hyperthymia, and cyclothymia (mild depressive, manic, and manic-depressive symptoms, respectively). In various studies, it's been found that manic temperaments—hyperthymia or cyclothymia—are present in about one-third of persons with recurrent unipolar depressive episodes. If so, these calculations would explain one-third or so of the 35% of remaining persons with depressive episodes (i.e., about 12%). We now have explained 77% of all persons traditionally diagnosed with severe clinical depressive episodes (50% + 15% + 12%). This would be almost four out of five of such persons.

Affective temperaments appear to predispose one to a later risk of depressive episodes. Often these depressive episodes are mixed with manic symptoms, in the case of cyclothymia and hyperthymia, because the baseline manic symptoms of those temperaments remain and are mixed with new onset depressive episodes. Sometimes people with cyclothymia and hyperthymia have pure depressive episodes, not mixed states. Often these depressive episodes are of the melancholic type.

Thus, affective temperaments are relevant in two ways: (1) If present, patients often have mixed states when they become depressed; (2) many people with pure or melancholic depressive episodes have manic temperaments before or after their depressive states. In the latter case, Koukopoulos would argue that long-standing hyperthymic or cyclothymic temperaments predispose such persons to depressive episodes. Again, manic symptoms cause depressive symptoms.

This leaves 23% of people with clinical depression. As noted in Chapter 19, "MDD" is not the same thing as unipolar depression. Unipolar depression was seen always as a subtype of MDI: it was severe, episodic, recurrent, highly genetic, and biological. In contrast, neurotic depression was mild, chronic, and not highly genetic. The remainder of depressed persons could be of the neurotic variety, with brief, severe exacerbations leading to clinical attention. This group of depressed patients does *not* have mixed states. They are notably anxious, but they are not markedly agitated, and not rageful or impulsive.

In DSM-5, there is acknowledgment of much of this work demonstrating that mixed states occur in depressive episodes that are diagnosed as MDD, without full DSM-based manic episodes allowing the diagnosis of bipolar illness. Thus, "mixed episodes" as a subtype of bipolar disorder was removed from DSM-5, and replaced with "mixed features," which could be applied to both bipolar disorder and MDD. "MDD with mixed features" was limited, however, on conceptual grounds, to "non-overlapping" symptoms. Thus, if a patient has depression, they cannot be diagnosed as having mixed features according to DSM-5 if they also have psychomotor agitation, irritable mood, or distractibility. Those manic symptoms are excluded from the mixed features definition in MDD. The only manic symptoms that can be used are classic euphoric ones, such as euphoric mood, grandiosity, flight of ideas, along with evidence of increased energy, such as increased goal-directed activities. The problem with this DSM-5 approach is that it excludes the most common manic symptoms that occur in mixed states; namely, psychomotor agitation, marked anger/irritability, and distractibility. This would be like excluding pain in the head from a diagnosis of migraine. Thus, the DSM-5 mixed concept has been criticized by the primary researchers in mixed states as being, as is typical with DSM, based on conceptual concerns (a narrow definition to avoid "over-diagnosis") as opposed to following the empirical scientific evidence (allowing the symptoms that are most common in mixed states to be included in the diagnosis).

CLINICAL SCENARIOS

So what are the clinical scenarios of these different kinds of mixed states? Here are typical examples of how patients would present:

Bipolarity specifier (Angst and Benazzi): These patients have brief manic periods, lasting hours to days, as part of a longer depressive episode. Thus, a person might be severely depressed for two months, with low sleep, appetite, interest, and energy, and then suddenly for a weekend he has high energy and is sexually impulsive and talking fast; then he has another two months of low sleep, appetite, interest, and energy.

Mixed depression (Koukopoulos): These patients are markedly agitated, highly angry and rageful, and very labile in mood, alternating from angry, to sad, to tearful. These symptoms are constant for months on end, along with classic depressive symptoms (low energy, appetite, interest, sleep, concentration).

Mixed hypomania (DSM-5): MDD with mixed features excludes the classic irritability and agitation of Koukopoulos's mixed depression. It also excludes the brief manic states of Angst and Benazzi's bipolarity specifier. In effect, it represents a hypomanic state with some depressive symptoms, rather than a depressive state with some manic symptoms (as in the other two mixed states just described). These patients are energetic, grandiose, and highly active most of the time, but they have dysphoric mood and some depressive symptoms like poor appetite and guilt.

In summary, mixed states are an important concept to understand when thinking about "depression." The DSM approach to life tries to force all patients into one of two categories: depression or mania. (Hypomania is just mild mania, and captured in the same category, just as mild depression—to be consistent, we should speak of "hypodepression"—is part of the category of depression). Instead, a large clinical and scientific literature supports the view that most mood states are mixed states, not purely depression or mania, but both. Often the depressive features predominate, but notable manic symptoms of psychomotor excitation are present. In the DSM-based ideology, mania is restricted to a very small definition, excluding the classic psychopathology of psychomotor excitation (often referred to colloquially as "agitation" or "stimulation," but then not seen as "manic"). The classic pre-DSM tradition in psychiatry, dating to Kraepelin, can be supported with newer research by thinkers like Koukopoulos. This literature resuscitates the concept of psychomotor excitation as being diagnostically very important, and as identifying mixed states. Furthermore, Koukopoulos's hypothesis that mania causes depression can be supported by the high frequency of manic states occurring either just before or during depressive states, as reviewed before (with the proviso that neurotic depression is a different condition in which manic states are not present).

As discussed in Chapter 19, mixed states are misdiagnosed only as "depression" and treated with so-called antidepressants. The latter agents worsen these mixed states while dopamine blockers and second-messenger modifiers (mood stabilizers) improve mixed states. This issue emphasizes the point that these mixed states occur primarily in patients diagnosed with "MDD," not in bipolar illness. This key point is central to understanding the diagnosis and treatment of mixed states.

BY THE NUMBERS

Here is a summary of the frequency of mixed states, defined as a full clinical depression with some manic symptoms ("mixed depression" or the "depressive mixed state"). Percentages refer to the frequency of all "major" depressive episodes (MDEs; percentages are rounded):

In DSM-defined "MDD": 50%
In DSM-defined bipolar disorder type I: 50%
In DSM-defined bipolar disorder type II: 60%

Most common manic symptoms in mixed depression:

Psychomotor agitation: >90%
Marked anger/rage/irritability: 80%
Flight of ideas/racing thoughts: 50%

Distractibility: 50%
Grandiosity: 20%
Euphoric mood: 10%
Frequency of DSM-5 defined "MDD with mixed features," as percentage of all MDEs: 10%
Frequency of "mixed depression," (using bipolarity specifier or Koukopoulos's criteria), as percentage of all MDEs: 50%

Frequency of mood episodes in unipolar depression and bipolar illness combined:

Pure depression: 20%
Pure mania: 20%
Mixed states (mixed depression and dysphoric mania): 60%

BOTTOM LINE

- Mixed states are the most common type of mood states.
- They occur in about one-half of depressive episodes, even in patients diagnosed with "MDD," i.e., not bipolar illness.
- Mixed states may reflect the primacy of mania, meaning that manic symptoms or episodes caused depressive symptoms or episodes.
- Neurotic depression may be an exception to the concept of the primacy of mania.
- Manic temperaments are common in persons with depressive episodes, often leading to mixed states.
- MDD with mixed features in DSM-5 is narrow on conceptual grounds, while broader mixed state definitions have stronger research evidence for them.
- Mixed states are key to the proper diagnosis and treatment of "depression."

SELECTED REFERENCES

Angst, J., Azorin, J. M., Bowden, C. L., et al. (2011). Prevalence and characteristics of undiagnosed bipolar disorders in patients with a major depressive episode: The BRIDGE Study. *Archives of General Psychiatry, 68*(8), 791–798.

Koukopoulos, A., & Ghaemi, S. N. (2009). The primacy of mania: A reconsideration of mood disorders. *European Psychiatry, 24*(2), 125–134.

Appendix II

Bipolar or Borderline?

The differential diagnosis of bipolar illness and borderline personality is important, controversial, and difficult. Some claim that bipolar illness is over-diagnosed and that borderline personality is under-diagnosed. Others claim the reverse. Those who argue that bipolar illness is over-diagnosed often assert that those patients instead have borderline personality. Others claim the reverse. The most common approach to this controversy is to focus on the overlap between the syndromes and then to assert that one merely represents the other. It also would seem to make sense to focus on areas of difference, if indeed these are different conditions.

Borderline personality and bipolar illness have features in common, just as schizophrenia and anxiety conditions can also have symptoms in common (e.g., insomnia). One question is whether the similarities between borderline personality and bipolar illness are central to those conditions, or peripheral and secondary features.

This clinical overview gives a clinical and conceptual examination of how they are similar and how they differ (Table AII.1).

The classic diagnostic validators used in psychiatric nosology research are: symptoms, genetics, course, treatment response, and biological markers. The scientific literature on borderline personality and bipolar illness can be examined for these features. These are summarized in the table and are presented based on the diagnostic validators of symptoms (mood lability, impulsivity, parasuicidal self-harm, mania), genetics, course (sexual abuse), treatment response, and neurobiology.

MOOD LABILITY

The diagnostic validator of symptoms or phenomenology can also be examined regarding the most common psychopathology discussed in the literature on bipolar versus borderline differential diagnosis: mood lability. Mood lability is here defined as rapid alternations or fluctuations in mood over minutes to hours. It should be noted that mood

TABLE AII.1 Differences Between Bipolar and Borderline

	Bipolar	Borderline
Symptoms	Euphoric mood, increased activities	Dissociative symptoms Parasuicidal behavior
Genetics	Very strong	Non-specific
Course	Severe recurrent mood episodes	High prevalence of sexual abuse
Treatment	Biological cure in 1/3	Modest drug effects
Biology	Hippocampal atrophy Amygdala enlargement	Non-specific

lability is a DSM-5 criterion for borderline PD, but not for bipolar illness. It is common in bipolar illness, however.

One study of 29 subjects reported being able to distinguish mood lability between these two conditions, based on type and intensity of mood shifts; it was small and based on self-report, however. Another study, of 55 subjects, did not have a bipolar illness alone group (only one comorbid with personality disorders) and thus could not address the question.

In sum, small differences in intensity or frequency may exist, but mood lability is common in both conditions, and is not a strong distinguishing feature between them.

IMPULSIVITY

The symptom of impulsivity is closely allied to mood lability, and is often seen as manifesting as sexual impulsivity in these two conditions, although it can also be physical, aggressive, or financial. There are many studies demonstrating high impulsivity in both conditions separately, but very few have directly compared the two conditions, and in most of those studies, adequate comparison was not made between subjects who met only criteria for one or the other condition, as opposed to comparing one diagnosis versus a comorbid control group. Thus, as with mood lability, impulsivity seems to be common in both conditions and has not been shown to be distinctly different in one condition versus the other.

PARASUICIDAL SELF-HARM

Another key differentiating feature is parasuicidal self-harm. A recent systematic review of 51 articles found that self-mutilation is common in borderline personality (50–80% of cases) and is frequently repetitive (41% of patients have more than 50 self-mutilation acts). The largest study of parasuicidal behavior in bipolar illness, and the only such study in an unselected non-clinical population (i.e., a general population sample) is found in the National Comorbidity Survey (NCS) (n = 5,877). In that study, the prevalence of self-harm among patients with type I bipolar illness was only 0.9%. The importance of the NCS data is that they are epidemiological, not clinical. They are based on determining prevalence of parasuicidal behavior in persons with bipolar illness who are in the community, not those who seek treatment in clinicians' offices. By using clinically selected samples, higher rates of parasuicidal behavior are seen, even in bipolar type I illness, in some studies, but these samples involve a selection bias of those who seek help, and do not generalize to the entire bipolar population. Even with this limitation, the highest parasuicidal behavior rate reported in clinical studies is 36%, which remains two-fold less frequent than in borderline personality. In contrast, the NCS study does generalize to the whole bipolar population and is probably the most valid data on which to base judgments about parasuicidal self-harm prevalence. In the general population, self-mutilation is reported to occur in only about 4% of non-clinical samples, compared with 21% of clinical samples (patients with psychiatric diagnoses of varied types). Hence, the rate of parasuicidal behavior in the NCS non-clinical sample of bipolar illness is similar to the general population's, even slightly lower, and comparable to other clinical samples of psychiatric conditions (excluding borderline personality).

In sum, compared to bipolar illness, borderline personality involves at least a two-fold increased relative risk of parasuicidal self-harm in clinical samples. In the general population, this difference is immense, about a 50–80-fold higher rate in borderline personality. This difference compares favorably to the classic association of cigarette smoking and lung cancer, in which a five- to eight-fold effect size has been considered to be quite large and convincing. Given the literature reviewed here, similar judgments would seem to be reasonable in the case of parasuicidal self-harm and borderline personality.

MANIC SYMPTOMS

The most straightforward diagnostic validators may be symptoms. A few studies have assessed whether the presence of manic symptoms or manic/hypomanic episodes can distinguish bipolar illness from borderline personality. The largest study (n = 5,635), which assessed an unselected mood population with depressive episodes, examined mixed states, defined as the presence of three or more DSM-IV-defined manic symptoms, of any duration, along with a major depressive episode. This definition of "mixed depression" differs from the DSM-IV definition of a full manic episode lasting at least one week in duration, co-occurring with a full depressive episode. This definition of "mixed depression" included patients who would meet DSM-IV-defined bipolar disorders, type I or II, or DSM-IV-defined MDD. In other words, "mixed depression" reflects a mood disorder population. The question was whether manic symptoms in this mood disorder population were also found in subjects who met DSM-IV criteria for borderline personality disorder. Using this broad "mixed depression" definition, DSM-IV-defined manic symptoms occurred much more frequently in "mixed depression" than in borderline personality. In contrast, borderline personality had more of the following DSM-IV features than did patients with "mixed depression": fears of abandonment, identity disturbance, recurrent suicidal or self-mutilating behavior, and dissociative symptoms.

In short, the literature on presence or absence of manic symptoms supports the view that manic symptoms distinguish bipolar illness from borderline personality.

GENETICS

The most definitive review of the immense genetic literature on bipolar illness compared to personality disorders and other conditions is a systematic review of twin studies of genetic heritability. In that systematic review, bipolar illness was found to be one of the two very heritable mental illnesses, along with schizophrenia, both having about 80% heritability, similar to Alzheimer's dementia. This rate is about twice as much as found in that systematic review for borderline personality or other personality traits or disorders, which tend to have about 40% heritability. For instance, in a study of 2,794 Norwegian twins, the genetic heritability of borderline personality was only 37%; in fact, all DSM-IV-defined personality disorders fell into the 20–41% heritability range, with the highest being for antisocial personality disorder. Environmental heritability, in contrast, was 63–79%, which indicated that it was the major causative feature for these conditions. These studies used personal clinical interviews to assess personality disorders using DSM-IV criteria. It has been reported, using the same Norwegian sample, that the addition of self-report evaluations leads to higher heritability assessments, reaching 69% for borderline personality disorders, and generally in the 60–70% range for all personality disorders. Whether it is legitimate to add self-report to clinical interview in assessing personality disorders is a methodological question that remains to be answered. But if one accepts clinical interviews as the gold standard, and thus compares personality disorders using that method that is the standard approach in genetic twin research, then the genetic heritability of borderline personality disorder is much lower than that of bipolar illness.

It should be noted that 40% heritability is not zero; it indicates a modest genetic effect. But it is half as much as 80%, which is similar to the heritability of traits that are widely accepted to be mostly genetic, such as physical height.

In sum, using currently accepted standards of genetic twin research, bipolar illness is almost completely genetic in causation, with a small environmental component. In contrast, borderline personality is mostly environmental in causation, with a small genetic component.

COURSE OF ILLNESS

A key course feature that potentially could differentiate bipolar illness from borderline personality is a history of sexual abuse. In a commonly cited meta-analysis of 21 studies, 50–76% of patients with borderline personality disorder had experienced sexual trauma. In contrast, sexual abuse occurs in less than 30% of bipolar subjects. These prevalence rates are based on a number of different studies with large samples, including systematic reviews. For instance, a recent systematic review including 3,407 bipolar patients found a 24% prevalence of sexual trauma in bipolar illness. According to one of the most extensive national studies of the topic, the U.S. Department of Health and Human Services reported a prevalence of childhood sexual abuse in the general population of 9.2%.

In sum, there is a consistent frequency of sexual abuse in bipolar illness that is similar to the general population rate in some studies, or possibly higher than in the general population. Yet the frequency of childhood sexual abuse is consistently at least two-fold higher in borderline personality than in bipolar illness or the general population.

It has been noted the average effect size for the association between childhood sexual abuse and borderline personality is only moderate ($r = 0.279$), but this way of assessing the data does not contradict the frequency noted here. It merely addresses the fact that other causative factors also exist for borderline personality. In this setting, the question is whether this specific risk factor is common in borderline personality, not whether other risk factors also might be common.

NEUROBIOLOGY

In bipolar illness, numerous consistent neurobiological changes are reported in dozens of studies. Although a range of abnormalities is found, two of the most consistent abnormalities found are hippocampal atrophy and amygdalar enlargement. These differences are shown in studies that compare bipolar illness both to normal controls and often to other psychiatric conditions, like schizophrenia.

In contrast, there are fewer studies of neurobiological changes in borderline personality, and some abnormalities found compared to normal controls, such as deficits in integration between cognition and emotional processing stimuli, are not unique to borderline personality but are also found in other neuropsychiatric syndromes, including schizophrenia and bipolar illness.

TREATMENT RESPONSE

Treatment response has generally been seen as the least specific diagnostic validator, as medications can affect varied diagnoses. However, certain treatment effects may be diagnostically specific. Regarding bipolar illness versus borderline personality, there is a strong consensus after a century of practice and research that psychotherapies alone are not effective in bipolar illness. They may be effective adjunctively with medications, but not by themselves. In contrast, there is a similar strong clinical consensus for decades that psychotherapies are central to the treatment of borderline personality; many experts in borderline personality see medications as adjunctive treatments for that condition. Many RCTs of bipolar illness exist, and demonstrate good efficacy with various agents, like lithium, in prophylaxis of that condition, sometimes with complete remission. In contrast, fewer RCTs exist of treatment with medications for borderline PD, and they tend to demonstrate modest symptomatic benefits with psychotropic medications.

In sum, it would seem to be a fair reflection of a long-held clinical consensus that treatment response in bipolar illness versus borderline personality tends to be inverse: in bipolar illness, appropriate psychotropic medications are necessary, with psychotherapies being adjunctive; in borderline personality, appropriate psychotherapies are seen as necessary, with psychotropic medications being adjunctive.

DISCUSSION OF DIAGNOSTIC VALIDATORS

Reviewing the empirical evidence on classic diagnostic validators, it appears that bipolar illness and borderline personality are distinguishable and different. The clearest differentiating features appear to be a family history of bipolar illness, parasuicidal self-harm, and past sexual abuse, each of which is at least twice as frequent in one condition as in the other. Treatment response also appears to differ markedly, with medication efficacy much stronger and central to treatment of bipolar illness, whereas psychotherapies are not effective alone; in borderline personality, medication effects are modest at best, while psychotherapies are central to its treatment. Symptom features do not differentiate between these conditions as clearly as these genetic, course, and treatment validators. Mood lability and impulsivity are not different in any clearly proven and replicated manner between these conditions; manic symptoms and manic episodes may differentiate between them, but directly comparative studies are few. A large neurobiological literature also exists that finds abnormalities in bipolar illness to a more consistent and definitive degree than in borderline personality. A number of direct comparisons exist that demonstrate more neurobiological abnormalities, and often of different kind, in bipolar illness than borderline personality. In short, these conditions appear to be different in a number of major diagnostic validators.

To summarize: bipolar illness is a very genetic condition, with a large amount of neurobiological abnormalities, that requires medication treatment as central to its management. In contrast, borderline personality is a mostly environmental condition, with fewer neurobiological abnormalities, that requires psychotherapies as central to its management.

One way of summarizing the proposed interpretation given in this review is that while there are superficial similarities between bipolar illness and borderline personality, there are profound differences. The comparison is between red apples and red skies; redness is shared, but these are two very different entities.

"COMORBIDITY"?

Even if borderline personality and bipolar illness can be distinguished, it may sometimes be the case that they can occur together. For instance, since bipolar illness is a genetic and biological condition, persons who are genetically predisposed to it are also likely to be at higher risk of sexual impulsivity being present in family members with bipolar illness; sometimes this may lead to sexual trauma that can derail personality development and eventually lead to borderline personality. This kind of co-occurrence of different conditions is what was meant by the introduction of the term "comorbidity" by Feinstein in 1970. In contrast, as the leadership of DSM-IV has explicitly stated, the DSM psychiatric nosology has been set up allowing for extensive overlap in diagnostic criteria so as to encourage diagnosis of multiple conditions at once. This "comorbidity" could rationally be attributed to our DSM system, rather than nature. Hence the application of DSM criteria and report of high comorbidity rates between bipolar disorder and borderline personality disorder does not imply that those conditions are highly similar.

A final historical point is that bipolar illness is derived from MDI, which has been well defined in the scientific literature for over a century, if not much longer—dating to ancient Rome. Borderline personality, in contrast, was first clearly defined in the psychoanalytic literature in the late 1960s, and thus is a more recent construct. Bipolar illness is based on standard medical methods: observation of signs and symptoms and course of illness. Borderline personality is partly based on such standard medical observation, and DSM criteria are not specifically psychoanalytic in nature, but the most prominent borderline experts emphasize that this condition is also centrally determined by certain psychoanalytic concepts, such as splitting, projection, and countertransference. Hence, the evaluation of the empirical literature here is consistent with historical and conceptual differences in how these conditions have been came to be conceived and continue to be understood.

AFFECTIVE TEMPERAMENTS MISINTERPRETED AS BORDERLINE PERSONALITY

Historically, it should be noted that the concept of MDI as used by Kraepelin included depressive and manic episodes as part of the same illness, merely as gradations of severity, rather than as two separate illnesses. It can further be added that Kraepelin and Kretschmer held the view that even milder versions of mania and depression; namely, hyperthymic and cyclothymic temperaments, were also part of MDI. Recent clinical and genetic studies find high rates of these temperaments in persons with bipolar illness and their relatives. Since hyperthymia and cyclothymia are seen as mood temperaments, part of personality, they can appear to be similar to clinical features that are often viewed as borderline personality traits, such as mood lability and impulsivity, which this review found to be non-specific diagnostically. If the concept of mood temperaments is scientifically valid, it would require even more caution in making the borderline personality diagnosis in such persons who may not have bipolar illness type I or type II (i.e., full manic or hypomanic episodes) but have hyperthymic or cyclothymic temperament along with other features of MDI (such as a family history of bipolar illness and severe recurrent depressive episodes).

Often it is emphasized that bipolar illness involves severe episodes. If symptoms are constant or chronic, borderline personality is presumed. But this conclusion ignores the concept of affective temperament. If sexual trauma and self-cutting are absent, then cyclothymia often is misdiagnosed as borderline PD, since DSM criteria easily diagnose the latter in persons with constant mood swings and anger.

BOTTOM LINE

- Borderline personality and bipolar illness are distinguishable clinically and diagnostically.
- Bipolar illness can be seen as a genetically based biological disease, while borderline personality can be interpreted as a psychosocially caused clinical picture.

- The two illnesses should be treated distinctly, with appropriate medications emphasized for bipolar illness, and psychotherapies emphasized in borderline personality.
- Borderline personality may be misdiagnosed in persons with cyclothymic or hyperthymic affective temperaments.

SELECTED REFERENCES

The material cited in this Appendix can be examined in the references of the review paper from which this appendix was derived:

Ghaemi, S. N., et al. (2014). Bipolar or borderline: A clinical overview. *Acta Psychiatrica Scandinavica, 130*(2), 99–108.

APPENDIX III

Attention Deficit Disorder in Children and Adults

Attention deficit disorder (ADD) is a common diagnosis made in children and, increasingly, in adults. In this appendix, a diagnostic examination of the validity and scope of this concept will be provided.

PART I: CHILDHOOD ATTENTION DEFICIT DISORDER

A first basic idea is to drop the "H" which is commonly used in the term "ADHD" (attention-deficit hyperactivity disorder). Hyperactivity is a common misconception in the diagnosis of ADD, especially in children. If one says a child is "hyperactive" and thus has ADHD, one would diagnose every manic child with ADHD. Of course, that's another debate, which many proponents of ADHD solve by denying that there is any, or much, bipolar illness in children. (That's a separate topic, discussed in Chapter 28). For now, let us ask the question: What do we mean by "hyperactivity"? Do we mean increased energy? If so, increased energy is not a diagnostic criterion of ADHD, and it never has been. But it is a core diagnostic criterion for mania. Do we mean a decreased need for sleep? This is not a diagnostic criterion for ADHD, but it is a central diagnostic criterion of mania. Does increased energy happen as a diagnostic criterion of any psychiatric diagnosis besides mania/hypomania?

No.

So the problem with the word "hyperactivity" is that it frequently connotes increased energy, which is usually part of a decreased need for sleep, and these symptoms are not part of the ADD syndrome, but rather only occur in bipolar illness as part of manic or hypomanic episodes. So what is meant by hyperactivity in ADHD, if we can't use the term to refer to increased energy? What seems to be meant is psychomotor agitation: children don't sit still. Why don't they sit still? Is it because they have increased energy? We already established this is not the case, because increased energy would define them as having mania, not ADHD. Instead, the general view is that children don't sit still because they can't focus, they're distractible: that's the first "D" in ADHD. They're in school for six to eight hours a day, expected to sit at a desk and focus on a teacher, and they can't focus, so they have a hard time sitting at the desk. In other words, the apparent "hyperactivity" isn't hyperactivity at all, but rather psychomotor agitation that's an effect of the main psychopathological problem: distractibility. And this psychomotor agitation isn't always present. Some children can't focus, but they manage to stay seated. In adults, since they are no longer in schools and are not usually forced to sit at a desk for six to eight hours daily, there is no "hyperactivity" or psychomotor agitation in most people. ADD is distractibility, pure and simple, in adults, with the associated cognitive impairment of executive dysfunction and disorganization. So, an initial common error is to diagnose "ADHD" in children mainly based on "hyperactivity" without asking whether this reflects increased energy, in which case the diagnosis should be mania instead, not ADHD. One way to avoid this common error is to refuse to go along with the unscientific insistence of DSM on using the term "ADHD" and instead to use the term "ADD" so as to put the emphasis of the diagnosis where the science shows it to be: in cognitive impairment, not increased energy.

Another benefit of realizing that "hyperactivity" is not a scientifically sound aspect of ADD is that it is no longer "paradoxical" that "stimulants" reduce hyperactivity. There is no paradox to decrease of hyperactivity with stimulants because (a) there is no hyperactivity, and (b) "stimulants" aren't stimulants.

It just was explained how there is no hyperactivity in ADD, if by that term is meant increased energy. There is psychomotor agitation in some children secondary to being unable to sit still for long periods of time, usually in school settings, as a result of their marked cognitive impairment of distractibility.

Now one can add that "stimulants" aren't stimulants. What do they stimulate? How do they stimulate anything? The reference here is to amphetamines, including methylphenidate, which is an amphetamine. These agents are dopamine agonists (and some also have norepinephrine agonism). This is a kind of biological "stimulation," but we don't call SRIs serotonin "stimulants" because they increase serotonin activity. Instead, the term "stimulants" seems to imply a clinical meaning. Patients feel stimulated. What does this mean? They have more energy. That's right; we know that amphetamines increase energy even in normal persons. But we also know that amphetamines markedly improve attention. So is there any paradox to their benefit in ADD, a condition of poor attention? If you have poor attention, and you take a drug that improves attention, and then you sit still because now you can focus, where is the paradox? Since these children are not high in energy to begin with, there is no paradox that a drug that increases energy makes them less agitated. It makes sense when we realize that the agitation is secondary to poor attention, which is improved by the dopamine agonists.

The presence of a diagnosis doesn't entail the presence of a disease. This is especially the case with DSM, where hundreds of diagnoses are included but the majority are not diseases of the body or brain. A diagnosis, if valid scientifically, basically reflects a clinical syndrome that can be distinguished from other clinical syndromes. This scientific validity is based on the classic diagnostic validators of symptoms, genetics, course, and treatment response. Childhood ADD can be claimed to differ from other childhood clinical syndromes based on these diagnostic validators. It may be a valid diagnosis, but is it a disease of the body?

One should note that it isn't enough to show changes in the brain. There are changes in the brain with any clinical presentation because all thoughts and feelings are mediated by the brain. Positron emission tomography (PET) scans and even structural MRIs of Republicans and Democrats, of men and women, differ; but political preference and gender are not diseases. A special danger exists in assuming disease processes in children since childhood is a period of biological and psychological development. The child is a runner in motion; taking a picture at one point in time to claim a disease process may not hold true a year later. The importance of development in understanding ADD is brought out by some excellent work examining the brain in children with ADD using MRI and PET scans, not just cross-sectionally but prospectively. In that study, compared to matched controls, children with ADD showed evidence of brain abnormalities (decreased blood flow, reduced cortical thickness) in some regions (like dorsolateral prefrontal and ventromedial frontal cortex). These abnormalities were present around age 7–8 but then normalized by about age 11–12.

In sum, there was a two- to three-year delay in cortical maturation, especially in the prefrontal cortex, in ADD children versus matched non-ADD controls. The straightforward interpretation of this research is that ADD is a developmental delay, not a permanent disease. It represents normal childhood, slowed down by a few years.

Readers probably wonder about the effects of treatments in this research. Medication effects were not examined, nor would they be definitive since these studies are not randomized trials. About half of children diagnosable with ADD are treated with medications, thus one cannot assume that the improvement seen in this study was due to medication effects. It could be due to natural history as well, or solely. If so, then the question is raised whether the main thing to do with this developmental phase delay is to help symptomatically for a brief period of time, not more than two or three years, and then leave these children alone.

This evidence for developmental delay also is consistent with the older ADD literature (before the introduction of Strattera, atomoxetine, and the subsequent rise of adult ADD) that indicated that about 90% of children diagnosable with ADD were no longer diagnosable by age 18. In other words, since this is not a disease but a developmental delay in which there is natural recovery, the vast majority of children with ADD will "grow out of it." This concept contrasts with popular belief in the existence of adult ADD, which is addressed next.

The clinical relevance of this discussion is the following:

> When diagnosing ADD in children, do not focus on hyperactivity. Rather, the central clinical diagnostic feature should be inattention. Even then, the diagnosis shouldn't be made in the setting of other conditions that cause inattention: most importantly, anxiety, depression, mania, and psychosis. The most common symptom in children that produces inattention is anxiety. Anxiety itself often is an early prodrome to other conditions, such as mood and psychotic illnesses.

Both of the latter conditions are worsened with amphetamines, so careful attention should be given to recognizing anxiety in children as an important cause of inattention. Since most clinicians avoid benzodiazepines in children, SRIs are commonly used for anxiety, but SRIs can worsen mood and psychotic conditions, thus they should be used in low doses and not continued long-term, meaning for years and years, if possible. Long-term use produces major problems with serotonin withdrawal syndrome when the child ultimately needs to come off those agents someday. Furthermore, the long-term effects of SRIs on sexual development, if continued throughout adolescence, are not known. In short, with children, don't routinely diagnose ADD with inattention, and certainly not for hyperactivity. Consider anxiety and other syndromes, but even then, minimize dosing and duration of medication treatment as much as possible. In this view, it is a developmental delay, not a permanent disease. Medication treatment is not always necessary, especially for the long term.

Bottom Line

- ADD is characterized by the core feature of inattention. Increased energy is not a feature of the syndrome.
- Hence there is no "paradoxical" effect of "stimulants." These agents simply improve attention, which improves behavior.
- Childhood ADD is a developmental delay, not a permanent disease.
- Treatment for ADD can be given for short duration, if at all, in childhood and need not be continued into adulthood in most persons.

PART II: ADULT ATTENTION DEFICIT DISORDER

Diagnostic Considerations

Turning to adult ADD, it is worth noting that the concept hardly existed before a pharmaceutical company marketed the drug Strattera (atomoxetine) for this indication in the United States in 2003. Before then, the general consensus of researchers was that ADD did not persist into adulthood in the vast majority of persons. Nine prospective studies were conducted before 2003; in a total of 718 persons followed for 13–25 years from childhood into adulthood, from a mean of age 10 to age 25, the prevalence of ADD fell by 90%. In other words, only 10% of children with ADD continued to have it in their mid-20s. This observation contrasts with the common opinion these days that the majority of children with ADD will continue to have it as adults. Post-Strattera research, often funded by pharmaceutical companies marketing adult ADD medications, report higher rates of persistence into adulthood, but even then, the full ADD syndrome is reported to be present in only about 40% of children followed to age 18–20. In other words, the majority still lose the diagnosis by early adulthood. Now the claim is made that, despite syndromic remission, ADD symptoms still persist and cause functional impairment. But, even if so, it is worth noting that all studies show that the majority of children with ADD have syndromal remission by about age 18: they no longer meet ADD criteria.

Again, the question of treatment comes up. In general, in these studies, some children are treated and some are not, and the studies do not assess outcomes based on treatment in any systematic fashion, nor are they randomized. Thus they cannot answer this question, but since a good number of the study subjects are untreated, it cannot be assumed that the results are the effect of treatment. Natural history still remains an important possible interpretation of the results.

The most cited recent data represent the National Comorbidity Survey (NCS) epidemiological study in the United States, which found that about 3% of adults are diagnosable with ADD, which means that they meet criteria as adults in a current cross-sectional assessment as part of the NCS study, and that they retrospectively met those criteria as children.

It has been found that 45% of those who met adult ADD criteria also met bipolar disorder criteria, and 39% of those who met adult ADD criteria also met MDD criteria. In other words, 84% of those who can be diagnosed with current adult ADD are also diagnosable with current bipolar disorder or MDD. Here is the question: What causes what? Are they just unlucky, and every time they have one disease they have two diseases? Or does the ADD cause depression, as many ADD experts assume? Does ADD also cause recurrent manic episodes? This would seem biologically implausible.

At least in the case of bipolar illness, the proponents of the adult ADD diagnosis haven't explained why almost half those patients also have manic episodes. They haven't explained why we should believe they have two diseases, when one disease could explain all the symptoms, since a cardinal feature of mania is distractibility. Why should pneumonia always happen with "fever disorder"?

One of the most interesting studies (R. G. Klein et al., Dec. 2012, *Archives of General Psychology*, 69, 1295–1303) that can add to this literature was a recent publication that represents the longest prospective outcome of ADD: a 33-year outcome study following children diagnosed with ADD at age eight, and compared with matched controls who did not have ADD. They were all followed to age 41. Here is an interesting observation: ADD was diagnosable in the control group in 5% as adults. These were children who were carefully assessed and found *not* to have ADD as children, but then they met the criteria 30 years later. How is this possible? This is not adult ADD, because the diagnosis is supposed to reflect persistence of childhood ADD, but this group did not have childhood ADD, and yet it is almost twice as large as the prevalence claimed in the NCS study for adults who had persistence of childhood ADD.

Here is one potential explanation: the 5% who did not have ADD in childhood but met adult criteria are simply adults who have statistically abnormal attention spans. They don't have a disease, and they don't have a developmental delay of the maturing brain; they are just at an extreme of the normal curve for the cognitive trait for attention. Recall that most psychological and biological traits are distributed on a normal curve in the general population. Most of us are at or near the 50th percentile. At two standard deviations from the middle of the curve, on each end, there is about 2% of the population. This is not disease, and it is not "disorder." Some people are short, some are tall; some are skinny, some are not; some are shy, some are extroverted; some are hyper-focused in attention, some are distractible: 4–5%, in fact.

So what is "adult ADD"? Could it just be the extreme of the psychological trait of attention, which is not a bad thing?

If one thinks about attention as a cognitive trait with a normal curve, one might ask the question: Are we humans supposed to be highly attentive? Nature seems to have evolved in such a way that many of the "symptoms" we treat are in fact quite normal when present to a mild to moderate degree. It's normal to be somewhat anxious. It's normal at times to be sad. It's normal even to be somewhat illogical in our thought processes. These are all proven to be common traits in the normal population. All are distributed as in an inverted U-shaped curve. What about attention? Is it normal to be a little inattentive?

Of course it is. What would life be like if you focused on every little thing that crossed your mind? You would have this idea, then that, then another; you would focus on one, then the other, then the next. It is normal to filter sensations and thoughts, and focus on some but not others. Inattention is normal. When we have no filter, and attend too much to all our thoughts and feelings, we are psychotic. That is the nature of the thought disorder of schizophrenia. It is not an accident that amphetamines are used as an animal model of psychosis. Too much attention is psychotic. That's why we are selected to be normally inattentive. And some people are more inattentive than others. That is expected for any normal psychological trait. It's not a disease; it's an extreme of a natural trait.

One might say that even if this is the case, inattention should be treated if it is causing functional impairment. This may be defensible, or perhaps not. We treat the extreme of the normal trait of blood pressure, but not because it causes functional impairment. In fact, it is famous for having no symptoms at all, for being "silent." We treat high blood pressure because it later causes certain diseases, like coronary artery disease or stroke. What future diseases does inattention cause? None that we know of.

Still, one might argue for treatment for current functional impairment. But as shown in the longest randomized trial of amphetamines in childhood ADD (the MTA study, even if this is the case, non-medication treatments are as effective as medication treatments for functional improvement of ADD.

A final comment: In the 33-year prospective study, 78% of subjects with childhood ADD were no longer diagnosable with it as adults. Again, the older literature seems closer to the truth that the majority of children with ADD (about 80% in this study) will not have it as adults. Clinicians need not feel impelled, as is the case these days, to continue amphetamine medications for decades and decades, on the assumption that once the ADD diagnosis is made, then long-term treatment is entailed.

A final important clinical consideration in analyzing apparent adult ADD is the concept of mood temperaments. As noted previously in Chapter 19, mood temperaments are highly under-appreciated in contemporary psychiatry. The terms dysthymia and cyclothymia are in the DSM, and are thus known, but they are misused or not used at all. Most commonly, dysthymia is used as a "comorbidity" along with MDD or other conditions. In contrast, cyclothymia is not used as a comorbidity, but is thought to be exclusive of the diagnoses of MDD or bipolar illness. The mood temperament of "hyperthymia," or mild constant manic symptoms, is not known by most clinicians, mainly because it is not included in the DSM. All three terms, described in more detail in Chapter 19, are not comorbidities because mood temperaments are not diseases in themselves; they are personality traits in persons, or their relatives, who have mood diseases.

New research suggest that it is commonly the case that adult ADD is mistakenly diagnosed in persons with cyclothymia, most commonly, or with hyperthymia. The affective manic symptoms are chronic, hence the attentional impairment is constant. But the causal source may be the affective temperament, not a separate disease of "adult ADD." Observational data suggest that patients improve in their affective symptoms, including inattention, with low-dose mood stabilizers, whereas amphetamines either provide only partial or inconsistent benefit.

Bottom Line

- Adult ADD probably reflects an extreme of the natural trait of attention.
- The best evidence that adult ADD is not likely to be a valid independent disease entity is that it almost always occurs with mood illnesses, which themselves cause inattention.
- In the longest follow-up into middle age, similar inattention is seen in adults without past ADD as in adults with childhood ADD.
- Apparent adult ADD often reflects mood temperaments, like hyperthymia and cyclothymia.

SELECTED REFERENCES

Many of the citations in this Appendix can be accessed in the reference list of the following review paper:

Vergne, D. E., Whitham, E. A., Barroilhet, S., Fradkin, Y., & Ghaemi, S. N. (2011). Adult ADHD and amphetamines: A new paradigm. *Neuropsychiatry (London)*, *1*(6), 591–598. doi:10.2217/npy.11.63

Other specific citations are as follows:

Jensen, P. S., et al. (1999). A 14-month randomized clinical trial of treatment strategies for attention-deficit/hyperactivity disorder. The MTA Cooperative Group. Multimodal Treatment Study of Children with ADHD. *Archives of General Psychiatry*, *56*(12), 1073–1086.

Shaw, P., et al. (2007). Attention-deficit/hyperactivity disorder is characterized by a delay in cortical maturation. *Proceedings of the National Academy of Sciences*, *104*, 19649.

Appendix IV

Schizoaffective Illness

The understanding of schizoaffective disorder can be organized in five different theories. One approach holds that schizoaffective disorder is its own illness, separate from others, as appears to be the case superficially by its separate diagnostic criteria in DSM-IV. A second model holds that schizoaffective disorder represents a middle clinical picture on a psychotic continuum that extends from bipolar disorder to schizophrenia; in other words, this model rejects the Kraepelinian dichotomy of bipolar disorder and schizophrenia. A third model argues that schizoaffective disorder represents the comorbidity of affective disorders and schizophrenia, thereby maintaining the Kraepelinian dichotomy and explaining overlap symptoms as chance co-occurrence. A fourth theory views schizoaffective disorder as basically a variant of bipolar disorder, and a fifth sees schizoaffective disorder as a variant of schizophrenia.

Many clinicians unconsciously take the first approach. They assume that since "schizoaffective disorder" represents two words, and they exist on a page of paper, especially in the DSM criteria, then those two words must represent a "real" thing, a real illness in the real world, separate and apart from other illnesses. This common human conclusion flows from the assumption that once you name something, it exists. Of course we name many things that don't exist, sometimes fantasies, sometimes mere falsehoods.

In Chapter 16, this text reviews the rationale for why many DSM labels do not correspond to "real" diseases or illnesses, but rather represent social constructs of the American psychiatric profession. Separate from this fact, we should keep in mind that any diagnostic label represents only a clinical picture, first and foremost. Whether that clinical picture is a different disease or illness from another clinical picture—that's a different question.

So readers should understand that this chapter is about a "clinical picture": we see patients who have mixtures of delusions/hallucinations along with mood. What this clinical picture means—is it a separate illness or not?—is another question.

PHENOMENOLOGY

At the level of observation, the term "schizoaffective" simply applies to individuals with continuous psychotic and mood symptoms. Unlike mood disorders, psychotic symptoms are not brief. And unlike in schizophrenia, mood symptoms are not absent. Clinically, many patients seem to fall into this overlap region. In fact, the original paper describing the occurrence of such patients with such overlap was published in 1933. Indeed, Kraepelin himself observed that a good number of patients had such an overlap of manic-depressive and dementia praecox symptoms. Hence, the fact that such an overlap occurs is almost universally accepted, even by Kraepelin, who originated the idea that mood and psychotic disorders differ.

By itself, the presence of overlap doesn't invalidate the diagnoses of schizophrenia and MDI. This is partly because phenomenology is only one of four diagnostic validators (along with genetics, course of illness, and treatment effects/biological markers). This is also partly because a difference in symptoms is not an all-or-nothing phenomenon. In other words, to say that schizophrenia and mood disorders differ in symptoms is not to say that they *never* overlap. It only means that they *usually* don't overlap. And indeed, some well-done symptom prevalence studies have shown that patients with mood and psychotic symptoms tend to differentiate into two big groups, one with mainly mood symptoms and one with mainly psychotic symptoms, although there is some overlap (Figure AIV.1).

It is sometimes argued that the mere existence of schizoaffective disorder is a counter-example to the Kraepelinian dichotomy of schizophrenia and affective illness. As should be clear from the preceding considerations, this is not the case. Some overlap is expected; and symptoms are only one aspect of diagnostic validation. To refute the Kraepelinian diagnostic schema, one would also need to look at genetic, course, and treatment response data.

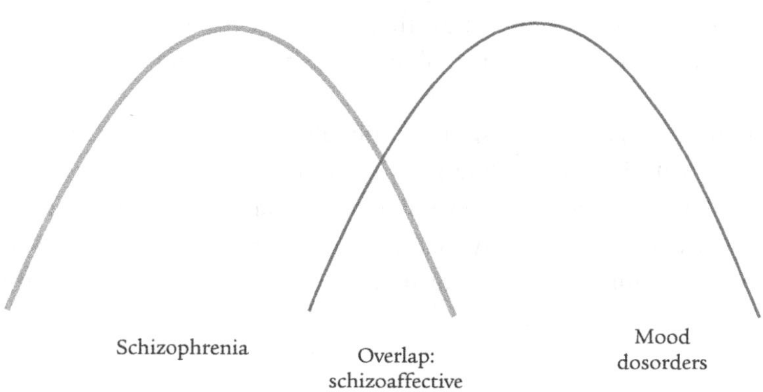

FIGURE AIV.1 *Schizoaffective illness as an overlap condition.*

GENETICS

If schizoaffective disorder is a separate illness in its own right, one would expect that it would breed true in families. However, almost all genetic studies are consistent in demonstrating that it doesn't breed true. Schizoaffective disorder isn't found mainly in families of persons with schizoaffective disorder. Rather, various studies suggest a unique pattern. In some studies of families of persons with bipolar disorder, there is an increased prevalence of schizoaffective disorder, bipolar type. In some studies of families of persons with schizophrenia, there is an increased prevalence of schizoaffective disorder, depressed type. And in a number of well-executed studies comparing both major groups, schizoaffective disorder is more prevalent in families of persons with schizophrenia or bipolar disorder than in control populations or in families of persons with schizoaffective disorder.

These results are consistent with a number of possibilities. In some persons, schizoaffective disorder, bipolar type, appears to be a more severe variant of bipolar disorder. In others, schizoaffective disorder, depressed type, appears to be a less severe variant of schizophrenia. And in still others, since it seems to run in families of persons with both schizophrenia and bipolar illness, only two explanations seem possible: (1) either schizoaffective illness may indeed be the counter-example to the Kraepelinian dichotomy between manic-depressive illness and schizophrenia; no distinction between any psychotic disorders can be made and they should all be seen as one continuum; or (2) schizoaffective disorder may simply represents the comorbidity of having, by chance, schizophrenia and bipolar disorder (or unipolar depression) *at the same time*, just as one might have diabetes and asthma at the same time.

The genetics of schizoaffective disorder argues against the concept of a separate illness, but the four other possibilities remain open.

COURSE OF THE ILLNESS

Studies of the course of schizoaffective disorder tend to be rather consistent: the course of the illness is more severe than in bipolar disorder, but less severe than in schizophrenia. Furthermore, schizoaffective disorder, depressed type, appears to demonstrate less recovery than schizoaffective disorder, bipolar type.

These findings again are consistent with the four remaining models. If there is only one continuum of psychotic illness, bipolar disorder may lie at the less extreme end, schizophrenia at the more extreme end, and schizoaffective disorder in between. Hence schizoaffective disorder might have an intermediate course. On the other hand, if it represents a comorbidity, it may be that the more severe outcome of schizophrenia is leavened by the coexistence of bipolar disorder so that an intermediate outcome would be observed in schizoaffective disorder. Furthermore, if the bipolar type of schizoaffective disorder is a variant of bipolar disorder, it would be expected to have a worse outcome than bipolar disorder, but better than schizophrenia. Also, if the unipolar depressed type of schizoaffective disorder is a variant of schizophrenia, one would expect a better outcome than schizophrenia, given the more responsive affective illness factor.

In short, the course studies are similar to the genetic studies in supporting all of the models except the concept of a separate illness.

TREATMENT RESPONSE

This is the least specific diagnostic validator, but it still can be useful. There are few studies of treatment of schizoaffective disorder, but it is generally thought that these patients require long-term treatment with antipsychotic agents, as in schizophrenia, and long-term treatment with either mood stabilizers (bipolar type) or antidepressants (unipolar depressed type), as in the corresponding affective disorders. Again, this treatment response pattern is consistent with all four models except the separate illness model.

AND THE ANSWER IS . . .

It appears clear that, its appearance in DSM-III–5 notwithstanding, there is no evidence that schizoaffective disorder is a separate illness distinct from schizophrenia and bipolar disorder. Studies of symptomatology vary, but some important and well-done studies tend to find a difference in symptoms in psychotic and affective populations that more or less falls along the lines of Kraepelin's dichotomy of schizophrenia and affective disorders. While there are overlapping areas, such overlapping is empirically expected in a real-world population of persons (or animals, or any other grouping). Therefore, studies of phenomenology can be interpreted as leaning against the single psychosis continuum model.

If schizoaffective disorder represents a comorbidity of schizophrenia and bipolar disorder, one would expect an epidemiological prevalence that is significantly lower than that of the other two. In other words, schizoaffective disorder should be very infrequent, since comorbidity should not be overly frequent by chance. Clinical impressions to the contrary notwithstanding, epidemiological prevalence studies indeed demonstrate that schizoaffective disorder appears to be very infrequently diagnosable in the general community, at a level of less than 0.5%, which is much lower than accepted prevalence rates for schizophrenia (1%) and bipolar disorder (2–4%).

THREE FINAL MODELS

These considerations suggest that the remaining three models are consistent with the available diagnostic research (Figure AIV.2):

- Some persons experience mainly bipolar mood symptoms, with only some excess of psychosis. These persons are diagnosable with schizoaffective disorder, bipolar type, seen as a severe variant of bipolar disorder. By and large, they need aggressive mood stabilizer treatment and perhaps somewhat less aggressive antipsychotic treatment. They have a relatively good prognosis.

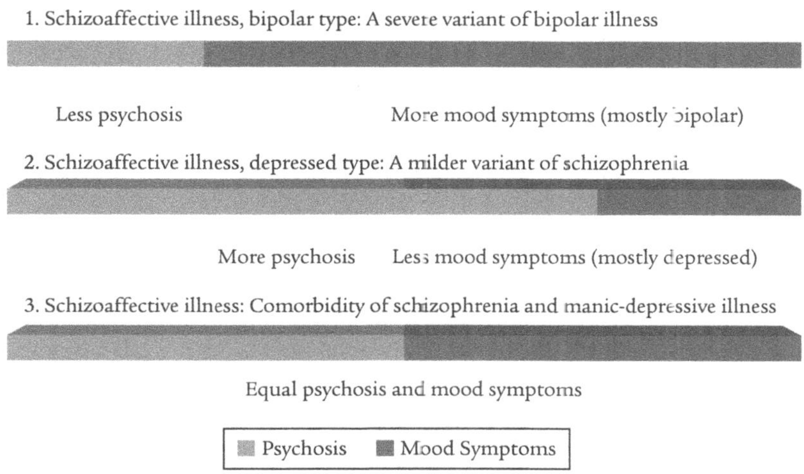

FIGURE AIV.2 *Three varieties of schizoaffective illness.*

- Some persons experience mainly psychotic symptoms, with only some excess of unipolar depressive symptoms. These persons are diagnosable with schizoaffective disorder, depressed type, seen as a somewhat less severe variant of schizophrenia. By and large, they need aggressive antipsychotic treatment, and perhaps somewhat less aggressive antidepressant treatment. Their prognosis, though better than in schizophrenia, is usually only fair.
- Some persons appear to be truly schizoaffective: they experience psychotic and affective symptoms in more or less equal amounts. This group represents the true comorbidity of schizophrenia and affective disorders, has an intermediate outcome, and requires aggressive, persistent, long-term treatment with both antipsychotic agents and either mood stabilizers or antidepressants.

If clinicians try to differentiate apparently schizoaffective patients in this manner, they will encounter these three groupings.

BOTTOM LINE

- Schizoaffective disorder isn't a valid separate illness.
- When defined strictly, it probably represents the chance comorbidity of schizophrenia and MDI in the same person.
- When mood symptoms predominate, it represents a more severe version of MDI.
- When delusional/hallucinatory symptoms predominate, it represents a less severe version of schizophrenia.
- Treatments should target mainly the mood, or mainly delusions/hallucinations, depending on which of the last two variants are present.

SELECTED REFERENCES

Goodwin, F. K., & Ghaemi, S. N. (2010). The conundrum of schizoaffective disorder: A Review of the literature. *Psychiatric Annals, 40,* 168–171.

Maier, W. (2006). Do schizoaffective disorders exist at all? *Acta Psychiatrica Scandinavica, 113,* 369–371.

Marneros, A. (2003). The schizoaffective phenomenon: The state of the art. *Acta Psychiatrica Scandinavica, 108,* 29–33.

Index